Fundamentals of Urine and Body Fluid Analysis

Fundamentals of Urine and Body Fluid Analysis

Nancy A. Brunzel, C.L.S., M.T.

Laboratory Manager
Division of Medical Technology
Department of Laboratory Medicine and Pathology
University of Minnesota
Minneapolis, Minnesota

SAUNDERS
An Imprint of Elsevier Science

SAUNDERS
An Imprint of Elsevier Science

The Curtis Center
Independence Square West
Philadelphia, Pennsylvania 19106

Library of Congress Cataloging-in-Publication Data

Brunzel, Nancy A.
    Fundamentals of urine and body fluid analysis./Nancy A. Brunzel.
      p. cm.
    ISBN 0-7216-3976-3
    1. Urine–Analysis.   2. Body fluids–Analysis.   3. Clinical chemistry.   I. Title.
    DNLM: 1. Body Fluids–chemistry.   @. Urinalysis.   3. Urine–chemistry.
QY 185 B911f 1994]
RB53.B86   1994
616.07′56–dc20
DNLM/DLC   92-48472

Fundamentals of Urine and Body Fluid Analysis   ISBN 0-7216-3976-3

Permissions may be sought directly from Elsevier's Health Sciences Rights Department in Philadelphia, USA: phone: (+1)215-238-7869, fax: (+1)215-238-2239, email: healthpermissions@elsevier.com. You may also complete your request on-line via the Elsevier Science homepage (http://www.elsevier.com), by selecting 'Customer Support' and then 'Obtaining Permissions'.

Printed in China

Last digit is the print number: 9   8   7   6   5   4

Dedication

To John, Gloria, Nathan, and Xavier

Preface

The purpose of this textbook is to present the fundamental principles of urine and body fluid analysis in a format suitable for all students of clinical laboratory science, regardless of academic background or primary field of study—medical technology, medicine, nursing, or other allied health professions. A major goal of this text is to go beyond the mere presentation of factual information for memorization by the reader. It strives to teach how to correlate data with one's knowledge of basic anatomy and physiology in order to understand pathologic processes. To achieve this goal, the anatomic and physiologic processes involved in the formation of each body fluid are presented and provide a framework on which to evaluate each body fluid.

To serve as a straightforward, in-depth teaching and reference text for the study of urine and body fluids (i.e., feces, seminal fluid, amniotic fluid, cerebrospinal fluid, synovial fluid, and serous fluids) encountered in the clinical laboratory, each chapter begins with an outline of the material to be discussed. In addition, learning objectives focus on important concepts to be learned. A list of key terms assists in the understanding of new terminology and concepts as they are introduced. At the end of each chapter a series of study questions is provided to enhance comprehension and reader participation. Diagrams and tables are used extensively throughout the text to clarify concepts and to reinforce the content. The final chapter (16) is devoted to the evaluation of case studies involving each of the body fluids. This chapter enables the reader to apply the fundamental principles obtained throughout the text, as well as to develop problem-solving skills (i.e., integration and correlation of data).

The initial chapters of this text cover topics that are common to the study of all body fluids. Chapter 1 provides basic information that all microscope users need: the description and function of each component of a microscope; principles of operation; adjustment optimization for Köhler illumination; and microscope troubleshooting, care, and preventive maintenance. Brightfield, phase contrast, polarizing, and interference contrast microscopy are compared and contrasted in text and tabular form, as well as visually represented in photomicrographs. The principle of each microscope technique along with its advantages and disadvantages is discussed.

Chapter 2 covers quality assurance and safety in the laboratory, especially when dealing with urine and body fluids. This chapter includes a discussion of preanalytical, analytical, and postanalytical variables of quality assurance and a discussion of the identification, handling, storage, and use of biological and chemical hazardous materials. Because adherence to established laboratory protocols and guidelines helps to ensure a safe working environment and the consistent generation of accurate test results, this chapter emphasizes the need for procedural standardization of all aspects of the clinical laboratory. This standardization ranges from protocols for specimen procurement and the handling of biological and chemical substances, to the reporting of test results.

In Chapter 3, the attention of the text shifts to the study of urine, the most frequently analyzed body fluid other than blood. Different urine specimen types are discussed, including guidelines and techniques for the proper collection of each. In this as well as in subsequent chapters, the emphasis is on providing procedural principles, rather than actual step-by-step procedures. This approach is taken because actual procedures can vary among institutions, while the basic principle remains the same (e.g., to measure the amount of glucose in urine or to determine the L/S ratio in amniotic fluid). In other words, the principle or purpose of a procedure is more important than the specific process used.

Chapters 4 and 5 describe renal anatomy, physiology, and function and provide the groundwork for understanding the importance of each parameter reported in the routine urinalysis. In Chapter 6, an in-depth discussion of the physical examination of urine is provided. Of particular note is an overview of the methods used for the assessment of urine concentration, namely specific gravity and osmolality. These parameters are compared, and the various methods available to determine them are presented.

Chapter 7 discusses the principles involved in the chemical examination of urine when using the three most popular commercial reagent strips, including their advantages and disadvantages, and the possible interferences that can affect each reagent strip. Straightforward explanations facilitate understanding and meet the needs of the student as well as the experienced clinical laboratory scientist. This chapter also includes a discussion of semiautomated reagent strip readers and a urinalysis workstation. The basic principles and limitations of each instrument are described and compared.

Chapter 8 describes the microscopic examination of urine. It begins with a discussion of the importance of standardized procedures and presents techniques that can be used to enhance the visualization of urine sediment. Over 120 photomicrographs accompany a comprehensive discussion of urine sediment components in order to 1) describe the microscopic appearance of each sediment component, 2) correlate each component with the physical and chemical examination of urine, and 3) explain the clinical significance of each component. Several tables enhance this section; for instance, Table 8–5 compares epithelial cells in urine sediment based on size, shape, and other characteristics.

Chapter 9 describes the pathophysiology of renal and metabolic diseases and integrates urinalysis findings with various disease states. In this chapter, renal disease is subdivided according to primary origin (e.g., glomerular, tubular, tubulointerstitial, or vascular) to facilitate understanding the disease process involved and the laboratory results obtained. The role of the urinalysis laboratory in the diagnosis of selected amino acid, carbohydrate, and metabolic disorders is also discussed.

Chapters 10 through 15 are individual discussions of feces, seminal fluid, amniotic fluid, cerebrospinal fluid, synovial fluid, and serous fluids (i.e., pleural, pericardial, and peritoneal). These chapters present the physiology and composition of each fluid and the physical, chemical, and microscopic examinations routinely performed, including the clinical significance of each parameter.

In my attempt to fulfill the needs of students with diverse academic backgrounds, I have faced the constant challenge of achieving a balance in the depth and breadth of the anatomy, physiology, and chemistry presented, while at the same time maintaining a readable format. My intent has been to present the content in a manner that arouses interest, promotes understanding, and facilitates the correlation of data with physiologic and pathologic processes. The analysis of urine and body fluids is a fascinating and crucial area within clinical laboratory science. It is my hope that this text promotes the study of urine and body fluids by students and serves as a resource for clinical laboratory scientists and other health professionals.

Acknowledgements

So many people have provided me with support, guidance, and encouragement throughout the course of writing this book—I wish I could name them all. First, I want to thank my family and friends for their loving patience and constant support, without which this task would not have been possible.

Second, I want to extend special thanks to Karen Karni for being my mentor, critic, and friend (she is truly responsible for the birth of this project); Karen Lofsness for always having a moment and for her many varied resources; Carol Wells for her expertise and assistance in photomicroscopy; and all my colleagues and students in clinical laboratory science for having contributed to me as an individual, and hence to this book.

To Scott Weaver, my Associate Developmental Editor, special thanks and a gold star for his constant guidance and steadfast support throughout this project. I want to thank Chris King for reviewing the content—her ideas and expertise were greatly appreciated—and to thank Selma Ozmat, Acquisitions Editor, for the opportunity to work on this challenging project. Many other people at W.B. Saunders Company are responsible for the quality of this text, and among them I'd like to thank Linda R. Garber, Production Manager; Paul Fry, Designer; and Andrea Mina, Copy Editor. I am truly grateful to you all.

NANCY A. BRUNZEL
Minneapolis, Minnesota

Contents

14

Synovial Fluid Analysis 385

15

Pleural, Pericardial, and Peritoneal Fluid Analysis 401

16

Case Studies 415

Glossary of Terms 445

Answers to Study Questions 463

Appendix A 471

Nomogram for the Determination of Body
Surface Area of Children and Adults

Appendix B 472

An Example of a Material Safety Data
Sheet

Appendix C 478

Cell Counts Using a Hemacytometer

Appendix D 484

Reference Ranges

Index 489

1

Microscopy

LEARNING OBJECTIVES

After studying this chapter, the student should be able to

1. Identify and explain the functions of the following components of a microscope:
   - aperture diaphragm
   - condenser
   - eyepiece (ocular)
   - field diaphragm
   - mechanical stage
   - objective

2. Describe Köhler illumination and the microscope adjustment procedure used to ensure optimal specimen imaging.

3. Describe the daily care and preventive maintenance routines for microscopes.

4. Compare and contrast the principles of the following types of microscopy:
   - brightfield
   - phase contrast
   - polarizing
   - interference contrast
   - darkfield
   - fluorescence

5. List an advantage of and application for each type of microscopy discussed.

KEY TERMS

aperture diaphragm: the microscope component that regulates the angle of light presented to the specimen. It is located at the base of the condenser and changes the diameter of the opening that the source light rays must pass to enter the condenser.

birefringent (also called **doubly refractile**): the ability of a substance to refract light in two directions.

brightfield microscopy: type of microscopy that produces a magnified image that appears dark against a bright or white background.

chromatic aberration: the unequal refraction of light rays by a lens because the different wavelengths of light refract or bend at different angles. As a result, the image produced has undesired color fringes.

condenser: the microscope component that gathers and focuses the illumination light onto the specimen for viewing. It is a lens system (either a single lens or combination of lenses) and is located beneath the microscope stage.

darkfield microscopy: type of microscopy that produces a magnified image that appears brightly illuminated against a dark background. A special condenser presents only oblique light rays to the specimen. The specimen interacts with these rays (e.g., refraction, reflection), causing visualization of the specimen. It is used on unstained specimen preparations and is the preferred technique for identification of spirochetes.

eyepiece (also called **ocular**): the microscope lens or system of lenses located closest to the viewer's eye. It produces the secondary image magnification of the specimen.

field diaphragm: the microscope component that controls the diameter of the light beams that strike the specimen and hence reduces stray light. It is located at the light exit of the illumination

2

source. With Köhler illumination, the field diaphragm is used to appropriately adjust and center the condenser.

fluorescence microscopy: type of microscopy modified to visualize fluorescent substances. It employs two filters: one to select a specific wavelength of illumination light (excitation filter) that is absorbed by the specimen, and another filter (barrier filter) to transmit the different, longer-wavelength light emitted from the specimen to the eyepiece for viewing. The selection of these filters is determined by the fluorophore (natural or added) present in the specimen.

interference contrast microscopy: type of microscopy in which the difference in optical light paths through the specimen is converted into intensity differences in the specimen image. Three-dimensional images of high contrast and resolution are obtained, without haloing. Two types available are modulation contrast (Hoffman) and differential interference contrast (Nomarski).

Köhler illumination: type of microscopic illumination in which a lamp condenser (located above the light source) focuses the image of the light source (lamp filament) onto the front focal plane of the substage condenser (where the aperture diaphragm is located). The substage condenser sharply focuses the image of the field diaphragm (located at or slightly in front of the lamp condenser) at the same plane as the focused specimen. As a result, the filament image does not appear in the field of view, and bright, even illumination is obtained. Köhler illumination requires appropriate adjustments of the condenser and both the field and aperture diaphragms.

mechanical stage: the microscope component that holds the microscope slide with the specimen for viewing. It is adjustable, front to back and side to side, to enable viewing of the entire specimen.

numerical aperture (NA): a number that indicates the resolving power of a lens system. It is derived mathematically from the refractive index (N) of the optical medium (for air, N = 1) and the angle of light (μ) made by the lens: $NA = N \times \sin \mu$.

objective: the lens or system of lenses located closest to the specimen. It produces the primary image magnification of the specimen.

parcentered: describing objective lenses that retain the same field of view when the user switches from one objective to another of a differing magnification.

parfocal: describing objective lenses that remain in focus when the user switches from one objective to another of a differing magnification.

phase contrast microscopy: type of microscopy in which variations in the specimen refractive index are converted into variations in light intensity or contrast. Areas of the specimen appear light to dark with haloes of varying intensity related to the thickness of the component. Thin, flat components produce less haloing and the best-detailed images. It is ideal for viewing low-refractile elements and living cells.

polarizing microscopy: type of microscopy that illuminates the specimen with polarized light. It is used to identify and classify birefringent substances (i.e., substances that refract light in two directions) that shine brilliantly against a dark background.

resolution: the ability of a lens to distinguish two points or objects as separate. The resolving power (R) of a microscope is dependent on the wavelength of light used (λ) and the numerical aperture (NA) of the objective lens. The greater the resolving power, the smaller the distance distinguished between two separate points.

spherical aberration: the unequal refraction of light rays when they pass through different portions of a lens, such that the light rays are not brought to the same focus. As a result, the image produced is blurred or fuzzy and unable to be brought into sharp focus.

A high-quality brightfield microscope is required for the microscopic examination of urine and other body fluids. Considerable care must be given to its selection because its use is an integral part of laboratory work and microscopes with quality objective lenses are costly. Because some brightfield microscopes can be modified to allow several types of microscopy from a single instrument—brightfield, phase contrast, polarization—good planning ensures selection of the most appropriate instrument. Whereas acquiring a suitable microscope is of utmost importance, appropriate training on its use as well as proper maintenance and cleaning of the microscope is crucial to ensure maximization of its potential. The user must be familiar with each microscope component and its function, as well as the proper microscope adjustment and alignment procedures.

The Brightfield Microscope

A brightfield microscope (Fig. 1–1) produces a magnified specimen image that appears dark against a brighter background. A simple brightfield microscope consisting of only one lens is known as a magnifying glass. In the clinical laboratory, however, compound brightfield microscopes predominate and consist of two lens systems. The first lens system, located closest to the specimen, is the **objective** mounted in the nosepiece. It produces the primary image magnification and directs this image to the second lens system,

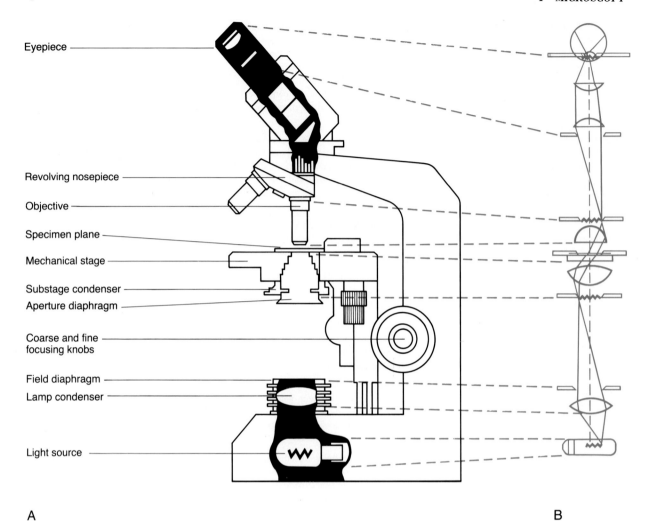

Eyepiece

Revolving nosepiece

Objective

Specimen plane

Mechanical stage

Substage condenser

Aperture diaphragm

Coarse and fine
focusing knobs

Field diaphragm

Lamp condenser

Light source

A   B

FIGURE 1–1. *A,* A schematic representation of a brightfield microscope and its components. *B,* Path of illumination using Köhler illumination.

the **eyepiece,** or ocular. The eyepiece further magnifies the image received from the objective lens. Total magnification of a specimen is the product of these lens systems, i.e., the multiplication of the objective lens magnification times the eyepiece lens magnification. For example, a 10× objective with a 10× eyepiece results in a 100× magnification. In other words, the viewed image is 100× larger than its actual size.

The purpose of the lens system is to sufficiently magnify an object for viewing with maximum resolution. **Resolution,** or resolving power, describes the ability of the lens system to reveal fine detail. Stated another way, it is the smallest distance between two

points or lines at which they are distinguished as two separate entities. Resolving power (R) is dependent on the wavelength (λ) of light used and the numerical aperture (NA) of the objective lens, according to Equation 1–1:

(1–1)

$$R = \frac{0.612 \times \lambda}{NA}$$

where

R = resolving power or resolvable
distance in microns
λ = wavelength of light
NA = numerical aperture of
objective

Because the light source on a microscope remains constant, as the NA of the objective lens increases, the resolution distance gets smaller. In other words, one can distinguish a smaller distance between 2 distinct points.

Numerical aperture (NA) is a designation engraved on objective lenses and condensers that indicates the resolving power of each specific lens. The NA is derived mathematically from the refractive index (N) of the optical medium (e.g., air has an N value of 1.0) and the angle of light made by the lens (μ) (i.e., the aperture angle).

(1–2)

$$NA = N \times \sin \mu$$

The NA of a lens can be increased by changing the refractive index of the optical medium or by increasing the aperture angle. For example, immersion oil has a greater refractive index (N = 1.515) than air and also increases the magnitude of the aperture angle (Fig. 1–2). As a result, use of immersion oil effects a greater NA (e.g., 100×, NA = 1.2) than is possible with high-power dry lenses. An increase in NA equates with greater magnification and resolution.

As previously discussed, the ability of a lens to resolve two points increases with the increase of its NA. However, one can achieve maximal resolution of the microscope only if the NA of the microscope condenser is equal to or slightly greater than the NA of the objective lens used. This requirement is neces-sary to ensure adequate illumination to the objective lens and can be better understood by reviewing the dynamics involved. Illumination light from the light source is presented to the condenser. The condenser lens system, along with the aperture diaphragm, is adjustable and serves to converge the illumination light into a cone-shaped focus on the specimen for viewing. If the condenser NA is less than the objective NA, inadequate illumination light will be presented to the objective lens and maximal resolution cannot be attained. In contrast, objective lenses with NAs less than the condenser NA are used optimally on the microscope. This is accomplished by making routine condenser and diaphragm adjustments that effectively reduce the condenser NA to match that of the objective NA (see Microscope Adjustment Procedure). Condenser height adjustments serve to focus the light specifically on the specimen plane and thus achieve maximal resolution. Optimal field diaphragm adjustments diminish stray light, thereby increasing the image definition and contrast. Adjustment of the aperture diaphragm to approximately 75 percent of the objective's NA is necessary to achieve increased image contrast, increased focal depth, and a flatter field of view.

The body or frame of the microscope serves to hold its four basic components in place: 1) the optical tube with its lenses (eyepieces and objectives); 2) a stage upon which to place the specimen for viewing; 3) a condenser to focus light onto the specimen; and 4) an illumination source. Each component and its unique features are discussed below.

Eyepiece

Whereas some microscopes have only one eyepiece (monocular), those used in most clinical laboratories have two eyepieces (binocular). However, with a monocular microscope, it is important to always view with both eyes open to reduce eyestrain. Initially this may be difficult, but with practice the image seen by the unused eye will be sup-

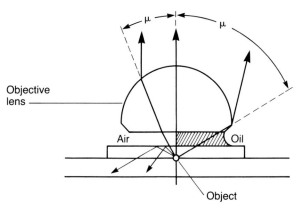

FIGURE 1–2. A drawing of a numerical aperture. Note the gain in the numerical aperture when immersion oil is used.

pressed. With a binocular microscope, adjustments to the oculars are necessary to ensure optimal viewing. The *interpupillary distance* of the eyepiece tubes must be adjusted by simply sliding them together or apart until perfect binocular vision is obtained. Because vision in both eyes is not always equivalent, the individual eyepieces are adjusted to compensate using the *diopter adjustment*. To adjust the eyepieces, view the image using only the right eyepiece and the right eye and sharply focus the specimen using the fine adjustment knob. Next, while looking through the left eyepiece with the left eye, rotate the diopter adjustment ring on this eyepiece until the specimen is also in sharp focus with this eye (Fig. 1–3). Each technologist must make both the interpupillary and diopter adjustments to suit his or her eyes. To eliminate eyestrain or tired eyes when performing microscopic work, always look through the microscope with relaxed eyes. Focus the microscope, not your eyes, by constantly using the fine adjustment control.

Eyeglass wearers should consider keeping their glasses on when performing microscopic work. Rubber guards are available that fit over the eyepieces and prevent scratching of the eyeglasses. Individuals with only spherical corrections (nearsighted or farsighted) can work at the microscope without their glasses. The microscope's focus adjustments will compensate for these visual defects. However, individuals with an astigmatism that requires a toric lens for correction should do microscopic work wearing their eyeglasses because the microscope cannot compensate for this. To determine if eye-

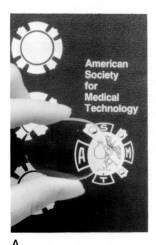 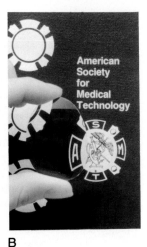

A   B

FIGURE 1–4. A test to check eyeglasses for toric correction. *A*, Note the length and width of the lettering behind the lens. *B*, After the lens is rotated 45 degrees, the length and width of the lettering changes.

glasses have any toric correction in them, hold the glasses in front of some lettering at arm's length. The eyeglass will either magnify or reduce it. Now rotate them 45 degrees. If the lettering changes in length and width, the glasses contain toric correction and should be worn when one uses the microscope (Fig. 1–4); if the lettering does not change, the eyeglasses have only spherical correction and do not need to be worn for microscopic work.

Mechanical Stage

The microscope **mechanical stage** is designed to hold firmly in place the slide to be examined. It has conveniently located adjustment knobs to move the slide front to back and side to side. When viewing the slide, the user views the image upside down. Moving the slide in one direction causes the image to move in the opposite direction. Some stages have a vernier scale on both a horizontal and a vertical edge to facilitate relocation of a particular field of view. By recording both the horizontal and vertical vernier scale values, one can remove and later replace the slide on the stage for re-examination of the same field.

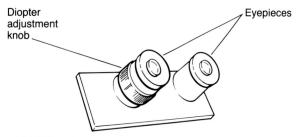

Diopter adjustment knob   Eyepieces

FIGURE 1–3. A schematic representation of a binocular eyepiece showing the location of the diopter adjustment ring.

Condenser

The **condenser,** located beneath the mechanical stage, consists of two lenses (Fig. 1–5). Its purpose is to evenly distribute and optimally focus the light from the illumination source onto the specimen. This is achieved by adjusting the condenser up or down using the condenser adjustment knob. The correct position of the condenser is always at its uppermost stop; it is slightly lowered only with **Köhler illumination.** The **aperture diaphragm,** located at the base of the condenser, regulates the beam of light presented to the specimen. The aperture diaphragm is usually an iris diaphragm made up of thin metal leaves that can be adjusted to form an opening of various diameters. Some microscopes employ a disc diaphragm, consisting of a movable disc with openings of various sizes, for placement in front of the condenser (Fig. 1–6). The purpose of the aperture diaphragm is to control the angle of the illumination

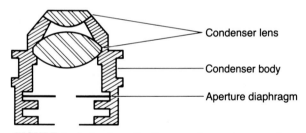

FIGURE 1–5. A schematic diagram of a condenser and an aperture diaphragm located beneath the mechanical stage of the microscope.

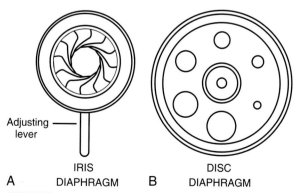

FIGURE 1–6. Two types of aperture diaphragms. *A,* An iris diaphragm. *B,* A disc diaphragm.

light presented to the specimen and objective lens. When the user properly adjusts the aperture diaphragm, he or she achieves maximal resolution, contrast, and definition of the specimen. One of the most common mistakes made is to use the aperture diaphragm to reduce the brightness of the image field; in so doing resolution is lost. Instead, the user should decrease the light source intensity or place a neutral density filter over the source.

Illumination System

Microscopes today usually have a built-in illumination system. The light source is either a tungsten or a tungsten-halogen lamp located in the microscope base. These lamps are often manufactured specifically to ensure alignment of the lamp filament when a bulb requires changing. Dual controls are usually available: one to turn the microscope on and another to adjust the intensity of the light. Adjustment of the illumination intensity should be done at the light source. This can be accomplished in two ways, either by turning down the lamp intensity or by placing neutral density (ND) filters over the source. Neutral density filters do not change the color of the light but reduce its intensity. The filters are marked to indicate the reduction made: e.g., an ND of 25 allows 75 percent of the light to pass. Some microscopes come with a daylight blue filter that makes the light slightly bluish. It has been found that this color is restful to the eyes and is desirable for prolonged microscopic viewing.

Most clinical microscopes have a **field diaphragm** located at the light exit of the illumination source. The purpose of this diaphragm is to control the diameter of the light beam that strikes the specimen. It is an iris-type diaphragm that when properly adjusted is just slightly larger than the field of view and serves to reduce stray light. Proper adjustment is outlined in the microscope adjustment procedure found in this chapter.

Objectives

The objectives are the most important optical components of the microscope because they produce the primary image magnification. The objectives are located on a rotatable nosepiece; only one objective is used at a time. They are easily changed by simple rotation of the nosepiece; however, each objective has a different "working distance," i.e., the distance between the objective and the coverslip on the slide. This working distance decreases as the magnification of the objective used increases; for example, a 10X objective has a working distance of 7.2 mm, whereas a 40X objective has only 0.6 mm clearance. Therefore, to prevent damage to the objective or to the slide being observed, care must be taken when objectives are changed or focused.

Both coarse and fine focus adjustment knobs are provided on the microscope. The user can focus the microscope by moving the mechanical stage holding the specimen up and down. Once the initial coarse focusing adjustments have been made, fine adjustments are done.

Various engravings found on the objective indicate its magnification power, the numerical aperture, the optical tube length required, the coverglass thickness to be used, and the lens type (if not an achromat). Most often the uppermost or largest number inscribed on the objective is the objective's magnification power. Following this number is the numerical aperture, inscribed on the same line or just beneath it (Fig. 1–7). As already discussed, the objective produces the primary magnification of the specimen and the numerical aperture mathematically expresses the objective's resolving power. Most objectives, designed for use with air between the lens and the specimen, are called dry objectives. In contrast, some objectives require immersion oil to achieve their designated numerical aperture. These objectives are inscribed with the term "oil" or "oel."

The optical tube length—the distance between the eyepiece and the objective in use—can differ depending on the microscope. If the microscope has a fixed optical tube length (usually 160 mm), the objectives used should have "160" engraved on them (see Fig. 1–7). On some microscopes, the tube length can be changed when devices such as

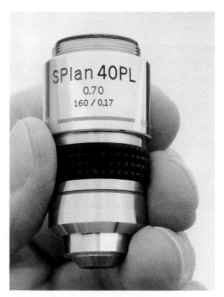

FIGURE 1-7. The engravings on this objective indicate that it is a planachromat lens (SPlan); the initial magnification is 40X; the numerical aperture is 0.70; it is designed for a microscope with an optical tube length of 160 mm; and the coverslip thickness should be 0.17 ± 0.01 mm.

a polarizer or a Nomarski prism are placed between the objective and the eyepiece. Using these devices requires the use of objectives designed for infinity correction or requires correcting lenses to maintain the tube length of 160 mm optically. Objectives designed for infinity correction have an infinity symbol (∞) engraved on them.

Some objectives are designed to be used with a coverglass. If a coverglass is required, its thickness is engraved on the lens after the optical tube type (e.g., 160/0.17). Objectives that do not use a coverglass are designated with a dash (e.g., ∞/− or 160/−). A third type of objective is designed to be used either with or without a coverglass. These objectives have no inscription for coverglass thickness; rather, they have a correction collar on them with which to adjust and fine-focus the lens appropriately for either application.

Objectives are corrected for two types of aberrations: chromatic and spherical. **Chromatic aberration** occurs because different wavelengths of light bend at different angles after passing through a lens (Fig. 1–8). This

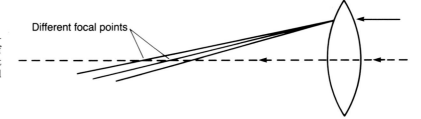

FIGURE 1-8. An illustration of chromatic aberration. Each wavelength of light is bent to a different focal point after passing through an uncorrected lens.

results in a specimen image with undesired color fringes. Objectives corrected to bring the red and blue components of white light to the same focus are called achromats and may not have a designation engraved on them. Objectives that bring red, blue, and green light to a common focus are termed apochromats and are identified by the inscription "apo". **Spherical aberration** occurs when light rays pass through different parts of the lens and therefore are not brought to the same focus (Fig. 1-9). As a result, the specimen image appears somewhat blurred and cannot be sharply focused. Objectives are corrected to bring all light entering the lens, regardless if it is at the center or the periphery, to the same central focus. Achromat objectives are spherically corrected for green light, whereas apochromats are spherically corrected for both green and blue light.

Other abbreviations may be engraved on the objective to indicate specific lens types. For example, "Plan" indicates that the lens is a planachromat, both achromatically corrected and designed for a flat field of view over the entire area viewed. "Ph" indicates that it is an objective lens for phase contrast microscopy. Regardless of the manufacturer, the same basic information is engraved on all objective lenses, with only the format varying slightly. To ensure a compatible system, it is advisable to use objectives and eyepieces

designed by the same manufacturer that designed the microscope.

Two final features of objective lenses need to be discussed. The first characteristic is termed **parcentered** and relates to the ability of objective lenses to retain the same central field of view when the user switches from one objective to another. In other words, when an objective is changed to one of higher magnification for a closer look, the object does not move from the center of the field of view. The second feature, termed **parfocal,** refers to the ability of objectives to remain in focus regardless of the objective used. This allows initial focusing at low power; changing to other magnifications requires only minimal fine focus adjustment. Whereas both of these features are taken for granted today, in the recent past each objective required individual centering and focusing.

When the microscope is used, adjustments must be made with each objective to produce optimal viewing. These adjustments strive to equate the NA of the objective lens in use (e.g., 10×, NA 0.25) with the condenser NA (NA 0.9) and thereby achieve maximal magnification and resolution. On current microscopes that utilize Köhler illumination, the condenser height adjustment once made remains unchanged regardless of the objective used. The user lowers the effec-

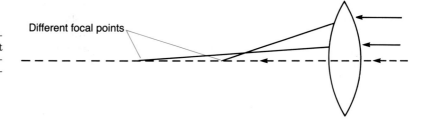

FIGURE 1-9. An illustration of spherical aberration. Each light ray is bent toward a different focal point depending on where the ray enters an uncorrected lens.

tive NA of the condenser by decreasing the light the condenser receives (i.e., closing the field diaphragm) and by adjusting the aperture diaphragm for the objective. On microscopes with which Köhler illumination is not possible, using low-power objectives may require 1) reducing the illumination source light, if possible; 2) slightly lowering (approximately 1.0 mm) the condenser from its uppermost position; or 3) minimally closing the aperture diaphragm. An adjustment error that users frequently make is lowering the condenser too much, resulting in loss of resolution as the contrast increases.

When high-power dry objectives (e.g., 40×, NA 0.65) are used, the NA is closer to that of the condenser (NA 0.9). Therefore, the condenser NA needs less reduction to achieve maximal viewing. Because going from a low-power to a high-power objective means changing from a low NA to a higher NA, more illumination is required. Microscopes using Köhler illumination require only field and aperture diaphragm adjustments with each objective change. When using high-power objectives on a microscope without Köhler illumination, the user should put the condenser all the way up and close the aperture diaphragm just enough for effective contrast. Never use the condenser or aperture diaphragm to reduce image brightness; rather, decrease the illumination intensity or use neutral density filters.

Microscope Adjustment Procedure

· ·

Clinical microscopes today primarily use Köhler illumination. With this type of illumination, the light source image (light filament) is focused onto the front focal plane of the substage condenser at the aperture diaphragm by a lamp condenser, located just in front of the light source. The substage condenser then focuses this image onto the back of the objective in use (see Fig. 1–1). As a result, this illumination system produces bright, uniform illumination at the specimen plane even when a coil filament light source

is used. The proper use of this illuminating system is just as important as the selection of a microscope and its objectives. To use a microscope with Köhler illumination the microscopist must know how to set up and optimally adjust the condenser and the field and aperture diaphragms. Manufacturers supply instructions with the microscope that are usually clear and easy to follow. Table 1–1 gives a basic procedure for the adjustment of a typical binocular microscope with a Köhler illumination system. Whereas initially these steps may feel cumbersome, with use they will become routine. When other types of microscopy are used, additional adjustment procedures may be necessary to ensure optimal viewing. For example, phase contrast microscopy requires that the phase rings be checked and aligned, if necessary.

Each day, before setting up and adjusting the microscope, the user should check it over and ensure that it is clean. The microscopist should look for dust or dirt on the illumination source port, the filters, and the upper condenser lens. Check the eyepiece and the objectives, especially any oil immersion objective, to be sure they are clean and free from oil and fingerprints. By routinely inspecting the microscope and optical surfaces before adjustment, one can save valuable time in microscope setup and in troubleshooting problems. In laboratories where the entire staff uses the same microscope, inspection before use allows one to identify individuals who need to be reminded of proper microscope care and maintenance.

Care and Preventive Maintenance

· ·

The microscope is a precision instrument. Therefore, ensuing long-term mechanical and optical performance requires care, including routine cleaning and maintenance. Dust is probably the greatest cause of harm to both the mechanical and optical components of a microscope. It settles in mechanical tracks and on lenses. Although dust can be removed from lenses by cleaning, the less cleaning of

**TABLE 1–1.   BINOCULAR MICROSCOPE ADJUSTMENT PROCEDURE
WITH KÖHLER ILLUMINATION**

PREPARING THE MICROSCOPE
1. Turn on the light source. Adjust the intensity to a comfortable level.
2. Position the low-power (10×) objective in place by rotating the nosepiece.
3. Place a specimen slide on the mechanical stage. Be sure the slide is firmly seated in the slide holder. Position the specimen on the slide directly beneath the objective using the mechanical stage adjustment knobs.

Interpupillary Adjustment
4. Looking through the eyepieces with both eyes, adjust the interpupillary distance until perfect binocular vision is obtained (i.e., the left and right images are fused together). Using coarse and fine adjustment knobs, bring the specimen into focus.

Diopter Adjustment
5. Closing the left eye, look through the right eyepiece with the right eye and bring the specimen into sharp focus using the fine adjustment knob.
6. Now using only the left eye, bring the image into sharp focus by rotating the diopter adjustment ring located on the left eyepiece. (Do not use the adjustment knobs.)

CONDENSER ADJUSTMENT
(NOTE: If at any point during adjustment the light intensity is very bright and uncomfortable, decrease the lamp voltage or insert a neutral density filter.)

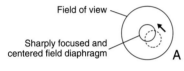

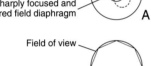

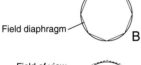

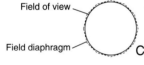

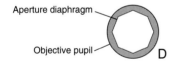

Condenser Height and Centration
1. Close the field iris diaphragm.
2. Using the condenser height adjustment knob, bring the edges of the diaphragm into sharp focus.
3. Center the condenser, if necessary, using the condenser centration knobs (see Figure *A*).

Field Iris Diaphragm Adjustment
4. Open the field iris diaphragm to just inside the edges of the field of view to confirm adequate centration (see Figure *B*). Recenter if necessary.
5. Open field iris diaphragm until it is slightly larger than the field of view (see Figure *C*).

Condenser Aperture Diaphragm Adjustment
6. Remove one eyepiece from the observation tube.
7. Looking down the tube at the back of the objective, close the aperture diaphragm.
8. Open the aperture diaphragm until 70% to 80% of the field is in view (approximately 25% less than fully opened). See Figure *D*.
   Alternatively, on microscopes with a scale of numerical apertures on the condenser, adjust the aperture to 70% to 80% of the objective's NA (e.g., for 80% of 40× NA 0.65, adjust condenser aperture to 0.52).
9. Each time an objective is changed, both the field and aperture diaphragms should be readjusted.

lenses the better. To remove dust, dirt, or other particulate matter, the microscopist should use a grease-free brush (camel hair) or an air syringe (e.g., an infant's ear syringe). If compressed air is used, it should be filtered (e.g., with cotton wool) to remove any contaminating residues or moisture. Using a microscope dust cover when the instrument is not in use or placing it in a storage cabinet eliminates dust buildup.

On microscopes, all mechanical parts are lubricated with special long-lasting lubricants. Therefore, the user should never use grease or oils to lubricate the microscope. When mechanical parts are dirty, cleaning and regreasing should be performed by the manufacturer or a professional service representative.

In climates where the relative humidity is consistently greater than 60 percent, precautions must be taken to prevent fungal growth on optical surfaces. In these areas, a dust cover or a storage cabinet may reduce ventilation and enhance fungal growth. Therefore, microscopes may require storage with a desiccant or in an area with controlled temperature and air circulation. In addition to high humidity, microscopes should also be protected from direct sunlight and high temperatures.

When handling the microscope, such as removing it from a storage cupboard or changing work areas, the user must always carry it firmly using both hands and avoid abrupt movements. The counter upon which the microscope is placed should be vibration free. This eliminates undesired movement in the field of view as well as the detrimental effects long-term vibration can have on precision equipment.

All optical surfaces must be clean to provide crisp brilliant images. Because the nosepiece is rotated by hand, the objectives are constantly in danger of becoming smeared with skin oils. The user should avoid all handling of optical surfaces with the fingers. Should a lens need cleaning, the user should follow the manufacturer's suggested cleaning protocol. Optical lenses are easily scratched; therefore, all particulate matter must be removed from the lens before cleaning. Some residues may be removed simply by breathing on the lens surface and polishing with lens paper. Others may require a commercial lens cleaner. The microscopist should never use gauze, facial tissue, or lint-free tissue to clean optical surfaces. After using oil immersion objective lenses, the microscopist should carefully remove the oil using a dry lens paper. This should be repeated using a lens paper moistened with lens cleaner. The microscopist must store oil immersion objectives dry, because oil left on the lens surface can impair its optical performance. Whereas some manufacturers suggest the use of xylene to clean oil immersion lenses, this practice is not recommended for several reasons. If residual xylene is left on the objective, it destroys the adhesive that holds the lens in place. In addition, xylene fumes are toxic and should be avoided.

The eyepiece is particularly susceptible to becoming dirty, especially when the user wears mascara. Therefore, when performing microscopy, individuals should avoid wearing mascara. If an eyepiece is removed for cleaning, care must be taken to prevent dust from entering the microscope tube and settling on the back lens of the objective.

When the specimen image shows a visual aberration and a dirty lens is suspected, the following procedure can help identify which lens needs attention. Specks appearing in the field of view are most often on the eyepiece or coverglass. The user should rotate the eyepiece; if the speck moves, the lens should be cleaned. If the specks move when the slide position is changed, the coverglass is dirty. If the objective lens is dirty, the speck will not be present when a different objective is used. Often a blurred or hazy image (i.e., decreased sharpness or contrast) is obtained when an objective is dirty, such as from a fingerprint on the objective lens.

Removal of the microscope base to replace the light source is easily performed following the manufacturer's directions. Only replacement lamps designated by the manufacturer should be used; this ensures compatibility and proper light source alignment. Any other repair that requires microscope disassembly should be performed only by a professional service representative. As with other instrumentation, microscope cleaning, maintenance, and problems should be routinely documented. In addition, service to clean, lubricate, and align its components should be performed annually by the manufacturer or a professional service representative.

Table 1-2 lists the do's and don'ts of good microscope care. A good demonstration of the appropriate technique for cleaning optical surfaces, as well as a microscope troubleshooting guide, is available from the National Committee for Clinical Laboratory Standards in Physician's Office Laboratory Guidelines, Tentative Guideline, document POL1-T (1989). As with any precision instrument, the microscope will give long-lasting and optimal performance if it is maintained and cared for properly.

TABLE 1–2. MICROSCOPE DO'S AND DON'TS

DO'S	DON'TS
• Always use lens paper on optical surfaces.	• Never use gauze, facial tissue, or lint-free tissue on lens surfaces.
• Always use a commercial lens cleaner to clean optical surfaces.	• Never touch optical surfaces with fingers or hands.
• Protect microscope from dust when not in use. Avoid temperature extremes and direct sunlight.	• Never wipe off dust or particulate matter; remove using suitable brush or air syringe.
• Document all cleaning and maintenance; have microscope professionally serviced annually.	• Never wear mascara while performing microscopy.
	• Never clean the back lens of the objectives.
	• Never use grease or oil on mechanical parts.
	• Never disassemble microscope for repair; call service representative.
	• Never leave microscope tubes without eyepieces; insert dust plugs if necessary.

Types of Microscopy

· ·

All types of microscopy (with the exception of electron microscopy) use the same basic magnification principles employed in the compound brightfield microscope. Different types of microscopy—phase contrast, polarizing, interference contrast, darkfield, and fluorescence—are achieved by changing the illumination system or the character of the light presented to the specimen. In research and in the clinical laboratory, some of these techniques are being used for new applications. As their usage grows, the different types of microscopy become increasingly more commonplace.

Brightfield Microscopy

Brightfield microscopy is the oldest and most common type of illumination system used on microscopes. The name refers to the dark appearance of the specimen image against a brighter background. This remains the principal type of microscopy employed in the clinical laboratory. Historically, room light was used as the illumination source. A major disadvantage to this procedure was uneven and variable illumination of the field of view. Now, with Köhler illumination, the light is focused not at the specimen plane but at the condenser aperture diaphragm. This allows for bright, even illumination of the

specimen field despite the use of a coil filament lamp.

Phase Contrast Microscopy

Often in the clinical laboratory, a microscopist encounters components with a low refractive index (e.g., hyaline casts in urine) that are difficult to view without staining. With **phase contrast microscopy,** variations in refractive index are converted into variations in light intensity or contrast. This permits detailed viewing of low-refractile components as well as of living cells (e.g., trichomonads). In equivalent detailed imaging using other techniques, cells are no longer living because normal fixation and staining has killed them.

Briefly, phase microscopy is based on the wave theory of light. If light waves are in "phase," the intensity of the light observed is the sum of all the individual waves (Fig. 1–10*A*). If some of the light waves are slowed, such as from passing through an object, the light intensity observed will be lower (Fig. 1–10*B*). If some waves are retarded exactly one-half of a wavelength, they will completely cancel out an unaffected light wave, thereby reducing further the light intensity (Fig. 1–10*C*).

Components retard light to different degrees depending on their unique shape, refractive index, and absorbance properties.

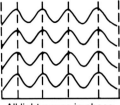

All light waves in phase.

Net intensity observed

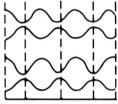

Some light waves partially
out of phase.

Net intensity observed

Equal number of light waves
in phase and out of phase.

Net intensity observed ───── 0

FIGURE 1–10. The effect of the phase of light waves upon the light intensity observed. *A,* All light waves are in phase and light intensity is maximal. *B,* Some light waves are slower or partially out of phase, resulting in a decrease in the light intensity observed. *C,* Equal numbers of light waves are in phase and out of phase. As a result, the net intensity observed is zero (i.e., the light waves cancel each other).

The best contrast is achieved when light retardation is one-quarter of a wavelength; however, this retardation is not possible without modification to the brightfield microscope.

Converting a brightfield microscope for phase contrast microscopy requires changes in both the condenser and the objective. The condenser must be fitted with an annular diaphragm either in the condenser itself or below it. Depicted in Figure 1–11, the annular diaphragm resembles a target and produces a light annulus or ring. Illumination light can pass through only this central clear ring of the diaphragm before penetrating the specimen. The objective used must be fitted with a phase-shifting element, also depicted

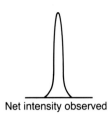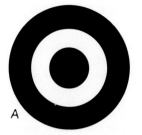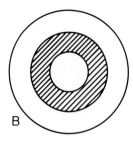

FIGURE 1–11. A schematic representation of *A,* an annular diaphragm (placed below the condenser) and *B,* the phase-shifting element (placed in back of the objective).

in Figure 1–11. Note that it too resembles a target. However, its central ring retards light by one-quarter of a wavelength, producing a dark annulus or ring. Both the light and dark annuli produced can be viewed on the back of the objective by removing an eyepiece. This enables proper alignment of the condenser and objective; i.e., the light annulus of the condenser is adjusted until the light and dark annuli are concentric and superimposed (Fig. 1–12).

Normally in brightfield microscopy, undiffracted and diffracted light rays are superimposed to produce the magnified image. In phase contrast microscopy, light is presented to the specimen only from the central light annulus of the condenser's annular diaphragm. After passing through the specimen, diffracted light enters the clear rings of the phase-shifting element, while all undiffracted light is shifted one-quarter of a wavelength out of phase. These light rays are recombined, producing varying degrees of

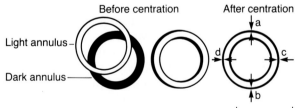

Before centration   After centration

Light annulus

Dark annulus

$a = b = c = d$

FIGURE 1–12. Phase ring alignment. A schematic representation of the view at the back of the objective when one is looking down the eyepiece tube with the eyepiece removed. The dark annulus is formed by the phase-shifting element in the objective; the light annulus is formed by the annular diaphragm. One can achieve phase ring alignment by adjusting the light annulus until it is centered and superimposed on the dark annulus.

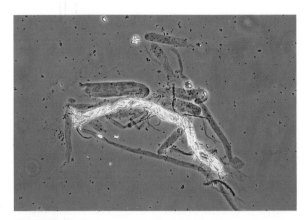

FIGURE 1-13. An example of phase contrast microscopy. This low-power (100X) view of urine sediment includes a highly refractile fiber revealed by its brightly haloed image. The hyaline casts and mucus threads are less refractile and have haloes of decreased intensity in comparison to the highly refractile fiber.

contrast in the specimen image (Fig. 1-13). Areas of the specimen appear light and dark with haloes of various intensities. Thin, flat specimens that produce less haloing are viewed best by this technique. The bright haloes produced by the optical gradient of some components can reduce visualization of the object's detail and dimension. Unstained specimens, especially living cells and low refractive index components, result in more detailed images than are possible with bright-field microscopy.

Polarizing Microscopy

Understanding the principle of **polarizing microscopy** requires a fundamental knowledge of polarized light. It can best be explained by comparison. Regular or unpolarized light vibrates in every direction perpendicular to its direction of travel; in contrast, polarized light vibrates in only one direction or plane (Fig. 1-14). When polarized light is passed through an optically active substance, it is split into two beams. One beam follows the original light path, while the other is rotated 90 degrees. Substances that are not optically active simply permit the light to pass through unchanged.

Polarizing microscopy has widespread applications in the clinical laboratory, as

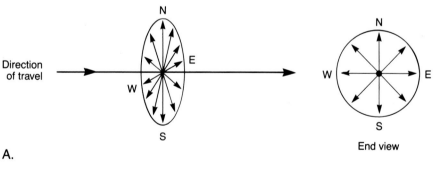

A.

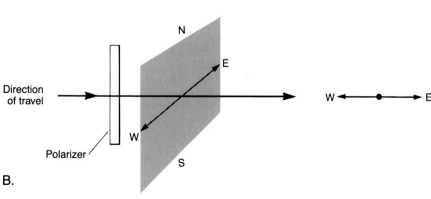

B.

FIGURE 1-14. Comparison of light ray orientation in *A*, regular light (vibrating in all directions) and *B*, polarized light (vibrating in only one plane).

well as in pharmaceuticals, forensics, pathology, geology, etc. *Anisotropic* or birefringent substances such as crystals, fibers, bones, or minerals can be identified based on their effect on polarized light. Anisotropic is a general term that refers to the ability of a substance to exhibit properties (e.g., refractive index, heat conduction) with different values when measured along axes in different directions. The term **birefringent** is more specific and refers to the ability of a substance to refract light in two directions (at 90 degrees). Substances need only very small differences in refractive indices to appreciably change the rotation of light. Birefringence can be of two types, negative and positive. If the optically active substance rotates the plane of polarized light clockwise (when looking toward the light source), the substance has positive birefringence; if the rotation is to the left or counterclockwise, the substance is said to have negative birefringence. This optical rotation characteristic provides a means of identifying and distinguishing birefringent substances. For example, monosodium urate crystals exhibit negative birefringence, whereas calcium pyrophosphate crystals are positively birefringent.

To convert a brightfield microscope to a polarizing one, two filters are required. One filter, called the polarizing filter, is placed below the condenser. Whether placed in a holder below the condenser or directly on the built-in illumination port, it is easily added and removed. This filter is adjusted to allow only light vibrating in an east-west direction perpendicular to the light path to pass to the specimen (Fig. 1–15). The second filter, called the analyzer, is placed between the objective and the eyepiece. Its orientation is such that only light vibrating in the north-south direction can pass. When both filters are in place—and in opposite orientation—they are said to be in a "crossed" position or "crossed pols." With no optically active specimen in place, the field of view will appear black because no light is passing through the analyzer. However, if an optically active specimen is in place, the incident polarized light will be refracted by the specimen into two rays vibrating at 90 degrees to each other. These rays pass through the analyzer and appear as white light.

Many substances found in clinical laboratory specimens are birefringent. Some chemical analyte crystals (e.g., amino acid crystals) have clinical importance in urine, and others (e.g., monosodium urate) have clinical importance in synovial fluid. Because other birefringent substances may be encountered (e.g., drugs, dyes, starch), technical expertise and training are necessary to ensure proper identification.

In order to identify a crystal based on its negative or positive birefringence, a first-order red compensator or a full wave plate is used. This compensator is placed in the light path between the "crossed pols." When the compensator is in place, the field of view is no longer black but red-violet—hence the name red compensator. This color results from the removal of the blue-green color component of white light. Besides changing the background color, the red compensator splits the polarized light into slow and fast rays. The direction of vibration of the slow rays is indicated by an inscription on the compensator. This inscription enables the microscopist to orient the birefringent substance parallel and perpendicular to the slow ray component for observation of the substance's characteristic birefringence. The refracted rays originating from a birefringent substance can be additive with the slow rays produced by the red compensator, causing the substance to appear blue-green (positive birefringence) against the red-violet background; or the refracted rays can be subtractive with the slow rays of the red compensator, causing the substance to appear yellow (negative birefringence). In the clinical laboratory, this microscopic technique is used primarily for urine and synovial fluid microscopic examinations. For gout studies, the use of a red compensator predominates in the differentiation of monosodium urate crystals from calcium pyrophosphate crystals in synovial fluid.

Interference Contrast Microscopy

This section covers two types of **interference contrast microscopy,** modulation contrast

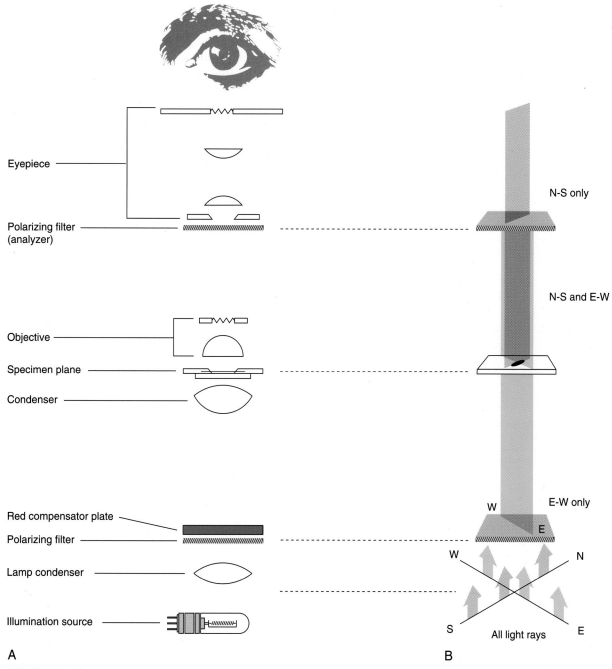

FIGURE 1–15. A schematic diagram of *A*, a polarizing microscope and its components. *B*, The change in the polarized light rays caused by a birefringent specimen. Note that the polarizer and analyzer are in a "crossed" position.

(Hoffman) and differential interference contrast (Nomarski). In interference contrast microscopy, the microscope converts differences in the optical path through the specimen to intensity differences in the specimen image. Both techniques achieve specimen images of high contrast and resolution

without haloing, superior to those obtained with phase contrast microscopy. These methods also enable optical sectioning of a specimen because the image at each depth of field level is unaffected by material above or below the plane of focus (Fig. 1–16). Images have a 3-dimensional appearance that readily

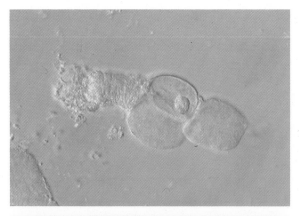

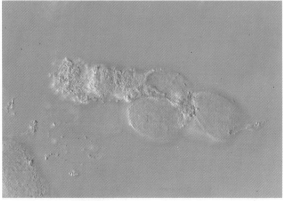

FIGURE 1–16. An example of differential interference contrast (Nomarski) microscopy and its optical sectioning ability. Note the different plane of focus captured in each photomicrograph, allowing for greatly detailed imaging.

reveals the contour detail of a specimen. Interference contrast microscopy is excellent for detailed viewing of unstained specimens. Its superior visualization of all components, including living cells and substances of low refractive indices, makes it particularly useful for microscopic examinations of wet preparations.

Modulation Contrast Microscopy (Hoffman)

Modulation contrast microscopy can be performed on a brightfield microscope with three modifications: 1) a special slit aperture is placed below the condenser; 2) a polarizer, to control contrast, is placed below this slit aperture; and 3) a special amplitude filter, called a modulator, is placed in the back of

each objective. Once the microscope has been adapted for modulation contrast microscopy, simply removing the slit aperture from the light path allows the instrument to be used for brightfield, darkfield, polarizing, or fluorescence techniques.

The basic principle of modulation contrast microscopy is schematically represented in Figure 1–17. Illumination light enters the polarizer, becomes polarized, and passes to the special slit aperture at the front focal plane of the condenser. This polarizer is rotatable and because the slit aperture is also partially covered with a second polarizer, rotating it achieves variations in contrast and spatial coherence (i.e., the reduction of scattering effects such as flare and fringes at specimen edges). The light rays proceed through and interact with the specimen. Where they enter the objective lens depends on their interaction (i.e., diffraction) with the specimen. As a result, they pass through different parts of the modulator located at the back of the objective. The modulator is divided into three regions of different size and light transmission (i.e., dark region, approximately 1 percent transmission; gray region, approximately 15 percent transmission; and bright region, 100 percent transmission). The modulator determines the intensity gradients of light to dark observed in the 3-dimensional image but does not effect a change in light phase. It is also the component from which this technique derives its name. "When light intensity varies above and below an average value the light is said to be modulated—thus the name modulation contrast." (Hoffman, 1977).

The microscope modifications made for modulation contrast are located at the same optical planes as in phase contrast microscopy. Both the modulator and the phase-shifting element are located at the back of their respective objectives, whereas the special slit aperture and the annular diaphragm (light annulus) are located in the condenser focal plane. Also, each system requires alignment of these conjugate planes for optimal specimen imaging. Modulation contrast produces 3-dimensional images that reveal contours and detail not possible with phase con-

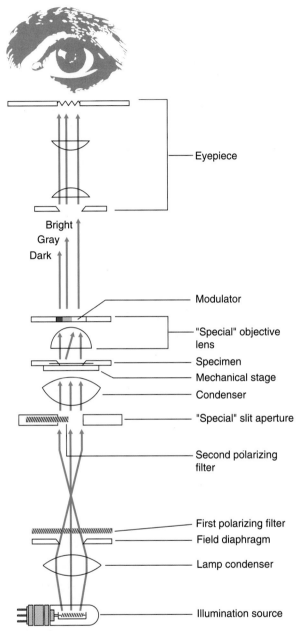

FIGURE 1–17. A schematic representation of a modulation contrast microscope and its components.

Labels (top to bottom): Eyepiece; Bright / Gray / Dark; Modulator; "Special" objective lens; Specimen; Mechanical stage; Condenser; "Special" slit aperture; Second polarizing filter; First polarizing filter; Field diaphragm; Lamp condenser; Illumination source

ever, because differential interference contrast uses polarization to achieve its 3-dimensional image, any birefringent substance present in the specimen plane will compromise the image obtained. In these latter situations, modulation contrast microscopy will produce an image of superior detail and contrast.

Differential Interference Contrast Microscopy (Nomarski)

In differential interference contrast microscopy, intensity differences in the specimen image are accomplished through the use of birefringent crystal prisms (i.e., modified Wollaston prisms) as beam splitters. One prism placed before the specimen plane splits the illumination light into two beams, while the second prism placed after the objective recombines them. The split beams follow different light paths through the specimen plane. They are rejoined before the eyepiece and a 3-dimensional image is produced (Fig. 1–18). The image obtained with differential interference contrast microscopy is similar to modulation contrast images and superior to phase contrast images because there is no halo formation. As with modulation contrast, optical sectioning or layer-by-layer imaging of specimens is possible because the depth of focus is small. Another characteristic of dif-

trast microscopy. However, for viewing essentially flat thin specimens, images using phase contrast microscopy—with which the halo effect is minimal—can be equivalent to those seen with modulation contrast. Differential interference contrast microscopy can produce specimen images comparable to those seen with modulation contrast. How-

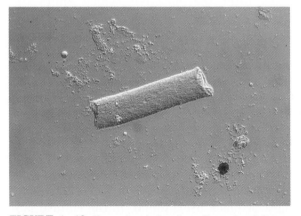

FIGURE 1–18. Example of the three-dimensional image produced by differential interference contrast (Nomarski) microscopy. This view shows a waxy cast at a magnification of 200×.

ferential interference contrast microscopy is that specimens with low or high refractive indices can produce equally detailed images.

Converting a brightfield microscope to differential interference contrast microscopy requires 1) a polarizer placed between the light source and condenser; 2) a special condenser containing modified Wollaston prisms for each objective; 3) a Wollaston prism placed between the objective and eyepiece; and 4) an analyzer (polarizing filter) placed behind this Wollaston prism and before the eyepiece (Fig. 1–19). Illumination light becomes polarized and enters the special condenser, where it is split into two beams. The two beams traverse slightly different parts of the specimen and are recombined at the prism located after the objective. From here the recombined rays (whose directions of vibration are perpendicular and do not interfere with each other) enter the analyzer. It is the analyzer that produces the interference image observed by changing the direction of vibration of the recombined rays, such that they interfere with each other. In reality two images are formed, but our eyes are unable to resolve them to produce a double image. As a result, the specimen image observed appears to be in relief, or 3-dimensional.

In differential interference contrast microscopy, the background field of view can be changed from black or dark gray to various colors (e.g., yellow, blue, magenta). This is achieved by rotating the prism located after the objective, which alters the path differences of the split light waves. In this way, specimen images similar to those achieved with darkfield microscopy can be obtained, as well as brilliantly colored ones. Gray backgrounds result in the most detailed 3-dimensional images.

Darkfield Microscopy

As the name implies, **darkfield microscopy** produces a bright specimen image against a dark or black background. In the clinical laboratory, this method is used only on unstained specimens and is the preferred technique for the identification of spirochetes. To obtain the specimen image, a special con-

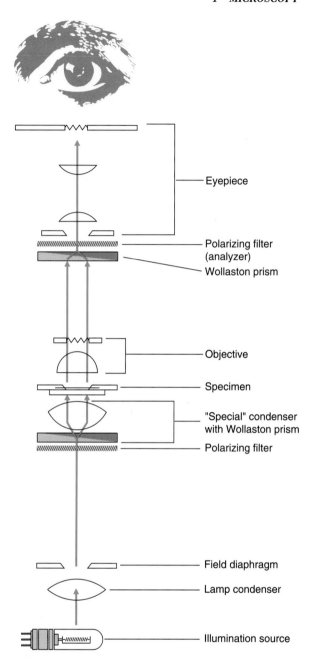

FIGURE 1–19. A schematic representation of a differential interference contrast (Nomarski) microscope and its components.

denser directs the illumination source light through the specimen plane only from oblique angles (Fig. 1–20). When light passes through a specimen, it interacts with it. This interaction, whether refraction, reflection, or diffraction, results in light entering the objective. The resultant image, a shining speci-

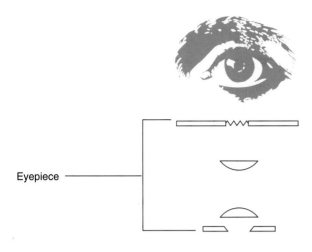

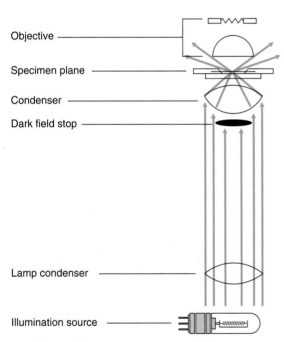

Eyepiece

Objective

Specimen plane

Condenser

Dark field stop

Lamp condenser

Illumination source

FIGURE 1–20. A schematic representation of a darkfield microscope and its components.

details. It is beneficial in clarifying edges and boundaries, but not as good as phase contrast microscopy or interference contrast microscopy in revealing internal structural detail. To convert a brightfield microscope for darkfield microscopy, the condenser must be replaced with a special darkfield condenser. Two types of darkfield condensers are available: one type uses air between it and the specimen slide as in brightfield microscopy, whereas the second, an immersion darkfield condenser, requires oil placed between the condenser and the specimen slide. The advantage of the immersion condenser is the ability to use objectives of high numerical apertures (NA values greater than 0.65) and therefore achieve greater magnification and resolution of the specimen.

By design, darkfield microscopy requires very bright illumination sources because only small amounts of light ever reach the objective lens. In addition, the glass slides used must be meticulously clean because any particles of dust or dirt present in the specimen plane will shine brightly against the dark background.

Fluorescence Microscopy

Fluorescence microscopy allows the visualization of fluorescent substances. Light of a selected wavelength is presented to the specimen. If a specific fluorescent substance is present in the specimen, the light is absorbed and emitted at a different, longer wavelength. Any emitted light is transmitted to the eyepiece for viewing. To accomplish this task, two filters are employed. The first filter, called the excitation filter, selects the wavelength of the excitation light presented to the specimen. The second filter, called the barrier or emission filter, selects a specific wavelength of emitted light from the specimen. Whereas some biological substances are naturally fluorescent (e.g., vitamin A), most applications of this technique require staining of the specimen with fluorescent dyes called fluorophores (e.g., quinacrine).

Each fluorophore has a unique excitation and emission wavelength. Consequently, the filters selected vary with the fluorophore

men on a black background, is visually enhanced by the increased contrast. If no specimen is present, the field of view appears black because no light is entering the objective lens.

Darkfield microscopy is a relatively inexpensive means of obtaining increased contrast to facilitate visualization of specimen

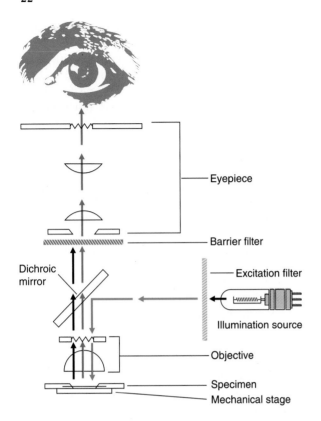

Eyepiece

Barrier filter

Dichroic mirror

Excitation filter

Illumination source

Objective

Specimen

Mechanical stage

FIGURE 1–21. A schematic representation of a reflected illumination fluorescence microscope and its components.

TABLE 1–3. COMPARISON OF MICROSCOPIC CAPABILITIES

				MICROSCOPY TYPES			
FEATURES	**Brightfield**	**Phase Contrast**	**Modulation Contrast**	**Differential Interference Contrast**	**Polarizing**	**Darkfield**	**Fluorescence**
Unstained Specimens:							
Resolution	Poor	Limited by contrast	Excellent	Excellent	Limited by contrast	Fair	NA*
Contrast	Poor	Optimal with thin flat structures†	Excellent for most specimens; adjustable	Excellent for most specimens; adjustable	Maximum for birefringent specimens	Good for most specimens	—
3-dimensional image	No	No	Yes	Yes	No	No	No
Halo	No	Yes, can be excessive	No	No	No	No	No
Optical sectioning	No	Limited by halo	Yes	Yes	No	No	No
Stained Specimens							
Resolution	Optimal	Often reduced	Optimal	Optimal	NA‡	NA‡	Adequate**
Image enhancement (compared to brightfield)	—	Only for faintly stained objects	At boundaries and gradients	At boundaries and gradients	—	—	Maximal, not visible otherwise
General Considerations							
Detailed imaging of birefringent specimens	Yes	Yes	Yes	Limited	Limited	Yes	No
Technical training required§	Minimal	Moderate	Moderate	Moderate	Moderate	Minimal	Minimal
Comparative cost	Low	Medium	Medium	Medium	Medium	Low	High (due to cost of source)

* Not applicable; technique requires staining with a fluorescent dye or the presence of a naturally occurring fluorophore.
† Contrast is optimal in thin sections, where structures are flat and differences in the refractive index are small.
** Stained with a fluorescent dye.
‡ Not applicable; technique used only to observe unstained specimens.
§ Training includes microscope set-up, alignment, and adjustment for optimized images.
Modified from Hoffman Modulation Contrast System, Modulation Optics, Inc., Greenvale, NY 11548.

used in the procedure. Historically, excitation and emission filters were made of glass and were not wavelength-selective enough for some applications. Today, selective interference filters made from metallic salts can be employed and greatly increase wavelength specificity.

Two types of illumination systems that differ in the path of the excitation light are available for fluorescence microscopy. A transmitted illumination system is similar to other microscopy systems in which the excitation light is presented to the condenser, focused, and passed through the specimen. In contrast, the excitation light in a reflected illumination system is presented to the specimen from above the specimen via the objective lens. Here, a dichroic mirror reflects excitation light from the illumination source, while the objective focuses it onto the specimen (Fig. 1–21). The dichroic mirror has a dual role: first, to reflect excitation light to the specimen, and second, to allow passage of emitted light to the selective barrier filter.

Reflected fluorescence microscopy is currently the method of choice. Its illumination sources vary from halogen-quartz lamps to mercury or xenon arcs. Fluorescence microscopy is very sensitive to extremely small quantities of fluorophores present on antibodies, antigens, viruses, or any other entity to which they become associated. As a result, fluorescence microscopy is frequently employed in microbiological and immunological procedures found in the clinical laboratory.

In summary, numerous microscopic techniques are available, and the method selected will depend on various factors. Obviously, specimen type plays an important role in determining the microscopic technique employed. Some techniques cannot produce detailed images of unstained living materials or of components with a low refractive index. Other methods require the presence of specific substances, such as a fluorescent dye or

a birefringent entity, to produce an image. The ability to produce a 3-dimensional image or to optically section a specimen may not be necessary in some applications. Each feature plays an important part in the selection of a microscope to suit each laboratory's needs: instrumentation cost, the amount of technical training required, the ability of the instrument to convert to other types of microscopy, and the need for adequate or more enhanced imaging. Table 1–3 lists each of the techniques discussed, compares the capabilities with different specimen types, and gives several general considerations.

Reference

. . . .

Hoffman R: The modulation contrast microscope: principles and performance. J Microsc *110:*205–222, 1977.

Bibliography

. . . .

Abramowitz MJ: Koehler illumination. American Laboratory *21*(4):106, 1989.

Abramowitz MJ: Microscope objectives. American Laboratory *21*(10):81, 1989.

Abramowitz MJ: The polarizing microscope. American Laboratory *22*(9):72, 1990.

Abramowitz MJ: The first order red compensator. American Laboratory *21*(11):110, 1989.

Abramowitz MJ: Darkfield illumination. American Laboratory *23*(11):60, 1991.

Abramowitz MJ: Fluorescence filters. American Laboratory *22*(3):168, 1990.

Brown B: Basic laboratory techyn iques. *In* Hematology: Principles and Procedures (5th ed.), Philadelphia, Lea & Febiger, 1988, pp. 11–17.

Leica Inc., Optical Products Division: Use and Care of the Microscope, Buffalo, NY, American Optical Instrument Division.

Mollring FK: Microscopy From the Very Beginning, Oberkochen, West Germany, Carl Zeiss, 1981.

Olympus Instruction Manual. Differential interference contrast attachment for transmitted light model BH2-NIC, AX5349, Tokyo, Olympus Optical Company, LTD.

Physician's Office Laboratory Guidelines, Tentative Guideline, POL 1-T, Villanova, PA, National Committee for Clinical Laboratory Standards, 1989.

Study Questions

1. **In a brightfield microscope, which lens produces the primary image magnification?**

    A. Condenser
    B. Eyepiece (ocular)
    C. Numerical aperture
    D. Objective

2. **A microscope has a 10× magnification eyepiece and a 100× objective lens. What is the total magnification of the specimen when viewed using this microscope?**

    A. 0.1×
    B. 10×
    C. 100×
    D. 1000×

3. **Select the numerical aperture that has the ability to distinguish the smallest distance between two distinct points, i.e., the greatest resolving power (R).**

    A. 0.25
    B. 0.65
    C. 0.85
    D. 1.25

4. **The numerical aperture of a lens can be increased by**

    A. decreasing the angle of light made by the lens.
    B. increasing the refractive index of the optical medium.
    C. increasing the illumination intensity.
    D. decreasing the interpupillary distance.

5. **Which parameter(s) will increase with an increase in the numerical aperture of an objective lens?**

   A. Magnification and resolution
   B. Field of view and resolution
   C. Magnification and field of view
   D. Magnification

6. **Match the microscope component with its primary function.**

Function	Microscope Component
____ A. Produces primary image magnification	1. Aperture diaphragm
____ B. Produces secondary image magnification	2. Condenser
____ C. Moves the specimen for viewing	3. Eyepiece
____ D. Optimally focuses light onto the specimen	4. Field diaphragm
____ E. Controls the angle of light presented to the specimen	5. Mechanical stage
____ F. Controls the diameter of light rays that strike the specimen.	6. Light source
	7. Objective

7. **Which of the following should be adjusted to decrease the illumination light or field brightness?**

   A. Aperture diaphragm
   B. Condenser
   C. Field diaphragm
   D. Light source

8. **Which lens characteristic is described as the ability to keep a specimen image in focus regardless of which objective lens is used?**

   A. Parcentered
   B. Parfocal
   C. Chromatic aberration
   D. Spherical aberration

9. **To achieve maximal image magnification and resolution**

   A. the condenser should be in its lowest position.
   B. the condenser numerical aperture must be equal to or greater than the objective numerical aperture.
   C. the aperture diaphragm should be used to decrease field brightness.
   D. the field diaphragm should be fully opened.

10. **Various inscriptions may be found on an objective lens. Select the objective lens inscription that indicates a numerical aperture of 0.25.**

   A. SPlan40PL
      0.65
      160/025

   C. E10
      0.25
      160/0.20

   B. 25
      0.10
      160/0.17

   D. DPlan25
      0.10
      25/160

11. **When a microscope with Köhler illumination is adjusted,**

   A. the condenser is adjusted up or down, until the field diaphragm is sharply focused.
   B. the field diaphragm is opened until it is slightly smaller then the field of view.
   C. the illumination intensity is adjusted using the field and aperture diaphragms.
   D. the aperture diaphragm is opened until 25% of the field is in view.

12. **Microscope lenses may be cleaned or polished using**

   1. gauze.
   2. facial tissue.
   3. lint-free tissues.
   4. lens paper.
      A. 1, 2, and 3 are correct.
      B. 1 and 3 are correct.
      C. 4 is correct.
      D. All are correct.

13. **When viewing a focused specimen in the microscope, the user sees a speck in the field of view. It remains in view when the objective is changed and when the specimen is moved. The speck is most likely located on the**

   A. condenser.
   B. eyepiece.
   C. objective.
   D. specimen coverslip.

14. **Which type of microscopy converts differences in refractive index into variations in light intensity to obtain the specimen image?**

   A. Brightfield microscopy
   B. Interference contrast microscopy
   C. Phase contrast microscopy
   D. Polarizing microscopy

15. **A birefringent substance is one that**

   A. vibrates light in all directions.
   B. vibrates light at two different wavelengths.
   C. refracts light in two different directions.
   D. shifts light one-half wavelength out of phase.

16. **Which type of microscopy is able to produce 3-dimensional images and perform optical sectioning?**

    A. Brightfield microscopy
    B. Interference contrast microscopy
    C. Phase contrast microscopy
    D. Polarizing microscopy

17. **The principle of fluorescence microscopy is based on**

    A. a substance causing the rotation of polarized light.
    B. differences in optical light path being converted to intensity differences.
    C. differences in refractive index being converted into variations in light intensity.
    D. the absorption of light and its subsequent emission at a longer wavelength.

18. **Converting a brightfield microscope for polarizing microscopy requires**

    A. two polarizing filters—one placed below the condenser and one placed between the objective and the eyepiece.
    B. a special condenser, two polarizing filters, and a Wollaston prism between the objective and eyepiece.
    C. an annular diaphragm in the condenser and a phase-shifting element in the objective.
    D. a slit aperture below the condenser, a polarizing filter, and a modulator.

19. **Which type of microscopy uses a special condenser to direct light onto the specimen from oblique angles only?**

    A. Darkfield microscopy
    B. Interference contrast microscopy
    C. Phase contrast microscopy
    D. Polarizing microscopy

20. **Match the type of microscopy to the characteristic.**

Characteristic	Microscopy Type
_____ A. Is the preferred technique for the identification of spirochetes.	1. Brightfield microscopy
_____ B. Is often used for the visualization of antigens, antibodies, and viruses.	2. Darkfield microscopy
_____ C. Enables three-dimensional viewing of unstained, low-refractile specimens.	3. Fluorescence microscopy
_____ D. Is used to identify negative and positive birefringence.	4. Phase contrast microscopy
_____ E. Produces less haloing with thin, flat specimens.	5. Polarizing microscopy
	6. Interference contrast microscopy

Quality Assurance and Safety

LEARNING OBJECTIVES

After studying this chapter, the student should be able to

1. Define and explain the importance of quality assurance in the laboratory.

2. Identify and explain preanalytical, analytical, and postanalytical components of quality assurance.

3. Differentiate between internal and external quality assurance and discuss how each contributes to an overall quality assurance program.

4. Define and discuss the importance of the following:
   - critical values
   - documentation
   - ethical behavior
   - preventive maintenance
   - technical competence
   - test utilization
   - turnaround time

5. Discuss the relationship of OSHA to safety and health in the workplace.

6. Define and give an example of the following terms:
   - biological hazard
   - chemical hazard
   - decontamination
   - protective barriers

7. Describe a Universal Precautions policy and state its purpose.

8. Discuss the three primary routes of transmission of infectious agents and a means of controlling each route in the clinical laboratory.

9. Describe appropriate procedures for the handling, disposal, decontamination, and spill control of biological hazards.

10. Discuss the source of potential chemical and fire hazards encountered in the laboratory and the procedures used to limit employee exposure to them.

11. State the purpose of and the information contained in a material safety data sheet.

KEY TERMS

biological hazard: a biological material or an entity contaminated with biological material that is potentially capable of transmitting disease.

Chemical Hygiene Plan (CHP): an established protocol developed by each facility for the identification, handling, storage, and disposal of all hazardous chemicals. It was established as a mandatory requirement for all facilities that deal with chemical hazards by the Occupational Safety and Health Administration (OSHA) in January 1990.

critical value: a patient test result representing a life-threatening condition that requires immediate attention and intervention.

decontamination: a process to remove a potential chemical or biological hazard from an area or entity (e.g., countertop, instrument, materials) and render the area or entity "safe." Various processes may be employed in decontamination, such as autoclaving, incineration, chemical neutralization, and disinfecting agents.

documentation: a written record. In the laboratory, it includes written policies and procedures, quality control, and maintenance records. It may encompass the recording of any action performed or observed including verbal correspondence, observations, and corrective actions taken.

external quality assurance: the use of materials (e.g., specimens, kodachrome slides) from an external unbiased source to monitor and determine if quality goals (i.e., test results) are being achieved. Results are compared to the results from other facilities performing the same function. Proficiency surveys are one form of external quality assurance.

infectious waste disposal policy: a procedure outlining the equipment, materials, and steps used in the collection, storage, removal, and decontamination of infectious material and substances.

material safety data sheet (MSDS): a written document provided by the manufacturer or distributor of a chemical substance listing information about that chemical's characteristics. An MSDS includes the chemical's identity and hazardous ingredients, its physical and chemical properties including reactivity, any physical or health hazards, and precautions for the safe handling, storage, and disposal of the chemical.

Occupational Safety and Health Administration (OSHA): established by Congress in 1970, OSHA is a division of the U.S. Department of Labor that is responsible for defining potential safety and health hazards in the work-

place, establishing guidelines to safeguard all workers from these hazards, and monitoring compliance with these guidelines. The intent is to alert, educate, and protect all employees in every environment to potential safety and health hazards.

preventive maintenance: the performance of specific tasks in a timely fashion to eliminate equipment failure. These tasks vary with the instrument and include cleaning procedures, inspection of components, and component replacement when necessary.

procedure manual: a written document describing in detail all aspects of each policy and procedure performed in the laboratory. For example, it includes supplies needed, reagent preparation procedures, specimen requirements, mislabeled- and unlabeled-specimen protocols, procedures for the storage and disposal of wastes, technical procedures, quality control criteria, reporting formats, and references.

protective barriers: items used to eliminate exposure of the body to potentially infectious agents. These barriers include protective gowns, gloves, eye and face protectors, biosafety cabinets (fume hoods), splash shields, and specimen transport containers.

quality assurance (QA): an established protocol of policies and procedures for all laboratory actions per-

formed to ensure the quality of services (i.e., test results) rendered.

quality control (QC) materials: materials used to assess and monitor the accuracy and precision (i.e., analytical error) of a method.

technical competence: the ability of an individual to perform a skilled task correctly. It also includes the ability to evaluate results, such as recognizing discrepancies and absurdities.

test utilization: the frequency with which a test is performed on a single individual and how it is used to evaluate a disease process. Repeat testing of an individual is costly and may not provide additional or useful information. Sometimes a different test may provide more diagnostically useful information.

turnaround time: to the laboratorian, it is the time that elapses from receipt of the specimen in the laboratory to the reporting of that specimen's test results. To physicians and nursing personnel, a broader time frame is assigned.

Universal Precautions (UP): a policy describing the procedures to employ when obtaining, handling, storing, or disposing of all blood, body fluid, or body substances regardless of patient identity or patient health status. All body substances should be treated as potentially infectious.

Quality Assurance (QA)

Quality Assurance — What Is It?

Quality assurance is a program of checks and balances designed to ensure the quality of a laboratory's services. All laboratorians must be aware of the impact their services have on the diagnosis and treatment of patients. These services must be monitored to ensure that they are appropriate and effective and that they meet the established standards for laboratory practice. The QA program must involve a mechanism for the detection of problems and provide an opportunity to improve services. In essence, "quality assurance is a broad spectrum of plans, policies, and procedures that together provide an administrative structure for a laboratory's efforts to achieve quality goals" (Westgard, 1987). Note that on a larger scale, all components of health care, including physicians, nurses, clinics, hospitals, and their services, are involved in QA. The laboratory is only part of a larger program to ensure quality health care.

QA has been an important part of the clinical laboratory since the first laboratory surveys of the 1940s. These early surveys revealed that not all laboratories reported the same results on identical blood specimens submitted for hematology and chemical analyses. Since the time of those first surveys, all sections of the clinical laboratory have become involved in assuring the quality, accuracy, and precision of the laboratory results they generate. The urinalysis laboratory is no exception.

A QA program encompasses all aspects of the urinalysis laboratory. Specimen collection, storage, and handling; instrumentation use and maintenance; reagent quality and preparation; and the laboratorian's knowledge and technical skills must meet specific minimum criteria to ensure the quality of the results generated. In order to achieve the goals set forth in a QA program, a commitment by all laboratory personnel, including administration and management, is necessary. This dedication must be evident in management decisions, including the allocation of laboratory space, the purchase of equipment and supplies, and the budget. Without adequate resources, the quality of laboratory services is compromised. Properly educated and experienced laboratory personnel with a high level of evaluative skills are essential to ensure the quality of laboratory results. "Many studies have shown that the standards of specimen collection technique and analytical performance are generally inferior to those obtained by skilled laboratorians" (Fraser, 1991). Because of the dynamic environment of clinical laboratory science, it is imperative that laboratorians acquire reference books and have opportunities for continuing education to assist them in skill maintenance and development. Not only do continuing education opportunities provide intellectual stimulation and challenges for laboratorians, but they also facilitate the development of quality employees and ensure that the maintenance of the urinalysis laboratory is kept abreast of technological advances.

A QA program for the urinalysis laboratory consists of three principal aspects: 1) the preanalytical components—procedures that occur before testing; 2) the analytical components—aspects that directly affect testing; and 3) the postanalytical components—procedures and policies that affect result reporting and interpretation. Because

an error in any component will directly affect the quality of results, each component must be monitored, evaluated, and maintained.

Preanalytical Components of QA

The preanalytical components involve numerous laboratory and ancillary staff, and in many instances, multiple departments. Because of the importance of cost-effective practices in test ordering, the laboratory plays a role in monitoring **test utilization**—i.e., avoiding duplicate testing and ensuring test appropriateness whenever possible. Each laboratory is unique; procedures designed to fit each laboratory's individual needs must be in place to intercept and eliminate unnecessary testing.

The importance of timely result reporting cannot be overemphasized. A delay in specimen transport and processing directly affects specimen **turnaround time.** The definition of turnaround time differs for the laboratorian as opposed to physicians or nursing personnel. For example, a laboratorian defines turnaround time as the time from the receipt of the specimen in the laboratory to the reporting of results either to a patient care area or into a data information system. In contrast, physicians view turnaround time as the time from when they write the order for the test until the result is communicated to them for action. To nursing personnel, it is the time that elapses from actual specimen collection until the results are communicated to them. To monitor and address potential delays that directly involve the laboratory, a policy for the documentation of specimen collection, receipt, and result report times is necessary.

Specimen collection techniques differ, are often controlled by medical personnel outside of the laboratory, and can have a direct impact on laboratory results. In addition, numerous factors can affect the urine specimen obtained (e.g., diet, exercise, hydration, medications), and appropriate patient preparation may be needed. To ensure an appropriate specimen, collection instructions (including special precautions and appropriate labeling) must be well written and must be

TABLE 2–1. CRITERIA FOR URINE SPECIMEN REJECTION

Insufficient volume of urine for requested test(s).
Inappropriate specimen type or collection.
Visibly contaminated (e.g., by fecal material, debris) specimen.
Incorrect urine preservative.
Specimen not properly preserved for transportation delay.
Unlabeled or mislabeled specimen or request form.
Request form incomplete or lacking.

distributed to and used by all personnel involved in specimen collection.

Laboratory staff who receive specimens must be educated to identify and handle inappropriate or unacceptable specimens. In addition, they must document any problems encountered, so that the problems can be ad-

dressed and corrected. The procedure the staff should follow involves 1) correlation of the patient's name on the request slip with the patient's name on the specimen container; 2) the evaluation of the elapsed time between the collection and the receipt of the specimen in the laboratory; 3) the suitability of specimen preservation, if necessary; and 4) the acceptability of the specimen—the volume collected, the container used, its cleanliness, any evidence of fecal contamination, etc. If the specimen is not acceptable, a procedure must be in place to ensure that the physician or nursing staff is informed of the problem, the problem or discrepancy is documented, and appropriate action is taken. Written guidelines that give the criteria for specimen rejection, as well as the procedure for the handling of mislabeled specimens, are

TABLE 2–2. DEFINITIONS AND AN EXAMPLE OF POLICY FOR HANDLING UNLABELED OR MISLABELED SPECIMENS

DEFINITIONS	
Unlabeled	No patient identification is placed directly on the container or the tube containing the specimen. It is inadequate to place the label on the plastic bag that holds the specimen.
Mislabeled	The name or identification number on the specimen label does not agree with that on the test request form.
POLICY FEATURES	
Notification	Contact the originating nursing station, clinic, etc. and indicate that the specimen must be recollected. Document the name of the individual contacted.
Document	Order the requested test and write CANCEL on the document with the appropriate reason for the cancellation, i.e., specimen unlabeled or specimen mislabeled, identification questionable. Initiate an incident report and include names, dates, times, and all circumstances.
Specimen	Do not discard the specimen. Process and perform analyses on those specimens that cannot be saved, but do not report the results. Properly store all other specimens. On specimens that *cannot* be recollected (e.g., cerebrospinal fluid): • The patient's physician must: contact the appropriate laboratory supervisor and request approval for the tests on the "questionable" specimen sign documentation of the incident • The individual who obtained the specimen must come to the laboratory to: identify the specimen properly label the specimen or correctly label the test request form sign documentation of the incident
Reporting Results	All labeling and signing of documentation must take place *before* results are released (except in cases of life-threatening emergencies, e.g., cardiac arrest, when a verbal specimen identification is acceptable and the documentation is completed later). All reported results must include comments describing the incident. For example, "Specimen was improperly labeled, but was approved for testing. The reported value may not be from this patient."
Quality Assurance Report	Forward a copy of the incident to the Quality Assurance committee and to the patient care unit involved (e.g., nursing station, clinic, physician's office).

required to ensure consistent treatment by all personnel (Tables 2–1 and 2–2).

The processing of urine specimens within the laboratory is another potential source of preanalytical problems. Routine urinalysis specimens should be processed immediately to prevent changes in specimen integrity; if delay at the reception area is unavoidable, the specimens must be protected from light and refrigerated. Timed urine collections require a written protocol to ensure adequate mixing, volume measurement, recording, aliquoting, and preservation if the specimen testing is to be delayed. With a written procedure for specimen processing in place, all personnel will perform these tasks consistently, eliminating unnecessary variables.

Because of the multitude of variables and personnel involved in urine specimen collection and processing, it is imperative that adequate training and supervision be provided. Written procedures must be available; equipment manuals and maintenance schedules must be adhered to; personnel must have had appropriate education regarding universal blood and body fluid precautions; and there must be consistent communication to the personnel of all procedure changes or introductions of new procedures. Preanalytical components are a dynamic part of the clinical laboratory and require adherence to protocol in order to ensure meaningful test results.

Analytical Components of QA

Analytical components are those variables that are directly involved in laboratory testing. They include reagents and supplies, instrumentation, analytical methods, monitoring the analytical methods, and the laboratory personnel's technical skills. Because each component is capable of affecting test results, procedures must be developed and utilized to ensure acceptable quality.

EQUIPMENT. All equipment, such as glassware, pipettes, analytical balances, centrifuges, refrigerators, freezers, microscopes, and refractometers, require routine monitoring to ensure appropriate function, calibration, and adherence to prescribed minimal standards. **Preventive maintenance** sched-

ules to eliminate equipment failure and "down time" are also important aspects of a QA program and should be included in the laboratory procedure manual. Use of instrument maintenance sheets for documentation provides a visual format to remind the staff of maintenance requirements and to record the performance of periodic maintenance (Fig. 2–1). Because the bench technologist is the first individual to be aware of an instrument failure, troubleshooting and "out-of-control" protocols including service and repair documentation should be readily available in the urinalysis laboratory.

The required frequency of maintenance differs depending on the equipment used, and the protocol should meet the minimal standards set forth by the Joint Commission on Accreditation of Health Care Organizations (JCAHO) or the College of American Pathologists (CAP) guidelines. Table 2–3 lists equipment found in the urinalysis laboratory with the frequency and types of performance checks that should be performed. For example, temperature-dependent devices are monitored and recorded daily, as are refractometers and osmometers. Whereas centrifuges should be cleaned daily, their revolutions per minute and timer checks can be performed periodically. Automatic pipettes, analytical balances, and fume hoods also require periodic checks, which are determined by the individual laboratory and often vary based on usage. Microscopes require daily cleaning and sometimes adjustments (e.g., illumination, phase ring alignment) to ensure optimal viewing. Microscopes and balances should have annual preventive maintenance and cleaning by professional service engineers to avoid potential problems and costly repairs. A current CAP inspection checklist is an excellent resource for developing an individualized procedure for performing periodic checks and routine maintenance on the equipment and for providing guidelines on the documentation necessary in the urinalysis laboratory.

REAGENTS. Reliable analytical results obtained in the urinalysis laboratory require the use of quality reagents. The laboratory must have an adequate supply of distilled or deionized water. Each urinalysis procedure

TABLE 2–3.   URINALYSIS EQUIPMENT PERFORMANCE CHECKS

EQUIPMENT	FREQUENCY	CHECKS PERFORMED
Automatic pipettes	Initially and periodically thereafter; varies with usage (e.g., monthly).	Check for accuracy and reproducibility.
Balances, analytical	Periodically (e.g., quarterly)	Check with standard weights (National Bureau of Standards Class S).
	Annually	Service and clean.
Centrifuges	Daily	Clean rotor, trunnions, and interior with suitable disinfectant.
	Periodically (e.g., annually)	Check revolutions per minute and timer.
	Periodically	Change brushes whenever needed; varies with centrifuge type and usage.
Fume hoods (i.e., biosafety cabinets)	Periodically (e.g., annually)	Air flow.
Microscopes	Daily	Clean and adjust if necessary (e.g., Köhler illumination, phase ring adjustment).
	Annually	Service and clean.
Osmometers	Daily	Determine and record osmolality of control materials.
Reagent strip readers	Daily	Calibrate reflectance meter with standard reagent strip.
	Daily (or periodically)	Clean mechanical parts and optics.
Refractometers	Daily	Read and record deionized water (SG 1.000) and at least one standard of known SG, e.g., NaCl, 3% (SG 1.015), 5% (SG 1.022), 7% (SG 1.035), or sucrose 9% (1.034).
Temperature-dependent devices, (e.g., refrigerators, freezers, water baths, incubators)	Daily (or when used)	Read and record temperature.
Thermometers used	Initially and annually thereafter	Check against National Bureau of Standards-certified thermometer.

should specify the type and quality of water required for tasks such as reagent preparation or reconstitution of lyophilized materials. Water quality requires periodic monitoring that varies with the source quality and the laboratory's needs. Routinely, resistivity (conductivity) and bacterial counts are performed and documented. In addition, because water loses its resistivity upon storage, it should be obtained fresh daily. Water quality tolerance limits and the action to be taken when these quality limits are exceeded must also be available in a written policy.

Reagent-grade or analytical reagent-grade (AR) reagents should be used when preparing reagent solutions for qualitative or quantitative procedures. Primary standards, if necessary for quantitative methods, must be made from chemicals of the highest grade available. These can be purchased from agencies such as the National Bureau of Standards (NBS) or CAP and can be accurately weighed to produce a standard of a known concentration. From these primary standards, secondary standards or calibration materials can be made. Any solvents used should be of suffi-

CLINITEK MAINTENANCE

MONTH ——— YEAR ———

DAILY MAINTENANCE (pp. 2, 3, 5 of Maintenance Guide)

	1	2	3	4	5	6	7	8	9	10	11	12	13	14	15	16	17	18	19	20	21	22	23	24	25	26	27	28	29	30	31
Clean blotter																															
Clean fixed platform and moving table																															
Clean read-head hold-downs																															
Wipe surface of instrument and printer with damp cloth																															
Run controls																															

WEEKLY MAINTENANCE (pp. 6–10 of Maintenance Guide)

	1	2	3	4	5	6	7	8	9	10	11	12	13	14	15	16	17	18	19	20	21	22	23	24	25	26	27	28	29	30	31
Remove hold-down assemblies and clean holddown retainers; check for bent retainers and pitting																															

Clean read-head grooves

Wash racks, centrifuge trunions and buckets

MONTHLY MAINTENANCE

Eye wash maintenance

PERIODIC MAINTENANCE

INITIALS

FIGURE 2–1. An example of an instrument maintenance chart. This chart incorporates the daily, weekly, and monthly maintenance for a Clinitek automated reagent strip reader on one chart. Other instrumentation may require several maintenance charts owing to the frequency, amount, and type of maintenance required. (Courtesy of University of Minnesota Hospital, Minneapolis, MN.)

37

cient purity to ensure appropriate reactivity and prevent interfering side reactions.

Standard laboratory practice is to check all newly prepared standards and reagents before using them. This is done by performing the assay on a control material using both the new and old reagents or standards. If the new standard or reagent performs equivalent to the old, it is acceptable and dated as approved for use; if the new performs inadequately, it should be discarded and a new reagent or standard made. New lot numbers of commercially prepared reagents and standards, as well as different bottles of a current lot number, must be checked against the old, proven reagents before being placed into use. Documentation of these reagent and standard checks must be made and maintained in the urinalysis laboratory. All standards, reagents, reagent strips, and tablets, whether laboratory-made or commercially prepared, must be dated when prepared or received and when checked out. Ensuring the quality of the commercial reagent strips and tablet tests used in the urinalysis laboratory is discussed specifically in Chapter 7.

PROCEDURE MANUALS. Procedure manuals must be available in the urinalysis laboratory and should comply with the National Committee for Clinical Laboratory Standards approved guideline, Clinical Laboratory Procedure Manuals (GP2-A, 1984). Each manual should be comprehensive, including details of all procedures performed, proper specimen collection and handling procedures, test principles, reagent preparation, control materials and acceptance criteria, step-by-step performance procedures, calculations, reporting of results, and references. Because the procedure manual is vital to the laboratory, it must be continually reviewed, updated, and adhered to in the performance of all tests. The manual must show documentation of any procedural changes and be reviewed annually. A well-written procedure manual provides a ready and reliable reference for the veteran technologist, as well as an informational training tool for the novice. The importance of procedure manuals cannot be overemphasized, because uniform perform-

ance of testing methods ensures accurate and reproducible results regardless of changes in personnel.

A routine urinalysis incorporates methods to ensure consistent quality in each of its components. The laboratory procedure manual details all examinations — physical, chemical, microscopic — and includes quality control checks, acceptable terminology, and tolerances for each. Steps to follow when tolerances are exceeded or results are questionable are also provided. In addition, procedures include criteria for the correlation of the physical, chemical, and microscopic examinations, as well as follow-up actions if discrepancies are discovered. (For instance, if the blood reagent strip is negative and the microscopic exam reveals red blood cells, check for ascorbic acid). Reference materials such as textbooks, atlases, and charts must be available for convenient consultation.

MONITORING. The microscopic examination requires the standardization of technique and adherence to the established procedure by all technologists to ensure consistency in results and reporting. This requires written step-by-step instructions of the volume of urine used, the centrifuge speed, the time of centrifugation, the sediment concentration, and the volume of sediment examined, as well as reporting format, terminology, and grading (Table 2–4). Several standardized urinalysis systems (e.g., Kova, Urisystem, Count-10) are available commercially; all are superior to the traditional glass slide and coverslip technique (Schumann, 1986).

Because many of the procedures performed in the urinalysis laboratory are manual, it is imperative to monitor **technical competence.** Uniformity of technique by all personnel is necessary and can be achieved through proper training, adherence to established protocols, and performance of quality control checks. New technologists should have their technical performance evaluated before they perform routine clinical tests. Similarly, new procedures introduced into the laboratory should be properly researched, written, and proven before being placed into use.

TABLE 2-4. GUIDELINES FOR STANDARDIZING MICROSCOPIC URINALYSIS

PROCEDURAL FACTORS

1. Volume of urine examined (10, 12, 15 mL)
2. Speed of centrifugation (400 × g, 600 × g)
3. Length of centrifugation (3, 5, 10 minutes)
4. Concentration of sediment (10:1, 12:1, 15:1)
5. Volume of sediment examined (0.4, 0.5, 1.0 mL)

REPORTING FACTORS

1. Each laboratory should publish its own normal values (based on system used and patient population).
2. All personnel must use same terminology.
3. All personnel must report results in standard format.
4. All abnormal results should be flagged for easy reference.

From Schweitzer SC, Schumann JL, Schumann GB: Quality assurance guidelines for the urinalysis laboratory. J Med Technol 3(11):570, 1986.

Before reporting results, technologists must be able to evaluate the results obtained, recognize absurdities or discrepancies, and seek answers or make corrections for those discrepancies encountered. Performing and recording results obtained, even when they differ from those expected or desired, is paramount. Because test results have a direct effect on patient diagnosis and treatment, the highest level of ethical behavior is required. Documentation of errors or problems and the action taken to correct them is necessary to 1) ensure communication to staff and supervisory personnel; 2) prevent the problem from recurring; and 3) provide a "paper trail" of actual circumstances and corrective actions taken as a result. These policies should be viewed as a means of guaranteeing the quality of the laboratory results.

Accurate results depend not only on the knowledge and technical competence of the technologist, but also on the technologist's integrity in reporting what is actually obtained. Circumstances can arise in laboratory testing that appear to contradict expected test results. When appropriately investigated, legitimate explanations that expand the technologist's scope of experience are obtained. For example, results can differ dramatically from those obtained previously. Investigation can reveal that a specimen mix-up occurred or that a drug the patient recently received is now interfering with testing. This highlights the need for good communication among all staff and supervisory personnel, as well as the need for a vehicle such as staff meetings or "quality circles" (i.e., a small team of individuals that meet to identify problems and discuss possible solutions) to ensure the dissemination of new information.

Monitoring Analytical Components of QA

For internal QA of testing methods, **quality control (QC) materials** are used to assess and monitor analytical error, i.e., the accuracy and precision of a method. These QC materials serve to alert the laboratorian of method changes that directly affect the quality of the results obtained. These materials can be prepared by the laboratory or purchased from commercial suppliers. They mimic patient samples in their physical and chemical characteristics; i.e., they have the same matrix. Some QC materials have their values assigned by the manufacturer. These values need to be confirmed and adjusted if necessary to reflect each laboratory's method and conditions.

Several urinalysis control materials are commercially available, including KOVA-Trol (ICL Scientific), CHEK-STIX (Miles, Inc.), and Quantscopics (Quantimetrix Corp.). These control materials are used to monitor the status of the qualitative chemical examination by reagent strips. Although they may be more costly than laboratory-made controls, these control materials are convenient and do not demand the time and expertise required to make good, stable control solutions. Also present in KOVA-Trol are stabilized red blood cells and organic particles (mulberry spores) to simulate white blood cells, whereas Quantiscopics currently includes only stabilized red blood cells, but plans to add stabilized white blood cells in the near future. Because of these microscopic constituents, these controls can be used to evaluate specimen processing steps and the microscopic examination. Another means of monitoring the entire urinalysis procedure is to aliquot a well-mixed urine specimen and have each technologist or shift of workers perform the procedure. Results should be recorded independently and evaluated. When multiple laboratories within a facility perform urinalyses, "in-house" laboratory testing can be done by having each laboratory test the same specimen and comparing results. If commercial control materials with sediment constituents are not used to evaluate the microscopic examination, this in-house duplicate testing can be instrumental in detecting subtle changes in the processing procedure, such as changes in centrifugation speed or time. The time and effort involved in intralaboratory testing are worthwhile because they ensure that each laboratory and all staff are consistently reporting equivalent results.

Results obtained on control materials, as well as from duplicate specimen testing, are recorded daily in either a tabular or graphic form. The tolerance limits for these results must be defined, documented, and readily available in the laboratory. When these tolerances are exceeded, corrective action must be taken and documented.

Whether the urinalysis laboratory performs quantitative urine procedures (e.g., total protein, creatinine) depends on the facility. In some settings, the urinalysis laboratory performs only the manual quantitative procedures, whereas the chemistry section performs those that are automated. Regardless, a brief discussion of the QC materials used for quantitative urine methods is necessary. The value assigned to commercial or homemade QC materials is determined in the laboratory by performing repeated analyses over different days. This enables variables such as personnel, reagents, and supplies to be represented in the data generated. After analyses are complete, the QC data are tabulated and control limits are determined using the mean ($\bar{x}$) and standard deviation (s). Initial control (or tolerance) limits can be established using a minimum of 20 determinations; as more data are accumulated, the limits can be revised. Because the error distribution is Gaussian, control limits are chosen such that

95 percent to 99 percent of the control values will be within tolerance. This corresponds to the mean value $\pm 2s$ or $\pm 3s$, respectively. Graphs of the QC values obtained over time are plotted and are known as Levey-Jennings control charts. They provide an easy, visual means of identifying changes in accuracy and precision. Changes in accuracy are evidenced by a shift in the mean, whereas changes in precision (random error) are manifested by an increase in scatter or a widening of the distribution about the mean (standard deviation).

There are also **external quality assurance** measures (e.g., proficiency surveys) to monitor and evaluate a urinalysis laboratory's performance compared with other facilities. These QA measures may be in the form of proficiency testing or participation in programs in which each laboratory utilizes the same lot of QC materials. The latter is used primarily with quantitative urine methods. Monthly, the results obtained by each laboratory are reported to the manufacturer of the QC material. Within weeks, reports summarizing the analytical methods used and the results obtained by each laboratory are distributed. These reports are very useful in detecting small continuous changes in systematic error in quantitative methods that may not be evident with the internal quality assurance procedures.

Interlaboratory comparison testing on a periodic basis, in the form of proficiency surveys, is required by CAP and more recently by the Clinical Laboratory Improvement Act (CLIA) of 1988. This comparison testing involves the performance of routine tests on survey samples provided to all participating laboratories. Each laboratory independently performs and submits the results to the survey agency for assessment and tabulation. Prior to the distribution of these survey samples, representative samples are assessed analytically by reference laboratories to establish the true or correct value. From the results submitted, the survey agency prepares extensive reports and charts of each analyte, the method used, and the values obtained. These surveys provide valuable information on laboratory performance and testing methods individually, by method, and as a whole.

Some urinalysis proficiency surveys include Kodachrome slides for the identification of sediment components, such as casts, epithelial cells, blood cells, and diaper fibers. One approach used to evaluate these slides is for each technologist in the laboratory to independently identify the sediment component. Results are shared and only one answer can be submitted to the survey agency. Although limited, this format does allow evaluation of competence in microscopic identification. In addition, if the process of arriving at an answer by consensus is used, it provides an opportunity to maintain and improve the competence of personnel.

Although QC materials help to detect decreased quality in laboratory testing, they do not pinpoint the source of the problem, nor do they solve it. Only with good communication and documentation can analytical problems be pursued and continuing education programs developed. Some problems encountered in the laboratory may best be approached by the development of a quality circle. The involvement of laboratorians in a problem-solving team reaffirms the technologists' self-worth and enhances their commitment to quality goals.

Postanalytical Components of QA

Urinalysis results can be communicated efficiently and effectively using a standardized reporting format and terminology. The report should include reference ranges as well as the opportunity to add additional informative statements if warranted, e.g., "glucose oxidase/reducing substances questionable owing to the presence of ascorbic acid" or "clumps of white blood cells present." Results should be quantitative (e.g., 100 mg/dL or 10 to 25 RBCs/HPF [red blood cells per high-power field]) wherever possible and standardized terminology used by all personnel (e.g., color or clarity terms).

The laboratory procedures should describe in detail the appropriate reporting for-

mat and also provide criteria for the reporting of any critical values. **Critical values** are significantly abnormal results that exceed either the upper or lower critical limit and are life-threatening. These results need to be relayed immediately to the physician for appropriate action. It is the laboratorian's responsibility to recognize them and communicate them in a timely fashion. Each institution must establish its own list of critical values. For example, the list might include as critical the presence of pathological urine crystals (e.g., cysteine, leucine, tyrosine); a strongly positive test for both glucose and ketones; and the presence of a reducing substance, other than glucose or ascorbic acid, in an infant.

QA measures, whether internal (QC materials) or external (proficiency surveys), require **documentation** and evidence of active review. When acceptable tolerances are exceeded, they must be addressed and corrective action taken. In the clinical laboratory, documentation is crucial, because an action that was not documented has essentially not been performed. The goal of an effective QA program is consistently accurate and reproducible results. In achieving this goal, test results reflect a patient's condition, rather than procedural or personnel variations.

Safety in the Urinalysis Laboratory

· ·

For years, the health care industry has been at the forefront in developing policies and procedures to prevent and control the spread of infection in all areas of the hospital to ensure both patient and employee safety. With the passage of the Occupational Health and Safety Act in 1970, formal regulation of safety and health for all employees, regardless of employer, officially began. This law is administered through the U.S. Department of Labor by the **Occupational Safety and Health Administration (OSHA).** As a result of the law, written safety manuals that define specific policies and procedures for all potential hazards are required in laboratories. Documentation of an annual review of this manual by all employees is mandatory. Because clinical laboratory employees are exposed to numerous workplace hazards in various forms — biological, chemical, electrical, radioactive, compressed gases, fires, and so on — safety policies are an integral part of the laboratory. This next section discusses those hazards frequently encountered in the clinical laboratory when working with urine and body fluids (e.g., feces, amniotic fluid, cerebrospinal fluid), as well as the policies and procedures necessary to ensure a safe and healthy working environment.

Biological Hazards

Biological hazards abound in the clinical laboratory. Any patient specimen or body substance (e.g., body fluid, fresh tissue, excretions, secretions, sputum, drainages, nonintact skin) must be treated as infectious, regardless of patient diagnosis. The transmission of diseases, especially hepatitis B virus (HBV) and human immunodeficiency virus (HIV), are of primary concern to health care workers. To prevent cross transmission and exposure to potentially infectious agents, **Universal Precautions (UP)** must be adhered to by all personnel. Initially published as recommendations by the Centers for Disease Control (CDC) in 1987, a UP policy describes the potential sources of infectious agents and the methods to be employed when handling and disposing of these agents, as well as precautions and techniques for working directly with patients. Although most institutions have an Infection Control Department, it is the responsibility of each laboratory to educate, implement, and monitor employee compliance to UP. In addition, this policy must be documented and available for reference in the laboratory.

Although urine, feces, and vomitus are body fluids, the 1988 CDC revision of these guidelines for the safety of laboratory workers excludes them from the requirement of UP unless the specimens are bloody. Identifying and separating specimens based on the presence of visible blood is time consuming and subjective, requires procedural variations,

and may promote laxity in processing and handling other specimen types. Although these body fluids may be unlikely sources of HBV or HIV, they can be a reservoir for other infectious agents. Therefore, most clinical laboratories employ UP when working with all body fluids.

The three primary routes of infection are 1) inhalation, 2) ingestion, and 3) direct inoculation or skin contact. Aerosols can be created when liquids (e.g., body fluids) are poured and pipetted, or spilled. The removal of tight-fitting caps from specimen containers and centrifugation are other sources of airborne transmission. Ingestion occurs when infectious agents are taken into the mouth and swallowed, such as from mouth pipetting; eating, drinking, or smoking in the laboratory; or hand-to-mouth contact following failure to appropriately wash one's hands. Direct inoculation involves parenteral exposure to the infectious agent as a result of a break in the technologist's skin barrier or contact with the mucous membranes. This includes skin punctures with needles, cuts or scratches from contaminated glassware, and splashes of specimens into the eyes, nose, and mouth. Although it is impossible to eliminate all sources of infectious transmission in the laboratory, they can be minimized through the use of protective barriers and adherence to UP.

When contact with urine or other body fluids is anticipated, appropriate **protective barriers** must be in place. Gloves should be worn when assisting patients in collecting specimens, when receiving and processing urine and body fluid specimens, when performing any testing procedure, and when cleaning equipment or work areas. In addition, they should be worn at all times in the laboratory where countertops, chairs, and other surfaces are exposed to these specimens. If the technologist is involved directly with patients, he or she should change gloves after each patient. In the laboratory, the gloves should be changed when they are visibly soiled or physically damaged. Gloves used in the urinalysis laboratory should not be worn outside of the area. Whenever gloves are removed or when contact with urine or other body fluids has occurred, hands should be washed with an appropriate antiseptic soap.

Protective laboratory coats must be worn in the laboratory. They should be changed daily or more often if soiled. These coats should not be worn outside of or removed from the laboratory area. If splashing of large volumes of urine or other body fluids is anticipated, a moisture-resistant apron or gown should be worn.

Because processing and performing procedures on urine and body fluids can often result in sprays or splatters, eyewear or headgear should be used to protect the eyes, nose, and mouth. Eyeglasses are usually sufficient for most situations in the laboratory; however, plexiglass shields, safety goggles, or hood sashes may be necessary for protection, depending on the procedure being performed and the substance being handled.

Specimen Processing

All specimens should be transported to the laboratory in sealed plastic bags, with the request slip placed on the outside of the bag. If the outside of the specimen container is obviously contaminated because of leakage or improper collection technique, the container's exterior may be cleaned using an appropriate disinfectant before processing; or it should be rejected and a new specimen requested. When removing lids or caps from specimens, the technologist should work behind a protective shield or cover the specimens with gauze or disposable tissues to prevent sprays and splatters. During centrifugation, specimens should be capped or placed in covered trunnions. Centrifuges should not be operated with their tops open, nor stopped by hand. If a specimen needs to be aliquoted, the technologist should use transfer pipettes or protective barriers if pouring from the specimen container.

Disposal of Waste

To protect all laboratory personnel, including custodial staff, adherence to an **infectious waste disposal policy** is necessary. Because all biological specimens and materials exposed to them (e.g., contaminated needles, glassware) are considered infectious, they must be disposed of properly. This requires leakproof well-constructed receptacles, clearly marked with the universal biohazard symbol, available in all laboratory areas (Fig. 2–2). These biohazard containers should not be overfilled. In addition, they should be adequately sealed and enclosed within a clean biohazard bag before removal from the laboratory area by custodial staff.

All biological specimens, except urine, must be sterilized or decontaminated before disposal. Both incineration and autoclaving are acceptable, with the latter usually being the most cost-effective. Urine, on the other hand, may be discarded directly down a sink or toilet, with caution taken to avoid splashing. When discarding urine down a sink, the technologist should rinse the sink well with water after specimens are discarded and at least daily with 0.5 percent bleach (sodium hypochlorite).

Contaminated sharps, such as needles, broken glass, or transfer pipettes, must be placed into puncture-resistant containers for disposal. These containers should not be overfilled. They should be securely sealed and enclosed in a clean infectious waste disposal bag to protect custodial personnel before removal from the laboratory area. Because contaminated sharps are considered infectious, they must also be incinerated or autoclaved before disposal.

Noninfectious glass, such as empty reagent bottles, and nonhazardous waste, such as emptied urine containers, are considered

BIOHAZARD

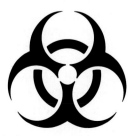

FIGURE 2–2. The universal biohazard symbol.

normal waste and require no special precautions for disposal.

Decontamination

Several agents are available for the daily **decontamination** of laboratory surfaces and equipment. Bleach or a phenolic disinfectant is used most often in the clinical laboratory. A 0.5 percent bleach solution, prepared by adding 1 part bleach to 9 parts water, is stable for 1 week. Phenolic disinfectants, a combination of phenolic compounds and detergents, are purchased commercially; appropriate dilutions are made according to the manufacturers' recommendations.

When spills occur, decontaminants are used to neutralize the biological hazard and to facilitate its removal. Because decontaminants are less effective in the presence of large amounts of protein, a body fluid spill should first be absorbed with a solid absorbent powder (e.g., Zorbitrol) or disposable towels. If an absorbent powder is used, the liquid will solidify and can be scooped up and placed into an infectious waste receptacle. If disposable towels are used, allow the spill to be absorbed and pour 0.5 percent bleach over the towels. Carefully pick up the bleach-soaked towels and transfer them to an infectious waste container. Decontaminate the spill area again using 0.5 percent bleach and clean with a phenolic detergent if desired. All disposable materials used to clean the spill area must be placed in infectious waste receptacles.

Chemical Hazards

Chemicals are ubiquitous in the clinical laboratory. Many are caustic, toxic, or flammable and must be specially handled to ensure the safety and well-being of laboratory employees. OSHA's rule of January 1990 requires each facility to have a **Chemical Hygiene Plan (CHP)** that defines the safety policies and procedures for all hazardous chemicals used in the laboratory. This plan includes the identification of a chemical hygiene officer; policies for the handling, storage, and use of chemicals; the use of protective barriers; criteria for monitoring overexposure to chemi-

cals; and provisions for medical consultations or examinations. Educating personnel about chemical safety policies and procedures is mandatory and requires a documented annual review. By developing and using a comprehensive CHP, chemical hazards are minimized and the laboratory becomes a safe environment in which to work.

The labeling of chemicals is fundamental to a laboratory safety program. Because hazardous chemicals can be classified into several categories, including caustic or corrosive materials, poisons, carcinogens, flammables, explosives, mutagens, and teratogens, each must be appropriately labeled to ensure proper handling. All chemicals are required to have descriptive warning labels on their shipping containers. These labels are color coded and include a pictorial representation of the hazard (see Fig. 2–1). However, when a chemical is removed from its original shipping container, its hazard identity is lost unless the laboratory appropriately relabels it. Although OSHA requires the labeling of hazardous chemicals, it does not mandate the type of labeling system to use. By using a consistent identification system, hazards can be identified readily and appropriate precautions taken. The National Fire Protection Association (NFPA) developed the 704-M Hazard Identification System, using bright, color-coded labels divided into quadrants. These labels are highly visible and identify the health (blue), flammability (red), and reactivity (yellow) hazard for each chemical, as well as any special considerations (white) (Fig. 2–3). The system also uses numbers from 0 to 4 to classify the hazard severity, with 4 representing extremely hazardous.

To limit employee exposure, appropriate usage and handling guidelines for each chemical type must be described in the laboratory safety manual. General rules such as prohibiting pipetting by mouth or sniffing of chemicals are mandatory. Because the greatest hazard encountered in the clinical laboratory is from the splattering of acids, alkalis, and strong oxidizers, appropriate use of protective barriers must be employed. Use of gloves, gowns, goggles, and a fume hood or safety cabinet will reduce the potential of injury. Chemical safety tips include the fol-

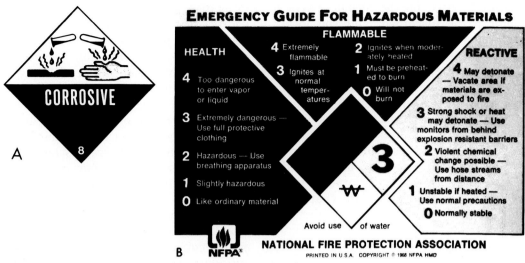

FIGURE 2–3. *A,* Labels used by the Department of Transportation to indicate hazardous chemicals. *B,* The label identification system developed by the National Fire Protection Association. (Reprinted with permission from NFPA, Copyright © 1986, National Fire Protection Association, Quincy, MA 02269.)

lowing: never grasp a reagent bottle by the neck or top, and always add acid to water; *never add water to concentrated acid.* Safety equipment such as an eyewash or shower must be readily available and accessible in case of accidental exposure.

The goal of OSHA's hazardous communication rule is to ensure that all employees are aware of potential chemical hazards in their workplace. This employee "right to know" required chemical manufacturers and suppliers to provide **material safety data sheets (MSDS).** These sheets, available for each chemical, include the chemical's identity information, hazardous ingredients, physical and chemical characteristics, physical hazards, reactivity, health hazards, precautions for safe handling and use, and regulatory information (see example in Appendix B). Whereas an MSDS for each hazardous chemical used in all laboratory areas must be available on site, each laboratory section should retain copies of the MSDS for chemicals frequently used in their areas for quick reference.

Handling Chemical Spills

In the event of a spill, the chemical's MSDS should be consulted for the appropriate action to be taken. Each laboratory should have available a chemical spill kit that includes absorbent, appropriate protective barriers (e.g., gloves, goggles), clean-up pans, absorbent towels or pillows, and disposal bags. Frequently, liquids may be contained by absorption using a spill compound (absorbent), such as ground clay or a sodium bicarbonate and sand mixture. The latter is generally appropriate for acid, alkali, or solvent spills. Following absorption, the absorbent is picked up and placed into a bag or sealed container for appropriate chemical disposal, and the spill area is thoroughly washed.

For emergency treatment of personnel affected by chemical splashes or injuries, clear instructions should be posted in the laboratory. Chemical spills of hazardous substances must be reported to supervisory personnel and appropriately documented. This permits a review of the circumstances and facilitates changes to prevent recurrence of the incident. Any injury or illness resulting from the spill or exposure also requires documentation and follow-up.

Disposal of Chemical Waste

All chemicals must be properly disposed of to ensure safety in the workplace and in the environment in general. Because chemical disposal differs based on the chemical type, the amount to be discarded, and the local laws, each laboratory must maintain its own policies for disposal. Following the performance of laboratory procedures, chemicals are often adequately diluted or neutralized, such that disposal in the sewer system is satisfactory. It is a good practice to always flush sinks and drains with copious amounts of water following the disposal of aqueous reagents. The appropriate steps to be followed must be available in a general laboratory policy or in the laboratory procedure that utilizes the chemical.

Other Hazards

Organic solvents used in the clinical laboratory represent both a health and a fire hazard. As a result, these flammable substances require special considerations regarding storage, use, and disposal. Appropriately vented storage cabinets are necessary to store solvents; the availability of the cabinets dictates the volume of flammables that are allowed to be stored on the premises. Because of potentially toxic vapors, adequate ventilation during solvent use, such as in a fume hood, is mandatory. Although small amounts of water-miscible solvents may be disposed of in the sewer system with copious amounts of water, disposal of flammable solvents in this fashion is dangerous. All solvent waste should be recovered following procedures in glass or other appropriate containers. Because not all solvents can be mixed together, a written laboratory protocol listing acceptable solvent combinations is necessary. After collection, each solvent waste container must be clearly marked with the solvent type and relative amount present and must be properly stored until disposal.

Other potential fire hazards in the laboratory include electrical hazards or hazards from flammable compressed gases. Laboratory personnel should report any deteriora-

tions discovered in equipment (e.g., electrical shorts) or their connections (e.g., a frayed cord). If a liquid spill occurs on electrical equipment or its connections, appropriate action must be taken to dry the equipment thoroughly, before it is placed back into use. Compressed gases must be secured at all times, regardless of their contents or the amount of gas in the tank. Their valve caps should be in place except when in use. A procedure for the appropriate transporting, handling, and storage of compressed gases is necessary to ensure proper usage. All laboratory personnel must be aware of the location of all fire extinguishers, alarms, and safety equipment; be instructed in the use of a fire extinguisher; and be involved in laboratory fire drills, at least annually.

References

Fraser CG, Petersen PH: The importance of imprecision. Ann Clin Biochem 28:207, 1991.

Schweitzer SC, Schumann JL, Schumann GB: Quality assurance guidelines for the urinalysis laboratory. J Med Technol 3(11):570, 1986.

Schumann GB, and Tebbs RD: Comparison of slides used for standardized routine microscopic urinalysis. J Med Technol 3:54–58, 1986.

Westgard JO, Klee GG: Quality assurance. In Tietz, NW (ed.): Fundamentals of Clinical Chemistry (3rd ed.), Philadelphia, W. B. Saunders Company, 1987, p. 238.

Bibliography

Hazardous Materials, Storage, and Handling Pocketbook, Alexandria, VA, Defense Logistics Agency, 1984.

National Fire Protection Association: Hazardous Chemical Data, Boston, MA, National Fire Protection Association, No. 49, 1975.

Occupational exposure to hazardous chemicals in laboratories, final rule. Federal Register 55:3327–3335, 1990.

Occupational safety and health standards, Federal Register 43, 1978.

Protection of laboratory workers from infectious disease transmitted by blood, body fluids, and tissue, Tentative Guidelines, M29-T, Villanova, PA, National Committee for Clinical Laboratory Standards, 1989.

Study Questions

1. **The ultimate goal of a quality assurance program is to**

    A. maximize the productivity of the laboratory.
    B. assure that patient test results are precise.
    C. ensure the appropriate diagnosis and treatment of patients.
    D. ensure the validity of the laboratory results obtained.

2. **Which of the following is a preanalytical component of a quality assurance program?**

    A. Quality control
    B. Turnaround time
    C. Technical competence
    D. Preventive maintenance

3. **Which of the following is a postanalytical component of a quality assurance program?**

    A. Critical values
    B. Procedure manuals
    C. Preventive maintenance
    D. Test utilization

4. **Analytical components of a quality assurance program are procedures and policies that affect**

    A. the technical testing of the specimen.
    B. the collection and processing of the specimen.
    C. the reporting and interpretation of results.
    D. the diagnosis and treatment of the patient.

5. **The purpose of quality control materials is to**

   A. monitor instrumentation to eliminate "down time."
   B. ensure the quality of test results obtained.
   C. assess the accuracy and precision of a method.
   D. monitor the technical competence of the laboratory staff.

6. **Why are written procedure manuals necessary?**

   A. To assist in the ordering of reagents and supplies for a procedure.
   B. To appropriately monitor the accuracy and precision of a procedure.
   C. To ensure that all individuals perform the same task consistently.
   D. To ensure that the appropriate test has been ordered.

7. **Which of the following is NOT considered to be an analytical component in quality assurance?**

   A. Reagents (e.g., water)
   B. Glassware (e.g., pipettes)
   C. Instrumentation (e.g., microscope)
   D. Specimen preservation (e.g., refrigeration)

8. **Which of the following sources should include a protocol for the way to proceed when quality control results exceed acceptable tolerance limits?**

   A. A reference book
   B. A procedure manual
   C. A preventive maintenance manual
   D. A specimen-processing protocol

9. **"Technical competence" is displayed when a laboratory practitioner**

   A. documents reports in a legible manner.
   B. recognizes discrepant test results.
   C. independently reduces the time needed to perform a procedure (e.g., by decreasing incubation times).
   D. is punctual and timely.

10. **Quality control materials should have**

   A. a short expiration date.
   B. a matrix similar to patient samples.
   C. their values assigned by an external and unbiased commercial manufacturer.
   D. the ability to test preanalytical variables.

11. **Within one facility, what is the purpose of performing duplicate testing of a specimen by two different laboratories (i.e., "in-house" duplicates)?**

    A. It provides little information because the results are already known.
    B. It saves money by replacing the need for internal quality control materials.
    C. It provides a means of evaluating the precision of a method.
    D. It can detect procedural and technical differences between laboratories.

12. **Interlaboratory comparison testing, such as proficiency surveys, provides a means to**

    A. identify critical values for timely reporting to clinicians.
    B. ensure that appropriate documentation is being performed.
    C. evaluate the technical performance of individual laboratory practitioners.
    D. evaluate a laboratory's performance compared to that of other laboratories.

13. **The primary purpose of a laboratory's Universal Precautions policy is to**

    A. ensure a safe and healthy working environment.
    B. identify processes (e.g., autoclaving) to be used to neutralize infectious agents.
    C. prevent the exposure and transmission of potentially infectious agents to personnel.
    D. identify patients with HBV, HIV, and other infectious diseases.

14. **Which agency is responsible for defining, establishing, and monitoring safety and health hazards in the workplace?**

    A. Occupational Safety and Health Administration (OSHA)
    B. Centers for Disease Control (CDC)
    C. Chemical Hygiene Agency (CHA)
    D. National Fire Protection Association (NFPA)

15. **Match the mode of transmission with the laboratory activity.**

	Laboratory Activity	Mode of Transmission
_____ A.	Not wearing gloves when handling specimens.	1. Inhalation
_____ B.	Centrifuging uncovered specimens.	2. Ingestion
_____ C.	Smoking in the laboratory.	3. Direct contact
_____ D.	Being scratched by a broken beaker.	
_____ E.	Having a specimen splashed into the eyes.	
_____ F.	Pipetting by mouth.	

16. **Which of the following is NOT considered a protective barrier?**

    A. Gloves
    B. Lab coat
    C. Disinfectants
    D. Eyeglasses

17. **Which of the following represents a good laboratory practice?**

    A. Washing hands frequently

    B. Wearing lab coats outside of the laboratory

    C. Removing lab coats from the laboratory for laundering at home in 2 percent bleach

    D. Wearing the same gloves to perform venipuncture on two different patients because the patients are in the same room

18. **Which of the following is NOT an acceptable disposal practice?**

    A. Discarding urine into a sink

    B. Disposing of used, empty urine containers with nonhazardous waste

    C. Discarding a used, broken specimen transfer pipette with noninfectious glass waste

    D. Discarding blood specimens into a biohazard container

19. **Which of the following is NOT part of a Chemical Hygiene Plan?**

    A. To identify and label hazardous chemicals

    B. To educate employees about the chemicals they work with (e.g., providing a material safety data sheet)

    C. To provide guidelines for the handling and use of each chemical type

    D. To monitor the handling of biological hazards

20. **Which of the following is NOT found on a material safety data sheet?**

    A. Exposure limits

    B. Catalog number

    C. Hazardous ingredients

    D. Flammability of the chemical

Urine Specimen Types, Collection, and Preservation

LEARNING OBJECTIVES

After studying this chapter, the student should be able to

1. State at least three clinical reasons for performing a routine urinalysis.

2. Describe four types of urine specimens and state at least one diagnostic use for each type.

3. Explain the importance of accurate timing and complete collection of timed urine specimens.

4. Describe the collection technique employed to obtain the following specimens:
   - random void
   - midstream "clean catch"
   - catheterized
   - suprapubic aspiration
   - pediatric collection

5. Describe materials and procedures used for the proper collection and identification of each type of urine specimen.

6. State the changes possible in unpreserved urine and explain the mechanism for each.

7. Name the most common method of urine preservation and discuss the advantages and disadvantages of other urine preservatives.

KEY TERMS

catheterized specimen: a urine specimen obtained using a sterile catheter (a flexible tube) that is inserted through the urethra and into the bladder. Urine flows directly from the bladder by gravity and collects in a plastic reservoir bag.

fasting specimen: a urine specimen collected after a fast and containing only those solutes and metabolites excreted during the fasting period.

first morning specimen: the first urine specimen voided after rising from sleep. The night before the collection, the patient voids before going to bed.

Usually the first morning specimen has been retained in the bladder for 6 to 8 hours and is ideal to test for substances that may require concentration (e.g., protein) or incubation for detection (e.g., nitrites).

fractional collection (also called **double-voided specimen**): a urine specimen collected after a specific time interval. The patient voids at the beginning of the collection. This initial specimen may be tested (e.g., fasting specimen of a glucose tolerance test) or discarded. At the end of the time interval, the patient voids and collects this

urine for testing (e.g., 2-hour postprandial [2 h PP] urine specimen for the detection of glucosuria). It is termed a double-voided specimen because, frequently, blood samples are drawn at the same time for comparison of the analyte of interest in the blood and urine.

midstream "clean catch" specimen: a urine specimen obtained after thorough cleansing of the glans penis in the male or the urethral meatus in the female. Following the cleansing procedure, the patient passes the first portion of the urine into the toilet, stops and collects the midportion in the specimen container, then passes any remaining urine into the toilet. Used for both routine urinalysis and urine culture, it is essentially free of contaminants from the genitalia and distal urethra.

random urine specimen: a urine specimen collected at any time, day or night, without prior patient preparation.

suprapubic aspiration: a technique used to collect urine directly from the bladder by puncturing the abdominal wall and distended bladder using a ster-

ile needle and syringe. It is used primarily to obtain sterile specimens for bacterial cultures from infants and occasionally from adults.

timed collection: a urine specimen collected throughout a specific timed interval. The patient voids at the beginning of the collection and discards this urine; then, all subsequent urine is collected. At the end of the time interval, the patient voids and includes this urine in the collection. This technique is used

primarily for quantitative urine assays because it allows comparison of excretion patterns from day to day; the most common are 12-hour and 24-hour collections.

urine preservative: a procedure or chemical substance used to prevent composition changes in a voided urine specimen (e.g., loss or gain of chemical substances, deterioration of formed elements). The most common form of urine preservation is refrigeration.

The purposes of performing a routine urinalysis are 1) to aid in the diagnosis of disease; 2) to screen for asymptomatic, congenital, or hereditary diseases; 3) to monitor disease progression; and 4) to monitor therapy effectiveness or complications (NCCLS, 1991). To obtain accurate urinalysis results, urine specimen integrity must be maintained. If the urine specimen submitted for testing is inappropriate (e.g., if a random specimen is submitted instead of a timed collection), or if the specimen has changed owing to improper collection or storage conditions, the testing will produce results that do not reflect the patient's condition. In such situations, the highest quality reagents, equipment, expertise, and personnel cannot compensate for the unacceptable specimen. Therefore, written criteria for urine specimen types, a description of their collection and preservatives, appropriate specimen labeling, and a handling timeline must be available to all personnel involved in urine specimen procurement.

Why Study Urine?

Urine is actually a fluid biopsy of the kidney and provides a "fountain" of information (Fig. 3–1). The kidney is the only organ with such a noninvasive means by which to directly evaluate its status. In addition, because urine is an ultrafiltrate of the plasma,

it can be used to evaluate and monitor body homeostasis and many metabolic disease processes.

Usually, urine specimens are readily obtainable, and their collection inconveniences the patient only briefly. Some individuals feel uncomfortable discussing body fluids and body function. Good verbal and written communication with each patient in a sensitive and professional manner ensures collection of the urine specimen desired. The ease with which urine specimens are obtained can lead to laxity or neglect in educating the patient and stressing the importance of a proper collection. If the quality of the urine specimen is compromised, however, so is the resultant urinalysis.

Specimen Types

The type of specimen selected and the collection procedure used are determined by the health care provider and depend on the tests to be performed. There are basically four types of urine specimens: first morning, random, fractional, and timed (Table 3–1). The ideal urine specimen is adequately concentrated to ensure, upon screening, the detection of analytes and formed elements of interest. These factors, in turn, depend on the patient's state of hydration and the length of time the urine is held in the bladder.

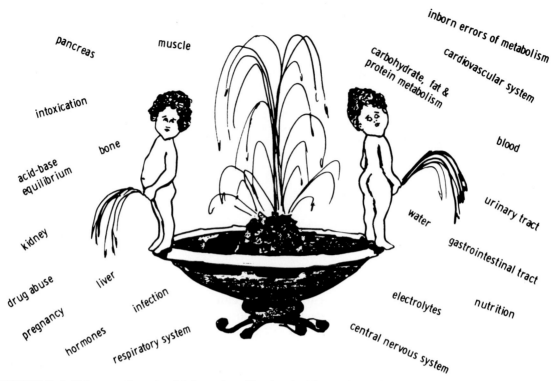

FIGURE 3–1. Urine as a fountain of information. (Reprinted with permission from Free AH, Free HM: Urinalysis in Clinical Laboratory Practice, West Palm Beach, Florida, CRC Press, Inc., 1975. Copyright CRC Press, Inc. Boca Raton, FL.)

First Morning Specimen

To collect a **first morning specimen,** the patient voids before going to bed and, immediately upon rising from sleep, collects a urine specimen. Because this urine specimen has been retained in the bladder for approximately 8 hours, it is ideal to test for substances that require concentration or incubation for detection (e.g., nitrites, protein) and to confirm orthostatic proteinuria. Formed elements such as white cells, red cells, and casts are more stable in these concentrated acidic urine specimens. However, these specimens are not suitable for cytology studies. Whereas the number of epithelial cells present may be high, their morphology is suboptimal owing to degeneration during the long retention. In addition, the highly concentrated salts in these specimens crystallize upon cooling to room temperature and cause adverse effects during processing for cytology studies.

Although the first morning urine is usually the most concentrated and is frequently the specimen of choice, it is not the most convenient to obtain. It requires that the patient pick up a container and instructions at least 1 day before his or her appointment; in addition, the specimen must be preserved if the specimen is not going to be delivered within 2 hours of collection.

Random Urine Specimen

For ease and convenience, routine screening is most often performed on **random urine specimens.** Random specimens can be collected at any time, usually during daytime hours, and without prior patient preparation. Because excessive fluid intake and exercise can directly affect urine composition, these specimens may not accurately reflect the patient's condition. Despite this, random specimens are usually satisfactory for routine

T A B L E 3 – 1.   SPECIMEN TYPES AND COLLECTION TECHNIQUES

SPECIMEN TYPES	USES
Random	Routine screening; cytology studies (with prior hydration).
First Morning	Routine screening, orthostatic proteinuria, cytology.
Fractional* (double-voided) fasting, 2 hour postprandial (2 h PP), glucose tolerance test (GTT), etc.	Diabetic screening and monitoring, fluid deprivation tests, etc.
Timed 2-hour, 12-hour, 24-hour, 2:00–4:00 PM, etc.	Quantitative assays, cytology, clearance tests, evaluation for fistula, etc.

COLLECTION TECHNIQUES	USES
Routine void	Routine screening.
Midstream "clean catch"	Routine screening, cytology, microbial culture.
Catheterized, urethral	Routine screening and microbial culture.
Catheterized, ureteral	Differentiation of bladder and kidney infections.
Suprapubic aspiration	Microbial culture, routine screening, and cytology.
Pediatric collection bags	Routine screening and quantitative assays.

* Blood samples are collected at the same time.

screening and are capable of detecting abnormalities indicating a disease process.

With prior hydration of the patient, a random "clean catch" urine specimen is ideal for cytology studies. Hydration consists of instructing the patient to drink 24 to 32 ounces of water each hour for 2 hours prior to urine collection. Most cytology protocols require collection of these specimens daily for 3 to 5 consecutive days. This increases the number of cells studied, thereby enhancing the detection of abnormality or disease. One method to increase the cellularity of the urine specimen is to have the patient exercise for 5 minutes by skipping or jumping up and down prior to specimen collection.

Fractional Collection

Fractional collections, also termed **double-voided specimens,** are used to compare the concentration of an analyte in urine to its concentration in the blood. Comparison of a series of urine specimens and blood samples, collected at specific timed intervals and tested for the presence of an analyte, can aid in the evaluation of renal threshold values and the diagnosis of disease. An example of a series of fractional collections is a glucose tolerance test (GTT). The first urine specimen collected in a GTT is a **fasting specimen.** This specimen does not contain any food solutes or metabolites from the time preceding the fast. To obtain this specimen, the patient is instructed to eat nothing after the evening meal. Upon rising in the morning, the first morning urine is discarded because it contains solutes and metabolites from the preceding evening meal. The second urine specimen excreted is a fasting urine specimen. It contains only those solutes and metabolites excreted since the last void and after the fasting period began.

Timed Collection

Due to the circadian or diurnal variation in excretion of many substances and functions (hormones, proteins, glomerular filtration rate, etc.), as well as to the effect of exercise, hydration, and body metabolism on excretion rates, quantitative urine assays often require a **timed collection.** These timed collections, usually 12-hour or 24-hour, eliminate the need to determine when excretion is optimal and allows comparison of excretion patterns from day to day. Timed urine specimens can be divided into two types: those collected for a predetermined length of time (e.g., 2 hours, 12 hours, 24 hours) and those collected during a specific time of day (e.g., 2:00 to 4:00 PM). For example, a 2-hour postprandial specimen for the determination of urinary glucose can be collected after any meal and is an ideal specimen to initially screen for glucosuria. In contrast, a 2-hour collection for the determination of urinary urobilinogen is preferably collected from 2 to 4 PM, the time when it is known to be maximally excreted.

Accurate timing and strict adherence to specimen collection directions are essential to ensure valid results from timed collections. For example, if two first morning specimens were included in a single 24-hour collection, the results would be in error from both the additional volume and analyte added. Table 3–2 summarizes a protocol for the timed collection of a 24-hour specimen. This same protocol is applicable to any timed collection. A rule of thumb is to empty the bladder and discard the urine at the beginning of a timed collection and to collect all urine subsequently passed during the collection period. At the end time of the collection, the patient must empty his or her bladder and include that urine in the timed collection.

Depending on the analyte being measured, a urine preservative may be necessary to ensure its stability throughout the collection. In addition, certain foods and drugs can affect the urinary excretion of some analytes. When this influence is known to be significant, the patient needs to be properly instructed to avoid these substances. Written instructions should include the test name, the preservative required, and any special instructions or precautions. The most common errors encountered in quantitative urine tests are directly related to specimen collection or to handling problems, such as loss of specimen, inclusion of two first morning samples, inaccurate total volume measurement, transcription error, or inadequate preservation.

TABLE 3–2.   COLLECTION PROTOCOL FOR A 24-HOUR (TIMED) URINE SPECIMEN

Discuss specimen collection procedure with patient, as well as provide him or her with written instructions.

On Day 1 at the start time (e.g., 8:00 AM), patient empties bladder in the toilet. *All* subsequent urine is collected for the next 24 h in the container provided.

On Day 2 at the end time (e.g., 8:00 AM), the patient empties bladder and includes this specimen in the collection.

After transportation to the laboratory, the entire specimen is mixed well, and the total volume excreted is accurately measured and recorded.

A sufficient aliquot, one that allows for repeat or additional testing, must be removed. The remaining urine may be discarded.

Collection Techniques

Routine Void

A routine voided urine specimen requires no patient preparation and is collected by having the patient urinate into an appropriate container. Normally, the patient requires no assistance other than clear instructions. These routine specimens—whether random, first morning, or fractional—can be used for routine urinalysis. For other collection procedures the patient may require assistance depending on the patient's age and physical condition or the technique to be used for collection (see Table 3–1).

Midstream "Clean Catch"

If there is the possibility of contamination (e.g., due to vaginal discharge) or if a bacterial culture is desired, a **midstream "clean catch" specimen** should be obtained. Collection of these specimens requires additional patient instructions, cleaning supplies, and perhaps assistance for elderly patients or young children. Prior to the collection of a midstream clean catch specimen, the glans penis of the male or the urethral meatus of the female is thoroughly cleansed and rinsed. Following the cleansing procedure, a midstream specimen is obtained when the patient first passes some urine into the toilet and then stops and urinates the midportion into the specimen container. Any remaining urine is passed into the toilet. To prevent contamination of the container and specimen, it is very important that the interior of the container does not come in contact with the patient's hands or perineal area. This midstream technique allows passage of the initial urine that contains any urethral washings (e.g., normal bacterial flora of the distal urethra) into the toilet and allows collection of a specimen that represents elements and analytes from the bladder, ureters, and kidneys. Because an informed patient can obtain these useful specimens with minimal effort, the midstream clean catch specimen is frequently collected. When done properly, it eliminates sources of contamination and provides an excellent specimen for both routine urinalysis and urine culture.

Catheterized Specimen

Both a routine voided or midstream clean catch specimen can be obtained by a well-instructed and physically able patient. In contrast, two collection techniques require medical personnel. A **catheterized specimen** is obtained following catheterization of the patient, i.e., insertion of a sterile catheter through the urethra into the bladder. Urine flows directly from the bladder through the indwelling catheter and accumulates in a plastic reservoir bag. A urine specimen can be collected at any time from this reservoir. Because urinary tract infections are common in catheterized patients, most often these urine specimens are sent for bacterial culture. However, if additional tests are ordered, the culture should always be performed first to prevent possible contamination of the specimen. Any of the specimen types discussed (e.g., random, timed) can be obtained from catheterized patients by following the appropriate collection procedure.

Suprapubic Aspiration

Another collection technique, **suprapubic aspiration,** involves collecting urine directly from the bladder by puncturing the abdominal wall and the distended bladder using a needle and syringe. The normally sterile bladder urine is aspirated into the syringe and sent for analysis. This procedure is principally used for bacterial cultures, especially for anaerobic microbes, and in infants, in whom specimen contamination is often unavoidable.

Pediatric Collections

Pediatric and newborn infants pose a challenge in collecting an appropriate urine spec-

imen. Because these patients are unable to urinate voluntarily, commercially available plastic urine collection bags with a hypoallergenic skin adhesive are used. The patient's perineal area is cleansed and dried before the specimen bag is placed onto the skin. The bag is placed over the penis in the male and around the vagina (excluding the rectum) in the female, and the adhesive is firmly attached to the perineum. Once the bag is in place, the patient is checked every 15 minutes to see if an adequate specimen has been collected. The specimen should be removed as soon as possible after collection and then labeled and transported to the laboratory. Because of the many possible sources of contamination despite the use of sterile bags and technique, urine for bacterial culture may need to be obtained by catheterization or suprapubic aspiration. However, when the patient is appropriately prepared, these "bag" specimens are usually satisfactory for routine screening and quantitative assays. The use of disposable diapers to collect urine for quantitative assay has also been reported (Roberts, 1985).

Collection Guidelines

Storing

Containers for urine specimen collections must be clean, dry, and made of a clear or translucent disposable material, such as plastic or glass. They should stand upright, have an opening of at least 4 cm to 5 cm, and have a capacity of 50 mL to 100 mL. To eliminate spillage, even if no transporting of the specimen is necessary, a cover should be provided. Those specimens requiring transporting need a firmly sealing lid that is easily placed onto and removed from the container and that provide a leakproof seal. Commercially available, disposable nonsterile containers are usually cost competitive, eliminating the need to reuse them. However, if a container must be reused, it must be adequately cleaned and rinsed such that it is equivalent to a new, unused container.

Sterile, individually packaged urine containers are also available from commercial sources for the collection of specimens for microbial culture. However, if a specimen must be stored for a period of time before testing (i.e., over 2 hours), the use of a sterile container is recommended, regardless of the tests ordered, owing to changes that can occur in unpreserved urine.

Various large containers are available for the collection of 12-hour and 24-hour urine specimens for quantitative analyses. These containers have a capacity of approximately 3000 mL and have a wide mouth and a leakproof screw cap. Usually made of a brown opaque plastic, they protect the specimen from ultraviolet and white light, and acid preservatives can be added to them.

Clear, pliable, polyethylene urine collection bags are available for collecting specimens from the pediatric patient. These collection bags can be purchased as nonsterile or sterile and can be self-sealed following collection for transportation to the laboratory. To collect a 24-hour specimen, some brands provide a tube attached to the bag base. This allows for easy transfer of urine to another collection container and eliminates the use of multiple bags. More importantly, this avoids repeated patient preparation and reapplication of adhesive to the child's sensitive skin.

Labeling

All specimen containers must be labeled before or immediately following collection. Because lids are removed, the patient identification label is always placed directly on the container holding the specimen. Under no circumstances should the label appear only on the removable specimen lid. This practice invites specimen mixups; once the lid is removed, such a specimen is technically "unlabeled."

Labels must have an adhesive that will resist moisture and adhere under refrigeration. The patient identification information required on the label may differ among laboratories. However, the following minimal information should be provided on all labels: the patient's full name, a unique identifica-

tion number, the date and time of collection, the patient's room number (if in-house), and the preservative used, if any.

Handling

CHANGES IN UNPRESERVED URINE. Urine specimens should be delivered to the laboratory immediately after collection. However, this is not always possible; if delay in specimen transportation is to be 2 hours or greater, precautions must be taken to preserve the integrity of the specimen, protecting it from the effects of light and room temperature changes. A variety of changes can occur in unpreserved urine (Table 3–3). These changes can potentially affect any aspect—the physical, chemical, or microscopic examinations—of a urinalysis. Changes in the physical examination result from 1) the alteration of the urine solutes to a different form, resulting in a color change; 2) bacterial growth causing an increased odor owing to their metabolism or proliferation; and 3) solute precipitation in the form of amorphous material, decreasing urine clarity. Individual components of the chemical examination (e.g., glucose, pH) can be affected. Most often these changes result in the removal of the chemical entity by various mechanisms, leading to false negative results.

In contrast, urinary nitrite and pH increase in unpreserved urine as bacteria proliferate, converting nitrate to nitrite and metabolizing urea to ammonia. The microscopic changes result from the disintegration of formed elements, particularly in hypotonic and alkaline urine, or from unchecked bacterial growth. In the latter case, it is impossible to determine if the large number of bacteria observed in these specimens results from improper storage or from a urinary tract infection.

In summary, changes will occur in unpreserved urine; which changes occur and their magnitude are variable and impossible to predict. Therefore, appropriate specimen collection, handling, and storage are necessary to ensure that these potential changes do not occur and that accurate results can be obtained.

TABLE 3–3.   POTENTIAL CHANGES IN UNPRESERVED URINE

PHYSICAL CHANGES

Color	Changes—due to oxidation or reduction of substances (e.g., bilirubin to biliverdin, hemoglobin to methemoglobin, urobilinogen to urobilin)
Clarity	Falsely decreased—due to bacterial proliferation, solute precipitation (crystals and amorphous materials).
Odor	Falsely increased—due to bacterial proliferation (e.g., *Pseudomonas* species) or to bacterial decomposition of urea to ammonia.

CHEMICAL CHANGES

pH	Falsely increased—due to bacterial decomposition of urea to ammonia; loss of CO_2.
	Falsely decreased—due to bacterial or yeast conversion of glucose to form acids.
Glucose	Falsely decreased—due to cellular or bacterial glycolysis.
Ketones	Falsely decreased—due to bacterial metabolism of acetoacetate to acetone.
	Falsely decreased—due to volatilization of acetone.
Bilirubin	Falsely decreased—due to photo-oxidation to biliverdin and hydrolysis to free bilirubin.
Urobilinogen	Falsely decreased—due to oxidation to urobilin.
Nitrite	Falsely increased—due to bacterial production following specimen collection.
	Falsely decreased—due to conversion to nitrogen.

MICROSCOPIC CHANGES

Red blood cells, white blood cells, and casts	Falsely decreased—disintegration of cellular and formed elements, especially in dilute alkaline urine.
Bacteria	Falsely increased—due to bacterial proliferation following specimen collection.

PRESERVATIVES. Unfortunately, no single **urine preservative** is available to suit all testing needs. Hence, the preservative used will depend on the type of collection, the tests to be performed, and the time delay before testing. The easiest and most common form of preservation, refrigeration at 4 degrees to 6 degrees Celsius, is suitable for the majority of specimens. Any urine specimen for microbiological studies should be promptly refrigerated if it cannot be transported directly to the laboratory. Refrigeration prevents bacterial proliferation, and the specimen remains suitable for culture up to 24 hours if necessary.

Although refrigeration is the easiest means of preserving most urine specimens, it is not recommended to refrigerate routine urinalysis specimens if they will be analyzed within 2 hours (NCCLS, 1985). Refrigeration can induce precipitation of amorphous urate and phosphate crystals that can interfere substantially with the microscopic examination. For routine urinalysis specimens that must be transported long distances, commercially prepared containers that use a boric acid preservative are available.

TIMED COLLECTIONS. Timed specimens, particularly 12-hour and 24-hour collections, may require the addition of a chemical preservative to maintain the integrity of the analyte of interest. Regardless of the preservative necessary, urine collections should be kept on ice or refrigerated throughout the duration of the collection.

The collection preservative needed for a particular analyte can differ among laboratories (Table 3–4). These variations stem from 1) different test methodologies, 2) how often the test is performed (i.e., turnaround time), and 3) time delays and transportation conditions (e.g., the sample is sent to a reference lab). Some laboratories may perform an assay daily in-house and require only refrigeration of the sample during the timed collection. In contrast, a small laboratory may send the assay to a reference facility that requires that a chemical preservative be used during the collection to ensure analyte stability. Each urinalysis laboratory must have in its procedure manual a protocol for the collection of all timed urine specimens. The protocol should include the name of the analyte, a description of the appropriate specimen col-

T A B L E   3 – 4.   COMMON URINE PRESERVATIVES

TYPE	COMMENTS	USED FOR*
Refrigeration	Does not interfere with routine screen. Acceptable for urine culture because bacterial growth is inhibited for approximately 24 hours. Precipitates urates and phosphates.	Electrolytes, creatinine, glucose, total protein, albumin, heavy metals, drug screens, follicle-stimulating hormone, estriol.
Freezing	Destroys formed elements. Preserves bilirubin and urobilinogen.	Bilirubin, urobilinogen.
Boric acid	Interferes only with pH of routine screen. Preserves protein and formed elements. Acceptable for urine culture since bacterial growth is inhibited for approximately 24 hours. Can precipitate urates.	Protein (albumin, amino acids, etc.), uric acid, 5-hydroxyindoleacetic acid, hydroxyproline, cortisol, estrogens, steroids.
Hydrochloric acid	Unacceptable for routine screen. Destroys formed elements; precipitates solutes. Bactericidal; hazardous.	Calcium, phosphorus, δ-aminolevulinic acid, oxalate.
Glacial acetic acid	Unacceptable for routine screen. Destroys formed elements; precipitates solutes. Bactericidal; hazardous.	Aldosterone, catecholamines, corticosteroids, cortisol, estrogens, metanephrines, vanillylmandelic acid, homovanillic acid, etc.
Sodium fluoride	Unacceptable for routine screen. Prevents glycolysis.	Glucose.
Sodium carbonate	Unacceptable for routine screen. Preserves porphyrins and porphobilinogen.	Porphyrins, porphobilinogen, urobilinogen, etc.
Formalin	Preserves formed elements. Interferes with chemical tests as a reducing substance.	Sediment preservation.
Thymol	Preserves formed elements. Interferes with protein precipitation tests. Inhibits bacteria and yeast.	Sediment preservation.
Saccomanno's fixative	Ideal preservation of cellular elements.	Cytology studies.

  * *Different urine preservatives may be used for certain analytes; therefore, the testing laboratory must be consulted before collection.*

lection technique, the appropriate preservative required, labeling requirements including precautions for certain chemical preservatives, the location at which the test is performed, reference ranges, and the expected turnaround time.

Timed urine collections should be transported to the laboratory as soon as possible after completion of the collection. The total volume is determined, the specimen is well mixed to ensure homogeneity, and aliquots are removed for the appropriate tests. Note that at no point in a timed collection can urine be removed or discarded, even if the volume is recorded. Because of diurnal variations, the concentration of the analyte in any

removed aliquot is unable to be determined and corrected for; thus, the collection would be invalidated.

References
· ·

National Committee for Clinical Laboratory Standards. Collection and transportation of single-collection urine specimens. Proposed Guideline. NCCLS Document GP8-P (ISBN 0273-3099), 5(7):161, 1985.

National Committee for Clinical Laboratory Standards. Routine urinalysis. Proposed Guideline. NCCLS Document GP16-P (ISBN 1-56238-125-3), 11(12):1, 1991.

Roberts SB, Lucas A: Measurement of urinary constituents and output using disposable napkins. Arch Dis Child 60:1021–1024, 1985.

Study Questions

1. **Which of the following is the urine specimen of choice for cytology studies?**

   A. First morning specimen
   B. Random specimen
   C. Fractional collection
   D. Timed collection

2. **Which of the following specimens usually eliminates contamination of the urine with entities from the external genitalia and distal urethra?**

   A. First morning specimen
   B. Midstream "clean catch" specimen
   C. Fractional collection
   D. Four-hour timed collection

3. **Substances that show a diurnal variation in their urinary excretion pattern are best evaluated using a**

   A. first morning specimen.
   B. midstream "clean catch" specimen.
   C. fractional collection.
   D. timed collection.

4. **Which of the following will NOT cause erroneous results in a 24-hour timed urine collection?**

   A. When the collection starts and ends in the evening
   B. When two first morning specimens are included in the collection
   C. When multiple collection containers are not mixed together prior to specimen testing
   D. When a portion of the collection is removed before total volume measurement

5. **A 25-year-old woman complains of painful urination and is suspected of having a urinary tract infection. Which of the following specimens should be collected for a routine urinalysis and urine culture?**

   A. Fractional collection
   B. Timed collection
   C. Midstream "clean catch" specimen
   D. Random specimen

6. **A 35-year-old pregnant woman is suspected of having gestational diabetes. However, a random urine specimen tests negative for glucose. Which of the following would be a better specimen to evaluate for glucosuria?**

    A. 2-hour postprandial
    B. 12-hour timed collection
    C. 24-hour timed collection
    D. Midstream "clean catch"

7. **An unpreserved urine specimen collected at midnight is kept at room temperature until the morning hospital shift. Which of the following changes will most likely occur?**

    A. Decrease in urine color and clarity
    B. Decrease in pH and specific gravity
    C. Decrease in glucose and ketones
    D. Decrease in bacteria and nitrite

8. **A urine specimen containing the substance indicated is kept unpreserved at room temperature for 4 hours. Identify the probable change to that substance.**

Substance	Change
_____ Bacteria	A. Decrease
_____ Bilirubin	B. No change
_____ Glucose	C. Increase
_____ Ketones	
_____ pH	
_____ Protein	
_____ Urobilinogen	

9. **Which of the following is the most common form of urine preservation?**

    A. Boric acid
    B. Sodium fluoride
    C. Freezing
    D. Refrigeration

10. **If refrigeration is used to preserve a urine specimen, which of the following may occur?**

    A. Cellular or bacterial glycolysis will be enhanced.
    B. Formed elements will be destroyed.
    C. Amorphous crystals may precipitate.
    D. Bacteria will proliferate.

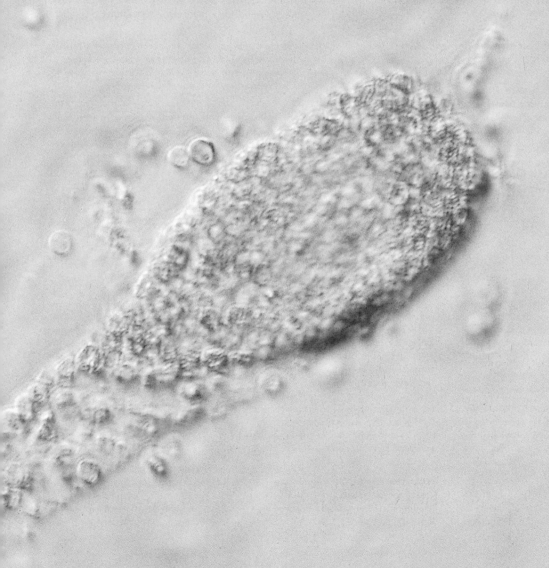

The Kidney

Renal Anatomy
....

Renal Circulation
....

Renal Physiology
....

Urine Formation

The Glomerulus

The Tubules

Tubular Function

. . . .

LEARNING OBJECTIVES

After studying this chapter, the student should be able to

1. Identify and state the primary functions of the macroscopic structures of the kidney and urinary tract.

2. Diagram the structure and state the function of each portion of the nephron.

3. Describe renal blood circulation and its role in renal function.

4. Discuss the components and the process of glomerular filtration and urine formation, including the anatomic structures, the filtration forces, and the substances involved.

5. Describe the transport mechanisms of tubular reabsorption and tubular secretion, including the substances involved.

6. Describe the three secretory mechanisms that the kidney employs to regulate the acid-base equilibrium of the body.

7. Explain tubular transport capacity (T_m) and discuss its relationship to renal threshold.

8. Compare and contrast the countercurrent multiplier mechanism, the countercurrent exchange mechanism, the urea cycle, and their roles in urine formation and concentration.

9. Briefly summarize the relationship of water reabsorption with antidiuretic hormone and the relationship of sodium reabsorption to renin and aldosterone.

. . . .

KEY TERMS

active transport: the movement of a substance (e.g., ion, solute) across a cell membrane and against a gradient, requiring the expenditure of energy.

afferent arteriole: a small branch of an interlobular renal artery that becomes the capillary tuft within a glomerulus.

antidiuretic hormone (ADH) (also called **vasopressin):** a hormone produced by the posterior pituitary that regulates the osmotic reabsorption of water by the collecting tubules. Without adequate ADH present, water is not reabsorbed.

basement membrane: a trilayer structure located within the glomerulus along the base of the epithelium (podocytes) of the urinary (Bowman's) space. The size-discriminating component of the glomerular filtration barrier, the basement membrane limits the passage of substances to those with an effective molecular radius less than 4 nm. Using electron microscopy, three distinct layers are evident in the basement membrane: the lamina rara interna (next to the capillary endothelium), the lamina densa (centrally located), and the lamina rara externa (next to the podocytes).

collecting duct: the portion of a renal nephron following the distal convoluted tubule. Many distal tubules empty into a single collecting duct. The collect-ing duct traverses both the renal cortex and the medulla and is the site of final urine concentration. The collecting ducts terminate at the renal papilla, conveying the urine formed into the renal calyces of the kidney.

countercurrent exchange mechanism: a passive exchange by diffusion of reabsorbed solutes and water from the nephron's medullary interstitium into the blood of its vascular blood supply (i.e., the vasa recta). A requirement of this process is that the flow of blood in the ascending and descending vessels of the U-shaped vasa recta be in opposite directions; hence the term *countercurrent.* The countercurrent exchange mechanism simultaneously supplies nutrients to the medulla and removes solutes and water reabsorbed into the blood. As a result, it assists in the maintenance of the medullary hypertonicity.

countercurrent multiplier mechanism: a process occurring in the loop of Henle of each nephron that establishes and maintains the osmotic gradient within the medullary interstitium. The medullary osmolality gradient ranges from being isoosmotic (~300 mOsm/kg) at its border with the cortex to approximately 1400 mOsm/kg at the inner medulla or papilla. A requirement of this process is that the flow of the ultrafiltrate in the descending and ascending limbs be in opposite directions; hence the name *countercurrent*. In addition, active sodium and chloride reabsorption in the ascending limb combined with passive water reabsorption in the descending limb are essential components of this process. The countercurrent multiplier mechanism accounts for approximately 50 percent of the solutes concentrated in the renal medulla.

distal convoluted tubule: the portion of a renal nephron immediately following the loop of Henle. It begins at the juxtaglomerular apparatus with the macula densa, a specialized group of cells located at the vascular pole. The distal tubule is convoluted and after two to three loops becomes the collecting tubule (or duct).

efferent arteriole: the arteriole exiting a glomerulus, the efferent arteriole is formed by the rejoining of the anastomosing capillary network within the glomerulus.

glomerular filtration barrier: the structure within the glomerulus that determines the composition of the plasma ultrafiltrate formed in the urinary space by regulating the passage of solutes. The glomerular filtration barrier consists of the capillary endothelium, the basement membrane, and the epithelial podocytes, each coated with a "shield of negativity." Solute selectivity by the barrier is based on the molecular size and the electrical charge of the solute.

glomerulus (also called renal corpuscle): a tuft or network of capillaries encircled by and intimately re-lated with the proximal end of a renal tubule (i.e., Bowman's capsule). The glomerulus is composed of four distinct structural components: the capillary endothelial cells, the epithelial cells (podocytes), the mesangium, and the basement membrane.

juxtaglomerular apparatus: a specialized area located at the vascular pole of a nephron. It is composed of cells from the afferent and efferent arterioles, the macula densa of the distal tubule, and the extraglomerular mesangium. The juxtaglomerular apparatus is actually an endocrine organ and the primary producer of renin.

kidneys: the organs of the urinary system that produce urine. Normally, each individual has two kidneys. The kidneys' primary function is to filter the blood, removing waste products and regulating electrolytes, water, acid-base balance, and blood pressure.

loop of Henle: the tubular portion of a nephron immediately following and continuous with the proximal tubule. Located in the renal medulla, the loop of Henle is composed of a thin descending limb, a U-shaped segment (also called a hairpin turn), and thin and thick ascending limbs. The thick ascending limb of the loop of Henle (sometimes called the straight portion of the distal tubule) ends as the tubule enters the vascular pole of the glomerulus.

maximal tubular reabsorptive capacity: denoted T_m, it is the maximal rate of *reabsorption* of a solute by the tubular epithelium per minute (mg/min). It varies with each solute and is dependent on the glomerular filtration rate.

maximal tubular secretory capacity: also denoted T_m, it is the maximal rate of *secretion* of a solute by the tubular epithelium per minute (mg/min). This rate differs for each solute.

mesangium: the cells that form the structural core tissue of a glomerulus, the mesangium lies between the glomerular capillaries (endothelium) and the podocytes (tubular epithelium). The mesangial cells derive from smooth muscle and have contractility characteristics and the ability to phagocytize and pinocytize.

nephron: the functional unit of the kidney. Each kidney contains approxi-mately 1.3 million nephrons. A nephron is composed of five distinct areas: the glomerulus, the proximal tubule, the loop of Henle, the distal tubule, and the collecting tubule or duct. Each region of the nephron is specialized and plays a role in the formation and final composition of urine.

osmosis: the movement of water across a semipermeable membrane in an attempt to achieve an osmotic equilibrium between two compartments or solutions of differing osmolality (i.e., an osmotic gradient). This mechanism is passive, i.e., it requires no energy.

passive transport: the movement of a substance (e.g., an ion, a solute) across a cell membrane along a gradient (e.g., concentration, charge). Passive transport does not require energy.

peritubular capillaries: the network of capillaries (or plexus) that forms from the efferent arteriole and surrounds the tubules of the nephron in the renal cortex.

podocytes: the epithelial cells that line the urinary (Bowman's) space of the glomerulus. These cells completely cover the glomerular capillaries with large finger-like processes that interdigitate to form a filtration slit. The name "podo," which is Greek for "foot," relates to the podocytes' foot-like appearance when viewed in cross section. Collectively, the podocytes comprise the glomerular epithelium that forms Bowman's capsule.

proximal tubule: the tubular part of a nephron immediately following the glomerulus. The proximal tubule has both a convoluted portion and a straight portion, the latter becoming the loop of Henle after entering the renal medulla.

renal threshold level: the plasma concentration of a solute above which the amount of solute present in the ultrafiltrate exceeds the maximal tubular reabsorptive capacity (T_m). Once the renal threshold level has been reached, increased amounts of solute are excreted (i.e., lost) in the urine.

renin: a proteolytic enzyme produced and stored by the cells of the juxtaglomerular apparatus of the renal nephrons. Secretion of renin results in the formation of angiotensin and the secretion of aldosterone; thus, it plays an important role in the control of blood pressure and fluid balance.

shield of negativity: a term describing the impediment produced by negatively charged components (e.g., proteoglycans) of the glomerular filtration barrier. Present on both sides of and throughout the filtration barrier, these negatively charged components effectively limit the filtration of negatively charged substances from the blood (e.g., albumin) into the urinary space.

titratable acids: a term representing H^+ ions (acid) excreted in the urine as monobasic phosphate (e.g., NaH_2PO_4). The urinary excretion of these acids results in the elimination of H^+ ions and the reabsorption of sodium and bicarbonate. The titration of urine using a standard base (e.g., NaOH) to a pH of 7.4 (normal plasma pH) will quantitate the amount of H^+ ions excreted in this form; hence the name *titratable acids.*

tubular reabsorption: the movement of substances (by active or passive transport) from the tubular ultrafiltrate into the peritubular blood or the interstitium by the renal tubular cells.

tubular secretion: the movement of substances (by active or passive transport) from the peritubular blood or the interstitium into the tubular ultrafiltrate by the renal tubular cells.

urea cycle: a passive process occurring throughout the nephron that establishes and maintains a high concentration of urea in the renal medulla. This process accounts for approximately 50 percent of the solutes concentrated in the medulla. With the countercurrent exchange mechanism, the urea cycle helps establish and maintain the high medullary osmotic gradient. Because urea can passively diffuse into the interstitium, as well as back into the lumen fluid, the selectivity of the tubular epithelium in each portion of the nephron plays an integral part in the urea-cycling process.

vasa recta: the vascular network of long U-shaped capillaries that forms from the peritubular capillaries and surrounds the loops of Henle in the renal medulla.

Renal Anatomy

The **kidneys** are bean shaped and are located on the posterior abdominal wall in the area known as the retroperitoneum (Fig. 4–1). An adult human kidney weighs approximately 150 g and measures roughly 12.5 cm in length, 6 cm in width, and 2.5 cm in depth. When the kidney is observed in cross section, two distinct areas are apparent: the cortex and the medulla. The outer cortex layer is approximately 1.4 cm thick and is somewhat granular in macroscopic appearance. Because all of the glomeruli are located there, the cortex is the exclusive site of the plasma filtration process. The inner layer, the medulla, consists of renal tissue shaped into pyramids. The apex of each of these pyramids is called a papilla; each contains a papillary duct that opens into a cavity called a calyx. The normal human kidney consists of about 12 minor calyces, which join together to form two to three major calyces. Each calyx acts as a funnel to receive urine from the collecting tubules and pass it into the renal pelvis.

The funnel-shaped renal pelvis emerges from the indented region of each kidney and narrows to join with the ureter, a fibromuscular tube, which is approximately 25 cm long. One ureter extends down from each kidney and connects to the base of the bladder, a muscular sac, which is shaped like a three-sided pyramid. The apex of this "bladder pyramid" is oriented downward and is where the urethra originates and extends to the exterior of the body. Reviewing briefly, urine forms as the plasma ultrafiltrate passes through the cortex and medulla. The minor and major calyces transfer the urine to the renal pelvis, where peristaltic activity by smooth muscle moves the urine down the ureters into the bladder. The bladder acts as a "holding tank" for temporary urine storage until the patient voids. When approximately 150 mL of urine accumulates, a nerve reflex is initiated. Unless the patient overrides it, this micturition reflex causes bladder muscular contraction and relaxation of the urinary sphincter, resulting in the passage of urine out through the urethra. The urethra, a canal connecting the bladder to the body exterior, is approximately 4 cm long in women and approximately 24 cm long in men.

Note that when an individual is healthy, the composition of urine is not altered appreciably at any point following its introduction into the minor and major calyces. The calyces and the subsequent anatomic structures serve

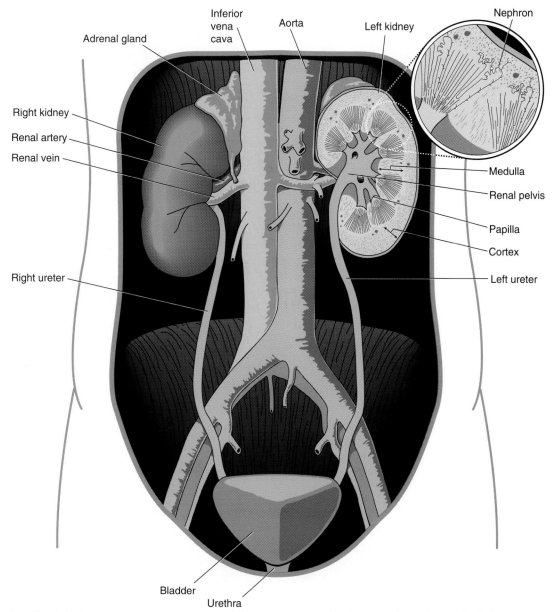

FIGURE 4–1. A schematic representation of the urinary tract, showing the relationship of the kidneys to the nephrons and the vascular system.

only as a conveyance for urine, the primary excretory product of the kidneys.

Each kidney contains approximately 1.3 million nephrons. It is the **nephron** that is the actual functional unit of the kidney. The nephron is composed of five distinct areas, each playing an important part in the formation and final composition of urine. Figure 4–2 shows the nephron, its component parts, and their physical interrelationship. The glomerulus consists of a capillary tuft surrounded by a thin epithelial layer of cells known as Bowman's capsule. Bowman's capsule is actually the proximal originating end of a renal tubule and its lumen is referred to as Bowman's space. The plasma filtrate of low-molecular-weight solutes initially collects in Bowman's space because of the hydro-

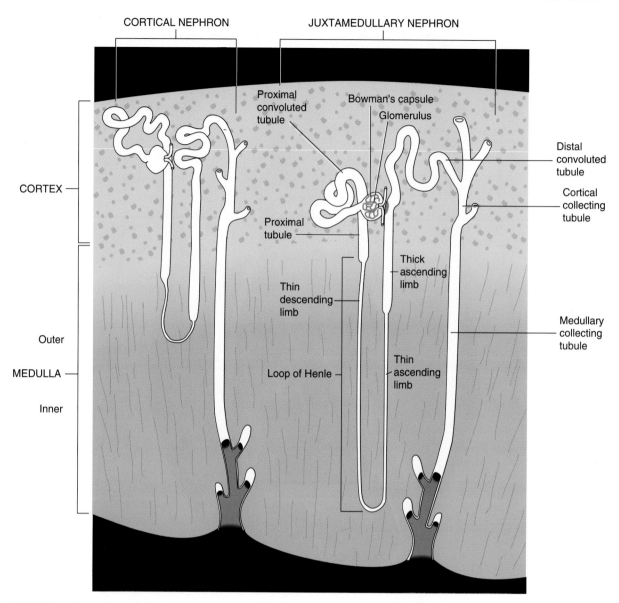

FIGURE 4–2. A schematic diagram showing the relationship of the nephron and its components to the renal cortex and the medulla.

static pressure difference between the capillary lumen and Bowman's space. (Fig. 4–4 shows the physical relationship of these two distinct lumens.)

The proximal convoluted tubule begins at the glomerulus and extends from it in a circuitous route through the cortex. Eventually the tubule straightens and turns downward, entering the medulla to become the **loop of Henle.** The loop of Henle has anatomically distinct areas: thin descending and ascending limbs that include a sharp hairpin turn, and thick descending and ascending limbs, which are actually the straight portions of the proximal and distal tubules (Table 4–1). Reentering the cortex at the macula densa—adjacent to the glomerulus—the straight distal tubule becomes the distal convoluted tubule. Note that up to this point, anatomically each nephron is structurally and functionally distinct. Each individual distal convoluted tubule joins to a "shared" collecting

TABLE 4–1. OUTLINE OF THE NEPHRON AND ITS COMPONENTS (AS USED THROUGHOUT THIS TEXT)

Glomerulus (or renal corpuscle)
1. Capillary tuft or glomerulus: often interchanged for entire entity.
2. Bowman's capsule

Tubules
1. Proximal tubule
   a. Convoluted portion – pars convoluta
   b. Straight portion – pars recta (or thick descending limb of the loop of Henle)
2. Loop of Henle
   a. Thin descending limb
   b. Thin ascending limb
   c. Thick ascending limb OR straight portion of distal tubule, terminates with macula densa
3. Distal tubule
   a. Straight portion, terminates with macula densa
   b. Convoluted portion
4. Collecting tubule (duct)
   a. Cortical collecting tubules
   b. Medullary collecting tubules

Modified from Koushanpour E, Kriz W: Renal Physiology (2nd ed.), New York, Springer-Verlag, 1986.

tubule or duct, which conveys the urine produced in several nephrons through the medulla for a second time. These collecting tubules fuse to become the larger papillary ducts, which empty into the calyces of the renal pyramids and finally into the renal pelvis. From the renal pelvis, the urine passes to the bladder to await excretion through the urethra.

Renal Circulation

The kidneys require a rich blood supply to execute their primary function of regulating the body's internal environment. In fact, despite their weight of only 300 g, or 0.5 percent of the total body weight, the kidneys receive 25 percent of the total cardiac output. This high degree of perfusion reflects the direct relationship of the kidneys' functional abilities to the blood supply they receive.

Each kidney is supplied by a single renal artery originating from the aorta. As the renal artery successively divides, it forms a distinct vascular arrangement, unique to and specifically adapted for the functions of the kidney. The kidney is the only human organ in which an arteriole subdivides into a capillary bed, becomes an arteriole again, and then for a second time subdivides into a capillary network. In addition, the renal arterioles are primarily end arteries that supply specific areas of renal tissue and do not interconnect. Therefore, disruption in the blood supply at the afferent arteriole or the glomerular tuft of a nephron will dramatically affect the blood supplied to the nephron's corresponding tubules in the cortex and medulla. Consequently, renal tissue is particularly susceptible to ischemia or infarction; the medulla is especially susceptible because it has no direct arterial blood supply. Should any vascular stenosis or occlusion occur, renal tissue damage will ensue dependent on the number and location of the blood vessels involved.

An **afferent arteriole** at the vascular pole supplies blood individually to the glomerulus of each nephron. Upon entering the glomerulus, the afferent arteriole branches into a capillary tuft, which is intimately related to the epithelial cells of Bowman's capsule. This branching and anastomosing capillary network comes together to become the **efferent arteriole** as it leaves the glomerulus. Subsequently, the efferent arteriole branches for a second time into a capillary plexus. The type of nephron the efferent arteriole is servicing determines the vascular arrangement of this second capillary plexus. The outer cortical nephrons have short loops of Henle and the efferent arteriole branches into a fine capillary plexus — the **peritubular capillaries** — which encompass the outer cortical tubules entirely. The mid- and deep-juxtamedullary nephrons have long loops of Henle. The efferent arterioles of these nephrons first branch into a peritubular capillary bed, which enmeshes the cortical portions of the tubules, and then divide into a series of long U-shaped vessels, the **vasa recta,** which descend deep into the renal medulla close to the loops of Henle (Fig. 4–3). The corresponding ascending vasa recta form the beginnings of the venous renal circula-

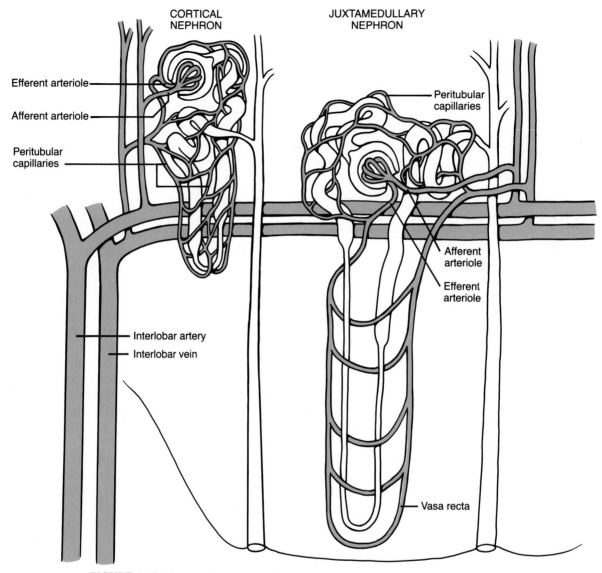

FIGURE 4-3. The vascular circulation of the nephrons in the renal cortex and medulla.

tion, emerging from deep in the medulla to form venules and drain into the renal veins. It is this close relationship between the peritubular capillary system and the renal tubules that enables the sequential processing and exchange of substances throughout the nephron.

The unique vascular arrangement of the renal circulation makes it possible for the kidney to function optimally. The comparatively wide-bore afferent arteriole allows for a high hydrostatic pressure at the glomeru-

lus. This pressure averages 55 mm Hg, approximately half of the mean arterial blood pressure, and is the driving force behind glomerular filtration. All other capillary beds have a narrower lumen, which provides a higher resistance to blood flow and consequently a low blood pressure within them. The ultrafiltrate, however, also affects the resultant filtration force across the filtration barrier. The plasma ultrafiltrate already in Bowman's space exerts a hydrostatic pressure of 15 mm Hg of opposing filtration. In addition, this ultrafiltrate is low in protein and high in water as compared to the plasma on the other side of the filtration barrier. Hence, water that freely passes the filtration barrier seeks to reenter the plasma from Bowman's space. As a result, an oncotic pressure of 30 mm Hg owing to this higher protein concentration in the plasma opposes glomerular filtration as well. The outcome of these pressure differences, however, is a net filtration pressure of 10 mm Hg, favoring the formation of plasma ultrafiltrate in Bowman's space of the renal tubule (Table 4–2). Note that the filtration barrier expends no energy in forming the plasma ultrafiltrate; rather, it is the cardiac output that provides the glomerular capillary blood pressure that drives the plasma ultrafiltration.

The afferent and efferent arterioles exit Bowman's capsule at the vascular pole in close proximity to each other. The vascular pole is also the site of the **juxtaglomerular apparatus.** The morphologically distinct structures that compose the juxtaglomerular apparatus are portions of the afferent and efferent arterioles, the extraglomerular mesangial cells (which are continuous with the supporting mesangium of the glomerulus), and the specialized area of the distal convoluted tubule (known as the macula densa). Characteristically, large amounts of secretory granules containing the enzyme renin are present in the smooth muscle cells of the afferent arteriole located in the juxtaglomerular apparatus. The juxtaglomerular apparatus, which is essentially a small endocrine organ, is the principal producer of renin in the kidney. **Renin** is an enzyme that, when

released into the blood stream in response to decreased blood volume, decreased arterial pressure, sodium depletion, vascular hemorrhage, or increased potassium, forms angiotensin and causes the secretion of aldosterone. This aldosterone secretion stimulates the kidneys to actively retain sodium and passively retain water. As a result, the volume of extracellular fluid expands, the blood pressure increases, and normal potassium levels, as well as normal renal perfusion, are restored. Conversely, an increase in blood volume, an acute increase in blood pressure, or the loss of potassium inhibits renin secretion and enhances sodium excretion. As a result of renin secretion, the juxtaglomerular apparatus and the kidneys play an important role in body fluid homeostasis through their ability to modify blood pressure and fluid balance.

Renal Physiology

Urine Formation

Urine formation is the primary excretory function of the kidneys. Urine formation consists of three processes: plasma filtration at the glomeruli followed by reabsorption and secretion of selective components by the renal tubules. It is through these processes that the kidneys play an important role in the removal of metabolic waste products, the regulation of water and electrolytes (e.g., sodium, chloride), and the maintenance of the acid-base equilibrium in the body. The kidneys are the body's "true regulators," determining which substances to retain and which to excrete regardless of what the body has ingested or produced.

The kidneys convert approximately 180,000 mL (125 mL/min) of filtered plasma each day into a final urine volume of 600 to 1800 mL. The largest component of urine is water. The principal solutes present are urea, chloride, sodium, and potassium, followed by phosphate, sulfate, creatinine, and uric acid. Other substances initially in the ultrafiltrate, such as glucose, bicarbonate, and albumin are essentially completely reabsorbed by the tu-

T A B L E 4 – 2.   FORCES INVOLVED IN GLOMERULAR FILTRATION

FORCE	MAGNITUDE
Hydrostatic (blood pressure)	+55 mmHg
Hydrostatic (ultrafiltrate in Bowman's space)	−15 mmHg
Oncotic (protein in blood and not in ultrafiltrate)	−30 mmHg
Net pressure	+10 mmHg

TABLE 4–3.   COMPARISON OF THE INITIAL ULTRAFILTRATE AND THE FINAL URINE COMPOSITION OF SELECTED SOLUTES PER DAY

COMPONENT	INITIAL ULTRAFILTRATE (mmol)	FINAL URINE (mmol)	PERCENT REABSORBED
Water (1.2 L*)	9,500,000.00	67,000.00	99.3
Urea	910.00	400.00	44.0
Chloride	37,000.00	185.00	99.5
Sodium	32,500.00	130.00	99.6
Potassium	986.00	70.00	92.9
Glucose†	900.00	0.72	100.0
Albumin	0.02	0.001	95.0

Data from First, 1984; Lehmann, 1991; Vander, 1985; O'Connor, 1982; and Tietz, 1987.
* Average 24 hour urine volume; glomerular filtration rate of 125 mL/min.
† Represents average glucose values.

bules. Consequently, the urine of normal healthy individuals does not contain these solutes in significant amounts. Table 4–3 presents a comparison of those selected solutes initially filtered by the glomerulus and those actually excreted after passage through the nephrons. Because normal urine output is approximately 1200 mL (approximately 1 percent of the filtered plasma volume), 99 percent of the initial ultrafiltrate volume is actually reabsorbed. In addition, the nephrons of the kidneys extensively and selectively reabsorb and secrete solutes as the ultrafiltrate passes through them.

The Glomerulus

The **glomerulus** is a tuft of capillaries encircled by and intimately related to Bowman's capsule, the thin epithelium-lined proximal end of a renal tubule. It forms a barrier that is specifically designed for plasma ultrafiltration. Although the glomerulus almost completely excludes proteins larger than albumin (MW 67,000), it is extremely permeable to water and low-molecular-weight solutes. From the capillary lumen to Bowman's space where the plasma filtrate first collects, four structural components are apparent by electron microscopy: the mesangium, consisting of mesangial cells and a matrix; the fenestrated endothelial cells of the capillaries; the podocytes or visceral epithelial cells of Bowman's capsule; and a distinct trilayer basement

membrane sandwiched between the podocytes of Bowman's capsule and the capillary endothelial cells or between the podocytes and the mesangium. Note that there is no basement membrane between the capillary endothelium and the mesangium, evidence of the basement membrane's role in ultrafiltration and not in structural anchoring. Knowledge of the structural composition of the glomerulus (Fig. 4–4) is important in understanding its function in health and in disease.

The **mesangium,** located within the anastomosing lobules of the glomerular tuft, forms the structural core tissue of the glomerulus. The glomerulus' mesangial cells are thought to be of smooth muscle origin, retaining contractility characteristics as well as a large capability for phagocytosis and pinocytosis, which helps to remove entrapped macromolecules from the filtration barrier. The mesangial cells' ability to contract suggests a role in regulating the glomerular blood flow. The matrix surrounding the mesangial cells is, as mentioned earlier, continuous with the extraglomerular mesangium of the juxtaglomerular apparatus.

The capillary endothelial cells of the glomerulus make up the first component of the actual filtration barrier. The endothelium is fenestrated, i.e., it has large open pores approximately 50 to 100 nm in diameter. When viewed from the lumen of the capillary, the endothelium takes on a "swiss dot" appearance (Fig. 4–5). In addition, the capillary en-

FIGURE 4–4. A schematic overview of a glomerulus. The afferent arteriole enters the glomerulus and the efferent arteriole exits the glomerulus at the vascular pole. Also at the vascular pole, a portion of the thick ascending limb of the distal tubule—the macula densa—is in contact with the glomerular mesangium. The Bowman's space is formed from specialized epithelial cells (Bowman's capsule) at the end of a renal tubule. At the urinary pole, Bowman's space becomes the tubular lumen of the proximal tubule. Podocytes are the epithelial cells that cover the glomerular capillaries and derive their name from their characteristic foot processes. The glomerular capillaries are lined with fenestrated endothelial cells (i.e., epithelium with pores). The basement membrane, which separates the capillary endothelium and the podocytes (the epithelium of Bowman's space), is continuous throughout the glomerulus. The basement membrane is absent between the capillary endothelium and the mesangium. The mesangial cells of the glomerular tuft form the structural core of the glomerulus and are continuous with the extraglomerular mesangial cells located at the vascular pole, between the afferent and efferent arterioles. The secretory granules of the granular cells contain large amounts of renin. The afferent arteriole is innervated by sympathetic nerves. The smooth muscle cells of the arterioles and all cells derived from smooth muscle, including the granular cells, are shaded.

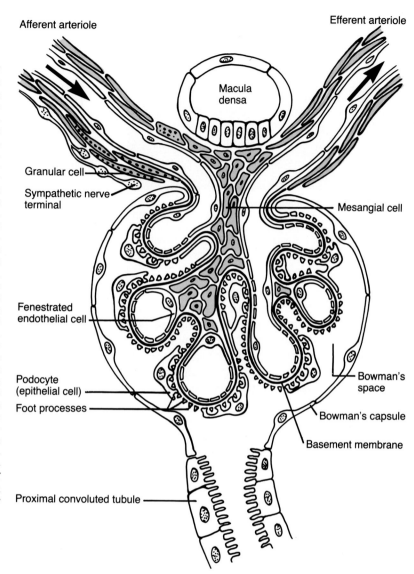

dothelium possesses a negatively charged coating that repels anionic molecules. Both the pores and the negative charge of the endothelium play an important role in the selectivity of plasma ultrafiltration.

The second component of the filtration barrier, the **basement membrane,** separates the epithelium of the urinary space from the endothelium of the glomerular capillaries. The basement membrane has three layers: the lamina rara interna lies adjacent to the capillary endothelium, the lamina densa (electrondense by electron micrograph) is centrally located, and the lamina rara externa is adjacent to the epithelium of the urinary space (Fig. 4–6). The basement membrane consistently courses below the epithelium of the urinary space and is absent between the capillary endothelium and the supporting mesangium. As mentioned previously, this trilayer structure is not the basement membrane of the glomerular capillaries; rather, it contributes specifically to the permeability characteristics of the filtration barrier. Composed principally of collagenous and noncollagenous proteins, the basement membrane of the filtration barrier is arranged in a matrix with hydrated interstices.

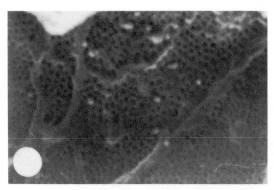

FIGURE 4–5. A scanning electron micrograph of the glomerular capillary endothelium as viewed from the capillary lumen. Note the "swiss dot" appearance of the fenestrated endothelium. (From Koushanpour E, Kriz W: Renal Physiology (2nd ed.), New York, Springer-Verlag, 1986. Used by permission.)

Nonpolar collagenous components concentrate in the lamina densa. An important polar noncollagenous component, heparin sulfate (a polyanionic proteoglycan), is located primarily in both lamina rara layers, endowing the layers with their strongly anionic character.

On the renal tubular side of the glomerulus, lining the urinary space, are the **podocytes.** Attached to the glomerular basement membrane, the podocytes constitute the third component of the filtration barrier. The name

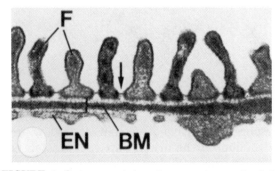

FIGURE 4–6. A transmission electron micrograph of the glomerular filtration barrier, consisting of the fenestrated capillary endothelium (EN), the basement membrane (BM), and the foot processes (F) of the podocytes. The basement membrane consists of three distinct layers: the lamina rara interna (next to the capillary endothelium), the lamina densa, and the lamina rara externa (next to the epithelium or podocytes). The arrow indicates the split diaphragm that lies between the interdigitating foot processes and on top of the basement membrane. (From Koushanpour E, Kriz W: Renal Physiology (2nd ed.), New York, Springer-Verlag, 1986. Used by permission.)

podocyte means foot cell and relates to their foot-like appearance when viewed in cross section (see Fig. 4–6). The podocytes completely cover the glomerular capillaries with extending finger-like processes and interdigitate with neighboring podocytes (Fig. 4–7). However, their processes do not actually touch each other; rather, a consistent space of approximately 20 to 30 nm separates them, forming a snakelike channel that zigzags across the surface of the glomerular capillaries (Koushanpour, 1986). This snakelike channel is called the filtration slit and covers only about 3 percent of the total glomerular basement membrane area. It is lined with a distinct extracellular structure known as the slit diaphragm. The substructure of the slit diaphragm consists of regularly arranged subunits with rectangular open spaces about the size of an albumin molecule. Often the slit diaphragm is considered part of the basement membrane, whereas it actually lies on it and is distinctly separate. The podocytes are metabolically active cells. They contain numerous organelles and extensive lysosomal elements that correlate directly to their extensive phagocytic ability. Macromolecules, which are unable to proceed through the slit diaphragm or return to the capillary lumen, are rapidly phagocytized by the podocytes to prevent occlusion of the filtration barrier. Like the capillary endothelium, all surfaces of the podocytes, filtration slits, and slit diaphragms that line the urinary space are covered with a thick, negatively charged coating.

In review, the three distinct structures that compose the **glomerular filtration barrier** are 1) the capillary endothelium with its large open pores; 2) the trilayer basement membrane; and 3) the filtration diaphragms located between the podocytes of the urinary space epithelium. Each component maintains an anionic charge on its cellular surface or within it, and each component is essential for proper functioning of the filtration barrier.

The selectivity of the filtration barrier is based on a solute's molecular size and charge. Water and small solutes rapidly pass through the filtration barrier with little or no resistance. In contrast, larger plasma molecules must overcome the negative charge present on the endothelium and be able to pass through the endothelial pores, which are 50 to 100 nm in diameter (Koushanpour, 1986). The endothelium's **shield of negativity** successfully repels the majority of plasma proteins, thereby preventing the filtration barrier from becoming congested with them. On the other hand, neutral and cationic molecules readily pass through the filtration barrier if they do not exceed the size restriction imposed by the basement membrane. In order to penetrate the basement membrane, the size discriminator, the neutral and cationic molecules must each possess an effective molecular radius of less than 4 nm. Approaching this radius, successful passage of the molecule decreases with its increasing size. Albumin has an effective radius of 3.6 nm (Cotran, 1989) and a molecular weight of approximately 67,000; if the shield of negativity that permeates the basement membrane and filtration slits were not present, albumin would readily pass through the filtration barrier. This is evidenced in glomerular diseases in which a loss of the shield of negativity (e.g., lipoid nephrosis) or an alteration in the filtration barrier structure (e.g., glomerulonephritis) results in proteinuria and hematuria.

The initial ultrafiltrate present in the urinary space differs from plasma in that it lacks all plasma cellular components and plasma proteins larger than albumin (including any protein-bound substances). The normal filtration rate of approximately 125 mL/min is dependent on body size and will be discussed at length in the section on glomerular filtration tests. Any condition that modifies the glomerular blood flow, the hydrostatic or oncotic pressures across the glomerular filtration barrier, or the structural integrity of the glomerulus will affect the glomerular filtration rate and ultimately the amount of urine produced.

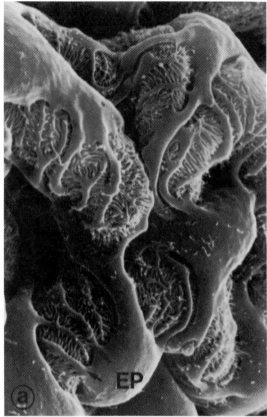

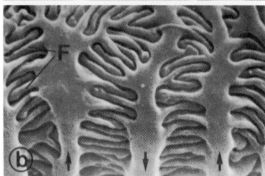

FIGURE 4-7. A scanning electron micrograph of podocytes and their interdigitating foot processes on glomerular capillaries as viewed from Bowman's space. *A,* Epithelial cells (EP), also called podocytes, giving rise to primary finger-like processes *(arrow). B,* An enlargement of the interdigitating foot processes (F) of adjacent epithelial cells. The arrows indicate primary processes and show the alternating pattern between epithelial cells. (From Koushanpour E, Kriz W: Renal Physiology (2nd ed.), New York, Springer-Verlag, 1986. Used with permission.)

The Tubules

The epithelium lining the renal tubules changes throughout the five distinct areas of the nephron. Looking at the diverse and specialized epithelial characteristics of each segment aids in understanding the various processes that take place.

Once the glomerular ultrafiltrate has been formed in the urinary space, hydrostatic pressure alone moves the ultrafiltrate through the remaining tubular portions of the nephron. Each tubular portion is distinctively different in its epithelium, relating directly to the unique and varied processes that occur there. The first section, the **proximal tubule,** consists of a large convoluted portion (pars convoluta) followed by a straight portion (pars recta). The proximal tubular epithelium consists of tall cells that extensively interdigitate with each other (Fig. 4–8). These intercellular interdigitations serve to increase the overall cellular surface area and are characteristic of salt-transporting epithelia. The cells' luminal surfaces exhibit a brush border owing to the abundant number of microvilli present (typical of absorbing epithelia, e.g., in the small intestine). These densely packed microvilli, by greatly increasing the luminal surface area, provide a maximal area for filtrate reabsorption. In addition, the proximal tubular cells also possess numerous mitochondria (evidence of their high metabolic activity) and are abundant in the enzymes necessary for active transport of various substances.

When the straight portion of the proximal tubule enters the outer medulla to become the thin descending limb of the loop of Henle, the tubular epithelium changes. At this point, the epithelium consists of flat, noninterdigitating cells that are simply organized (see Fig. 4–8). Depending on the length of the loop of Henle, the cellular organization may vary with the longest limbs—reaching deep into the medulla—showing increased cellular complexity. Regardless of the length of the limb, the epithelium changes again at the hairpin turn of the loop of Henle. The epithelial cells, although remaining flat, extensively interdigitate with each other. The interdigitating epithelium found at the hairpin turn continues throughout the thin ascending limb of the loop of Henle.

The thick ascending limb of the loop of Henle (or the straight portion of the distal tubule) is primarily characterized by tall, interdigitating cells (see Fig. 4–8). In the thick ascending limb, as in the proximal tubular epithelium, large numbers of mitochondria reside and there is a high level of enzymatic activity. In contrast to proximal tubular cells, distal tubular cells limit their interdigitation to their basal two-thirds, with the topmost portion exhibiting a simple polygonal shape and maintaining a smooth border with the neighboring cells. Following the macula densa or the juxtamedullary apparatus is the **distal convoluted tubule.** The amount of tubular convolution is less than that exhibited by the proximal tubule, and the distal convoluted tubule proceeds to a collecting duct after only two to three loops of convolution.

The **collecting duct** traverses both the renal cortex and medulla and is the site of final urine concentration. The epithelium of the collecting ducts consists of primarily polygonal cells with some small stubby microvilli and no intercellular interdigitations. These cells have intercellular junctions or spaces between them that span from their luminal surfaces to their bases (see Fig. 4–8). In the presence of **antidiuretic hormone (ADH),** the spaces between the cells dilate, rendering the epithelium highly permeable to water. In contrast, when ADH is absent, the spaces are tightly joined (Fig. 4–9). As the collecting duct approaches the papillary tip, the epithelial cells once again change, becoming taller and more columnar.

Tubular Function

The fact that only 1 percent (approximately 1200 mL) of the original plasma ultrafiltrate volume presented to the renal tubules is excreted as urine is evidence of the large amount of reabsorption that takes place within the renal tubules. In addition to this substantial volume change, the resultant solute makeup of the urine excreted differs dramatically from the original ultrafiltrate, un-

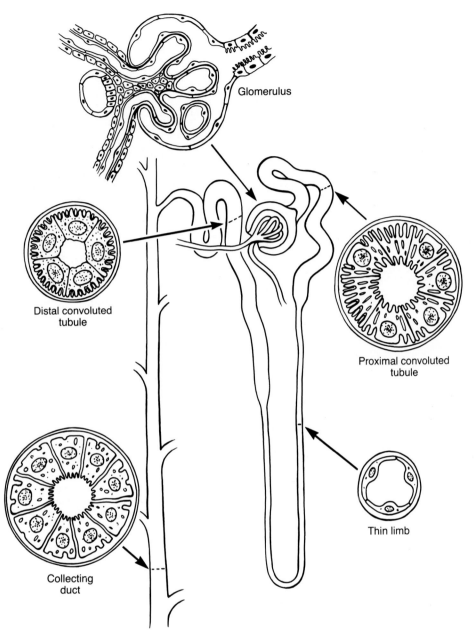

FIGURE 4–8. The general histologic characteristics of the renal tubular epithelium. Representative cross sections of the various tubular segments roughly indicate their cellular morphology, as well as the relative size of the cells, the tubules, and the tubular lumens.

derscoring the dynamic processes carried out by the renal tubules. By virtue of this renal tubular ability to adjust the excretion of water and solutes, the kidney is the most important organ involved in fluid exchanges. The mechanisms effecting these changes, namely **tubular reabsorption** and **tubular secretion,** are the same; it is the direction of substance movement that differs, moving the substance either from the tubular lumen into

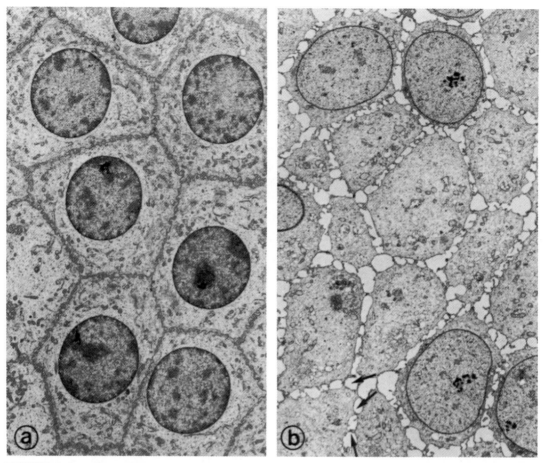

FIGURE 4–9. A transmission electron micrograph of cross sections of the medullary collecting duct epithelium. In *A*, the intercellular spaces are narrow; in *B*, the intercellular spaces are dilated *(arrows)*. The observed dilation is probably due to the effect of antidiuretic hormone (ADH) on the epithelium, inducing the reabsorption of water. (From Koushanpour E, Kriz W: Renal Physiology (2nd ed.), New York, Springer-Verlag, 1986. Used with permission.)

the peritubular capillary blood and interstitium (reabsorption) or from the peritubular capillary blood and interstitium into the tubular lumen (secretion).

Transport

The tubular transport mechanisms (i.e., reabsorption and secretion) are either active or passive. **Active transport** is the movement of a substance across cell membranes against a gradient (i.e., compartments differing in chemical or electrical composition). Such transport requires an expenditure of energy, either directly or indirectly. Active transport, in which substances are moved directly as a result of expended energy (e.g., the exchange of potassium for sodium driven by adenosine triphosphate hydrolysis, the "sodium pump"), is called "direct" active transport. When the movement of one substance is coupled to the movement of another substance down a gradient (e.g., the indirect absorption of glucose with sodium in the proximal tubules), it is called "indirect" active transport or cotransport.

Active transport occurs across the cell (transcellularly) and involves specific protein binding sites that span the cell membrane. In active transport, 1) the substance binds to its specific membrane binding site; 2) it is passed through the cell membrane; and 3) it is released within or out of the cell as the binding site undergoes a conformational change.

Passive transport, on the other hand, requires no energy and is characterized by the movement of a substance along a gradient, or, in other words, from an area of higher concentration to one of lower concentration, such as the movement of urea. This type of transport may be either transcellular or paracellular (i.e., between cells through junctions and intercellular spaces).

Each solute has a specific transport system. Cellular protein binding sites may be unique for a particular solute — transporting only that solute across the membrane — or they may transport several solutes, often exhibiting preferential transport of one analyte over another. In addition, the mode of transport, whether active or passive, is not always the same; it differs depending on the tubular location, e.g., chloride is reabsorbed actively in the ascending loop of Henle and passively in the proximal tubule (Table 4–4).

Reabsorption

Tubular function is selective, reabsorbing the substances necessary for the maintenance of body homeostasis and function such as water, salts, glucose, amino acids, and proteins, while excreting waste products such as creatinine and metabolic acids. Table 4–4 summarizes some important ultrafiltrate components according to the location of tubular reabsorption. The table also indicates the primary mode of transport of the components. This summary, however, refers to the major overall transport of the analyte; in reality, the reabsorption of some solutes actually involves several mechanisms. In this section, the principal interactions of the major solutes and their transport processes are discussed.

Secretion

As with tubular reabsorption, tubular secretion takes place throughout the nephron. The principal roles of the renal secretory process are 1) to eliminate metabolic wastes and those substances not normally present in the plasma and 2) to adjust the acid-base equilibrium of the body. These two functions overlap in that many metabolic by-products and foreign substances are weak acids and bases, thereby directly affecting the body's acid-base equilibrium. Table 4–5 summarizes

TABLE 4–4. SUMMARY OF TUBULAR REABSORPTION OF SOME IMPORTANT ULTRAFILTRATE COMPONENTS

LOCATION	MODE OF REABSORPTION	SUBSTANCE
Proximal tubule (convoluted and straight portions)	Passive	H_2O, Cl^-, K^+, urea
	Active	Na^+, HCO_3^-, glucose, amino acids, proteins, phosphate, sulfate, Mg^{++}, Ca^{++}, uric acid
Loop of Henle		
Thin descending limb	Passive	H_2O, urea
"U" turn and thin ascending limb	Passive	Na^+, Cl^-, urea
Thick ascending limb (medullary and cortical)	Passive	Urea
	Active	Na^+, Cl^-
Distal tubule (convoluted portion)	Active	*Na^+, Cl^-, sulfate, uric acid
Collecting tubules		
Cortical	Passive	†H_2O, Cl^-
	Active	*Na^+
Medullary	Passive	H_2O, urea

* Reabsorption under aldosterone control by the renin-angiotensin-aldosterone system.
† Reabsorption under ADH control.

T A B L E 4 – 5.   SUMMARY OF TUBULAR SECRETION OF SOME IMPORTANT ULTRAFILTRATE COMPONENTS

LOCATION	SUBSTANCE
Proximal tubule	H^+, NH_3, weak acids and bases
Loop of Henle	—
Distal tubule	H^+, NH_3, K^+
Collecting tubule	H^+, NH_3, K^+

some of the important secreted ultrafiltrate components and the location of their tubular secretion.

Most of the substances secreted, other than hydrogen ions, ammonia, and potassium, are weak acids or bases. These weak acids and bases originate from either metabolic or exogenous sources. They are 1) substances incompletely metabolized by the body (e.g., thiamine); 2) substances not metabolized at all and secreted unchanged (e.g., radiopaque contrast media, mannitol); or 3) substances not normally present in the plasma (e.g., penicillin, salicylate). In addition, some of these same substances are simply unable to pass through the glomerular filtration barrier for excretion because they are bound to plasma proteins, primarily albumin (e.g., unconjugated bilirubin, various drugs). As a result of being carried by plasma proteins, their overall size is dramatically increased and their original charge characteristics are modified. Tubular secretion, however, provides a means for the elimination of these substances. As these protein-bound substances flow through the peritubular capillaries, they interact with endothelial binding sites, are transported into the renal tubular cells, and are ultimately secreted into the tubular lumen.

Regulation of Acid-Base Equilibrium

To better understand the role of tubular secretion in the regulation of the body's acid-base equilibrium, a basic knowledge of the endogenous production of acids and bases is needed. In health, the normal blood pH is alkaline and ranges from 7.35 to 7.45; however, in pathologic disease states, the pH may be as low as 7.00 or as high as 7.80. The blood is alkaline and is constantly threatened by the endogenous production of acids from normal dietary metabolism. These endogenous acids are formed from 1) the production of carbon dioxide owing to oxidative metabolism of foods, with the resultant formation of carbonic acid; 2) from the catabolism of dietary proteins and phospholipids; or 3) from the production of acids in certain pathologic or physiologic conditions (e.g., acetoacetic acid in uncontrolled diabetes mellitus or lactic acid in exercise).

Three body systems are involved in maintaining the blood pH at a level compatible with life: 1) the blood buffer system: the substances involved are inorganic phosphates, bicarbonate, proteins, and hemoglobin; 2) the pulmonary system; and 3) the renal system. Although all three systems work in concert to maintain homeostasis, the blood buffer and the pulmonary systems are able to respond immediately, although only partially to pH changes. The renal system, on the other hand, despite its comparatively slow response, is capable of completely correcting deviations in the blood pH.

In response to changes in the blood pH, the kidneys selectively excrete acid or alkali into the urine. Whereas excess alkali is eliminated by the excretion of sodium salts, such as disodium phosphate (Na_2HPO_4) and sodium bicarbonate ($NaHCO_3$), excess acids are eliminated by the excretion of ammonium salts (e.g., NH_4Cl and $[NH_4]_2SO_4$) and titratable acids (monosodium phosphate, NaH_2PO_4).

Three secretory mechanisms are employed in maintaining the blood pH and each relies directly or indirectly on the tubular secretion of H^+ ions. In acidotic conditions, H^+ ions (acids) are secreted in exchange for sodium and bicarbonate ions (alkali), whereas in alkalotic conditions, the tubular secretion of H^+ ions is minimized and additional alkali is eliminated from the body.

In the first secretory mechanism, H^+ ions are secreted into the proximal tubule, directly preventing the loss of bicarbonate, a vital component of the blood-buffer system. In Figure 4–10, bicarbonate ions (HCO_3^-),

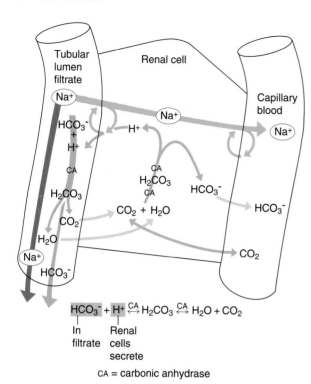

$$HCO_3^- + H^+ \overset{CA}{\Leftrightarrow} H_2CO_3 \overset{CA}{\Leftrightarrow} H_2O + CO_2$$

In
filtrate

Renal
cells
secrete

CA = carbonic anhydrase

FIGURE 4-10. H$^+$ ion secretion and the mechanism of filtered bicarbonate reabsorption in the proximal tubule.

lumen of the nephrons, secreted hydrogen ions exchange with the sodium ions, and disodium phosphate (Na_2HPO_4) becomes monosodium phosphate (NaH_2PO_4). These monobasic phosphates—specifically combined with hydrogen ions and excreted in the urine—are referred to as **titratable acids.** The name derives from the ability to titrate urine to a pH of 7.4 (pH of normal plasma), using a standard base (e.g., NaOH), to determine the amount of acid present as a result of these monobasic phosphates. Hydrogen ions combined with other solutes are not measured.

(4-1) In blood:

$$H_3PO_4 + 6\ Na^+ \longrightarrow 3\ Na_2HPO_4$$

In ultrafiltrate:

$$Na_2HPO_4 + H^+ \longrightarrow NaH_2PO_4 + Na^+$$

$$Na^+ + HCO_3^- \longrightarrow NaHCO_3$$
$$\text{(reabsorbed)}$$

As a direct result of these phosphates present in the ultrafiltrate, acid is removed from the body and the urine is acidified; in

which readily pass the glomerular filtration barrier, react with the secreted H$^+$ to form carbonic acid (H_2CO_3) in the tubular lumen. This carbonic acid, however, is rapidly catalyzed to carbon dioxide and water, owing to the high concentration of the enzyme carbonic anhydrase present in the brush border of the proximal tubular cells. The carbon dioxide diffuses into the proximal cell, where once again, by the action of carbonic anhydrase, it is converted to HCO$_3^-$ and H$^+$. As a result, H$^+$ ions are available once more for renal tubular secretion and HCO$_3^-$ ions are reabsorbed from the tubular lumen. This reabsorbed bicarbonate diffuses back into the peritubular capillary blood, resupplying the blood-buffer system.

The second secretory mechanism, illustrated in Figure 4-11, depends on the amount of phosphate present in the ultrafiltrate. Phosphoric acids produced by dietary metabolism are rapidly converted in the blood to neutral salts (e.g., Na_2HPO_4) and are transported to the kidney. In the tubular

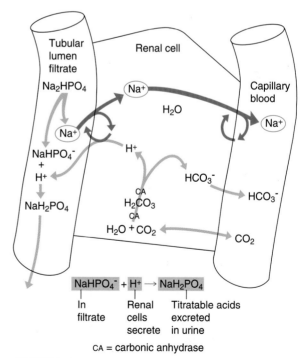

$$NaHPO_4^- + H^+ \longrightarrow NaH_2PO_4$$

In
filtrate

Renal
cells
secrete

Titratable acids
excreted
in urine

CA = carbonic anhydrase

FIGURE 4-11. H$^+$ ion secretion and the formation of titratable acids. This is a mechanism of urine acidification in the collecting ducts.

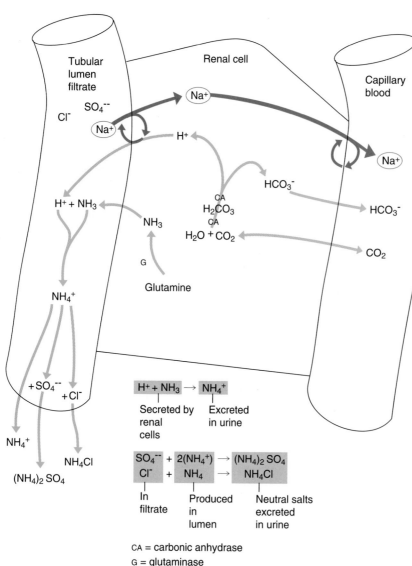

FIGURE 4–12. H^+ ion secretion and the formation of ammonium ions. This is a mechanism of urine acidification in the collecting ducts.

addition, sodium and bicarbonate ions are returned to the peritubular capillary blood.

The third secretory mechanism for acid removal, illustrated in Figure 4–12, depends on ammonia secretion and the subsequent exchange of sodium ions for ammonium ions. Ammonia (NH_3) is produced in the renal tubular cells by the action of the enzyme glutaminase on the substrate glutamine, obtained from the peritubular capillary blood. Because NH_3 is not ionized, it is lipid soluble and readily diffuses across tubular cell membranes into the tubular lumen. Once in the lumen, it rapidly combines with H^+ ions to form ammonium ions (NH_4^+). These ions, essentially nondiffusible because of their charge, remain in the tubular lumen and may combine with neutral salts such as sodium chloride or sodium sulfate, a metabolic by-product. Equations 4–2 and 4–3 depict the chemical reactions taking place in the tubular lumen.

(4–2)

$$NH_3 + H^+ \longrightarrow NH_4^+$$

$$NH_4^+ + NaCl + HCO_3^- \longrightarrow NH_4Cl + NaHCO_3$$
$$\qquad\qquad\qquad\qquad\qquad \text{(excreted)} \quad \text{(reabsorbed)}$$

(4–3)

$$NH_3 + H^+ \longrightarrow NH_4^+$$

$$2NH_4^+ + Na_2SO_4 + 2HCO_3^- \longrightarrow$$
$$(NH_4)_2SO_4 + 2NaHCO_3$$
$$\text{(excreted)} \qquad \text{(reabsorbed)}$$

Note that in both reactions, bicarbonate and sodium are again available for tubular reabsorption.

The ammonia (NH_3) excreted in urine is primarily derived from renal tubular synthesis. Both the proximal and collecting duct cells are responsible for ammonia production; however, it is in the collecting ducts where final urine acidification principally occurs. In addition, the rate of ammonia synthesis is regulated, responding directly to the systemic acid-base status (e.g., production of ammonia increases in response to acidotic conditions).

In summary, the kidney regulates the acid-base equilibrium of the body by three renal secretory mechanisms: 1) H^+ ion secretion to recover bicarbonate; 2) H^+ ion secretion to yield urine titratable acids (e.g., monosodium phosphate); and 3) H^+ ion and NH_3 secretion to yield ammonium salts (e.g., ammonium chloride and ammonium sulfate). In each of these mechanisms, the hydrogen ion secretion (i.e., the loss of acid) results in sodium or bicarbonate reabsorption (i.e., the gain of alkali). Therefore, the kidney will modulate its secretion of hydrogen ions and ammonia based on the dynamic acid-base needs of the body.

Tubular Transport Capacity

The capacity of the renal tubules for reabsorption as well as secretion varies depending on the substance being transported. For some substances, as the amount of solute presented to the renal tubules increases, the rate of tubular reabsorption will also increase until a maximal rate of reabsorption is attained. This maximal rate of reabsorption will remain constant despite any further increases in the solute's tubular concentration and results in the excess solute appearing in the urine. This reabsorptive characteristic of the renal epithelium is known as the **maximal tubular reabsorptive capacity.** Denoted

T_m, it represents the amount of solute (mg) reabsorbed per minute. The T_m varies depending on the specific solute being reabsorbed, as well as on other factors, such as the glomerular filtration rate. Glucose, amino acids, proteins, phosphate, sulfate, and uric acid are a few of the solutes that exhibit a T_m-limited tubular reabsorptive capacity. In addition, these substances will have a plasma blood concentration, known as the **renal threshold level,** which relates specifically to their T_m. For example, the T_m for glucose is approximately 350 mg/min (when corrected to 1.73 m² body surface area) and the corresponding plasma renal threshold level is 160 to 180 mg/dL. Stated another way, regardless of the amount of glucose present in the renal tubular lumen, a maximum of 350 mg can be reabsorbed per minute. Plasma blood glucose levels exceeding 160 to 180 mg/dL will result in the ultrafiltrate concentration exceeding the ability of the tubules to reabsorb (T_m) and the additional glucose being observed in the urine.

Similarly, some solutes secreted by the tubules have a **maximal tubular secretory capacity,** also denoted T_m, (e.g., *p*-aminohippurate, a weak organic acid). Note that the same designation, T_m, is appropriate because both processes refer to the maximum capacity for the active transport of a substance, and the direction of movement—whether into or out of the tubular lumen—is immaterial.

In contrast, some solutes are not limited in the amount that may be reabsorbed (e.g., sodium) or secreted (e.g., potassium). For these substances, other factors influence their rate of transport, such as the tubular flow rate, the amount of time the solute is in contact with the renal epithelium, the concentrations of other solutes in the filtrate, the presence of transport inhibitors, or changes in hormone levels (e.g., ADH).

Proximal Tubular Reabsorption

The proximal tubule reabsorbs more than 66 percent of the filtered water, sodium, and chloride. In addition, essentially 100 percent of the glucose, amino acids, and proteins are reabsorbed by a cotransport mechanism coupled to sodium. Other solutes such as bicarbonate, phosphate, sulfate, magnesium, calcium, and uric acid are reabsorbed in the proximal tubule as well (see Table 4–4). Although these reabsorptive processes significantly reduce the fluid volume and the concentrations of specific solutes, the proximal tubular filtrate remains osmotically unchanged. In other words, despite the proximal tubule's substantial reabsorption of solutes and water, the absolute number of solute particles (osmoles) present per kg of water remains identical to that of the original ultrafiltrate, which is identical to the plasma (if made protein-free) in the peritubular capillaries. Also, the solute particles in this filtrate differ significantly (e.g., less sodium and more chloride) from those in the original ultrafiltrate.

In summary, as the filtrate leaves the proximal tubule, the fluid volume has been reduced by over two-thirds; significant reabsorption of salts, glucose, proteins, and other important solutes has taken place either actively or passively and the osmolality remains unchanged. Osmolality—a measurable, physical characteristic of urine, used to evaluate the renal tubules' ability to concentrate urine—will be discussed further in Chapter 5.

Water Reabsorption

Water is reabsorbed throughout the nephron except in the ascending limbs (thin and thick) of the loops of Henle, located in the renal medulla (Fig. 4–13). In the ascending limbs, the tubular epithelium is selectively impermeable to water, despite the large osmotic gradient that exists between the tubular lumen fluid and the medullary interstitium. In all other areas of the nephron, osmosis in synergy with the tubular epithelium is responsible for water reabsorption. It is the epithelium that provides the membrane or barrier retarding the diffusion of water into the interstitium (paracellularly) or into the cells themselves (transcellularly). The anatomic structure of the tubular epithelium—specifically, the characteristics of its intercellular spaces—changes throughout the

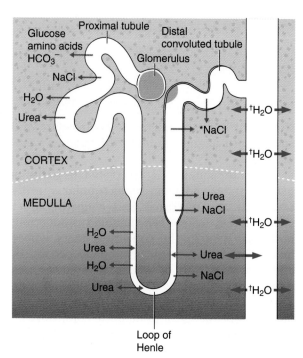

FIGURE 4–13. A schematic representation of the solute and water transport processes occurring in various segments of the nephron. * indicates that sodium absorption is under aldosterone control; † indicates that water absorption is under ADH control.

nephron (as previously discussed). These epithelial characteristics, regulated by bodily needs and hormonal control, dictate when, where, and how much water is ultimately reabsorbed by the nephron.

Osmosis is the movement of water across a membrane from a solution of low osmolality to one of higher osmolality. The cell membrane is semipermeable, allowing some but not all solutes to cross it. An osmolality gradient (i.e., two areas differing in the number of solute particles present per volume of solvent), induces the diffusion of water across the membrane in an attempt to reach an osmotic equilibrium. This passive mechanism is solely responsible for the massive reabsorption of water by the renal tubules. Critical to this process is the high solute concentration or hypertonicity of the renal medulla, which establishes the necessary osmotic gradient.

Renal Concentration Mechanism

The only tissue in the body that is hypertonic with respect to normal plasma (i.e., its osmolality is greater than 290 mOsm/kg), is the renal medulla. In the medulla, the hypertonicity progressively increases, being lowest at its border with the iso-osmotic cortex and greatest in the papillary tips of the renal pyramids. In addition, this increased hypertonicity is shared by all components in the medullary interstitium, including tissue cells, interstitial fluid, blood vessels, and blood.

The gradient hypertonicity of the medullary interstitium is established and maintained by two countercurrent mechanisms: 1) an "active" **countercurrent *multiplier* mechanism,** occurring in the loops of Henle; and 2) a "passive" **countercurrent *exchange* mechanism** involving the vasa recta. The loops of Henle and the vasa recta are ideally configured—they are parallel structures close to each other with the fluid in the ascending and descending segments flowing in opposite directions; hence the name "countercurrent" mechanism. The ascending limb of the loop of Henle actively reabsorbs sodium and chloride into the medullary interstitium, and this limb is essentially impermeable to water (see Fig. 4–13). As this active process occurs, the interstitium increases in tonicity (i.e., the solute concentration increases), whereas that of the ascending tubular fluid decreases. At the same time in the descending limb, water (but not solutes) readily passes into the interstitium. The reabsorption of sodium and chloride in the ascending limb continues until an osmotic equilibrium is attained between the medullary interstitium, with the reabsorbed solutes from the ascending limb, and the descending tubular fluid, with water passively diffusing out into the interstitium. In other words, the osmolality of the descending limb fluid and the interstitium become equal and greater than the fluid in the ascending limb. As this process continues, a gradient of hypertonicity develops with the descending tubular fluid and the interstitium becomes progressively more concentrated (Fig. 4–14). Note that the intratubule osmolality difference from cortex to medulla is significantly greater than that laterally (i.e., at the same level in descending and ascending tubules). Essentially, the osmotic gradient within the tubule from cortex to medulla has been "mul-

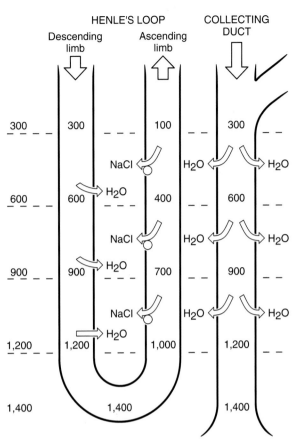

FIGURE 4–14. A schematic representation of the countercurrent multiplier mechanism producing hypertonic urine. Osmolality values are in mOsm/kg H_2O. Note that the maximum urine osmolality possible is the same as that of the renal medulla, approximately 1400 mOsm/kg.

tiplied," owing to the countercurrent processes in which sodium and chloride are actively reabsorbed in the ascending limb and water is passively reabsorbed in the descending limb of the loop of Henle.

Initially, it appears as if the countercurrent multiplier mechanism has accomplished little because the tubular lumen fluid becomes concentrated in the descending limb only to become diluted owing to solute removal in the ascending limb of the loop of Henle. The net result is a tubular lumen fluid slightly hypotonic to that originally presented to the loop of Henle (Table 4–6). However, the primary purpose of the countercurrent "multiplier" mechanism is not to concentrate the lumen fluid, but to establish and maintain the gradient hypertonicity in the medullary interstitium. Subsequently, when the tubular lumen fluid enters the col-

TABLE 4–6.   TUBULAR LUMEN FLUID OSMOLALITY* THROUGHOUT THE NEPHRON

TUBULE SEGMENT	OSMOLALITY CHANGE
Proximal tubule	Enters: iso-osmotic, Exits: iso-osmotic
Loop of Henle	Enters: iso-osmotic
Thin descending limb	Becomes progressively hyperosmotic
"U" turn	Maximally hyperosmotic
Thick ascending limb (medullary and cortical)	Becomes progressively hypo-osmotic
	Exits: slightly hypo-osmotic
Distal tubule (convoluted portion)	Enters: slightly hypo-osmotic
	Exits: iso-osmotic
Collecting tubules	Enters: iso-osmotic
	Exits: adjustable, under ADH control; may be hyper-, hypo-, or iso-osmotic.

* Iso-osmotic = plasma osmalality ≃ 290 mOsm/kg.

lecting tubules, which traverse all areas of the renal cortex and medulla, it will become concentrated or diluted to form the final urine.

In contrast, the second countercurrent mechanism is a passive exchange process occurring in the vascular bed deep in the renal medulla, where reabsorbed solutes and water in the medullary interstitium are passively exchanged by diffusion into the vasa recta. Like the tubular lumen fluid, the blood becomes progressively concentrated as it flows toward the papillary tip and progressively diluted after it turns and ascends to the renal cortex. This vascular countercurrent mechanism provides a means to supply nutrients to the medulla and remove reabsorbed water, thereby maintaining the medullary hypertonicity.

Because the lumen fluid leaving the distal tubules is iso-osmotic, the concentration of or the dilution of the final urine must take place within the collecting tubules. In the collecting tubules, processes involving solute exchange and water reabsorption occur simultaneously and often under hormonal control. It is also interesting to note that water is never secreted; rather, it is selectively not reabsorbed.

When the iso-osmotic lumen fluid enters the cortical collecting tubules, sodium and water reabsorption is hormonally controlled by two distinct and independent processes. The renin-angiotensin-aldosterone system is responsible for sodium reabsorption. Briefly described in the renal circulation section and depicted in Figure 4–15, the juxtaglomerular apparatus releases renin into the bloodstream in response to decreased sodium, blood volume, or blood pressure. Angiotensin II forms rapidly, which stimulates the adrenal cortex to secrete the hormone aldosterone. Subsequently, aldosterone activates sodium reabsorption by the distal and cortical collecting tubules.

On the other hand, water reabsorption in the collecting tubules requires the presence of ADH or vasopressin. The posterior pituitary continuously produces and releases ADH into the blood stream, while vascular baroreceptors located in the heart monitor arterial blood pressure. When an increase in arterial blood pressure occurs, the hypothalamus is signalled and it in turn inhibits the production of ADH by the posterior pituitary cells. This interactive process is called a "negative feedback" mechanism and is outlined in Figure 4–16. As the plasma level of ADH decreases, the collecting tubule epithelium changes (see Fig. 4–9) and the osmosis of water from the lumen fluid also decreases. Sodium reabsorption is unaffected; however, water is not reabsorbed, resulting in a large volume of dilute (hypo-osmotic) urine. In contrast, a decrease in blood pressure sensed by the baroreceptors would stimulate an increase in the production of ADH. As a direct result, the collecting tubule epithelium allows

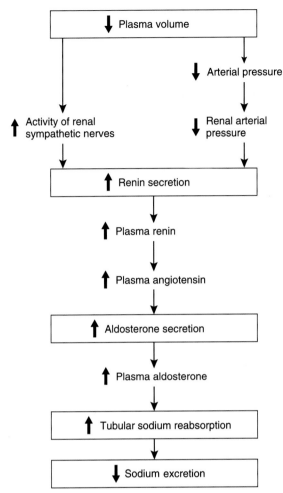

FIGURE 4–15. A schematic representation of the renin-angiotensin-aldosterone system and its role in the tubular reabsorption of sodium.

The other 50 percent of the solutes are due to the high medullary concentration of urea maintained by a process called the **urea cycle** (see Fig. 4–13). Urea, a by-product of protein catabolism, freely penetrates the glomerular filtration barrier, passing into the tubules as part of the ultrafiltrate. Despite the fact that it is a metabolic waste product and the body has no use for it, 40 percent to 70 percent of urea is passively reabsorbed into the medullary interstitium. It subsequently diffuses along its concentration gradient into the lumen fluid in the loops of Henle. When the lumen fluid enters the cortical collecting tubules, water is reabsorbed in the presence of ADH, whereas the epithelium

increased water reabsorption by osmosis. Again, sodium reabsorption is not affected; however, the increased amount of water reabsorbed results in a concentrated (hyperosmotic) final urine. Owing to the substantial osmolality gradient that exists between the medullary interstitium and the collecting tubular fluid, the osmotic force is great and progressively increases as the lumen fluid proceeds to the papillary tips. Because of this tremendous gradient, the original ultrafiltrate osmolality of 290 mOsm/kg can be concentrated to 900 to 1400 mOsm/kg in the final urine.

Normally, the countercurrent multiplier mechanism accounts for about 50 percent of the solutes concentrated in the renal medulla.

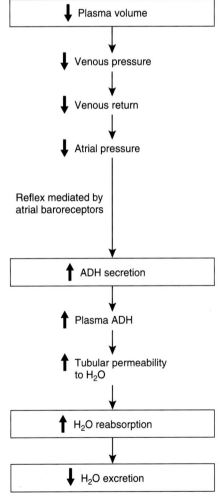

FIGURE 4–16. A schematic representation of the mechanism controlling antidiuretic hormone secretion.

in the cortical collecting tubules is impermeable to urea. Any water reabsorption serves to further concentrate the amount of urea present in the lumen fluid. When the lumen fluid reaches the medullary collecting tubules, both water (under ADH influence) and urea readily diffuse into the interstitium. In other words, the cortical epithelium of the collecting tubule is never permeable to urea, whereas the medullary epithelium is readily permeable. Therefore, in the medullary collecting tubules, urea diffuses along its concentration gradient from the concentrated lumen fluid into the interstitium until the urea concentration in both these areas is equal. As a result of this urea equilibrium, 1) the sodium salts in the hypertonic medulla serve to osmotically balance all the "non-urea" solutes in the final urine and 2) the concentration of urea in the final urine is actually determined by urea itself. Another factor affecting urea concentration in the final urine is the urine flow rate and its affect on urea reabsorption. Slow urine flow rates of less than 2 mL/min result in a larger amount of urea reabsorbed, whereas flow rates exceeding 2 mL/min allow minimal and constant urea reabsorption.

In summary, the hypertonicity of the medullary interstitium results from the countercurrent multiplier mechanism and the urea cycle. The hypertonic medulla established by these two processes provides a massive osmotic force for water reabsorption from the collecting tubules and is regulated by the presence of ADH in response to bodily needs. Despite the fact that solutes such as sodium —under aldosterone control—can be selectively reabsorbed or excreted in the distal and collecting tubules, it is the regulation of water content by the collecting tubules that ultimately determines the concentration of the final urine. Stated another way, as the iso-osmotic fluid from the distal tubule enters the collecting tubule, solute exchange may occur; however, the total number of solutes (i.e., osmoles) remains unchanged. It is the volume of water in which these solutes are excreted that varies. Therefore, the selective reabsorption of water by the collecting tubules determines whether a concentrated (hypertonic) or a dilute (hypotonic) final urine is produced.

References

Cotran RS, Kumar V, Robbins SL: Robbins Pathological Basis of Disease (4th ed.), Philadelphia, W. B. Saunders Company, 1989, pp. 1011–1014.
Koushanpour E, Kriz W: Renal Physiology (2nd ed.), New York, Springer-Verlag, 1986, pp. 53–72.

Bibliography

Cotran RS, Leaf A: Renal Pathophysiology (3rd ed.), New York, Oxford University Press, 1985, pp. 1–47.
First MR: Renal function. *In* Kaplan LA, Pesce AJ (eds.): Clinical Chemistry Theory, Analysis, and Correlation, St. Louis, The C. V. Mosby Company, 1984, pp. 403–410.
Klahr S, Weiner ID: Disorders of acid-base metabolism. *In* Chan JCM, Gill JR, Jr (eds.): Kidney Electrolyte Disorders, New York, Churchill Livingstone, 1990, pp. 1–15.
Lehmann HP, Henry JB: SI units. *In* Henry JB (ed.): Clinical Diagnosis and Management by Laboratory Methods (18th ed.), Philadelphia, W. B. Saunders Company, 1991, pp. 1373–1375.
O'Connor WJ: Normal Renal Function, New York, Oxford University Press, 1982, p. 212.
Tietz NW: Reference ranges. In Tietz NW (ed.): Fundamentals of Clinical Chemistry (3rd ed.), Philadelphia, W. B. Saunders Company, 1987, pp. 944–968.
Vander AJ, Sherman JH, Luciano DS: Human Physiology (4th ed.), New York, McGraw-Hill Book Company, 1985, pp. 423–446.

Study Questions

1. **Beginning with the glomerulus, number the following structures in the order the ultrafiltrate travels for processing and excretion in the kidney.**

   _____ A. bladder
   _____ B. calyces
   _____ C. collecting tubule
   _____ D. distal tubule
   _____ E. glomerulus
   _____ F. juxtaglomerular apparatus
   _____ G. loop of Henle
   _____ H. proximal tubule
   _____ I. renal pelvis
   _____ J. ureter
   _____ K. urethra

2. **How many nephrons are found in an average kidney?**

   A. 13,000
   B. 130,000
   C. 1.3 million
   D. 13 million

3. **The ultrafiltration of plasma occurs in glomeruli located in the renal**

   A. cortex.
   B. medulla.
   C. pelvis.
   D. ureter.

4. **Which component of the nephron is located exclusively in the renal medulla?**

   A. The collecting tubule
   B. The distal tubule
   C. The loop of Henle
   D. The proximal tubule

5. **Which of the following is NOT a vascular characteristic of the kidney?**

   A. The afferent arteriole has a narrower lumen than the efferent arteriole.
   B. The arteries are primarily end arteries, supplying specific areas of tissue, and do not interconnect.
   C. The arterioles subdivide into a capillary network, rejoin as an arteriole, and subdivide into a second capillary bed.
   D. The vasa recta vessels deep in the renal medulla form the beginning of the venous renal circulation.

6. **The formation of the ultrafiltrate in the glomerulus is driven by the**

   A. hydrostatic blood pressure.
   B. oncotic pressure of the plasma proteins.
   C. osmotic pressure of the solutes in the ultrafiltrate.
   D. pressures exerted by the glomerular filtration barrier.

7. **Which of the following is a characteristic of renin, an enzyme secreted by specialized cells of the juxtaglomerular apparatus?**

   A. It stimulates the diffusion of urea into the renal interstitium.
   B. It inhibits the reabsorption of sodium and water in the nephron.
   C. It regulates the osmotic reabsorption of water by the collecting tubules.
   D. It causes the formation of angiotensin and the secretion of aldosterone.

8. **The glomerular filtration barrier is composed of the**

   A. capillary endothelium, basement membrane, and podocytes.
   B. mesangium, basement membrane, and shield of negativity.
   C. capillary endothelium, mesangium, and juxtaglomerular apparatus.
   D. basement membrane, podocytes, and juxtaglomerular apparatus.

9. **The ability of a solute to cross the glomerular filtration barrier is determined by its**

   1. molecular size.
   2. molecular radius.
   3. electrical charge.
   4. plasma concentration.
      A. 1, 2, and 3 are correct.
      B. 1 and 3 are correct.
      C. 4 is correct.
      D. All are correct.

10. **The epithelium characterized by a brush border owing to numerous microvilli is found in the**

    A. collecting tubules.
    B. distal tubules.
    C. loops of Henle.
    D. proximal tubules.

11. **The kidneys play an important role in the**

    1. excretion of waste products.

    2. regulation of water and electrolytes.

    3. maintenance of acid-base equilibrium.

    4. control of blood pressure and fluid balance.

        A. 1, 2, and 3 are correct.

        B. 1 and 3 are correct.

        C. 4 is correct.

        D. All are correct.

12. **What percent of the original ultrafiltrate formed in the urinary space is actually excreted as urine?**

    A. 1%

    B. 10%

    C. 25%

    D. 33%

13. **What differentiates tubular *reabsorption* from tubular *secretion* in the nephron?**

    A. The direction of movement of the substance being absorbed or secreted is different.

    B. Reabsorption is an active transport process, whereas secretion is a passive transport process.

    C. Cell membrane binding sites are different for the reabsorption and secretion of a solute.

    D. The location of the epithelium in the nephron determines which process will occur.

14. **During tubular transport, the movement of a solute against a gradient**

    A. is called passive transport.

    B. requires little to no energy.

    C. involves specific cell membrane binding sites.

    D. may occur paracellularly, i.e., between cells through intercellular spaces.

15. **Substances bound to plasma proteins in the blood can be eliminated in the urine by**

    A. glomerular secretion.   C. tubular secretion.

    B. glomerular filtration.   D. tubular reabsorption.

16. **Which statement characterizes the renal system's ability to regulate blood pH?**

    A. It has a slow response with complete correction of the pH to normal.

    B. It has a fast response with complete correction of the pH to normal.

    C. It has a slow response with only partial correction of the pH toward normal.

    D. It has a fast response with only partial correction of the pH toward normal.

17. **The kidneys excrete excess alkali (base) in the urine as**

    A. ammonium ions.
    B. ammonium salts.
    C. sodium bicarbonate.
    D. titratable acids.

18. **Which of the following substances is secreted into the tubular lumen to eliminate hydrogen ions?**

    A. Ammonia (NH_3)
    B. Ammonium ions (NH_4^+)
    C. Disodium phosphate (Na_2HPO_4)
    D. Monosodium phosphate (NaH_2PO_4)

19. **Urine titratable acids can form when the ultrafiltrate contains**

    A. ammonia.
    B. bicarbonate.
    C. phosphate.
    D. sodium.

20. **The renal threshold level for glucose is 160 to 180 mg/dL. This corresponds to**

    A. the rate of glucose reabsorption by the renal tubules.
    B. the concentration of glucose in the tubular lumen fluid.
    C. the plasma concentration above which tubular reabsorption of glucose occurs.
    D. the plasma concentration above which glucose will be excreted in the urine.

21. **When too much protein is presented to the renal tubules for reabsorption, it is excreted in the urine because**

    A. the renal threshold for protein has not been exceeded.
    B. the maximal tubular reabsorptive capacity for protein has been exceeded.
    C. protein is not normally present in the ultrafiltrate and it cannot be reabsorbed.
    D. the glomerular filtration barrier will allow only abnormal proteins to pass.

22. **More than 66% of the filtered water, sodium, and chloride and 100% of filtered glucose, amino acids, and proteins are reabsorbed in the**

    A. collecting tubules.
    B. distal tubules.
    C. loops of Henle.
    D. proximal tubules.

23. **Water reabsorption occurs throughout the nephron EXCEPT in the**

   A. cortical collecting tubules.
   B. proximal convoluted tubules.
   C. ascending limb of the loops of Henle.
   D. descending limb of the loops of Henle.

24. **The process solely responsible for water reabsorption throughout the nephron is**

   A. osmosis.
   B. the urea cycle.
   C. the countercurrent exchange mechanism.
   D. the countercurrent multiplier mechanism.

25. **Hypertonicity of the renal medulla is maintained by**

   1. the countercurrent multiplier mechanism.
   2. the countercurrent exchange mechanism.
   3. the urea cycle.
   4. osmosis.
      A. 1, 2, and 3 are correct.
      B. 1 and 3 are correct.
      C. 4 is correct.
      D. All are correct.

26. **Which of the following is NOT a feature of the renal countercurrent multiplier mechanism?**

   A. The ascending limb of the loop of Henle is impermeable to water.
   B. The descending limb of the loop of Henle passively reabsorbs water.
   C. The descending limb of the loop of Henle actively reabsorbs sodium and urea.
   D. The fluid in the ascending and descending limbs of the loop of Henle flows in opposite directions.

27. **The purpose of the renal countercurrent *multiplier* mechanism is to**

   A. concentrate the tubular lumen fluid.
   B. increase the urinary excretion of urea.
   C. preserve the gradient hypertonicity in the medulla.
   D. facilitate the reabsorption of sodium and chloride.

28. **Which vascular component is involved in the renal countercurrent *exchange* mechanism?**

   A. The afferent arteriole
   B. The efferent arteriole
   C. The glomerulus
   D. The vasa recta

29. Antidiuretic hormone (ADH) regulates the reabsorption of

    A. water in the collecting tubules.

    B. sodium in the collecting tubules.

    C. sodium in the distal convoluted tubule.

    D. water and sodium in the loop of Henle.

30. Which of the following describes the tubular lumen fluid that enters the collecting tubule as compared to the tubular lumen fluid in the proximal tubule?

    A. Hypo-osmotic

    B. Iso-osmotic

    C. Hyperosmotic

    D. Counterosmotic

31. The final concentration of the urine is determined within the

    A. collecting ducts.

    B. distal convoluted tubules.

    C. loops of Henle.

    D. proximal convoluted tubules.

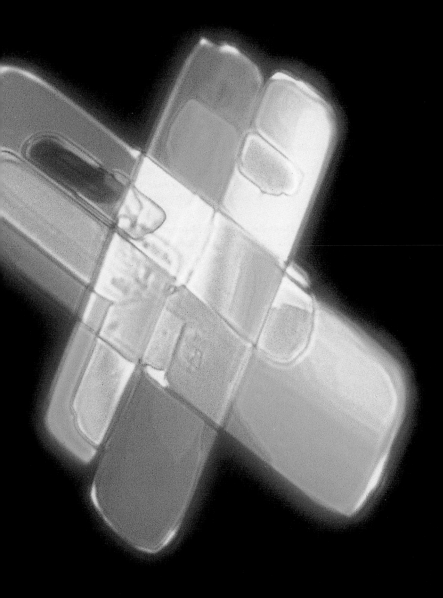

5

Renal Function

LEARNING OBJECTIVES

After studying this chapter, the student should be able to

1. State the volume and the solute composition of normal urine.

2. Differentiate between the solute amount (osmolality) and the solute mass (specific gravity) in urine and the ways in which they are measured.

3. Discuss the effects that diet, disease, and some exogenous substances (e.g., x-ray contrast media) have on solute composition measurements.

4. Discuss the physiologic factors involved in determining the volume of urine that is excreted.

5. Describe a protocol and one purpose for each of the following procedures:
   • a fluid deprivation test
   • an osmolar clearance determination
   • a free-water clearance determination

6. Calculate osmolar clearance and free-water clearance results using data provided.

7. Compare and contrast the creatinine clearance test and the inulin clearance test for the assessment of glomerular filtration.

8. Describe a protocol for a creatinine clearance test and discuss factors that can influence the results obtained.

9. Calculate creatinine clearance results using data provided.

10. Describe the *p*-aminohippurate (PAH) clearance test for the assessment of renal plasma flow.

11. Discuss briefly the relationship of renal tubular secretory function to the urinary excretion of acids.

12. Describe the oral ammonium chloride test for the assessment of tubular function.

anuria (also called **anuresis**): the absence or cessation of urine excretion.

creatinine clearance: a renal clearance test that measures the volume of plasma cleared of creatinine by the kidneys per unit of time. Reported in milliliters per minute, it is determined by the equation $C = U \times V/P$, in which U and P are the urine and plasma concentrations of creatinine, respectively, and V is the volume of urine excreted in a timed collection, usually 24 hours.

free water clearance (also called **solute-free water clearance**): the volume of water cleared by the kidneys per minute in excess of that necessary to remove solutes. Denoted C_{H_2O} and reported in milliliters per minute, it is determined using the equation $C_{H_2O} = V \times C_{Osm}$. V is the volume of urine excreted in a timed collection (mL/min), and C_{Osm} is the osmolar clearance (mL/min).

glomerular filtration rate (GFR): the rate of plasma cleared by the glomeruli per unit of time (mL/min). This rate is determined using clearance tests of substances that are known to be exclusively removed by glomerular filtration and that are not reabsorbed or secreted by the nephrons (e.g., inulin).

nocturia: excessive or increased frequency of urination at night (i.e., the patient excretes greater than 500 mL per night).

oliguria: a significant decrease in the volume of urine excreted (less than 400 mL/d).

osmolality: an expression of concentration in terms of the total number of solute particles present per kilogram of solvent, denoted $Osm/kg\ H_2O$.

osmolar clearance: the volume of plasma water cleared by the kidneys each minute that contains the same amount of solutes that are present in the blood plasma (i.e., the same osmolality). Stated another way, osmolar clearance is the volume of plasma water necessary for the rate of solute elimination. Reported in milliliters per minute, it is determined by the equation $C = U \times V/P$, in which U and P are the urine and plasma osmolalities, respectively, and V is the volume of urine excreted in a timed collection, usually 24 hours.

polydipsia: intense and excessive thirst.

polyuria: the excretion of large volumes of urine (greater than 3 L/d).

renal blood flow (RBF): the volume of blood that passes through the renal vasculature per unit of time. The RBF normally ranges from 1000 to 1200 mL/min.

renal clearance: the volume of plasma cleared of a substance by the kidneys per unit of time. Reported in milliliters per minute, it is determined by the equation $C = U \times V/P$, in which U and P are the urine and plasma concentrations of the substance, respectively, and V is the volume of urine excreted in a timed collection, usually 24 hours. The most common renal clearance test is the creatinine clearance test.

renal plasma flow (RPF): the volume of plasma that passes through the renal vasculature per unit of time. The RPF normally ranges from 600 to 700 mL/min.

specific gravity: a measure of a solution's concentration based on its density. The solution's density is compared to the density of an equal volume of water at the same temperature. Specific gravity measurements are affected by both solute number and solute mass.

Urine Composition

The volume and solute composition of urine can vary greatly depending on an individual's diet, physical activity, and health. Because of these variables, normal (i.e., reference) urine values for each organic and inorganic component are difficult to establish. Urine is an ultrafiltrate of plasma with selected solutes reabsorbed, other solutes secreted, and the final water volume determined by the body's state of hydration; therefore, when an individual is healthy, the final urine contains essentially those solutes the body does not need, diluted in the volume of water the body does not need. Although the final urine is normally 94 percent water and 6 percent solutes, the kidney's ability to adjust its excretion of these components (as discussed in Chapter 4) makes it the principal organ involved in the regulation of body fluids.

Solute Elimination

Besides being able to selectively conserve electrolytes and water, renal excretion is also the primary mode for the elimination of soluble metabolic wastes (e.g., organic acids and bases) and exogenous substances (e.g., radiographic contrast media, drugs). Carbon dioxide and water, the normal by-products of carbohydrate and triglyceride metabolism, do not require renal excretion. In contrast, the metabolism of proteins and nucleic acids yields soluble substances, such as urea, creatinine, uric acid, and other inorganic solutes, which can be eliminated from the body only in urine. Of these substances excreted exclusively by the kidneys, urea and creatinine in particular provide a means of monitoring and evaluating renal function, specifically glomerular filtration. In addition, because of their characteristically high concentration in urine, these substances provide a means of positively distinguishing urine from other body fluids.

Table 5–1 compares the amounts and weights of the principal urine components. Note that the "amount" of a component in millimoles relates to the number of particles present, whereas the "weight" of the component relates to its mass. For example, the number of inorganic phosphate molecules present is less than that of potassium molecules; however, the weight of inorganic phosphate present is actually greater than that of potassium. The importance of making this distinction between the number of solute particles present and the weight of particles present relates directly to osmolality and

specific gravity measurements, respectively. Both osmolality and specific gravity measurements are used to assess the quantity of solutes present or the ability of the kidneys to concentrate urine.

Measurements of Solute Composition

Osmolality

Osmolality, denoted Osm/kg, is the concentration of a solution expressed in osmoles of solute particles per kilogram of solvent. An osmole is the amount of a substance that dissociates to produce 1 mole of particles (6.023×10^{23} particles, Avogadro's number) in a solution. A milliosmole (mOsm) is 1 millimole (mmol) of particles in a solution and is the term most frequently used when discussing body fluid solute compositions. For example, urea in solution does not dissociate; therefore, 1 mmol of urea (60 mg) equals 1 mOsm. In contrast, NaCl dissociates into two particles, Na^+ ions and Cl^- ions; therefore, 1 mmol of NaCl (58 mg) equals 2 mOsm. Consequently, the osmolality of a 1-mmol/L NaCl solution is greater (approximately two times greater because of essentially complete disso-

T A B L E 5 – 1.   COMPOSITION OF SELECTED COMPONENTS IN AN AVERAGE 24-HOUR URINE COLLECTION

COMPONENT	AVERAGE AMOUNT (mmol)	AVERAGE WEIGHT (mg)
Water (1.2 L*)	67,000.00	1,200,000.0
Urea	400.00	24,000.0
Chloride	185.00	6,570.0
Sodium	130.00	2,990.0
Potassium	70.00	2,730.0
NH_4	40.00	720.0
Inorganic PO_4	30.00	2,850.0
Inorganic SO_4	20.00	1,920.0
Creatinine	11.80	1.335.0
Uric acid	3.00	505.0
Glucose	0.72	130.0
Albumin	0.001	90.0

Data from First, 1984; Preuss, 1991; Vander, 1985; O'Connor, 1982; and Rock, 1987.
* The average 24-hour urine volume with a glomerular filtration rate of 125 mL/min.

ciation) than a 1 mmol/L urea solution. In urine, the solvent is water and the solute particles are those that pass the filtration barrier and are not reabsorbed, plus those additional solutes secreted by the tubules.

As previously discussed, the concentration and type of solutes in the filtrate change continuously throughout its passage through the nephron. In contrast, the osmolality remains unchanged (i.e., iso-osmotic) until the solute reaches the thin descending limb of the loop of Henle. The filtrate becomes progressively hyperosmotic in the descending limb and hypo-osmotic in the ascending limb of the loop of Henle owing to the countercurrent mechanism. As a result, the filtrate enters the distal tubule slightly hypo-osmotic but becomes iso-osmotic before entering the collecting tubule. It is in the collecting tubule that the osmolar concentration gradient of the surrounding hypertonic medullary interstitium and the reabsorption of water determine the final osmolality of the urine. Note that the maximum urine osmolality possible —1400 mOsm/kg—equals that of the medullary interstitium because the collecting tubule can passively reabsorb water only until osmotic equilibrium is attained.

The osmolality of a random urine specimen may be as low as 50 mOsm/kg or as high as 1400 mOsm/kg. Under normal circumstances, however, urine osmolality ranges from one to three times (275 to 900 mOsm/kg) that of serum (275 to 300 mOsm/kg). Often the urine-to-serum osmolality ratio (U/S) is used as an indicator of the renal tubules' ability to concentrate or dilute the urine. In normal individuals with an average fluid intake, the U/S ratio is between 1.0 and 3.0.

The kidneys actually change the urine osmolality by adjusting the volume of water the solutes are excreted in. With the typical American diet, an individual needs to eliminate 100 to 1200 mOsm of solutes each day. With diets high in salt and protein, however, the solute load can be substantially greater, requiring a larger volume of urine for excretion. Diseases that present an abnormally large number of solutes for renal excretion (e.g., glucose in diabetes mellitus) can pro-

duce as much as 5000 mOsm/d of solutes needing elimination. This magnitude of solutes requires significant amounts of water for elimination. Because the kidneys have no direct means of replacing excessive water loss, adequate fluid intake is mandatory. Hence, these individuals experience an intense thirst, known as **polydipsia,** in order to maintain water homeostasis and to excrete the solutes necessary.

Specific Gravity

Specific gravity relates the density of urine to the density of an equal volume of water. Because it is a ratio—comparing the weight of the solutes present in urine to pure water —the value for specific gravity will always be greater than 1.000. Normal specific gravity values for urine range from 1.002 to 1.035, reflecting the kidneys' dilution or concentration of the final urine. The specific gravity of the initial ultrafiltrate in Bowman's space is 1.010, the same as that of protein-free plasma. Normally, as the filtrate passes through the tubules and solute exchanges take place, the filtrate's specific gravity also changes. Therefore, when an individual is healthy, the final urine specific gravity—like osmolality—depends on the volume of water in which the solutes are eliminated, which is directly dependent on the individual's fluid intake and the body's state of hydration.

Because density is dependent on both the number of solute particles present and their relative mass, the relationship of specific gravity to osmolality is close but not linear (Fig. 5–1). This relationship is relatively constant in health; however, in certain conditions this relationship may be nonexistent owing to the excretion of high-molecular-weight substances such as glucose, urea, or proteins. Table 5–2 shows specific gravity values of water with NaCl, urea, and glucose added. Each solute addition represents essentially the same number of particles in the solution, approximately 5.2×10^{23} particles. Note that the specific gravity differs despite the presence of the same number of particles

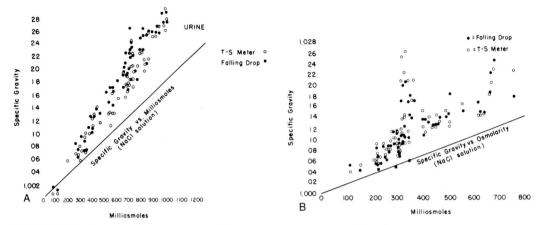

FIGURE 5–1. A comparison of urine specific gravity and urine osmolality. Specific gravity measurements were determined by both a direct (falling drop) and an indirect (refractometry) method. The straight lines represent the specific gravity and osmolality results obtained with solutions of varying sodium chloride concentrations. *A,* A comparison of urines obtained from healthy medical students; *B,* A comparison of urines obtained from patients on renal service. (From Holmes JH: Workshop on Urinalysis and Renal Function Studies, Chicago, American Society of Clinical Pathologists, 1962. Used with permission.)

—evidence of the effect that solute mass has on some specific gravity measurements. In addition, note that the specific gravity values also depend on the specific gravity method employed. The urinometer is a direct measure of density, whereas refractive index or reagent strip determinations are indirect measurements. Regardless of the measurement method employed, increases in large urinary solutes such as glucose, urea, or protein will increase the "true" specific gravity dramatically compared to an equivalent increase in small solutes such as sodium or chloride ions.

Occasionally, urine specimens may give an extremely high specific gravity value (i.e., greater than or equal to 1.050) that exceeds the specific gravity physiologically possible (1.040). With these specimens, excretion of a high-molecular-weight substance, such as ra-

diopaque contrast media (x-ray dye) or mannitol should be suspected. Both of these substances are exogenous and are infused into the patient. The substances are "contaminating" the urine specimen and are not indicative of a disease or a disease process. Although these urine specimens give physiologically impossible specific gravity values, their urine osmolalities are normal. Osmolality is affected only by the number of solutes present; even though the contaminating substances are high-molecular-weight solutes, their numbers are too few to affect the osmolality of urine when compared to the total number of the solutes present (e.g., sodium, urea). In other words, the mass of the solutes present is significant enough to affect the urine's specific gravity, but the number of solute particles present is too small to signif-

TABLE 5–2.   COMPARISON OF SPECIFIC GRAVITIES OF DIFFERENT SOLUTIONS

| | SOLUTE CHARACTERISTICS | | | SPECIFIC GRAVITY | |
Solution	Number of Solute Particles Added	Amount of Solute (mol/L)	Density	Refractive Index	Ionic (Reagent Strip)
Water	0.0	0.	1.000	1.000	1.000
Water and NaCl	5.2×10^{23}	0.43	1.017	1.012	1.005
Water and urea	5.2×10^{23}	0.86	1.012	1.020	1.000
Water and glucose	5.2×10^{23}	0.86	1.056	>1.050	1.000

icantly affect the urine's osmolality. In such cases, the urine specimens are considered contaminated and unacceptable for analysis; therefore, a new specimen should be collected at an appropriate time when the exogenous substance is no longer being excreted.

In summary, urine specific gravity measurements change with respect to both solute number and solute mass, whereas urine osmolality measurements change with respect only to solute number, regardless of the solute type. Both specific gravity and osmolality are physical properties of urine. The various methods available to perform these determinations are discussed at length in Chapter 6.

Urine Volume

. . . .

Normally for the kidneys to eliminate the average daily load of solutes (600 to 700 mOsm), they produce a minimum urine vol-

ume of approximately 500 mL per day. The kidneys achieve water homeostasis, however, by producing a volume of urine that exactly balances the volume of water intake and water from metabolic production. When the body is water-deprived or dehydrated, the kidneys excrete the solutes necessary in as small a urine volume possible, whereas when the body is excessively hydrated, the kidneys excrete the solutes in a large volume of urine (i.e., as much as 25 L/d may be produced).

Polyuria is the excretion of excessive amounts of urine (greater than 3 L/d). The causes of polyuria can be divided diagnostically into two types: 1) conditions that result in water diuresis (having a urine osmolality of less than 200 mOsm/kg); and 2) conditions that are due to solute diuresis (having a urine osmolality of approximately 300 mOsm/kg) (Walmsley, 1988). Figure 5–2 is a flowchart for the evaluation of polyuria. Conditions characterized by water diuresis

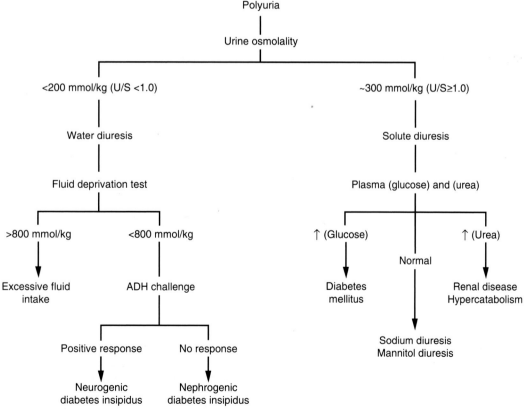

FIGURE 5–2. A flowchart for the evaluation of polyuria. (Redrawn from Walmsley RN, White GH: A Guide to Diagnostic Clinical Chemistry, Melbourne, Blackwell Scientific Publications, 1983.)

TABLE 5–3.   DIFFERENTIATION OF POLYURIA

I. Water diuresis (urine osmolality is less than 200 mOsm/kg)
   A. Decreased ADH secretion
      1. Excessive fluid intake (physiologic)
      2. Neurogenic diabetes insipidus
   B. Ineffective response by kidney to ADH— nephrogenic
      1. Congenital nephrogenic diabetes insipidus
      2. Acquired nephrogenic diabetes insipidus
         a. Renal diseases
         b. Drugs
II. Solute diuresis (urine osmolality is 300 ± 50 mOsm/kg)
   A. Sodium
      1. Increased intake
      2. Diuretic therapy
      3. Renal salt losing disorders
   B. Urea
      1. Hypercatabolic states
      2. Chronic renal failure
      3. Post-obstructive nephropathy
      4. Post-acute tubular necrosis
   C. Glucose
      1. Diabetes mellitus

Modified from Walmsley RN, White GH: A Guide to Diagnostic Clinical Chemistry, Melbourne, Blackwell Scientific Publications, 1988, pp. 160–161.

have a common link: antidiuretic hormone (ADH). With these disorders, either inadequate ADH is secreted or ADH's action on the renal receptors is ineffective. In contrast, conditions characterized by solute diuresis have no common feature. The solute involved also differs, being principally glucose, urea, or sodium (Table 5–3).

Diabetes mellitus and diabetes insipidus derive the name "diabetes" from the fact that both disorders produce copious amounts of urine. Despite being entirely different conditions, both diabetes mellitus and diabetes insipidus are characterized by an intense thirst (polydipsia) and the excretion of a large volume of urine (polyuria). Diabetes mellitus is a disorder of carbohydrate metabolism characterized by inadequate secretion or utilization of insulin, whereas diabetes insipidus is a disorder characterized by the decreased production or function of ADH.

In contrast, various conditions such as urinary obstruction, renal tubular dysfunction, or additional fluid loss can result in a decrease in the amount of urine produced. These conditions are often described by the term **oliguria,** defined as a total urine volume of less than approximately 400 mL/d. Note that this volume would not allow the elimination of the normal daily solute load; consequently, if oliguria is prolonged, death will ensue. In conditions in which no urine is excreted from the body, termed **anuria,** death is imminent unless intervention occurs. Anuria usually develops gradually, initially presenting as oliguria in progressive renal diseases. Anuria may occur suddenly, however, as a result of a dramatic decrease in renal perfusion (e.g., hemorrhage) or because of sudden extensive renal damage.

In conclusion, normal urine volume varies from approximately 500 to 1800 mL/d. This final urine volume reflects the daily solute load ingested, the fluid intake, and the activity of ADH as discussed in Chapter 4. With renal and metabolic diseases, however, the urine volume can decrease to zero output or increase as much as 15 times.

Assessment of Renal Concentrating Ability— Tubular Reabsorptive Function
. . . .
Osmolality vs. Specific Gravity

Both osmolality and specific gravity are measurements that express the solute composition of a fluid. With urine, these parameters change as the tubules actively adjust the volume of water the solutes are eliminated in. Therefore, an easy test to assess the renal capacity to conserve water (i.e., tubular reabsorptive function) is to demonstrate the tubules' ability to produce a concentrated urine specimen: a specimen whose osmolality exceeds 800 mOsm/kg or a specific gravity greater than 1.025.

Although specific gravity determinations are easier and require less time to perform, osmolality determinations are preferred when evaluating renal concentrating ability. Osmolality is considered to be more accurate because, as previously discussed, each solute particle present in the urine contributes equally to the final osmolality value. In contrast, the specific gravity is affected more by some solutes than by others because it is a density comparison. Recall from Table 5–1 that the three most prevalent urinary solutes excreted are urea, chloride, and sodium. Chloride and sodium are selectively reabsorbed, both actively and passively, at various segments throughout the nephrons. Therefore, monitoring the concentration of chloride and sodium in the urine reveals the kidneys' ability to concentrate the ultrafiltrate in the tubules. Urea, on the other hand, while present in large amounts, is passively reabsorbed and secreted throughout most of the nephron (i.e., urea cycle), and the magnitude of the exchange is variable. As a result, urea is not an accurate indicator of the kidneys' ability to concentrate the urine. Another reason that osmolality determinations are better than specific gravity determinations for assessing the concentrating ability of the kidneys is that specific gravity measurements are affected by small amounts of high-molecular-weight solutes (e.g., glucose, protein), whereas osmolality measurements are not. Glucose and protein are solutes that are actively and, essentially, completely reabsorbed in the proximal tubules; their presence in urine indicates disease process, not a change in the ability of the tubules to concentrate the urine (see Fig. 5–1). In contrast to specific gravity measurements, the osmolality of a urine that contains glucose and protein will remain relatively constant, because even though the "density" increases significantly owing to the relatively high molecular weight of these solutes, the actual increase in particle numbers is relatively small. Note that a change in specific gravity indicates a change in the density of the solutes present and that this change does not necessarily reflect a change in the renal concentrating ability. Therefore, in evaluating renal concentrating ability, osmolality is preferred over specific gravity because its value increases in direct proportion to the increase in the solute number, regardless of the solute type.

With some chronic renal diseases, the tubular concentrating ability slowly diminishes until the specific gravity and the osmolality of the excreted urine remain fixed. In other words, the tubules are unable to actively reabsorb and secrete selected solutes from the ultrafiltrate as it passes through the nephron. As a result, the solute concentration of the ultrafiltrate remains unchanged, and the osmolality and specific gravity of the final urine excreted will be the same as that of the initial ultrafiltrate in Bowman's space, namely a specific gravity of 1.010 and an osmolality of approximately 290 mOsm/kg (i.e., the same specific gravity and osmolality of protein free plasma). This "fixation" of the urine solute composition, a common feature of chronic renal diseases, causes an individual to experience polyuria. In addition, these patients also experience **nocturia**: excessive urination at night.

Nocturia, often a hallmark of renal disease, also occurs in those conditions that reduce the capacity of the bladder (e.g., pregnancy, bladder stones, prostate enlargement) or simply following excessive fluid intake at night.

Both specific gravity and osmolality are nonspecific tests used to assess the concentration of the urine. They can only indicate or confirm suspected decreased renal function. The underlying problem, whether it be diabetes insipidus, the effect of diuretic therapy, or renal disease, is not usually discernible using these tests.

Fluid Deprivation Tests

A fluid deprivation test is performed to assess renal concentrating ability or to investigate the cause of polyuria. The patient is allowed to eat a normal evening meal. From 1800 h (6:00 PM) until 0800 h (8:00 AM) the next day, the patient is allowed no water or fluid intake. Beginning at 0800 h, a urine specimen is collected and its osmolality is determined. If the osmolality exceeds 800 mOsm/kg, the patient is considered to have normal renal concentrating ability and the test is ended.

If the osmolality does not exceed 800 mOsm/kg, fluid deprivation continues until 1000 h (10:00 AM), at which time both a urine and a serum specimen are collected for osmolality determinations. If the urine osmolality exceeds 800 mOsm/kg or the ratio of urine osmolality to serum osmolality (U/S) exceeds 3.0, the patient is considered to have normal renal concentrating ability and the test is ended. If neither condition is met, however, ADH (vasopressin) is administered subcutaneously. Osmolality determinations on both urine and serum are repeated at 1400 h and 1800 h (20 hours and 24 hours, respectively, after the test's beginning). Regardless of the patient's response, the test is terminated at 1800 h or after 24 hours. A positive response to the ADH administration is a urine osmolality exceeding 800 mOsm/kg or a U/S ratio equal to or greater than 3.0. These results indicate that the patient's kidneys can respond to ADH but that inadequate ADH is being produced by the patient (i.e., a neurogenic problem). On the other hand, a negative response to ADH indicates that the patient's renal receptors for ADH are dysfunctional and the problem is nephrogenic (see Fig. 5–2).

Several tests use urine specific gravity measurements to evaluate renal concentrating ability. In the Fishberg concentration test, after the patient undergoes fluid deprivation regimens as previously described, a series of urine specimens are collected for specific gravity determinations. A specific gravity of 1.025 or greater indicates a normal renal concentrating ability. Mosenthal's test differs from those already discussed in that patients are allowed to maintain a normal diet and fluid intake. After this test, both the urine specific gravity and the urine volume are evaluated. Mosenthal's test requires the collection of a 24-hour urine specimen as well as the separation of the 12-hour day portion from the 12-hour night portion. A normal Mosenthal's test is indicated by a daytime urine volume that exceeds the nighttime urine volume, as well as a nighttime urine specific gravity equal to or greater than 1.020.

Osmolar and Free Water Clearance

Just as simultaneous determinations of the serum and urine osmolalities aid the clinician in the differential diagnoses of various diseases (e.g., neurogenic diabetes insipidus vs. nephrogenic diabetes insipidus), determinations of the amounts of water and solutes that are not reabsorbed by the kidney are of diagnostic value. These determinations are made by measuring the renal clearance of solutes and comparing it to the renal clearance of solute-free water. This determination requires a timed urine collection and a serum specimen. The U/S multiplied by the timed urine volume gives the **osmolar clearance,** designated C_{Osm}:

(5–1)

$$C_{Osm} \text{ (mL plasma/min)} = \frac{U_{Osm} \text{ (mOsm/kg)}}{S_{Osm} \text{ (mOsm/kg)}} \times V \text{ (mL/min)}$$

Normally, fasting osmolar clearance values vary from 2 to 3 mL/min and are not dependent on the urine flow (Koushanpour, 1986). The osmolar clearance is the volume of plasma water cleared by the kidneys each minute, containing the same amount of solutes as the blood plasma and therefore having the same osmolality. In other words, the osmolar clearance is the rate of solute elimination from plasma that, along with the volume of water necessary, makes a tubular lumen fluid that is iso-osmotic with the plasma. Any additional water in the tubular lumen fluid would exceed that necessary for solute removal and is considered solute-free water. Therefore, the total urine volume (V) actually consists of two separate volumes, the solute-free water (C_{H_2O}) and the osmolar clearance water (C_{Osm}):

(5–2)

$$V \text{ (mL/min)} = C_{Osm} \text{ (mL/min)} + C_{H_2O} \text{ (mL/min)}$$

Rearranging Equation 5–2, the **free water clearance** (C_{H_2O}) becomes:

(5–3)

$$C_{H_2O} \text{ (mL/min)} = V \text{ (mL/min)} - C_{Osm} \text{ (mL/min)}$$

From this rearrangement and Equation 5–1,

one can see that for the excreted urine to be iso-osmotic with the plasma ($U_{Osm} = S_{Osm}$), the total urine volume must equal the osmolar clearance volume ($V = C_{Osm}$). Consequently, the solute-free water clearance would be zero.

If the urine is dilute owing to excessive water ingestion or diuresis, the U_{Osm} would be smaller than the S_{Osm}. In addition, the total urine volume (V) would be larger than the osmolar clearance water (C_{Osm}), and the solute-free water clearance (C_{H_2O}) would be a positive number. A positive free water clearance value indicates that water is not reabsorbed and that the urine is hypo-osmotic or hypotonic. In contrast, when the U_{Osm} is greater than the S_{Osm}, such as when the body is dehydrated, the total urine volume (V) would be less than the osmolar clearance water (C_{Osm}), and the solute-free water clearance (C_{H_2O}) would be a negative number. This negative free water clearance value indicates that additional water is reabsorbed and that the urine is hyperosmotic or hypertonic.

Keep in mind, however, that the urine osmolality is due principally to urea, whereas the serum osmolality is due primarily to sodium and chloride. Therefore, the applicability of the osmolar and free water clearance is limited to indicating the urine solute concentration and volume; it is of no value in determining the cause of polyuria or diuresis (O'Connor, 1982).

In summary, to maintain overall body fluid homeostasis, the kidneys manipulate the amount of water excreted to eliminate unwanted solutes. Any additional water can be eliminated or reabsorbed. The kidneys' ultimate goal—to maintain a normal plasma osmolality—is achieved by selectively eliminating or reabsorbing solutes and water.

Assessment of Glomerular Filtration

Renal Clearance

In order for the kidneys to remove metabolic wastes and selectively reabsorb solutes and water, they require an adequate renal plasma flow (RPF) through the glomerulus. It is this RPF that determines the amount of plasma ultrafiltrate formed in Bowman's space and, therefore, the amount of plasma processed by the kidneys. The volume of renal plasma actually filtered at the glomerulus directly affects the final urine volume and composition. The portion of the plasma that is not filtered flows into the peritubular capillaries, where the tubules actively and selectively remove limited plasma solutes for excretion. A large amount of a particular solute excreted in the urine indicates that a volume of plasma that contained that same quantity of the solute must have been processed. This is often referred to as the "clearance" of the solute or substance. Stated another way, the renal clearance is the volume of plasma in milliliters completely cleared of a substance per unit of time.

Because renal disease can be a slow process, with a significant loss of renal tissue before detection of the disease by other methods (e.g., routine urinalysis, blood chemistry results), renal clearance tests provide a means of evaluating a patient's renal status. By measuring the amount of a substance in the plasma and in a timed urine specimen, one can determine the ability of the kidney to remove this substance from the blood. It is called a **renal clearance** (C) and is determined as follows:

(5–4)

$$C_{(mL/min)} = \frac{U_{(mg/dL)} \times V_{(mL/min)}}{P_{(mg/dL)}}$$

U and P are the urine and plasma (or serum) concentrations of the substance (measured in milligrams per deciliter); V is the volume of urine excreted in a timed collection (measured in milliliters per minute), and C is the renal clearance of that substance (measured in mL/min). Note that the units for the urine and plasma concentrations must be the same. It does not matter if the units are in milligrams per deciliter or millimoles per liter (SI units), as long as they cancel each other out in the renal clearance calculation. A 24-hour timed collection is preferred for most substances, and it is mandatory for those analytes or functions that demonstrate a diurnal variation.

Inulin Clearance

A clearance test does not tell whether a substance has been filtered, secreted, or reabsorbed, or has undergone a combination of these processes. Evaluating these specific renal functions requires substances whose mode of excretion is known and strictly limited. For example, some substances are known to be removed by the glomerulus only and are not secreted (e.g., inulin), whereas others are exclusively removed by renal tubular secretion (e.g., *p*-aminohippurate, or PAH; phenolsulfonphthalien, or PSP). Hence, evaluating glomerular filtration, tubular reabsorption, and tubular secretion, as well as renal blood flow, is possible.

Hypothetically, any substance that 1) maintains a steady plasma level; 2) is solely excreted by glomerular filtration; and 3) is not reabsorbed or secreted by the tubules could be used to determine the **glomerular filtration rate (GFR).**

The best assessment of glomerular filtration uses inulin, an *exogenous* nontoxic fructo-polysaccharide (MW 5200). Inulin is neither created nor destroyed by the body; it readily passes the glomerular filtration barrier and is not reabsorbed or secreted by the renal tubules. Thus, it is considered the reference method for the determination of GFR.

For routine clinical use, however, performing an inulin clearance test has several drawbacks. First, special patient preparations must be made because inulin must be infused throughout the duration of the test to maintain a constant plasma level. Second, the current methods available for the analysis of inulin in urine and plasma are difficult and time consuming. Third, in patients suspected of having renal disease, the GFR is assessed frequently to aid in its diagnosis and treatment. Consequently, the inulin clearance test is not practical for routine GFR measurement.

Creatinine Clearance

In order to eliminate the problems posed by inulin, an *endogenous* substance whose renal clearance approximates that of inulin has been sought. Both urea and creatinine, because of their large urinary concentrations and ease of measurement, were considered. Urea, however, is reabsorbed by the tubules, and its concentration is directly affected by the urine flow rate. In addition, plasma urea levels are affected by diet. As a result, urea clearances are rarely performed (Koushanpour, 1986). On the other hand, creatinine is not reabsorbed by the renal tubules or affected by the urine flow rate, nor are plasma levels altered by a normal diet. As a result, the **creatinine clearance** is the most commonly used clearance test for the routine assessment of the GFR.

Since 1938 it has been known that the creatinine clearance closely approximates that of inulin (Miller, 1938). Creatinine is a by-product of muscle metabolism formed from creatine and phosphocreatine (Fig. 5–3). It is produced at a steady rate, resulting in a constant plasma concentration, as well as a constant urinary excretion rate. Because creatinine production is directly dependent on individual muscle mass, production varies with the patient's sex, physical activity, and age: male patients and muscular athletes (both male and female) produce more creatinine than do nonathletic female patients, children, or elderly patients. Because of this dependence on individual muscle mass, creatinine clearance values are normalized to the external body surface area (SA) of an "average" individual: 1.73 m². In the calculation for the normalized clearance, Equation 5–5, the factor 1.73 m²/SA denotes the body surface area of the "average" individual divided by the calculated body surface area of the patient.

(5–5)

$$C\ (\text{mL/min}) = \frac{U \times V}{P} \times \frac{1.73\ \text{m}^2}{\text{SA}}$$

The body surface area of an individual is easily determined using the patient's height and weight and a nomogram (Appendix A).

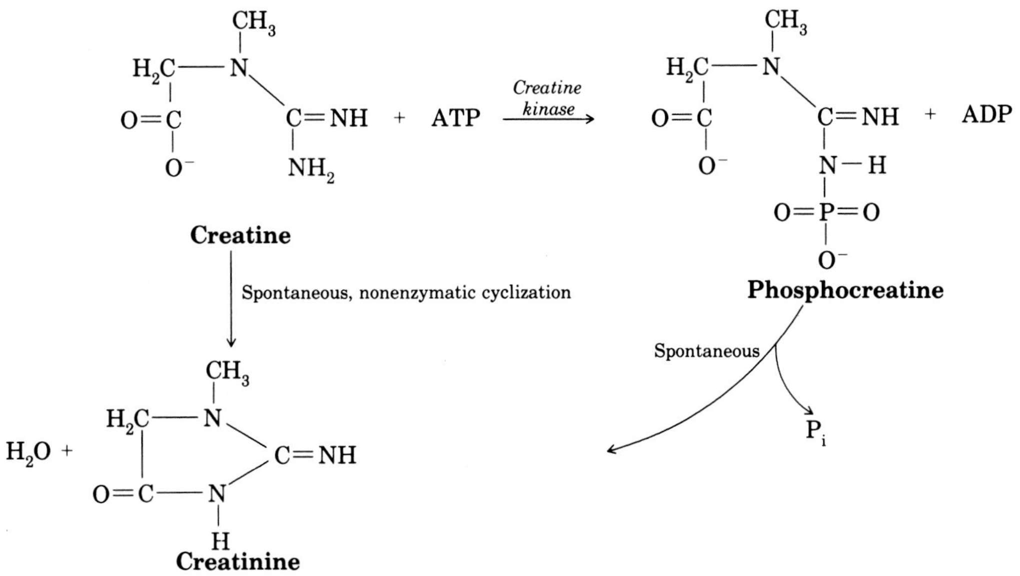

FIGURE 5–3. The formation of creatinine from creatine and phosphocreatine.

Normalization allows the comparison of the clearance results or the GFR with those of other individuals, regardless of the patient's body surface area. Creatinine clearance data for individuals according to age and sex are listed in Table 5–4.

Advantages and Disadvantages

The measurement of creatinine in urine and plasma is rapidly and easily performed; in addition, the precision and reliability of each measurement method are known and well documented. Despite its advantages, the creatinine clearance has several shortcomings that need to be addressed in order to ensure the correct interpretation of results. In reality, a small amount of creatinine is secreted by the renal tubules (approximately 7 percent to 10 percent) (Rock, 1984). This secretion results in an elevated urine excretion concentration (U in Equation 5–4), which would result in an overestimation of the GFR. This increase is offset, however, when the popular, nonspecific alkaline picrate method (Jaffé's reaction) is used for creatinine measurement. Owing to the reaction of plasma noncreatinine chromogens by this method, the plasma creatinine result (P in

equation 5–4) is also overestimated. Fortunately, these two factors offset each other, and the creatinine clearance correlates well with the inulin clearance. When more specific creatinine methods (e.g., enzymatic) are used, these factors do not offset each other.

TABLE 5–4. VARIATION IN REFERENCE INTERVALS FOR SERUM CREATININE AND CREATININE CLEARANCE ACCORDING TO AGE AND SEX

	AGE (yrs)	SERUM CREATININE (mg/L)	CREATININE CLEARANCE (mL/min/ 1.73 m²)
Males	10	5–8	60–130
	20	8–13	80–135
	40	9–14	75–130
	60	10–14.5	45–100
	80	7–14	30–80
Females	10	5–8	60–130
	20	7–11	70–120
	40	8–12	60–110
	60	8–12.5	45–95
	80	8–13	30–80

The factor 1.73 m² normalizes clearance for average body surface area.

From Lente FV: "Creatinine" in analytes. Clin Chem News 16(10):8, 1990.

In these latter instances, the measured plasma creatinine is not overestimated but the urine creatinine is because of the tubular secretion. As a result, the creatinine clearance (C in Equation 5–4) is overestimated, and these clearances do not compare as well with the inulin clearance.

Patients with diminished renal function (i.e., their plasma creatinine concentration is increased) may also be difficult to evaluate using the creatinine clearance. In these patients, the renal tubular secretion of creatinine (a T_m-limited process) is increased because of the elevated plasma concentration; this results in an increased concentration in the urine (U in Equation 5–4), and again an erroneous GFR is obtained. Other factors known to interfere with the renal secretion of creatinine are exogenous agents such as salicylate, trimethoprim, and cimetadine. These drugs inhibit the tubular secretion of creatinine, thereby lowering the urine creatinine concentration and causing a falsely low creatinine clearance or GFR.

Thus, several factors can affect the tubular secretion of creatinine. In addition, the methodology employed for creatinine quantitation will directly affect the creatinine clearance results. Despite these shortcomings, however, an estimation of the GFR by the creatinine clearance provides the clinician with valuable information. Because creatinine methodologies have been extensively researched and have proven reliability, the performance of creatinine clearances at regular intervals provides valuable diagnostic and prognostic information about a patient's ongoing renal status.

Importance of Time Interval

In order to perform a creatinine clearance test, a timed urine specimen must be obtained. The time interval over which the urine collection takes place must be provided with the specimen. Because of the diurnal variation in the GFR, a 24-hour urine collection is considered the specimen of choice for creatinine clearance determinations. The plasma specimen for the clearance determination may be sampled anytime during the 24-hour period. Shorter collection intervals (e.g., 12-hour or 2-hour intervals) may be used, especially with patients requiring repeated GFR determinations to monitor their renal status. In these cases, the patient must be kept well-hydrated throughout the test; the urine collection should be performed at the same time of day for comparison purposes; and the plasma sample is usually collected midway through the collection. Because creatinine clearance results can vary as much as 15 percent to 20 percent within a single individual, 24-hour collections are preferred (Rock, 1987). Collections taken over a shorter time interval can increase this variability even more. See Chapter 3 for more detailed information regarding the collection of timed urine specimens.

The importance of the urine collection and its timing cannot be overemphasized. Using the time interval and the total volume of urine collected, the amount of urine excreted (V) in milliliters per minute is calculated for insertion into the clearance equation. From this equation, one can see that both the volume of urine (V) and its creatinine concentration (U) directly affect the magnitude of the clearance results.

It is important to look at some factors that can affect these parameters. Improper storage of the urine specimen with subsequent bacterial proliferation can result in creatinine breakdown to creatine (owing to pH changes) or creatinine's degradation by bacterial creatinases. Either case leads to a falsely decreased urine creatinine value (U). On the other hand, if the urine volume (V) used for the clearance determination is in error, the clearance results are also invalid. Practically speaking, it is impossible for the laboratorian to evaluate the acceptability of information (urine volume and collection interval) submitted with a specimen for a creatinine clearance. However, evaluating the individual plasma and urine creatinine results and determining what they indicate about renal status and the clearance equation can alert the laboratorian to inconsistencies in the information provided. The following example highlights the importance of 1) evaluating the individual plasma and urine

CREATININE CLEARANCE

EXAMPLE:

The laboratory receives a 24-h urine specimen from a 26-year-old male (6′4″ or SA = 2.34 m²; 230 lb.), and the specimen volume measures 800 mL. After the creatinine determinations were performed by the alkaline picrate method, the clearance results were calculated:

Plasma creatinine (P) 1.2 mg/dL
Urine creatinine (U)   150 mg/dL
Urine volume (V)   800 mL

$$C = \frac{U \times V}{P}$$

$$= \frac{(150\ \text{mg/dL}) \times (800\ \text{mL/24 h} \times 1\ \text{h/60 min})}{1.2\ \text{mg/dL}}$$

C = 69 mL/min (abnormally low clearance result despite a normal plasma level)

$$C_{corrected} = 69\ \text{mL/min} \times \frac{1.73\ \text{m}^2}{2.34\ \text{m}^2}$$

$$C_{corrected} = 51\ \text{mL/min}$$

DISCUSSION:

From these data, the normalized creatinine clearance is extremely low compared to a reference range of 80 to 125 mL/min/1.73 m² (Preuss, 1991). Note that even correction for the patient's height and weight does not bring the GFR closer to "normal." This abnormally low GFR is unusual because the patient's plasma creatinine is normal (reference range: 0.8 to 1.3 mg/dL). All specimen identifications were checked, and the creatinine determinations were repeated, with the same results. The plasma creatinine value agreed with previous determinations.

The best explanation points to a problem with the urine collection. Most likely, 1) some urine was lost or discarded during the 24-hour collection; 2) the time interval for the collection is incorrect; or 3) the specimen was improperly preserved and the creatinine has degraded.

creatinine results used in the clearance equation and 2) being aware of the potential problems that may occur during specimen collection, information recording, etc.

In summary, the determination of the GFR by the creatinine clearance provides a convenient diagnostic tool for the evaluation of a patient's renal status. Despite its disadvantages, the creatinine clearance test remains the method of choice for routine clinical assessment and the monitoring of glomerular filtration. Pathologic conditions that cause alterations in the glomerular filtration barrier will be reflected in the GFR. Similarly, changes in the renal blood flow to the glomerulus are reflected in the GFR; for example, if a decreased amount of blood plasma is presented to the glomerulus for processing, the GFR will decrease. Note that the GFR itself is never adjusted by the kidney. Instead, the blood flow to the glomerulus is adjusted by the afferent and efferent arterioles in response to changes in renal hemodynamics. Maintaining a constant blood flow maintains a constant GFR. This close relationship between the GFR and renal

blood flow allows the use of the easily obtainable measurement, the creatinine clearance, to be used routinely to monitor renal function.

Assessment of Renal Blood Flow and Tubular Secretory Function

Determination of Renal Plasma Flow and Renal Blood Flow

Normal renal function depends on adequate **renal blood flow (RBF).** If the blood flow to the kidney should change for any reason, a change in renal function occurs. Not only is glomerular filtration affected, but so is the tubules' ability to reabsorb and secrete. The glomerulus produces an ultrafiltrate from only the plasma portion of the circulating blood. The portion of the blood plasma that is not filtered enters the peritubular capillaries and is processed by the tubules. Not all the blood that flows into the kidney is processed, however; approximately 8 percent of the RBF never comes into contact with functional renal tissue (Duston, 1955). Note that renal plasma flow (RPF) is different from renal blood flow (RBF). They are related to each other, however, as described in Equation 5–6, in which Hct denotes the hematocrit (Koushanpour, 1986).

(5–6)

$$RBF = \frac{RPF}{1 - Hct}$$

The ideal clearance substance to measure RPF and subsequently RBF must 1) reside exclusively in the plasma portion of the blood; 2) be primarily removed from the plasma by renal tubular secretion rather than by glomerular filtration; and 3) be completely removed from the plasma in its first pass through the kidney, resulting in essentially zero concentration in the venous renal blood. By fulfilling these criteria, the measurement of RPF throughout the entire nephron may be accomplished. Because the substance is completely removed from the plasma after passage through the glomerulus and the peritubular capillaries, the actual plasma flow in milliliters per minute can be determined using the traditional clearance equation (Equation 5–4). Therefore, the renal tubules' secretory function must be normal in order to provide valid RPF results, and, conversely, the RPF must be normal to evaluate the tubular secretory function.

Clearance tests using p-aminohippurate (PAH) and phenolsulfonphthalein (PSP) are used to assess renal tubular secretory function. Both substances are actively secreted by the renal tubules; however, PSP is not completely removed as it passes through the kidney and is unsatisfactory for the assessment of the RPF. Although the RPF can be determined using the PAH clearance test, other techniques employing radioactive substances (e.g., ^{131}I orthoiodohippuran) have also been used. Regardless of the method employed to measure tubular secretory function or renal plasma flow, the substances used are exogenous, requiring infusion into the patient, and therefore these techniques are not routinely performed.

The PAH Clearance Test

The most common test used to measure **renal plasma flow (RPF)** is the PAH clearance test. PAH is an exogenous, nontoxic, weak organic acid that is almost exclusively secreted by the proximal tubules (a very small amount is filtered through the glomerulus). At certain plasma levels, PAH is secreted completely during its first pass through the kidneys. Hence, the PAH clearance test provides not only an excellent indicator of renal tubular secretory function, but also a means of determining the RPF and the RBF when normal secretory function is known. Although the PAH clearance test is the reference method for the measurement of the RPF, the current methods for the analysis of PAH in urine and plasma are difficult and time consuming. Because PAH is an exogenous substance, it must be infused—another drawback to its routine clinical use.

A normal RPF as determined by the PAH clearance test ranges from 600 to 700 mL/min. Assuming an average normal hematocrit of 0.42 (42 percent) and using Equation 5–6, normal values for the RBF range from approximately 1000 to 1200 mL/min. Using this information and a normal resting cardiac output of approximately 6 L/min, it can be calculated that the kidneys receive approximately 16 percent to 20 percent of the total cardiac output. This measurement does not account for the 8 percent of the RBF that never contacts functioning renal tissue. Adding in the 8 percent, the kidneys receive approximately 25 percent of the total cardiac output.

Assessment of Tubular Secretory Function for Acid Removal

As described in Chapter 4, the renal tubules actively secrete acids in response to changes in the body's acid-base equilibrium. The metabolism of proteins and phospholipids results in the formation of sulfuric and phosphoric acids. These acids are rapidly neutralized by bicarbonate into CO_2 and the neutral salts Na_2SO_4 and Na_2HPO_4. The CO_2 is excreted by the lungs, whereas the neutral salts are passed into the ultrafiltrate at the kidneys. As the renal tubules secrete ammonia and hydrogen ions, the neutral salts are further modified into ammonium salt (e.g., $(NH_4)_2SO_4$) or titratable acid (i.e., NaH_2PO_4) for excretion. Hence, the evaluation of the renal tubular ability to produce an acid urine involves the measurement of the ammonium salts and the titratable acids excreted. Normally 50 to 100 mmol of acid is excreted each day (Lennon, 1966).

Measurement of Titratable Acid vs. Urinary Ammonia

In urine, the amount of acid (H^+) combined with ammonia is normally twice that excreted as titratable acid. Titratable acid formation is limited by the concentration of phosphate ions in the ultrafiltrate. Because the plasma concentration of phosphate ions is normally small, the ultrafiltrate concentration is also small. On the other hand, ammonia is produced and secreted by the renal tubules in direct response to the need to eliminate acid from the body. Ammonia production is not limited, and healthy renal tubules will increase production to remove additional amounts of metabolic acids. For example, in patients experiencing diabetic ketoacidosis, the ammonium salt excretion can reach as much as 400 mmol/day, whereas their titratable acid excretion increases only to 100 to 200 mmol/day. In contrast, diseased tubules lose this ability to produce and secrete ammonia, as well as the ability to secrete hydrogen ions. In these cases, the amount of total acids excreted each day may decrease to only 3 to 35 mmol/day. At the same time, the amount of ammonium salts excreted compared to titratable acids may also decrease to the point where more acid is excreted as free titratable acid than that combined with ammonia.

Because the kidneys play a crucial role in maintaining a normal acid-base balance, systemic acidosis will occur if the tubular secretory function for acid removal is compromised. In fact, renal failure is usually associated with acidosis. In this regard, the measurement of the total hydrogen ion excretion in urine (titratable acid and ammonium salts) yields valuable information regarding the tubular secretory function.

Oral Ammonium Chloride Test

This test involves the oral administration of ammonium chloride, which metabolizes to urea and HCl. To adjust for this increased acid, the kidneys excrete increased amounts of titratable acid and ammonium salts, with the urine becoming more acid. Plasma bicarbonate measurements are made before and midway through the test to monitor the depletion of the bicarbonate pool. If the initial plasma bicarbonate is low (less than 20 mmol/L), the test should not be performed. An initial morning 2-hour urine specimen is collected prior to the test. If its pH is below 5.3, acid excretion is normal and the test need not be performed. During the test, urine is collected every 2 hours for 8 to 10 hours. Each 2-hour collection is measured for pH, titratable acid, and ammonium excretion.

Normal individuals are able to reduce the urine pH below 5.3, with a total hydrogen ion excretion (titratable acid plus ammonium salts) greater than 60 mmol/min. The titratable acid and the ammonium salt excretion should exceed 25 mmol per minute. At the same time, the plasma bicarbonate level should fall below 26 mmol/L. Failure to excrete an acid urine following this challenge test supports a diagnosis of renal tubular acidosis (RTA). RTA is a condition characterized by defective tubular hydrogen ion secretion, defective tubular ammonia production, or defective bicarbonate reabsorption in the proximal tubules. Regardless of the specific defect involved, patients with RTA excrete alkaline urine despite a systemic acidosis.

The measurement of titratable acids is performed by titrating a well-mixed aliquot of urine with 0.1 N NaOH to an endpoint pH of 7.4 using a pH meter. This endpoint corresponds to a blood pH of 7.4 and a urine pH of 4.4 (First, 1984). Subsequently, the ammonium concentration is calculated as the difference between the urine's total acidity and the acids present as titratable acids.

In conclusion, although measurements of localized functions of the nephron are possible, they are not routinely performed in a clinical setting. Instead, the most common and practical urine tests used to routinely evaluate renal function are the creatinine clearance test for assessment of the GFR; a urine osmolality determination for tubular concentrating ability; and a urinary protein electrophoresis to evaluate glomerular permeability to plasma proteins. In addition to these urine tests, the plasma creatinine—owing to its constancy of production and renal excretion—is a good indicator of compromised or changing renal function.

References

Duston H, Corcoran A: Functional interpretation of renal tests. Med Clin North Am *39:*947–956, 1955.

First MR: Renal function. *In* Kaplan LA, Pesce AJ (eds.): Clinical Chemistry: Theory, Analysis, and Correlation (2nd ed.), St. Louis, C. V. Mosby Company, 1989, pp. 349–351.

Koushanpour E, Kriz W: Renal Physiology (2nd ed.), New York, Springer-Verlag, 1986, p. 300.

Lennon EJ, Lemann J, Litzow JR: The effect of diet and stool composition on the net external acid balance of normal subjects. J Clin Invest *45:*1601–1607, 1966.

Miller BF, Winkler AW: The renal excretion of endogenous creatinine in man. Comparison with exogenous creatinine and inulin. J Clin Invest *17:*31–40, 1938.

O'Connor WJ: Normal Renal Function, New York, Oxford University Press, 1982, p. 212.

Preuss HG, Podlasek SJ, Henry JB: Evaluation of renal function and water, electrolyte, and acid-base balance. *In* Henry JB (ed.): Clinical Diagnosis and Management by Laboratory Methods (18th ed.), Philadelphia, W. B. Saunders Company, 1991, pp. 128–132, 1373–1375.

Rock RC, Walker WG, Jennings CD: Nitrogen metabolites and renal function. *In* Tietz NW (ed.): Fundamentals of Clinical Chemistry (3rd ed.), Philadelphia, W. B. Saunders Company, 1987, pp. 679–684, 944–968.

Vander AJ, Sherman JH, Luciano DS: Human Physiology (4th ed.), New York, McGraw-Hill Book Company, 1985, pp. 421–458.

Walmsley RN, White GH: A Guide to Diagnostic Clinical Chemistry (2nd ed.), Melbourne, Blackwell Scientific Publications, 1988, pp. 160–161.

Study Questions

1. **Which of the following solutes are present in the largest molar amounts in urine?**

   A. Urea, chloride, and sodium
   B. Urea, creatinine, and sodium
   C. Creatinine, uric acid, and ammonium
   D. Urea, uric acid, and ammonium

2. **Renal excretion is NOT involved in the elimination of**

   A. electrolytes and water.
   B. normal by-products of fat metabolism.
   C. soluble metabolic wastes (e.g., urea, creatinine).
   D. exogenous substances (e.g., drugs, x-ray contrast media).

3. **The concentration of which substances provides the best means of distinguishing urine from other body fluids?**

   A. Creatinine and urea
   B. Glucose and protein
   C. Uric acid and ammonia
   D. Water and electrolytes

4. **What is the definition of the "osmolality" of a solution?**

   A. The density of solute particles per liter of solvent
   B. The mass of solute particles per kilogram of solvent
   C. The number of solute particles per kilogram of solvent
   D. The weight of solute particles per liter of solvent

5. **The osmolality of a solution containing 1.0 mole of urea is equal to a solution containing**

   A. 1.0 mole of HCl.
   B. 1.0 mole of H_2PO_4.
   C. 0.5 mole of NaCl.
   D. 0.5 mole of glucose.

6. **The maximum osmolality that urine can achieve is determined by the**

   A. amount of solutes ingested in the diet.
   B. presence of ADH in the collecting tubules.
   C. osmolality of the medullary interstitium.
   D. osmolality of the fluid entering the collecting tubules.

7. **Serum osmolality remains relatively constant, whereas the urine osmolality ranges from**

   A. one-third to one-half that of serum.
   B. one-third to equal that of serum.
   C. one to three times that of serum.
   D. three to five times that of serum.

8. **Another name for excessive thirst is**

   A. polydipsia.
   B. polyuria.
   C. hydrophilia.
   D. hydrostasis.

9. **Specific gravity measurements are NOT affected by**

   A. temperature.
   B. solute charge.
   C. solute mass.
   D. solute number.

10. **Osmolality is a measure of solute**

   A. density.
   B. mass.
   C. number.
   D. weight.

11. **Which of the following solutes, if added to pure water, will affect the specific gravity more than it will affect its osmolality?**

   A. Sodium
   B. Chloride
   C. Potassium
   D. Glucose

12. **Occasionally the specific gravity of a urine specimen exceeds that physiologically possible (i.e., greater than 1.040). Which of the following substances when found in urine could account for such a high value?**

   A. Creatinine   C. Mannitol
   B. Glucose   D. Protein

13. **The excretion of large volumes of urine (greater than 3 L/d) is called**

    A. glucosuria.
    B. hyperuria.
    C. polydipsia.
    D. polyuria.

14. **The daily volume of urine excreted normally ranges from**

    A. 100 to 500 mL/d.
    B. 100 to 1800 mL/d.
    C. 500 to 1800 mL/d.
    D. 1000 to 3000 mL/d.

15. **When the body is dehydrated, the kidneys**

    A. excrete excess solutes in a constant volume of urine.
    B. excrete solutes in as small a volume of urine as possible.
    C. decrease the amount of solutes excreted and decrease the urine volume.
    D. increase the amount of solutes excreted while holding the urine volume constant.

16. **The excretion of less than 400 mL of urine per day is called**

    A. anuria.
    B. hypouria.
    C. nocturia.
    D. oliguria.

17. **The ultrafiltrate in the urinary space of the glomerulus has a**

    A. specific gravity of 1.005 and a lower osmolality than the blood plasma.
    B. specific gravity of 1.010 and the same osmolality as the blood plasma.
    C. specific gravity of 1.015 and a higher osmolality than the blood plasma.
    D. specific gravity of 1.035 and a higher osmolality than the blood plasma.

18. **All of the following conditions may produce nocturia EXCEPT**

    A. anuria.
    B. pregnancy.
    C. chronic renal disease.
    D. fluid intake at night.

19. **Which renal function is assessed using specific gravity and osmolality measurements?**

    A. Concentrating ability
    B. Glomerular filtration ability
    C. Tubular excretion ability
    D. Tubular secretion ability

20. **A fluid deprivation test is used to**

    A. determine renal plasma flow.
    B. investigate the cause of oliguria.
    C. assess renal concentrating ability.
    D. measure the glomerular filtration rate.

21. **A fluid deprivation test involves the measurement of serum and urine**

    A. density.
    B. osmolality.
    C. specific gravity.
    D. volume.

22. **The volume of plasma cleared per minute in excess of that required for solute elimination is called the**

    A. creatinine clearance.
    B. free water clearance.
    C. osmolar clearance.
    D. renal clearance.

23. **A free water clearance value of −1.2 would be expected from a patient experiencing**

    A. polyuria.
    B. dehydration.
    C. water diuresis.
    D. excessive fluid intake.

24. **Calculate the osmolar and free water clearances using the following patient data.**
    Serum osmolality = 305 mOsm/kg
    Urine osmolality = 250 mOsm/kg
    Urine volume = 300 mL/2 h

    A. Is this individual excreting more water than is necessary for solute removal? Yes/No
    B. Is the osmolar clearance "normal" (i.e., 2.0 to 3.0 mL/min)? Yes/No
    C. From the free water clearance result obtained, is the urine hypo-osmotic or hyperosmotic?

25. **Which of the following is an endogenous substance used to measure glomerular filtration rate?**

    A. Urea
    B. Inulin
    C. Creatinine
    D. Para-aminohippurate (*p*-aminohippurate)

26. **Renal clearance is defined as the**

    A. volume of urine cleared of a substance per minute.
    B. volume of plasma cleared of a substance in a time interval.
    C. volume of plasma flowing through the kidney per minute.
    D. volume of plasma containing the same amount of substance in 1 mL of urine.

27. **Creatinine is a good substance to use for a renal clearance test because it**

    A. is exogenous.
    B. is reabsorbed.
    C. is affected by fluid intake.
    D. has a constant plasma concentration.

28. **Which of the following groups would be expected to have the greatest 24-hour excretion of creatinine?**

    A. Infants
    B. Children
    C. Women
    D. Men

29. **Creatinine clearance results are "normalized" using an individual's body surface area to account for variations in the individual's**

    A. age.
    B. sex.
    C. dietary intake.
    D. muscle mass.

30. **The following data are obtained from a 60-year-old female who is 4′8″ tall and weighs 88 lbs.**
    Plasma creatinine = 1.2 mg/dL
    Urine creatinine = 500 mg/L
    Urine volume = 1440 mL/24 h

    A. Calculate the creatinine clearance.
    B. Calculate the normalized creatinine clearance. (Use Appendix A to determine the body's surface area.)
    C. Are these results normal for this patient? (Use reference intervals provided in Table 5–4.)

31. **A 24-hour urine collection is preferred for the determination of creatinine clearance because of the diurnal variation in the**

    A. glomerular filtration rate.
    B. plasma creatinine.
    C. creatinine excretion.
    D. urine excretion.

32. **Which of the following most often results in an erroneous creatinine clearance measurement?**

    A. A 24-hour urine collection from an individual on a vegetarian diet.
    B. A 24-hour urine collection maintained at room temperature throughout the collection.
    C. A plasma sample drawn at the beginning instead of during the 24-hour urine collection.
    D. Creatinine determinations made using the nonspecific alkaline picrate method (Jaffé's reaction).

33. **The glomerular filtration rate is controlled by**

    A. the renal blood flow.
    B. the renal plasma flow.
    C. the countercurrent mechanism.
    D. hormones (e.g., aldosterone and ADH).

34. **For the measurement of renal plasma flow, *p*-aminohippurate (PAH) is an ideal substance to use because it**

    A. is easily measured in urine and plasma.
    B. is endogenous and does not require an infusion.
    C. is completely secreted in its first pass through the kidneys.
    D. maintains a constant plasma concentration throughout the test.

35. **What percentage of the total cardiac output is received by the kidneys?**

    A. 8%
    B. 15%
    C. 25%
    D. 33%

36. **Measuring the amount of hydrogen ion excreted as titratable acids and ammonium salts in urine provides a measure of**

    A. tubular secretory function.
    B. tubular reabsorptive function.
    C. glomerular filtration ability.
    D. renal concentrating ability.

37. **The oral ammonium chloride test evaluates the ability of the tubules to secrete**

    A. ammonium and chloride.
    B. phosphate and sodium.
    C. bicarbonate and chloride.
    D. ammonia and hydrogen.

6

Physical Examination
of Urine

LEARNING OBJECTIVES

After studying this chapter, the student should be able to

1. State the importance of using established terminology for describing urine color and clarity.

2. Discuss the origin of the following pigments and their affect on urine color:
   • bilirubin
   • urobilin
   • urochrome
   • uroerythrin

3. List appropriate color terms and the substances that can produce the colors, and identify those substances that indicate a pathologic process.

4. List appropriate clarity terms, their definitions, and the substances that can cause clarity changes, and identify those substances that indicate a pathologic process.

5. Describe the effect that increased amounts of protein and bilirubin can have on urine foam.

6. Discuss the cause of normal urine odor, identify conditions that will change this urine characteristic, and list any odors associated with each condition.

7. Identify two variables involved in determining urine concentration.

8. Compare and contrast the specific gravity and osmolality determinations for the measurement of urine concentration.

9. State the principle of each of the following specific gravity determination methods:
   • the falling drop method
   • harmonic oscillation densitometry
   • the reagent strip method
   • refractometry
   • the urinometer method

10. Differentiate between direct and indirect measures of urine specific gravity and compare the limitations of each method.

11. State the principle of the following osmometry methods:
    • freezing point
    • vapor pressure

12. Discuss the factors that affect urine volume and the terms used to describe volume variations.

. . . .

KEY TERMS

clarity (also called **turbidity**): the transparency of a urine specimen. Clarity varies with the amount of suspended particulate matter in the urine specimen.

colligative property: a characteristic of a solution that depends only on the number of solute particles present, regardless of the molecular size or charge.

The four colligative properties are freezing point depression, vapor pressure depression, osmotic pressure elevation, and boiling point elevation. These properties form the basis of methods and instrumentation used to measure the concentration of solutes in body fluids (e.g., serum, urine, fecal supernates). (See **freezing point osmometer** and **vapor pressure osmometer**.)

density: an expression of concentration in terms of the mass of solutes present per volume of solution.

diuresis: an increase in urine excretion. Various causes of diuresis include increased fluid intake, diuretic therapy, hormonal imbalance, renal dysfunction, and drug ingestion (e.g., alcohol, caffeine).

freezing point osmometer: an instrument that measures osmolality based on the freezing point depression of a solution compared to that of pure water. It consists of a cooling bath that supercools the sample below its freezing point. Freezing of the sample is mechanically induced by a stir wire. As ice crystals form, a sensitive thermistor probe monitors the temperature until an equilibrium is obtained between the solid and liquid phases. This equilibrium temperature is

the sample's freezing point, from which the osmolality of the sample is determined. One osmole of solute per kilogram of solvent (1 Osm/kg) depresses the freezing point of water by $1.86\,°C$.

ionic specific gravity: the density of a solution owing to ionic solutes only. Nonionizing substances such as urea, glucose, protein, and radiographic contrast media are not detectable using ionic specific gravity measurements (e.g., specific gravity by commercial reagent strips).

refractive index: the ratio of light refraction in two differing media (N). It is mathematically expressed using either light velocity (V) or the angle of refraction ($\sin \theta$) in the two media, as $N_2/N_1 = V_1/V_2$ or $N_2/N_1 = \sin \theta_1/\sin \theta_2$. The refractive index is affected by the wavelength of light used, the solution's temperature, and the concentration of the solution.

refractometry: an indirect measurement of specific gravity based on the refractive index of light.

urobilin: an orange-brown pigment derived from the spontaneous oxidation of colorless urobilinogen

urochrome: a lipid-soluble yellow pigment that is continuously produced during endogenous metabolism. Present in plasma and excreted in the urine, urochrome gives urine its characteristic yellow color.

uroerythrin: a pink (or red) pigment in urine that is thought to derive from melanin metabolism. Uroerythrin deposits on urate crystals to produce a precipitate described as "brick dust."

vapor pressure osmometer: an instrument that measures osmolality based on the vapor pressure depression of a solution as compared to that of pure water. The dew point of the air in a closed chamber containing a small amount of a sample is measured and compared to that obtained using pure water. A calibrated microprocessor converts the change in the dew point observed into osmolality, which is read directly from the instrument readout.

· ·

The study of urine is the oldest clinical laboratory test still being performed. Historically, only the physical characteristics of urine were evaluated. Urine was evaluated by its color, clarity, odor, and taste. The latter characteristic—taste—has not been routinely performed for several centuries because of the advent of specific chemical methods that assess the "sweetness" of urine. The physical characteristics of urine continue to play an important part in a routine urinalysis. The presence of disease processes and abnormal urine components can be evident during the initial physical examination of urine.

Color

· ·

Urine color—normally different shades of yellow—can range from colorless to amber to orange, red, green, blue, brown, or even black. The color variations can indicate the presence of a disease process, a metabolic abnormality, or an ingested food or drug, or the variations may simply be due to excessive physical activity or stress. It is important to note that a change in urine color may often be the initial or only reason an individual seeks medical attention.

The characteristic yellow color of "normal" urine is due principally to the presence of the pigment **urochrome**. A product of endogenous metabolism, urochrome is a lipid-soluble pigment found in the plasma and excreted in the urine. Patients in chronic renal failure, with a decreased excretion of urochrome, may exhibit a characteristic yellow pigmentation of their skin because of urochrome's deposition in their subcutaneous fat. Because urochrome production and excretion are constant, the intensity of the urine color provides a crude indicator of urine concentration and the body's level of hydration. A concentrated urine is dark yellow, whereas a dilute urine is pale yellow or colorless. Also, urochrome, like other lipid-soluble pigments, darkens upon exposure to light (deWardener, 1985). This characteristic darkening is often observed in urine specimens that are improperly stored. Small amounts of **urobilin** (an orange-brown pigment) and **uroerythrin** (a pink pigment) also contribute to urine color. Urobilin and uroerythrin are normal urinary constituents; uroerythrin is most evident when it deposits on urate crystals, producing a precipitate often described as "brick dust."

The terminology used to describe urine colors often differs among laboratories. Regardless of the terminology used, an estab- lished list of terms should be available and used by all personnel in the laboratory. These terms should reduce ambiguity in color interpretation and improve consistency in the reporting of urine colors (Schweitzer, 1986). Such terms as "straw" and "beer brown" should be replaced with "light yellow" and "amber." The term "bloody" should be avoided. Although it is descriptive, it is not a color—red or pink would be more appropriate. Table 6–1 lists some appropriate urine color terms and the substances that may cause these colors.

An abnormal urine—one that reflects a pathologic process—may not have an abnormal color, whereas a normally colored urine may contain significant pathology. For example, a normal yellow or colorless urine may actually contain large amounts of glucose or

T A B L E   6 – 1.   COLOR TERMS

COLOR	CONSTITUENT	COMMENTS
Colorless, light yellow	Dilute urine	Fluid ingestion; polyuria
Yellow	Normal urine	
Amber	Concentrated urine	Dehydration, fever
	Urobilin	No yellow foam
Dark amber	Bilirubin	Yellow foam if sufficient bilirubin
	Biliverdin	Imparts green hue
Orange	Bilirubin	Yellow foam if sufficient bilirubin
	Urobilin	No yellow foam
	Medications (most often); see Table 6–2	
Red	Hemoglobin, red blood cells	
	Myoglobin	Muscle injury
	Porphyrins	
	Beets	Genetic
	Fuscin, analine dye	Foods, candy
Pink	Hemoglobin	
	Porphyrins	
Brown	Hemoglobin	
	Myoglobin	Muscle injury
	Methemoglobin	Acid pH
	Homogentisic acid	
	Melanin	
Black	Melanin	Upon standing; rare
	Homogentisic acid	Upon standing; alkaline urine
Green, blue	Indican	Infections of small intestine
	Chlorophyll	Breath deodorizers
	Pseudomonas infections	
	Dyes and medications; see Table 6–2	

porphobilinogen. In contrast, a red urine, often an indicator of the presence of blood, may simply be a result of the ingestion of beets by genetically disposed individuals. Nevertheless, urine color is valuable in the preliminary assessment of a urine specimen.

Many substances are capable of modifying the normal color of urine. These substances impart different colors to the urine depending upon 1) the amount of the substance present; 2) the urine pH; or 3) the structural form of the substance, which can change over time. Red blood cells provide an excellent example. In a fresh acidic urine, they produce a urine color ranging from a normal yellow to pink or red, varying with the number of red blood cells present. As the red blood cells disintegrate, their released hemoglobin oxidizes to methemoglobin and the urine turns brown or even black. This disintegration of cellular components is enhanced in alkaline urine. As a result, hemoglobin oxidation is promoted, and alkaline urines with blood often exhibit a red-brown color. Blood entering the urinary tract at the nephrons (e.g., owing to glomerular or tubular damage) can become oxidized before it collects in the bladder. The urine will appear brownish rather than the typical red associated with the presence of blood.

A fresh brown urine can indicate the presence of blood, hemoglobin, or myoglobin. It is difficult to distinguish among these substances, particularly between hemoglobin and myoglobin, because all three produce a positive chemical test for blood. Red blood cells are confirmed by a microscopic examination, whereas the discrimination between hemoglobin and myoglobin requires that the laboratorian perform additional urine chemical testing and possibly an evaluation of the blood plasma. Chapter 7 contains further discussion on the differentiation of hemoglobin and myoglobin.

Bilirubin is another substance that can contribute to urine color. It is a by-product of hemoglobin catabolism and has a characteristic yellow color. When present in sufficient amounts in the urine and the plasma, it imparts a distinctive amber coloration. However, upon standing or improper storage, bili-

rubin can oxidize to biliverdin, causing the urine to take on a greenish hue. Bilirubin is also susceptible to photo-oxidation by either artificial light or sunlight; therefore, specimens must be properly stored to avoid degradation of this component. This photosensitivity is temperature dependent; optimal specimen stability is obtained by storing the specimens at low temperatures in the dark.

Some substances are colorless and normally do not affect the color of urine; however, upon standing or improper storage, they can be converted to colored compounds. Urobilinogen, a normal constituent in urine, is colorless, whereas its oxidation product — urobilin — is orange-brown. Porphobilinogen, a colorless and chemically similar (tetrapyrroles) substance, is an abnormal urine component found in patients with abnormal porphyrin metabolism (heme synthesis). Porphobilin, porphobilinogen's oxidation product, imparts a red or purple color to urine. As a result, urines that contain these substances will change color over time. These color changes are strong indications of the presence of the colorless substances and can alert the laboratorian to the need for additional testing.

A multitude of urine colors result from ingested substances and often are of no clinical significance. Highly pigmented foods such as fresh beets, breath fresheners containing chlorophyll, candy dyes, and vitamins A and B can impart distinctive coloration to urine. Included in this group of ingested substances are numerous medications, some of which are used to specifically treat urinary tract infections. Other medications are present because they are eliminated from the body in the urine. Table 6–2 lists commonly encountered drugs and the colors they impart to the urine. It is worth noting that phenazopyridine, a urinary analgesic often encountered in the clinical laboratory, imparts a very distinctive yellow-orange coloration and a syrupy consistency to urine. This drug-produced color frequently interferes with the color interpretation of chemical reagent strip tests; alternative chemical testing methods must be employed on these urine specimens.

Pathologic conditions can be indicated by

T A B L E 6 – 2.   URINE COLOR CHANGES WITH COMMONLY USED DRUGS*

DRUG	COLOR
Alcohol, ethyl	Pale, diuresis
Anthraquinone laxatives (senna, cascara)	Reddish, alkaline; yellow-brown, acid
Chlorzoxazone (Paraflex) (muscle relaxant)	Red
Deferoxamine mesylate (Desferal) (chelates iron)	Red
Ethoxazene (Serenium) (urinary analgesic)	Orange, red
Fluorescein sodium (given intravenous)	Yellow
Furazolidone (Furoxone) (Tricofuron) (an antibacterial, anti-protozoal nitrofuran)	Brown
Indigo carmine dye (renal function, cytoscopy)	Blue
Iron sorbital (Jectofer) (possibly other iron compounds forming iron sulfide in urine)	Brown on standing
Levodopa (L-dopa) (for parkinsonism)	Red then brown, alkaline
Mepacrine (Atabrine) (antimalarial) (intestinal worms, *Giardia*)	Yellow
Methocarbamol (Robaxin) (muscle relaxant)	Green-brown
Methyldopa (Aldomet) (antihypertensive)	Darken; if oxidizing agents present, red to brown
Methylene blue (used to delineate fistulas)	Blue, blue-green
Metronidazole (Flagyl) (for *Trichomonas* infection, amebiasis, *Giardia*)	Darkening, reddish brown
Nitrofurantoin (Furadantin) (antibacterial)	Brown-yellow
Phenazopyridine (Pyridium) (urinary analgesic), also compounded with sulfonamides (Azo-Gantrisin, etc.)	Orange-red, acid pH
Phenindione (Hedulin) (anticoagulant) (important to distinguish from hematuria)	Orange, alkaline; color disappears on acidifying
Phenol poisoning	Brown; oxidized to quinones (green)
Phenolphthalein (purgative)	Red-purple, alkaline pH
Phenolsulfonphthalein (PSP, also BSP)	Pink-red, alkaline pH
Rifampin (Rifadin, Rimactane) (tuberculosis therapy)	Bright orange-red
Riboflavin (multivitamins)	Bright yellow
Sulfasalazine (Azulfidine) (for ulcerative colitis)	Orange-yellow, alkaline pH

Other commonly used drugs have been noted to produce color change once or occasionally: amitriptyline (Elavil)—blue-green; phenothiazines—red; triamterene (Dyrenium)—pale blue (blue fluorescence in acid urine). An extensive list may be found in Young et al.: Clin Chem 21:379. 1975.

From Henry B: Clinical Diagnosis and Management by Laboratory Methods (18th ed.), Philadelphia, W.B. Saunders Company, 1991.

the presence of certain analytes and components that color the urine. Substances such as melanin, homogentisic acid, indican, porphyrins, hemoglobin, and myoglobin or components such as red blood cells are evidence of a pathologic process taking place. In each case, urines suspected of containing these components require additional chemical testing and investigation. Many of these substances are discussed individually along with the metabolic disease that produces them in Chapters 7 and 9.

On the other hand, contaminants—substances not produced in the urinary tract—can also color the urine. Fecal material, menstrual blood, or hemorrhoidal blood will color the urine when present.

Urine color is actually a combination of the colors imparted by each constituent present. In order to consistently evaluate urine color, the criteria outlined in Table 6–3 are necessary. Without attention to these details and to the use of established terminol-

T A B L E 6 – 3.   RECOMMENDATIONS FOR THE EVALUATION OF URINE PHYSICAL CHARACTERISTICS

Use a well-mixed specimen.
View through a *clear* container—plastic or glass.
View against a white background.
Evaluate a consistent depth or volume of the specimen.
Maintain room lighting at a consistently adequate level.

ogy, consistent reporting of urine color is not possible.

Foam

. . . .

If a normal urine specimen is agitated sufficiently, a foam can be forced to develop at its surface and will readily dissipate upon standing. Certain substances, specifically protein and bilirubin, can change the characteristics of the urine foam. The foam's color and its ease of development and the amount of foam produced can be modified by the presence of a substance. Some substances that intensify or change the color of urine (e.g., hemoglobin), however, will not change the color or characteristics of the foam.

Moderate to large amounts of protein (albumin) in urine will cause a stable white foam to be produced upon pouring or agitation of the specimen. Like egg albumin, the foam that develops is thick and lasts noticeably longer than other foam. Much more foam is produced by the agitation of these urines than from agitating a normal urine.

Unlike protein, bilirubin, when present in sufficient amounts, causes the foam to become distinctly yellow. The yellowness is often observed as the urine is being processed and the physical characteristics recorded. Although not definitive, foam color provides preliminary supporting evidence for the suspected presence of bilirubin.

Foam characteristics noted in the physical examination are not reported in a routine urinalysis; instead, they serve as preliminary and supportive evidence for the presence of bilirubin and abnormal amounts of protein in the urine. These suspected substances must be detected and confirmed during the chemical examination before either constituent is reported.

Clarity

. . . .

Clarity, along with color, describes the overall visual appearance of a urine specimen. It is assessed at the same time as urine color and refers to the transparency of the speci-

men. Often called "turbidity," it describes the cloudiness of the urine owing to suspended particulate matter that scatters light. The criteria outlined in Table 6–3 for assessing urine color also apply when evaluating urine clarity. An established list of descriptive terms for clarity used by all laboratory personnel will assure consistency in reporting and will eliminate ambiguity. Table 6–4 defines common clarity terminology and provides a list of substances that produce these characteristics.

A normal "clean catch" urine is usually clear when freshly voided. If precautions are not made to eliminate potential contamination with squamous epithelial cells or mucus (especially in women), however, a normal specimen may appear cloudy. Likewise, if a specimen is improperly handled after its collection, bacterial growth can cause the specimen to become cloudy.

The precipitation of amorphous solutes, most commonly amorphous urates and phosphates, can also cause a normal urine specimen to appear cloudy. Amorphous phosphates and carbonates produce a white precipitate and are present only in alkaline urine. In acidic urine, a pinkish precipitate ("brick dust") results from the deposition of uroerythrin on amorphous urate and uric acid crystals. Indirectly, the white and pink precipitates indicate whether the urine pH is acid or alkaline.

A specific component may be evident on close inspection of the particulate matter present in urine; most commonly noted are red blood cells and small blood clots. Similarly, the excretion of fat or lymph should be suspected in a urine that appears opalescent or milky. Urine clarity provides a rapid quality check for the microscopic examination, i.e., a cloudy urine specimen should have significant numbers of components present when viewed microscopically.

Substances that cause urine turbidity can be pathologic or nonpathologic (Table 6–5). Principally, those substances considered nonpathologic are either contaminants or normal urine components. Spermatozoa and prostatic fluid are considered to be urine contaminants because they are not derived from the uri-

TABLE 6–4.   CLARITY TERMS

CLARITY	DEFINITION	CAUSES
Clear	No visible particulate matter present.	Normal urine. Constituents, if present, are soluble.
Slightly cloudy	Some visual particulate matter is present; newsprint is not obscured when viewed through urine.	Clarity will vary depending on the amount and constituent type: Urates, phosphates

Cloudy	Visible particulate matter; newsprint can be viewed through urine but is obscured or blurred.	Other crystals
		    White blood cells
		    Red blood cells ("smoky")

Turbid	Newsprint cannot be viewed through urine.	Bacteria, yeast
		    Epithelial cells
		    Fat (lipids, chyle)
		    Spermatozoa
		    Prostatic fluid
		    Mucus, mucin, pus
		    Calculi
		    Fecal contamination
		    Radiographic dye
		    Salves, lotions, creams
		    Powders, talc

Modified from Schweitzer SC, Schumann JL, Schumann GB: Quality assurance guidelines for the urinalysis laboratory. J Med Tech 3:11, 1986.

nary tract; rather, they use it as a conveyance. Radiographic contrast media present in the urine following an x-ray procedure are iatrogenic and not indicative of disease. The presence of fecal material and many squamous epithelial cells usually indicates the improper collection of the urine specimen. Pathologic conditions, however, such as a fistula between the bladder and colon can also result in the presence of fecal material in the urine and will cause a persistent urinary tract infection.

TABLE 6–5.   CLASSIFICATION OF SUBSTANCES CAUSING URINE TURBIDITY

PATHOLOGIC	NONPATHOLOGIC
Red blood cells	Normal crystals (e.g., urates, phosphates)
White blood cells	Radiographic media
Bacteria (fresh urine)	Mucus, mucin
Yeast, trichomonads	Squamous epithelial cells
Renal epithelial cells	Spermatozoa and prostatic fluid
Fat (lipids, chyle)	Fecal contamination
Abnormal crystals	Salves, lotions, creams
Calculi	Powders, talc
Pus	

Pathologic substances in the urine indicate 1) a deterioration of the barrier normally separating the urinary tract from the blood; 2) a disease process; or 3) a metabolic dysfunction. For example, the presence of red blood cells in the urine indicates damage to the urinary tract. At times the site of the injury can be localized, such as with the presence of dysmorphic red blood cells, which are highly indicative of glomerular damage, or with the presence of red blood cells in casts, indicating glomerular or tubular origin. White blood cells in the urine are indicative of an inflammatory process somewhere in the urinary tract. Although bacteria are the most common cause of urinary tract infections, other agents can produce inflammation without bacteriuria (see Chapter 9). The presence of bacteria, along with white blood cells and casts, in fresh urine indicates an infection of the upper urinary tract (e.g., renal pelvis, interstitium); whereas the presence of bacteria and white blood cells without casts implies a lower urinary tract infection (e.g., bladder, urethra). In contrast, yeast and trichomonads—although agents of infection—commonly originate from a vaginal infection and are often contaminants when present in a urine specimen. Regardless of their origin, these organisms are routinely reported when observed in the microscopic examination of a urine specimen.

In summary, a clear urine does not mean that it is normal. Abnormal amounts of glucose, protein, lysed red blood cells, or white blood cells may be present in a clear, "negative-appearing" urine. These components will be detected by a chemical examination. On the other hand, a freshly voided cloudy urine requires further investigation to identify the substance causing the turbidity.

Odor

. . . .

Historically, urine odor led to the research and discovery of the metabolic disease phenylketonuria (PKU). Currently, urine odors, unless remarkably strong or different, are not detected in a routine urinalysis. Because urine contains many organic and inorganic substances—by-products of metabolism—normal urine has a characteristic aromatic odor. This odor is normally faint and unremarkable; however, if normal urine is allowed to stand at room temperature and "age," it becomes particularly odorous and ammoniacal because of the conversion of urea to ammonia by the bacteria present. Normally, urine is sterile until it passes from the urethra out of the body, where it is easily contaminated by normal bacterial flora from the skin. In an improperly stored urine specimen, these contaminating organisms can proliferate. Because of this, urine odor can indicate that a specimen is old and not suitable for testing because of the many changes that occur in unpreserved urine (see Chapter 3). On the other hand, a patient with a urinary tract infection may also produce an ammonia-smelling urine owing to bacterial metabolism occurring within the urinary tract. The distinguishing factor is that, in the latter case, the urine smells distinctly ammoniacal even when it has been freshly voided. Severe urinary tract infections can also give rise to a strongly pungent or fetid aroma from pus, protein decay, and bacteria. Before proceeding with testing, it is important to determine that urines with strong odors are fresh specimens and that they have been properly stored.

The ingestion of certain foods or drugs can cause the urine to have a noticeably different odor. Foods such as asparagus and garlic or intravenous medications containing phenolic derivatives can result in urines with distinct aromas. Several metabolic disorders can also result in urine with unusual odors (Table 6–6). For example, the conditions of increased fat metabolism with the formation and excretion of aromatic ketone bodies can produce a sweet or fruity smelling urine. Of these conditions, the most common disorder is diabetes mellitus, in which the glucose present in the blood is unable to be utilized and the body fat is metabolized to compensate. Numerous amino acid disorders that produce noticeably odd urine odors are also listed in Table 6–6. Patients with these disorders exhibit clinical signs of metabolic dysfunction, and their diagnoses do not rely on the detection of urine odor (see Chapter 9). Various urine tests play an important role in the differential diagnosis of these metabolic disorders, however.

TABLE 6–6.   CAUSES OF URINE ODORS

ODOR	CAUSE
Aromatic, faintly	Normal urine
Ammoniacal	"Old" urine—improperly stored
Pungent, fetid	Urinary tract infection
Sweet, fruity	Ketone production owing to:
	Diabetes mellitus
	Starvation, dieting, malnutrition
	Strenuous exercise
	Vomiting, diarrhea
Unusual odors:	Amino acid disorders:
Mousy, barny	Phenylketonuria
Maple syrup	Maple syrup urine disease
Rancid	Tyrosinemia
Rotting/old fish	Trimethylaminuria
Cabbage, hops	Methionine malabsorption
Sweaty feet	Isovaleric and glutaric acidemias
	Ingested substances:
Distinctive	Asparagus, garlic, onions
Menthol-like	Phenol-containing medications
Bleach	Adulteration of the specimen or
	container contamination

On occasion, a urine specimen can smell strongly of bleach or other cleaning agents. Sometimes the agent was added to the urine specimen intentionally (i.e., the specimen was adulterated) to interfere with testing—particularly when the urine specimen was collected for the detection of suspected illegal drug use. If household containers are used to collect a specimen, however, it is possible for the cleaning agent to be present by accident, i.e., the container was contaminated prior to collection. Regardless of the cause of the contamination, the specimen is not acceptable for urinalysis testing.

Taste

Although historically (circa 1674) urine was tasted to detect the presence of urinary sugars, urine is no longer tasted. The terms *mellitus* meaning "sweet" and *insipidus* meaning "tasteless" were assigned to the disease *diabetes* based on the taste of the urine produced by these two different diseases. Both disorders produce copious amounts of urine, hence the name *diabetes;* however, the causes of the disorders are completely different.

Concentration

Another physical characteristic of urine is concentration—the amount of solutes present in the volume of water excreted. As discussed in Chapter 5, urine is normally 94 percent water and 6 percent solutes; the amount and type of solutes excreted varies with the patient's diet, physical activity, and health. A dilute urine has fewer solute particles present per volume of water; whereas a concentrated urine has more solute particles present per volume of urine. As previously mentioned, color provides a crude indicator of urine concentration. Dilute urine contains fewer of the solutes that impart color and is therefore light yellow or colorless. Similarly, a concentrated normal urine is dark yellow owing to an increase in these solutes without

a corresponding increase in the urine's water volume.

Urine concentration in the clinical laboratory is most often expressed as specific gravity or osmolality. As discussed previously in Chapter 5, these expressions of solute composition are similar and yet different. When an individual is healthy, a good correlation is maintained between the urine specific gravity and the urine osmolality; however, with disease, this relationship may not exist (see Fig. 5–1). In addition, methods available for determining the specific gravity and the osmolality differ with respect to instrumentation, complexity, and the time required to perform the determination. As a result, the specific gravity is most often used to rapidly screen urine concentration in the clinical laboratory, whereas the osmolality is used to obtain more accurate and specific information.

Specific Gravity

One expression of concentration is **density**—the mass of solutes present per volume of solution. The urine specific gravity, an expression of density, is the ratio of the density of urine to the density of an equal volume of pure water. Because specific gravity is a density measurement, it is affected by both the number of solutes present and the solutes' molecular size. Note from Equation 6–1 that as the density of urine approaches the density of pure water, the specific gravity approaches unity (1.000).

(6–1)

$$\text{Sp grav} = \frac{\text{Density of urine}}{\text{Density of equal volume of water}}$$

The greater the urine density, the larger the specific gravity value. It is physiologically impossible for the body to excrete pure water; as a result, the lowest urine specific gravity obtainable is 1.002. Conversely, the maximum specific gravity the urine can attain is exactly equal to that of the hyperosmotic renal medulla, approximately 1.040.

Several methods are available for the determination of the specific gravity in urine.

They can be divided into direct and indirect measurements. Direct measurements determine the urine density and relate it to pure water. Some direct measurements of specific gravity are: 1) the urinometer; 2) the falling drop method (employed in instrumentation by the Ames Corporation); and 3) the harmonic oscillation densitometric method (employed in instrumentation by International Remote Imaging Systems). Indirect measurements of specific gravity are refractometry and the reagent strip chemical method.

The direct specific gravity determinations measure normal renal solutes as well as glucose, protein, and radiographic media, if present. These high-molecular-weight substances are not a reflection of the body's renal concentrating ability. The substances are present owing to other processes unrelated to the concentrating ability. Therefore, when using direct specific gravity methods to assess this renal function, the presence of glucose and protein must be determined and corrections must be made to eliminate their significant contribution to the direct specific gravity measurement. On the other hand, radiographic contrast media cannot be corrected for; therefore, if such media are present, a new specimen must be obtained after a suitable timeframe, or an alternative measurement method must be used. If these high-molecular-weight solutes are not noted and accounted for, erroneous conclusions regarding the body's renal concentrating ability can be made.

Density is affected by temperature. Therefore, direct specific gravity methods must either control the temperature at which the measurements are performed or correct the results accordingly. In this regard, temperature control is easily obtained in the instrumentation employing the falling drop and harmonic oscillation densitometric measurement methods. In contrast, the urinometer method requires a manual correction of the results using temperature correction factors.

Urinometry

The urinometer, also known as a hydrometer (Fig. 6–1), is no longer considered to be an

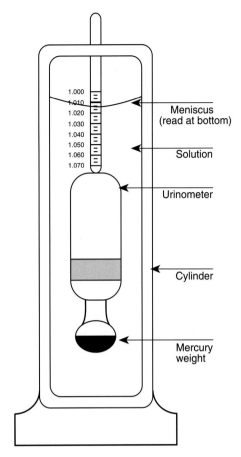

FIGURE 6–1. A schematic representation of a urinometer (hydrometer).

accurate device for the determination of urine specific gravity (NCCLS Document GP16-T, 1992). It is a weighted glass float with a long, narrow, calibrated stem. When placed in pure (distilled or deionized) water at a specific temperature, the urinometer sinks, displacing a volume of water equal to its weight. The meniscus of the water intersects the calibrated stem of the urinometer at the value 1.000. When placed in a solution of greater density than water (i.e., solutes are present), the urinometer displaces a smaller volume of liquid (it does not sink as deep) and the specific gravity read off the calibrated stem is greater than 1.000.

There are many disadvantages to using the urinometer; in particular, 1) a large volume (10 to 15 mL) of urine is required; 2) the urinometer must be calibrated daily; and 3) temperature corrections must be made for specimens whose temperature differs by greater than 3°C from the urinometer's calibrated temperature. In addition, the urinometer can be cumbersome and temperamental (e.g., inaccurate readings are caused by the float's touching the sides of the container or by excessive wetting of the calibrated stem above the water line).

Falling Drop Method

The falling drop method for the determination of the urine specific gravity was used by the Ames Corporation in the Clinitek Auto 2000, a semiautomated instrument (which is no longer being manufactured). In this direct measurement of density, a drop of urine is timed as it falls through a temperature-controlled column of a silicone-based oil. Two optical gates separated at a fixed distance record the elapsed time, which is directly related to the mass of solutes present in the urine. The microprocessor rapidly converts this time to the corresponding specific gravity value. The instrument requires daily calibration checks using standard solutions and is linear to 1.050.

Harmonic Oscillation Densitometry

Harmonic oscillation densitometry (i.e., soundwaves) is used by International Remote Imaging Systems on the Yellow IRIS, a semiautomated urinalysis workstation. This direct method uses soundwaves to measure urine density. During testing, a portion of the urine sample is held in a U-shaped glass tube that has an electromagnetic coil on one end and a motion detector on the other end. An electric current applied to the coil generates a soundwave of fixed frequency. This sonic oscillation is transmitted through the specimen, and the frequency attenuation is measured. The frequency (the oscillating cycle period) observed is directly proportional to the sample density; hence, the microprocessor converts this frequency to the corresponding specific gravity value. Because temperature affects the density, a thermistor monitors the sample temperature in the tube

and supplies this information to the microprocessor for correction, if necessary. The instrument is calibrated daily during its self-test and is linear to a specific gravity of 1.080.

Refractometry

Refractometry, an indirect measure of the specific gravity, is based on the refractive index of light. When light passes from air into a solution at an angle, the direction of the light beam is refracted and its speed decreases (Fig. 6–2). The ratio of the light refraction in the two differing media is called the **refractive index.** This refractive index (N) of the solution can be expressed mathematically using either the velocity of the incident and refracted light beams or their respective angles.

(6–2)

$$\frac{N_2}{N_1} = \frac{V_1}{V_2} \quad \text{or} \quad \frac{N_2}{N_1} = \frac{\sin \theta_1}{\sin \theta_2}$$

In Equation 6–2, N_1 is the refractive index of air, which by convention equals 1.0; N_2 is the refractive index of the solution being measured; V_1 is the velocity of light in air; V_2

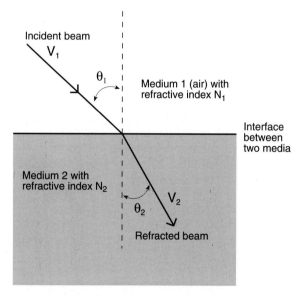

FIGURE 6–2. A schematic diagram illustrating the refraction (or bending) of light as it passes from one medium to another of differing density. Note that the velocity of the light beam also changes.

is the velocity of light in the solution; $\sin \theta_1$ is the angle of the incident beam of light, and $\sin \theta_2$ is the angle of the refracted beam of light. Although either velocity or the angles of refraction can be used to determine the refractive index, it is the measurement of angles that is the principle routinely employed in refractometers.

The refractive index of a solution is affected by three factors: 1) the wavelength of light used; 2) the temperature of the solution; and 3) the concentration of the solution. Both the temperature and the concentration of a solution affect its refractive index because they produce changes in the density of the solution. It is this direct relationship to solution density that allows the refractive index to be used as a measure of specific gravity. Stated another way, as the temperature changes or the amount of solutes in a solution changes, so does its density; hence, the refractive index changes. Like specific gravity measurements, refractometry measures all the solutes in solution, including any glucose and protein present. Therefore, results obtained by refractometry are comparable to those obtained by direct specific gravity methods.

Routinely, white light provides the radiant light beam used in refractometers. Isolation of a monochromatic light beam from polychromatic white light is managed by the design of the refractometer. Within the refractometer, a prism, a liquid compensator, and the chamber cover work together to direct only 589 nm of light onto the calibrated scale. Refractive index measurements differ depending on the wavelength used. Therefore, refractometers consistently use a single wavelength, most commonly 589 nm. Figure 6–3 shows a schematic of a refractometer widely used in the clinical laboratory.

The use of refractometry for the measurement of urine specific gravity has several advantages, most notably the small amount of the sample required and the ability to automatically make temperature compensations for specimens between 15°C and 37°C. One to two drops of urine placed between the cover plate and the prism cover glass rapidly temperature-equilibrate with the instrument. Within the instrument is a liquid reservoir whose refractive index varies with temperature. As the refracted light beam from the sample passes through this reservoir, it is corrected to the value that would be obtained at a temperature of 20°C. The refracted light beam makes several passes through the measuring prism before it is focused by a lens onto the calibrated scale. In the viewing field, a distinct edge between the light and dark areas is evident. This boundary is the point where the specific gravity value is read off the scale (Fig. 6–4). The scale is calibrated at the factory by measuring urines of known specific gravity. Similarly, refractometers are available with a second calibrated scale in the viewing field for the determination of serum or plasma protein concentration based on the refractive index.

In summary, refractometry compares the velocity or angle of refraction of light in a solution to that of light in the air. In a solution, as the number of solutes increases, the velocity of light decreases and the angle of light refraction increases. Refractometers automatically compensate for temperatures ranging from 15°C to 30°C; they are calibrated for both specific gravity and protein determinations; and they require a small sample volume. Like the direct specific gravity measurements, refractometry also measures any glucose and protein present in the urine, although to a lesser degree.

Specific Gravity by the Reagent Strip Method

The reagent strip chemical determination is an indirect colorimetric estimation of the specific gravity. This method detects only the *ionic* solutes present in the urine specimen. Hence, it will be referred to as the **ionic specific gravity** (SG_{ionic}). The concentration of the urine depends on the kidneys' ability to selectively reabsorb and secrete ionic solutes and water. The excretion of nonionic solutes, such as urea, glucose, protein, or radiographic media, does not reflect the status of this renal function. Therefore, the determination of the specific gravity by the re-

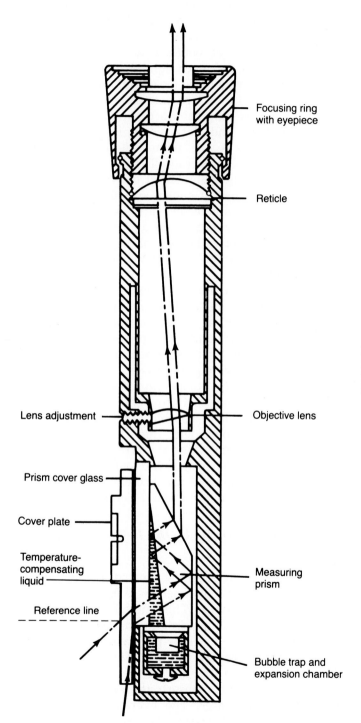

Focusing ring
with eyepiece

Reticle

Lens adjustment

Objective lens

Prism cover glass

Cover plate

Temperature-
compensating
liquid

Reference line

Measuring
prism

Bubble trap and
expansion chamber

FIGURE 6–3. A schematic representation of a refractometer (also called a total solids meter). (Courtesy of Leica, Inc., Buffalo, New York. Reprinted with permission.)

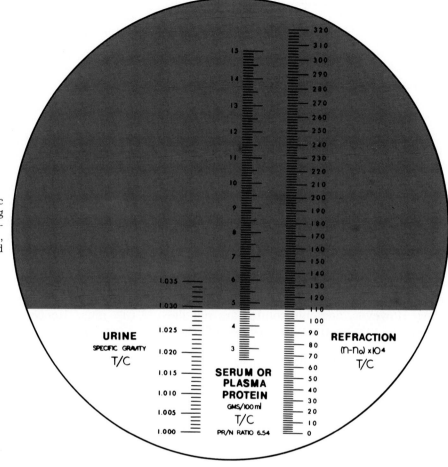

FIGURE 6-4. A schematic representation of the viewing field and scale in the refractometer. (Courtesy of Leica, Inc., Buffalo, New York. Reprinted with permission.)

agent strip method eliminates the need to correct the specific gravity measurements when significant numbers of nonionic solutes are present.

This chemical method consists of a reagent test pad adherent to an inert plastic strip. The test pad is impregnated with a polyelectrolyte, a pH indicator, and is maintained at an alkaline pH. When the strip is immersed in a urine sample, the pK_a of the polyelectrolyte will decrease proportionally to the "ionic" concentration of the specimen. As the pH of the test pad decreases, the bromthymol blue indicator changes color from dark blue-green (SG_{ionic} 1.000) to yellow-green (SG_{ionic} 1.030). Stated another way, as

more ions are present in the urine, more protons are released from the polyelectrolyte, resulting in a decrease in the test pad pH and a change in the indicator (Equation 6-3).

(6-3)

$$
\begin{array}{llllll}
C & C & C + \text{(urine ions)} & \xrightarrow{\text{alkaline}} & C & C & C & + H^+ \\
O & O & O & + - & & O & O & O \\
O & O & O & - + & & O^- & O & O^- \\
H & H & H & + - & & & H
\end{array}
$$

This indirect specific gravity method does not relay the "true" solute concentration because nonionic substances, regardless of their molecular size, go undetected. The "true" or total specific gravity (SG_T) of urine includes all solutes, both ionic and nonionic (Equation 6–4).

(6–4)

$$SG_T = SG_{ionic} + SG_{nonionic}$$

When an individual is healthy, the amount of nonionic solutes in urine relative to ionic solutes is insignificant. As a result, the ionic specific gravity (SG_{ionic}) is equal to the total specific gravity (SG_T) (Equation 6–5). This provides the basis for the efficacy of the reagent strip method for specific gravity determinations.

(6–5)

If $SG_{nonionic} <<< SG_{ionic}$; then, $SG_T = SG_{ionic}$

In summary, the SG_{ionic} determined by the reagent strip method is a rapid and useful tool to evaluate the ionic concentration of the urine. However, nonionic solutes are not detected by this method, regardless of their molecular weight.

Considering the different methods available for specific gravity determination, it is imperative that the limitations of each are known and understood in order to ensure proper interpretation of the results obtained. Table 6–7 summarizes the specific gravity methods discussed.

Osmolality

As described in Chapter 5, osmolality is the concentration of a solution expressed in terms of osmoles of solute particles per kilogram of water, denoted Osm/kg. An osmole is defined as the amount of a substance that dissociates to produce one mole of particles in a solution. For example, glucose in a solution does not dissociate; therefore, 1 mole of glucose equals 1 mole of particles or 1 osmole. In contrast, sodium chloride (NaCl) dissociates into two particles, Na^+ ions and Cl^- ions. Hence, 1 mole of NaCl produces 2 osmoles of particles in solution. Molecular weight (MW) does not play a role in osmolality; despite the relatively large molecular weight of glucose (MW 180), when sodium chloride (MW 58) is present in an equal

TABLE 6–7.   METHODS TO EVALUATE THE URINE CONCENTRATION

METHOD	PRINCIPLE	LIMITATIONS
Specific Gravity		
Direct Methods		
Urinometer	Density*	Values affected more by high-moleculer-weight solutes (e.g. glucose, protein, radiographic media) than by low-molecular-weight solutes and ions (e.g. urea, sodium, chloride).
Falling drop	Density*	
Harmonic oscillation densitometry	Density*	
Indirect Methods		
Refractometry	Refractive index*	Affect of high-molecular-weight solutes not as great as with the direct methods.
Reagent strip	pK$_a$ changes of a polyelectrolyte	Measures only ionic solutes (SG_{ionic}).
Osmolality†		
	Freezing point	More time-consuming than specific gravity methods; all solutes contribute equally.
	Vapor pressure	More time-consuming than specific gravity methods; all solutes contribute equally. Does *not* measure volatile solutes (e.g., ethanol, methanol, ethylene glycol).

* *Dependent on both solute size and number.*
† *Dependent on the number of solute particles only.*

molar amount, it will produce an osmolality double that of glucose.

Because the osmolality of biologic fluids such as urine and serum is low, the milliosmole is the unit of choice. In addition, the expression of concentration (mOsm/kg H_2O) is considered to be more precise because it is temperature independent, unlike its counterpart osmolarity (mOsm/L solution), in which the volume will vary directly with temperature. In urine, the solvent is water and the solute particles are those that pass the filtration barrier and are not reabsorbed by the tubules, plus those substances that are secreted by the tubules.

Osmolality is determined by measuring a **colligative property** of the sample, whether serum or urine. Colligative properties are those properties characteristic of a solution that depend only on the number of solute particles present. The particle size and ionic charge have no effect; only the number of particles present, either as ions or undissociated molecules, affect the colligative properties. The four colligative properties are 1) depression of the solvent freezing point; 2) depression of solvent vapor pressure; 3) elevation in osmotic pressure; and 4) elevation of solvent boiling point. These properties are interrelated and the value of one can be used to calculate each of the others. In the clinical laboratory, freezing point depression osmometry predominates for several reasons. It is sensitive to the presence of volatile solutes (e.g., ethanol, methanol, ethylene glycol); it produces accurate results even with lipemic serum samples (Tietz, 1987); and it has increased precision compared to vapor pressure osmometry.

Freezing Point Osmometry

A contemporary **freezing point osmometer** consists of four principal components: 1) a cooling bath thermostatically maintained at about $-7°C$ to slowly supercool the sample; 2) a stir wire to maintain the sample's homogeneity and to initiate freezing ("seeding") of the sample; 3) a thermistor probe to measure the sample's temperature; and 4) a direct readout display. Figure 6–5 is a simplified diagram of a freezing point osmometer.

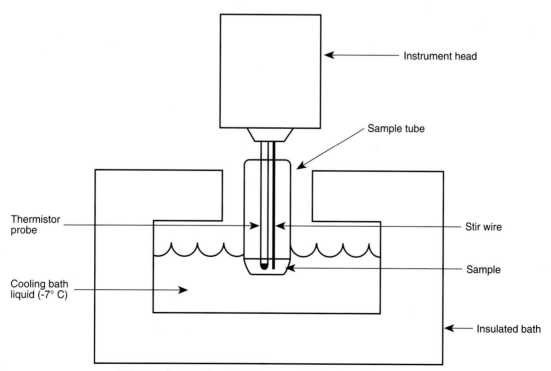

FIGURE 6–5. A simplified diagram of a freezing point osmometer.

The specimen—urine or serum—in a clean, dry sample tube is placed in the osmometer bath well. The instrument head, which holds the stir wire and the thermistor probe, is lowered into the sample tube and begins the cooling sequence depicted in Figure 6–6. The specimen is stirred constantly during the supercooling process (segment AB; Fig. 6–6) to prevent the freezing of the sample, because it is being cooled several degrees below its freezing point. As the sample temperature approaches that of the bath (−7°C), freezing of the sample is mechanically induced ("seeded") by a rapid vibration of the stir wire (point B). As ice crystals form, the heat of fusion released to the sample (segment BC) is detected by the sensitive thermistor probe. The sample temperature increases until an equilibrium between the solid and liquid phases is reached—by definition, the sample's freezing point (segment CD). This temperature plateau is maintained for 1 minute or more before it again decreases (segment DE) as the cooling bath begins to freeze the sample solid.

The measurement of freezing point depression is based on the fact that pure water freezes at 0°C and that adding 1 mole (1000 mOsm) of solute particles to 1 kg pure water will cause the freezing point to decrease by 1.86°C. This relationship is constant, and the proportionality formula given in Equation 6–6 is used to determine the osmolality once the freezing point of the sample is determined.

(6–6)

$$\frac{1000 \text{ mOsm particles}}{\begin{array}{c} \text{freezing pt.} \\ = -1.86°C \end{array}} = \frac{X \text{ mOsm particle}}{\begin{array}{c} \textit{measured} \text{ freezing} \\ \text{pt. of sample} \end{array}}$$

For example, the freezing point of a urine specimen is measured as −1.20°C by the thermistor probe. Inserting this value in the equation and solving for X, the osmolality of the urine sample is 645.2 mOsm/kg. In order to achieve the precision of ±2 mOsm/kg as seen with freezing point osmometers, accurate temperature measurements are crucial. These temperature measurements are obtained by the thermistor probe, which mea-

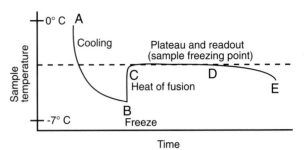

FIGURE 6–6. A time-temperature curve during freezing point depression osmometry.

sures the temperature very accurately and rapidly.

In order for osmolality results to be read directly from the instrument readout, the osmometer's microprocessor must be calibrated. It is calibrated using standard sodium chloride solutions of known osmolality. These sodium chloride solutions are either available commercially, in concentrations ranging from 50 to 1,500 mOsm, or are prepared by the laboratory. Following calibration, the osmometer measures the freezing point, converts it to the corresponding osmolality value, and displays it on the direct readout.

The sample size necessary for the osmolality determinations varies from 20 μL to 2.0 mL depending on the osmometer employed. After analysis, the osmolality samples can be thawed and used to perform other tests. Factors that interfere with freezing point osmometry measurements include 1) particulate matter in the sample that prevents proper supercooling and results in premature freezing of the sample, and 2) dirty or wet sample tubes that produce erroneous results.

Vapor Pressure Osmometry

Another method of determining osmolality is the **vapor pressure osmometer.** This instrument indirectly measures the decrease in vapor pressure owing to the solutes present in the sample by directly measuring the decrease in the dew point temperature from that of pure water. The smaller sample size (7 μL) required is an advantage; however, owing to its inability to detect volatile solutes or to achieve the precision of the freezing point osmometer, vapor pressure osmometry is not as popular in the clinical laboratory.

Normal serum osmolality values range from 275 to 300 mOsm/kg, whereas urine osmolality values vary from 1 to 3 times greater: 275 to 900 mOsm/kg. The kidneys excrete unwanted solutes in the volume of water that the body does not need. As a result, the urine osmolality varies greatly with the patient's diet, health, and physical activity, whereas the serum osmolality remains relatively constant.

The principal uses of osmolality measurements are to evaluate the kidney's renal concentrating ability, to monitor renal disease, to monitor fluid and electrolyte balance, and to differentially diagnose the causes of polyuria. For a discussion of osmolality and specific gravity measurements in the evaluation of renal function, see the Assessment of Renal Concentrating Ability section in Chapter 5.

In conclusion, osmolality expresses concentration as the number of solutes present, whereas specific gravity expresses concentration as the solutes' density (weight). Heavy molecules such as glucose, protein, and radiographic media will significantly affect specific gravity, whereas osmolality is unaffected because the osmolar amount of these substances is insignificant compared to other solutes. Because all solutes contribute to osmolality equally — regardless of their molecular size — osmolality is considered a better and more accurate assessment of the solute's concentration in serum and urine. See Table 6–7 for a summary of each of the methods discussed in the evaluation of urine concentration.

Volume

. . . .

Although the amount or volume of urine excreted per day is a physical characteristic of urine, urine samples are not assessed routinely for volume alone. Normally, urine volume varies from 600 to 1800 mL/d, with less than 400 mL excreted at night. When an individual excretes more than 500 mL of urine at night, the condition is termed nocturia and can be highly suggestive of chronic progressive renal failure. In chronic renal failure, the kidney has lost its ability to concentrate the urine, and the ultrafiltrate remains isoosmotic with the plasma. The urine specific gravity is 1.010, the same as that of the original plasma ultrafiltrate.

The daily urine volume is directly affected by an individual's diet, health, and exercise. The kidneys maintain a balance between fluid intake and excretion; however, their control is one-sided. Any excess fluid ingested but not needed can be excreted as urine, but the kidneys have a limited ability to compensate for the lack of adequate fluid intake. As the amount of metabolic solutes needing elimination from the body changes, so does the volume of water required to excrete the solutes. If the body lacks adequate hydration, solutes will accumulate in the body despite the kidney's best efforts to eliminate them.

Polyuria, the excessive excretion of urine (greater than 3 L/d), may be a complaint of patients; however, this alone rarely causes an individual to seek medical attention. Any increase in urine excretion is termed **diuresis** and may be due to excessive water intake (polydipsia), diuretic therapy, hormonal imbalance, renal dysfunction, or drug ingestion (e.g., alcohol, caffeine). Table 6–8 summarizes conditions of water and solute diuresis that result in polyuria.

Oliguria is a decrease in urine excretion (less than 400 mL/d) that can be caused by simple water deprivation, excessive sweating, diarrhea, or vomiting. Any condition that decreases the blood supply to the kidneys will also result in oliguria and eventually anuria if not corrected. Oliguric urines have an elevated specific gravity (approximately 1.030) as the kidneys maximally excrete solutes into the decreased water available. When plasma protein is lost and water shifts from the intravascular to the extravascular compartment as in conditions of edema, oliguria can result. Oliguria also develops in various renal diseases, ranging from urinary tract obstruction to end-stage renal disease.

T A B L E   6 – 8.   URINE VOLUME TERMS AND CAUSES

TERM	DEFINITION	CAUSES
Polyuria	Urine volume exceeds 3L/d	Water diuresis • Compulsive water intake • Diabetes insipidus • Renal disease • Drugs (e.g., lithium) Solute diuresis • Diabetes mellitus • Renal disease (e.g., salt-losing disorders) • Diuretic therapy, caffeine, alcohol
Oliguria	Urine volume less than 400 mL/d	Decreased renal blood flow • Water deprivation, dehydration • Shock, hypotension Renal disease • Urinary tract obstruction • Renal tubular dysfunction • End-stage renal disease Edema
Anuria	No urine excreted	Acute renal failure • Ischemic causes: shock, heart failure • Nephrotoxic causes: toxic agents, antibiotics Urinary tract obstruction Hemolytic transfusion reactions

Anuria is the complete lack of urine excretion. Anuria is fatal if not immediately addressed because of the accumulation of toxic metabolic by-products in the body. Any condition or disease, chronic or acute, that destroys functioning renal tissue can result in anuria. Principal among these are conditions that decrease the blood supply to renal tissue, such as hypotension, hemorrhage, shock, and heart failure. Toxic chemicals and nephrotoxic antibiotics induce acute tubular necrosis, which results in the loss of functional renal tissue and anuria (or oliguria). In addition, hemolytic transfusion reactions and urinary tract obstructions can also result in anuria.

In conclusion, urine volume measurements are not routinely performed. Although this information can be a valuable diagnostic aid, urine volume is usually determined with a timed urine collection and is used to calculate the concentration of various urine constituents or to assess the kidney's renal function, e.g., the glomerular filtration rate. Chapter 5 discusses renal function and its effect on urine volume. The terms polyuria, oliguria, and anuria are usually assigned based on a patient's health history and on clinical observation rather than on timed urine collections. These urine volume terms, their definitions, and their causes are outlined in Table 6–8.

References

deWardner HE: The Kidney (5th ed.), New York, Churchill Livingstone, 1985, p. 205.

National Committee for Clinical Laboratory Standards: Routine urinalysis. Tentative Guideline. NCCLS Document GP16-T (ISBN 1-56238-183-0), *12*(26):7, 1992.

Schweitzer SC, Schumann JL, Schumann GB: Quality assurance guidelines for the urinalysis laboratory. J Med Tech *3*(11), 569, 1986.

Tietz NW, Pruden EL, Siggaard-Andersen O: Electrolytes, blood gases, and acid-base balance. *In* Tietz NW (ed.), Fundamentals of Clinical Chemistry (3rd ed.), Philadelphia, W. B. Saunders Company, 1987, p. 620.

Study Questions

1. **The color of normal urine is due to the pigment**

   A. bilirubin.
   B. urobilin.
   C. uroerythrin.
   D. urochrome.

2. **A single substance can impart different colors to urine depending on**

   1. the amount of the substance present.
   2. the storage conditions of the urine.
   3. the pH of the urine.
   4. the substance's structural form.

      A. 1, 2, and 3 are correct.
      B. 1 and 2 are correct.
      C. 4 is correct.
      D. All are correct.

3. **Which of the following urine characteristics provides the best rough indicator of urine concentration and body hydration?**

   A. The urine's color
   B. The urine's clarity
   C. The urine's foam
   D. The urine's volume

4. **Which of the following pigments will deposit on urate and uric acid crystals to form a precipitate described as "brick dust"?**

   A. Bilirubin
   B. Urobilin
   C. Uroerythrin
   D. Urochrome

5. **Match the color to the urine pigment/substance. More than one color can be used for a single substance, e.g., 2 and 4.**

Urine Pigment/Substance	Color of Pigment/Substance
_____ A. Bilirubin	1. Colorless
_____ B. Biliverdin	2. Yellow
_____ C. Hemoglobin	3. Orange
_____ D. Myoglobin	4. Red
_____ E. Porphobilin	5. Pink
_____ F. Urobilin	6. Purple
_____ G. Urobilinogen	7. Brown
_____ H. Urochrome	8. Green
_____ I. Uroerythrin	

6. **Which of the following criteria should be used to evaluate urine color and clarity consistently?**

   1. Mix all specimens well.
   2. Use the same depth or volume of a specimen.
   3. Evaluate the specimens at the same temperature.
   4. View the specimens against a dark background with good lighting.

   A. 1, 2, and 3 are correct.
   B. 1 and 2 are correct.
   C. 4 is correct.
   D. All are correct.

7. **Select the urine specimen that does NOT indicate the possible presence of blood or hemoglobin.**

   A. A clear red urine
   B. A cloudy brown urine
   C. A clear brown urine
   D. A cloudy amber urine

8. **A urine that produces a large amount of white foam when mixed should be suspected to contain increased amounts of**

   A. bilirubin.
   B. protein.
   C. urobilin.
   D. urobilinogen.

9. **Which of the following substances will change the color of both the urine and its foam?**

   A. Bilirubin
   B. Hemoglobin
   C. Myoglobin
   D. Urobilin

10. **The clarity of a well-mixed urine specimen that has visible particulate matter and through which newsprint can be seen but not read should be described as**

    A. cloudy.
    B. flocculated.
    C. slightly cloudy.
    D. turbid.

11. **Classify each substance that can be present in urine as indicating a pathologic or nonpathologic condition.**

    Substance

    _____ A. Bacteria (fresh urine)
    _____ B. Bacteria (old urine)
    _____ C. Fat
    _____ D. Powder
    _____ E. Radiographic contrast media
    _____ F. Red blood cells
    _____ G. Renal epithelial cells
    _____ H. Spermatozoa
    _____ I. Squamous epithelial cells
    _____ J. Urate crystals
    _____ K. White blood cells
    _____ L. Yeast

    Condition

    1. Pathologic
    2. Nonpathologic

12. **Which of the following urine specimens is considered normal?**

    A. A freshly voided urine that is brown and clear.
    B. A freshly voided urine that is yellow and cloudy.
    C. A clear yellow urine specimen that changes color upon standing.
    D. A clear yellow urine specimen that becomes cloudy upon refrigeration.

13. **A white precipitate in a normal alkaline urine is most likely caused by**

    A. amorphous phosphates.
    B. amorphous urates.
    C. uric acid crystals.
    D. radiographic contrast media.

14. **Match the urine odor to the condition or substance that can cause it. More than one odor may be selected for a condition, e.g., 1 and 4.**

    Condition/Substance

    _____ A. Diabetes mellitus
    _____ B. Normal urine
    _____ C. Old, improperly stored urine
    _____ D. Specimen adulteration
    _____ E. Starvation
    _____ F. Urinary tract infection

    Urine Odor

    1. Ammonia-like
    2. Bleach
    3. Faintly aromatic
    4. Pungent, fetid
    5. Sweet, fruity

15. **Which of the following methods for determining the urine's specific gravity does NOT detect the presence of urinary protein or glucose?**

    A. The urinometer method
    B. The falling drop method
    C. The refractometer method
    D. The reagent strip method

16. **A small ion and a large uncharged molecule have the same effect when determining urine concentration by the**

    A. urinometer method.
    B. osmolality method.
    C. reagent strip method.
    D. refractometer method.

17. **Which of the following specific gravity values is physiologically impossible?**

    A. 1.000
    B. 1.010
    C. 1.020
    D. 1.030

18. **Match the principle to the specific gravity method. A principle may be used more than once.**

	Specific Gravity Method	Principle of Method
_____ A.	Falling drop	1. Density
_____ B.	Harmonic oscillation densitometry	2. Refractive index
_____ C.	Reagent strip	3. pK$_a$ changes
_____ D.	Refractometry	
_____ E.	Urinometer	

19. **Which of the following methods is an indirect measure of specific gravity?**

    A. The falling drop method
    B. Harmonic oscillation densitometry
    C. Refractometry
    D. The urinometer method

20. **The refractive index of a solution is affected by the**

    1. wavelength of light used.
    2. size and number of the solutes present.
    3. concentration of the solution.
    4. temperature of the solution.

       A. 1, 2, and 3 are correct.
       B. 1 and 2 are correct.
       C. 4 is correct.
       D. All are correct.

21. **Refractometry is preferred for specific gravity measurements because it**

    1. uses a small amount of sample.
    2. is fast and easy to perform.
    3. automatically compensates for temperature.
    4. measures only ionic solutes.

        A. 1, 2, and 3 are correct.
        B. 1 and 2 are correct.
        C. 4 is correct.
        D. All are correct.

22. **The principle of the reagent strip method for measuring specific gravity is based on**

    A. the pK_a of a polyelectrolyte decreasing in proportion to the ionic concentration of the specimen.
    B. the pH of a polyelectrolyte decreasing in proportion to the ionic concentration of the specimen.
    C. the pK_a of a polyelectrolyte increasing in proportion to the ionic concentration of the specimen.
    D. the pH of a polyelectrolyte increasing in proportion to the ionic concentration of the specimen.

23. **Ionic specific gravity (SG_{Ionic}) measurements using reagent strips provide useful clinical information because**

    A. all of the urinary solutes present are measured.
    B. the amount of nonionic solutes in urine relative to ionic solutes is significant.
    C. the excretion of nonionic solutes (e.g., urea, glucose, protein) does not reflect renal dysfunction.
    D. the kidneys' ability to concentrate urine is reflected in the reabsorption and secretion of ionic solutes.

24. **Which of the following as described is NOT a colligative property?**

    A. Boiling point elevation
    B. Freezing point depression
    C. Osmotic pressure depression
    D. Vapor pressure depression

25. **An advantage of freezing point osmometry over vapor pressure osmometry is**

    A. the increased precision of vapor pressure osmometry.
    B. the smaller sample size required for freezing point osmometry.
    C. the ability to detect volatile substances by freezing point osmometry.
    D. the ability to detect solutes based on the number of solutes present regardless of their size or charge.

26. **Osmolality measurements are considered to be a more accurate assessment of solute concentration in body fluids than are specific gravity measurements because**

    A. all solutes contribute equally.
    B. heavy molecules do not interfere.
    C. they are not temperature dependent.
    D. they are less time consuming to perform.

27. **The freezing point of a urine specimen is determined to be $-0.90°C$. What is the specimen's osmolality?**

    A. 161 mOsm/kg
    B. 484 mOsm/kg
    C. 597 mOsm/kg
    D. 645 mOsm/kg

28. **Which of the following will NOT influence the volume of urine produced?**

    A. Diarrhea
    B. Exercise
    C. Caffeine ingestion
    D. Carbohydrate ingestion

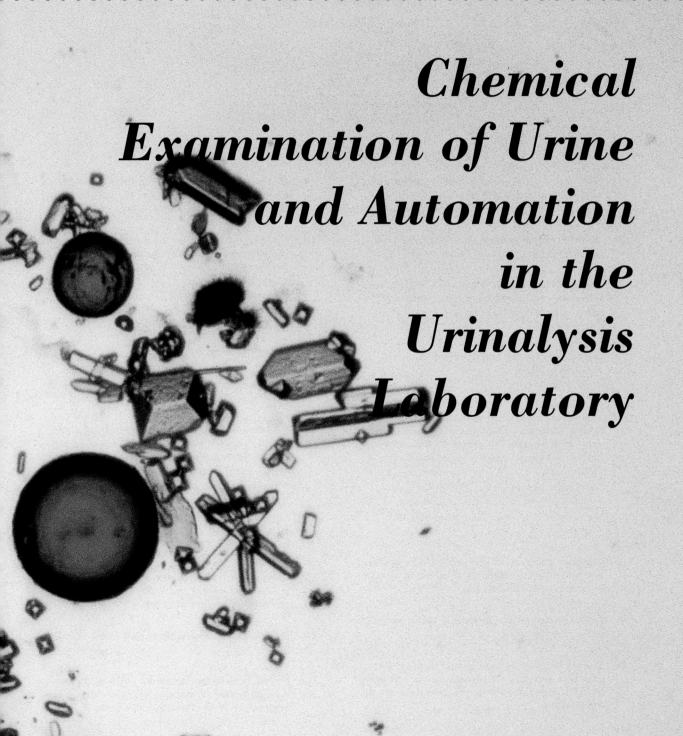

Chemical Examination of Urine and Automation in the Urinalysis Laboratory

Chemical Examination of Urine

Reagent Strips

Tablet and Chemical Tests

Chemical Testing Technique

Chemical Tests

Automation in the Urinalysis Laboratory

Reflectance Photometry

Instrumentation

Urinalysis Workstation

LEARNING OBJECTIVES

After studying this chapter, the student should be able to

1. State the proper care and storage of commercial reagent strip and tablet tests and cite at least three potential causes of their deterioration.

2. Describe quality control procedures for commercial reagent strip and tablet tests.

3. Discuss the appropriate specimen and testing techniques employed when using commercial reagent strip and tablet tests.

4. State the chemical principle employed on reagent strips for the measurement of
   - specific gravity
   - pH

5. Summarize the clinical significance of the following substances when they are found in the urine and describe the chemical principles employed on reagent strips to measure them:
   - blood
   - leukocyte esterase
   - nitrite
   - protein
   - glucose
   - ketones
   - bilirubin
   - urobilinogen
   - ascorbic acid

6. Compare and contrast the sensitivity, specificity, and potential interferences of each commercial reagent strip and tablet test.

7. Differentiate between hematuria and hemoglobinuria.

8. Discuss the clinical significance of myoglobin. Compare and contrast myoglobinuria and hemoglobinuria and describe a protocol for their differentiation.

9. Discuss the limitations of the leukocyte esterase and nitrite reagent strip tests for the detection of leukocyturia and bacteriuria.

10. Compare and contrast the mechanisms for and the clinical significance of the following types of proteinuria:
    - overflow proteinuria
    - glomerular proteinuria
    - postural proteinuria
    - tubular proteinuria
    - postrenal proteinuria

11. Discuss the clinical features of the nephrotic syndrome and Fanconi syndrome, including the specific renal dysfunctions involved.

12. Compare and contrast the chemical principle, sensitivity, and specificity of the following tests for the detection of proteins in the urine:
    - the reagent strip test
    - the sulfosalicylic acid precipitation test
    - the sensitive albumin tests

13. Describe two physiologic mechanisms that result in glucosuria.

14. Compare and contrast the glucose reagent strip test and the copper reduction test for the measurement of sugars in urine.

15. Describe three mechanisms that result in ketonuria.

16. Briefly explain the metabolic pathway that results in ketone formation; state the relative concentrations of the three ketones formed; and

discuss the reagent strip and tablet tests used to detect them.

17. Summarize the formation of bilirubin and urobilinogen, discuss their clinical significance, and describe three physiologic mechanisms that result in altered bilirubin metabolism.

18. Compare and contrast the principle, sensitivity, specificity, and limitations of the following methods for the detection of bilirubin in urine:
    * the physical examination
    * the reagent strip test
    * the tablet test

19. Describe two chemical principles employed on reagent strip tests for the detection of urinary urobilinogen and compare their sensitivity, specificity, and limitations.

20. Summarize the formation of porphobilinogen, discuss its clinical significance, and compare the principle, sensitivity, specificity, and limitations

of the following porphobilinogen screening methods:
    * the physical examination
    * the Hoesch test
    * the Watson-Schwartz test.

21. State the importance of ascorbic acid detection in urine; describe methods used to detect ascorbic acid; identify reagent strip tests that are adversely affected by ascorbic acid; and explain the mechanism of interference in each reagent strip test.

22. Describe the principle of reflectance photometry and briefly discuss the current reflectance photometry instrumentation available (i.e., reflectance photometers and a urinalysis workstation).

23. Identify at least two advantages of using semi-automated reagent strip readers (reflectance photometers).

24. Briefly discuss several advantages and disadvantages of a urinalysis workstation.

- -

KEY TERMS

albuminuria: the increased urinary excretion of the protein albumin.

ascorbic acid (also called **vitamin C**): a water-soluble vitamin; it is a strong reducing agent that readily oxidizes to its salt, dehydroascorbate.

ascorbic acid interference: the inhibition of a chemical reaction by the presence of ascorbic acid. As a strong reducing agent, ascorbic acid readily reacts with diazonium salts or hydrogen peroxide, removing these chemicals from intended reaction sequences. As a result, colorless dehydroascorbate is formed and no color change is observed.

bacteriuria: the presence of bacteria in urine.

bilirubin: a yellow-orange pigment resulting from heme catabolism. It causes a characteristic discoloration of urine, plasma, and other body fluids when present in the fluid in significant amounts. When exposed to air, bilirubin oxidizes to biliverdin, a green pigment.

Ehrlich's reaction: the development of a red- or magenta-colored chromophore as a result of the interaction of a substance (e.g., urobilinogen, porphobilinogen) with *p*-dimethylaminobenzaldehyde (also called Ehrlich's agent) in an acid medium.

Fanconi syndrome: a complication of inherited and acquired diseases characterized by generalized proximal tubular dysfunction, resulting in aminoaciduria, proteinuria, glucosuria, and phosphaturia.

glomerular proteinuria: increased amounts of protein in urine because of a compromised or diseased glomerular filtration barrier.

glucosuria: the presence of glucose in urine.

glycosuria: see **glucosuria.**

hematuria: the presence of red blood cells in urine.

hemoglobinuria: the presence of hemoglobin in urine.

hemosiderin: an insoluble form of storage iron. When renal tubular cells reabsorb hemoglobin, the iron is catabolized into ferritin (a major storage form of iron). Ferritin subsequently denatures to form insoluble hemosiderin granules (micelles of ferric hydroxide) that appear in the urine 2 to 3 days following a hemolytic episode.

hypersthenuric: the excretion of urine having a specific gravity greater than 1.010.

hyposthenuric: the excretion of urine having a specific gravity less than 1.010.

isosthenuria: the excretion of urine having the same specific gravity (and osmolality) as the plasma. Because the specific gravity of protein-free plasma and the original ultrafiltrate is 1.010, the inability to excrete urine with a higher or lower specific gravity indicates significantly impaired renal tubular function.

jaundice: the yellowish pigmentation of skin, sclera, body tissues, and body fluids owing to the presence of increased amounts of bilirubin. Jaundice appears when plasma bilirubin concentrations reach approximately 2 to 3 mg/dL, i.e., two to three times the normal bilirubin levels.

ketonuria: the presence of ketones (i.e., acetoacetate, β-hydroxybutyrate, acetone) in urine.

leukocyturia: the presence of leukocytes, i.e., white blood cells, in the urine. cf. **pyuria.**

myoglobinuria: the presence of myoglobin in urine.

nephrotic syndrome: a complication of numerous disorders characterized by the presentation of proteinuria, hypoalbuminemia, hyperlipidemia, lipiduria, and generalized edema.

overflow proteinuria: an increased amount of protein in urine owing to increased amounts of plasma proteins passing through a healthy glomerular filtration barrier.

porphobilinogen (PBG): an intermediate compound formed in the production of heme and a porphyrin precursor.

porphyrinuria: the presence of an increased amount of porphyrins or porphyrin precursors in urine.

postrenal proteinuria: an increased amount of protein in urine resulting from a disease process that adds protein to urine after its formation by the renal nephrons.

postural (orthostatic) proteinuria: an increased protein excretion in urine only when an individual is in an upright (orthostatic) position.

protein error of indicators: a phenomenon characterized by several pH indicators. These pH indicators undergo a color change in the presence of protein despite a constant pH. Described originally by Sorenson in 1909, the protein error of indicators now provides the basis of the protein screening tests employed on reagent strips.

proteinuria: the presence of an increased amount of protein in urine.

pseudoperoxidase activity: the action of heme-containing compounds (e.g., hemoglobin, myoglobin) to mimic true peroxidases by catalyzing the oxidation of some substrates in the presence of hydrogen peroxide.

pyuria: the presence of pus in urine. cf. **leukocyturia.**

reflectance: the scattering or reflecting of light when it strikes a matte or unpolished surface. The intensity and wavelength of the reflected light will vary depending on the color of the surface and the wavelength of the incident light used.

renal proteinuria: increased amounts of protein in urine as a result of impaired renal function.

tubular proteinuria: increased amounts of protein in urine owing to impaired or altered renal tubular function.

urinary tract infection (UTI): the invasion and proliferation of microorganisms in the kidney or urinary tract.

urobilinogen: a colorless tetrapyrrole derived from bilirubin. It is produced in the intestinal tract by the action of anaerobic bacteria and is later partially reabsorbed. The majority of the reabsorbed urobilinogen is reprocessed by the liver and re-excreted in the bile; the remainder passes to the kidneys for excretion in the urine. The portion of urobilinogen that is not reabsorbed becomes oxidized to the orange-brown pigment urobilin in the large intestine, which accounts for the characteristic color of feces.

Chemical Examination of Urine

Reagent Strips

Commercial reagent strips are currently used routinely for the chemical analysis of urine. Reagent strips provide a means of rapidly screening large numbers of urine specimens in a timely fashion for pH, protein, glucose, ketones, blood, bilirubin, urobilinogen, nitrite, and leukocyte esterase. In addition, specific gravity and ascorbic acid may also be screened by reagent strip depending on the brand of strip used. Three manufacturers of chemical reagent strips are 1) Miles Inc.,

Elkhart, IN, who manufacture Ames Multistix; 2) Boehringer Mannheim Corporation, Indianapolis, IN, who manufacture Chemstrip; and 3) Behring Diagnostics, Inc., Somerville, NJ, who manufacture Rapignost. Each of these products is available with single or multiple test pads on a reagent strip, allowing for flexibility in test selection and cost containment.

A reagent strip is an inert plastic strip onto which reagent-impregnated test pads are bonded (Fig. 7–1). Chemical reactions take place when the strip is wetted in a urine sample. These reactions result in a color change that can be visually or mechanically assessed. By comparing the color change observed to the color chart supplied by the

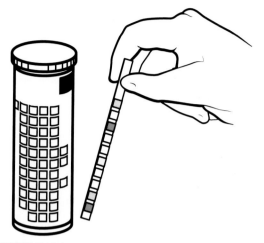

FIGURE 7–1. A commercial reagent strip for urine chemistry testing and its container with the color comparison chart. The reagent impregnated test pads are fixed to an inert plastic strip. Once the strip has been appropriately wetted in a urine sample, a chemical reaction causes the reagent pad to change color. Results are obtained by comparing the color of the reagent pad to the appropriate analyte on the color chart.

strip manufacturer, the laboratorian can determine qualitative results for each entity. Depending on the test performed, the results are reported 1) in concentration (mg/dL); 2) as small, moderate, or large; 3) using the plus system (1+, 2+, 3+, 4+); or 4) as positive, negative, or normal. The specific gravity and pH are exceptions; these results are estimated in their respective units. Manufacturers currently are not consistent in their reporting terminology. For example, Multistix strips report glucose values less than 100 mg/dL as negative, whereas Chemstrip and Rapignost strips report these glucose results as normal. Although these minor inconsistencies may be confusing, the amount present is clinically insignificant. More importantly, the laboratorian must be aware of the chemical principles involved and the specificity and the sensitivity of each test included on the particular reagent strips used in his or her laboratory.

The chemical principles employed on all reagent strips are essentially the same, with manufacturers differing only in the determination of urobilinogen (Table 7–1). Brands of reagent strips do differ, however, in the test or combination of tests available on them.

Only Rapignost strips include one test pad for the detection of ascorbic acid and one to account for urine color (used only when results are read by reflectance photometry). Rapignost strips, however, do not have a test pad for the assessment of specific gravity. Similarly, Chemstrip reagent strips have used iodate on the blood test pad to eliminate ascorbic acid interference; and recently, Multistix strips have been reformulated to reduce this interference. Because reducing agents such as ascorbic acid can adversely affect various reagent strip test results, it is important that this and other potential interferences be detected or eliminated. The presence of interferences must be known to enable alternative testing, if possible, or appropriate modification of the results reported. Common interferences encountered in the chemical examination of urine and the impact these interferences have on urinalysis results are discussed with each specific reagent strip test in this chapter.

Care and Storage

Chemical reagent strips or dipsticks are examples of "state-of-the-art" technology. Prior to the development of the first dry chemical dipstick test for glucose in the 1950s, all chemical tests were performed individually in test tubes. Reagent strips have significantly reduced the time required for testing and have reduced costs (e.g., reagents and personnel); enhanced test sensitivity and specificity; and reduced the amount of sample required for testing.

To ensure the integrity of reagent strips, their proper storage is essential, and the manufacturer's directions should be followed. Each manufacturer provides a comprehensive product insert that outlines the product's chemical principle, reagents, storage, use, sensitivity, specificity, and limitations. All reagent strips must be protected from moisture, chemicals, heat, and light. Any strips showing evidence of deterioration, contamination, or improper storage should be discarded. Tight-fitting lids, along with desiccants or drying agents within the product container, help eliminate reagent strip pad

T A B L E 7 – 1.   THE COMPARISON OF REAGENT STRIP PRINCIPLES

TEST	PRINCIPLE

Specific gravity	Ionic solutes present in the urine cause protons to be released from a polyelectrolyte. As the protons are released, the pH decreases and produces a color change of the bromthymol blue indicator from blue-green to yellow-green.
	BMC Chemstrip and Ames Multistix reagent strips only
	Polyelectrolyte used:
	    Chemstrip: ethyleneglycol-bis tetra-acetic acid
	    Multistix: polymethylvinyl ether/maleic acid

pH	Double indicator system. Indicator's methyl red and bromthymol blue are used to give distinct color changes from orange to green to blue (pH 5.0 to 9.0)
Blood	Pseudoperoxidase activity of the heme moiety. The chromogen reacts with a peroxide in the presence of hemoglobin or myoglobin to become oxidized and produce a color change from yellow to green. Chromogen used: tetramethylbenzidine

Leukocyte esterase	Action of leukocyte esterases to cleave an ester and form an aromatic compound. It is followed by an azo-coupling reaction of the aromatic amine formed with a diazonium salt on the reagent pad. The azo-dye produced causes a color change from beige to violet.
	Ester used:
	    Chemstrip and Rapignost: indoxylcarbonic acid ester
	    Multistix: derivatized pyrrole amino acid ester

Nitrite	Diazotization reaction of nitrite with an aromatic amine to produce a diazonium salt. It is followed by an azo-coupling reaction of this diazonium salt with an aromatic compound on the reagent pad. The azodye produced causes a color change from white to pink.
	Amine used:
	    Chemstrip: sulfanilamide
	    Multistix and Rapignost: *p*-arsanilic acid
	Aromatic compound:
	    Chemstrip and Multistix: tetrahydrobenzoquinolinol
	    Rapignost: naphthylethylenediamine

Protein	Protein "error of indicators." When the pH is held constant by a buffer (pH 3.0), indicator dyes release H^+ ions because of the protein present. Color changes range from yellow to blue-green. Indicator used: derivatives of tetrabromphenol blue

Glucose	Double-sequential enzyme reaction. Glucose oxidase on reagent pad catalyzes the oxidation of glucose to form hydrogen peroxide. The hydrogen peroxide formed in the first reaction oxidizes a chromogen on the reagent pad. The second reaction is catalyzed by a peroxidase provided on the pad. The color change differs with the chromogen used.
	Chromogen used:
	    Chemstrip: tetramethylbenzidine
	    Multistix: potassium iodide
	    Rapignost: tolidine hydrochloride

Ketones	Legal's test—nitroprusside reaction. Acetoacetic acid in an alkaline medium reacts with nitroferricyanide to produce a color change from beige to purple. The Chemstrip and Rapignost reagent strips include glycine in the reagent pad for the reaction and the detection of acetone. Multistix strips without glycine; Chemstrip and Rapignost strips with glycine

Bilirubin	Azo-coupling reaction of bilirubin with a diazonium salt in an acid medium to form an azodye. Color changes from light tan to beige or light pink are observed.
	Diazonium salt used:
	    Chemstrip: 2,6-dichlorobenzene diazonium tetrafluoroborate
	    Multistix: 2,4-dichloroaniline diazonium salt
	    Rapignost: 2,4-dichlorobenzene diazonium tetrafluoroborate

Urobilinogen	**Chemistrip and Rapignost strips: Azo-coupling reaction of urobilinogen with a diazonium salt in an acid medium to form an azodye. Color changes from light pink to dark pink are observed.**
	Diazonium salt used:
	    Chemstrip: 4-methoxybenzene-diazonium-fluoroborate
	    Rapignost: 3,2-dinitro-4-fluoro-4′-diazonium-diphenylamine tetrafluoroborate

T A B L E 7 – 1.   THE COMPARISON OF REAGENT STRIP PRINCIPLES *Continued*

TEST	PRINCIPLE
	Multistix strips: Modified Ehrlich's reaction. Urobilinogen present reacts with Ehrlich's reagent (*p*-dimethylaminobenzaldehyde) to form a red-colored compound. Color changes from light orange-pink to dark pink are observed.
Ascorbic acid	Ascorbic acid present reduces a dye impregnated in the reagent pad, causing a color change from blue to orange. Dye used: Rapignost: 2,6-dichlorophenolindophenol

deterioration resulting from moisture. Fumes from volatile chemicals, both acid and alkaline, can adversely affect the reagent test pads and should be avoided. All reagent strip containers protect the reagent strips from ultraviolet rays and sunlight; however, the containers themselves must be protected to prevent the fading of the color chart located on the outside of the container. Reagent strips should be stored at temperatures below 30°C (86°F) in their original containers; they are stable until the expiration date indicated on the label. To ensure accurate test results, all reagent strips—whether from a newly opened container or from one that has been opened for several months—must be tested daily using appropriate control materials.

Quality Control Testing

Quality control testing of reagent strips not only ensures that the reagent strips are functioning properly, but also confirms the acceptable performance and technique of the laboratorian using them. Multiconstituent controls at two distinct levels (e.g., negative, positive) for each test must be used to check the reagent strips daily. New containers or lot numbers of reagent strips must be checked when opened and daily thereafter.

Distilled water and commercial or laboratory-prepared materials can serve as acceptable negative controls. Similarly, positive controls can be purchased commercially or prepared by the laboratory. Because of the time and care involved in making a multiconstituent control material that tests each parameter on the reagent strip, most laboratories purchase control materials. Acceptable

test performance is indicated if the observed reaction is within one color block of the assigned target value. Negative results are acceptable only with the negative control material (NCCLS, 1992). Regardless of the control material used, care must be taken to ensure that the materials are within the critical detection levels for each parameter. For example, a protein control concentration of 1 g/dL far exceeds the desired critical detection level of 10 to 15 mg/dL and would be inappropriate as a control material.

An additional check on the precision of the chemical and microscopic examinations and on the procedural process used involves aliquoting a well-mixed specimen from the daily workload and having any ancillary testing laboratories (interlaboratory), or a technologist on each shift (intralaboratory), analyze the specimen. Interlaboratory duplicate testing checks the entire urinalysis procedure and detects such innocuous changes as variations in the speed of centrifugation and in centrifuge brake usage. Intralaboratory duplicate testing primarily monitors the precision among laboratorians from different shifts, assuming that the reagents, the supplies, and the equipment adjustments are maintained at the appropriate level.

Tablet and Chemical Tests

Care and Storage

Commercial tablet tests (e.g., Ictotest, Clinitest, Acetest) must be handled and stored according to the inserts provided by the manufacturers. These products are susceptible to deterioration owing to exposure to light, heat, and moisture. Hence, commercial tablets should be inspected before each use and discarded if any of the following changes are noted: tablet discoloration, contamination, incorrect storage or spoilage, or a past due expiration date. The stability of the tablets can decrease after opening because of repeated exposure to atmospheric moisture; therefore, the tablets should not be stored for an extended period of time. To ensure tablet integrity, an appropriate quality control program must be employed.

Chemical tests such as the sulfosalicylic acid precipitation test (SSA), the Hoesch test, the Watson-Schwartz test, or any other test performed requires "fresh," appropriately made and tested reagents. When new reagents are prepared they should be tested in parallel with the old reagents to ensure equivalent performance. Chemical tests must also be checked daily according to a quality control program to ensure the reliability and reproducibility of the test results obtained.

Quality Control Testing

As with reagent strips, tablet or chemical tests performed in the urinalysis laboratory must have quality control materials run to ensure the integrity of the reagents and the technique used in testing. Some commercial controls for reagent strips can also be used to check the integrity of the Clinitest, Ictotest, and Acetest tablets. In addition, lyophilized chemistry controls or "laboratory-made" control materials can be used. For example, a chemistry albumin standard at an appropriate concentration (approximately 30 to 100 mg/dL) provides a satisfactory control for the performance of the SSA protein precipitation test.

Quality control materials, both positive and negative, must be run daily with these tests. New tablets and reagents must be checked before being placed into use, and according to the daily protocol thereafter.

Chemical Testing Technique

Reagent Strips

Although reagent strips are easy to use, proper technique is imperative to ensure ac-

curate test results. The manufacturer's instructions provided with the reagent strips and the tablet tests should be followed; these instructions can vary among different manufacturers and among the products themselves. Because technology is always advancing and changing, the inserts from new lots of strips received must be checked for any procedural changes. Table 7–2 summarizes the reagent strip testing technique that should be used.

A fresh, well-mixed, uncentrifuged specimen should be used for testing. It should be at room temperature and tested less than 2 hours after collection. The specimen may be tested in the original collection container or after pouring an aliquot into a labeled centrifuge tube. The laboratorian should dip the reagent strip *briefly* into the urine specimen, wetting all test pads. Excess urine should be drained from the strip by drawing the edge of the strip along the rim of the container or by placing the strip edge on an absorbent paper. Inadequate removal of excess urine from the strip can cause contamination of one test pad with the reagents from another, whereas prolonged dipping of the strip in the specimen causes the chemicals to leach from the test pad into the specimen. Both of these actions can produce erroneous test results.

The time required before full color development and reading of the reaction varies with each test parameter on the reagent strip. To obtain reproducible and reliable results, the timing instructions provided by the

T A B L E 7–2. THE SUMMARY OF REAGENT STRIP TESTING TECHNIQUE

Use a well-mixed, uncentrifuged urine specimen at room temperature and less than 2 hours old.

Dip the reagent strip *briefly* into the specimen.

Remove excess urine by running the edge of the strip along the rim of the container or placing the edge of the strip on absorbent paper.

Time according to manufacturer's recommendations using a timing device with a second hand.

Read color reactions visually with the pad placed close to the color chart in a well-lit area.

Know the sensitivity, specificity, and interferences for each test.

manufacturer must be followed. These timing intervals can differ among reagent strips from the same manufacturer and among different manufacturers of the same test. For example, when using the Ames Multistix strips, the ketone test pad is read at 40 seconds; however, when using Ames Ketostix strips, the test area is read at 15 seconds. Some reagent strips have the flexibility of reading all test pads, except leukocytes, at any time between 60 and 120 seconds (e.g., Rapignost and Chemstrip strips), whereas others require the exact timing of each test pad for semiquantitated results (e.g., Multistix strips).

The visual interpretation of color varies slightly among individuals; therefore, reagent strips should be read in a well-lit area with the strip held close to the color chart on the strip container. The strip must be properly oriented to the chart before the laboratorian reads the results. Because of similar color changes by several of the test pads, improper orientation of the strip to the color chart is a potential source of error. Those color changes that appear only along the edge of the reaction pad or after 2 minutes are diagnostically insignificant and should be disregarded. When reagent strips are read by automated instruments, the timing intervals are set by the factory. The advantage of the automated instruments in reading reagent strips is their consistency in timing and color interpretation regardless of the room lighting or testing personnel. Some instruments, however, are unable to identify and compensate for urines that are highly pigmented because of medications; false positive reagent strip test results follow because of the masking of the "true" color reaction by a drug pigment. Highly pigmented urine specimens must be identified by the laboratorian and manually tested using reagent strips or alternative methods. Table 7–3 summarizes the sensitivity and specificity of three brands of commercial reagent strips.

Tablet and Chemical Tests

No standard technique encompasses the performance of all tablet and chemistry tests performed in the urinalysis laboratory. With each test, the manufacturer's directions must be followed exactly to ensure reproducible and reliable results. All chemical tests, such as the SSA precipitation test for protein or the Watson-Schwartz test for urobilinogen and porphobilinogen, must be performed according to established written laboratory procedures. As with reagent strips, the laboratorian must know the sensitivity, specificity, and potential interferences for each test. Chemical and tablet tests are generally performed 1) to confirm results already obtained by the reagent strip test, 2) as alternative testing methods for highly pigmented urines; 3) because they are more sensitive for the substance of interest than the reagent strip test (e.g., Ictotest tablets); or 4) because the specificity of the test differs from the specificity of the reagent strip test (e.g., SSA test, Hoesch test).

Chemical Tests

Specific Gravity

Specific gravity is a physical property of urine and an expression of concentration. It is discussed at length in Chapters 5 and 6. It is briefly included here because the reagent strip methodology available is actually a chemical means of indirectly determining specific gravity.

CLINICAL SIGNIFICANCE. The ultrafiltrate entering Bowman's space in the glomerulus has the same specific gravity as protein-free plasma (i.e., 1.010). As this ultrafiltrate passes through the nephron, solutes and water are selectively absorbed and secreted. If the tubules are unable to perform these functions, the specific gravity of the urine excreted will be identical to that of the original ultrafiltrate. This condition, termed **isosthenuria,** implies significant renal tubular dysfunction. Patients exhibiting this condition—a fixed specific gravity of 1.010, regardless of hydration—also experience nocturia because the kidneys are unable to selectively retain solutes and water adequately. Urine specimens with a specific gravity below 1.010 can be termed **hyposthenuric,** whereas those with a specific gravity above 1.010 are termed **hypersthe-**

TEST	SENSITIVITY	SPECIFICITY
Specific gravity	Chemstrip: 1.000 to 1.030 Multistix: 1.000 to 1.030	Detects only ionic solutes *Falsely low* owing to: • glucose and urea concentrations > 10 g/dL • a pH ≥ 6.5; add 0.005 *Falsely high* owing to: • protein approximately equal to 100 to 500 mg/dL • ketoacids: lactic acid, ketones, etc.
pH	Chemstrip: 5.0 to 9.0, in 1.0 pH increments Multistix: 5.0 to 8.5, in 0.5 pH increments Rapignost: 5.0 to 9.0, in 1.0 pH increments	pH; hydrogen ion concentration No interferences known; unaffected by protein concentration
Blood	Chemstrip: 0.02 to 0.03 mg/dL Hgb (5 to 10 RBCs/μL) Multistix: 0.02 to 0.06 mg/dL Hgb (6 to 20 RBCs/μL) Rapignost: 0.02 to 0.03 mg/dL Hgb (5 to 10 RBCs/μL)	Equally specific for hemoglobin and myoglobin Intact RBCs are lysed on reagent pad *False positive* results owing to: • menstrual contamination • microbial peroxidases • strong oxidizing agents *False negative* results owing to: • ascorbic acid with Multistix "new formulation" (≥ 9 mg/dL); with Rapignost (≥ 5 mg/dL); Chemstrip unaffected • high nitrite (≥ 10 mg/dL) reduces strip reactivity
Leukocyte esterase	Chemstrip: approximately 10 WBCs/μL Multistix: approximately 5 to 15 WBCs/per high-power field (~10 to 25 WBCs/μL) Rapignost: approximately 20 WBCs/μL in 90% of urines tested	Detects only granulocytic leukocytes *False positive* results owing to: • substances that induce color mask results, e.g., drugs (phenzopyridine), beet ingestion • vaginal contamination of urine *False negative* results owing to: • lymphocytes present are not detected • increased glucose (> 3 g/dL), protein (> 500 mg/dL) • high specific gravity • strong oxidizing agents • drugs, e.g., gentamicin, cephalosporins
Nitrite	Chemstrip: 0.05 mg/dL nitrite ion in 90% of urines tested Multistix: 0.06 mg/dL nitrite ion Rapignost: 0.05 mg/dL nitrite ion in 90% of urines tested	*False positive* results owing to: • substances that induce color mask results, e.g., drugs (phenazopyridine), beet ingestion • improper storage with bacterial proliferation *False negative* results owing to: • ascorbic acid (≥ 25 mg/dL) interference • various factors that inhibit or prevent nitrite formation despite bacteriuria
Protein	Chemstrip: 6.0 mg/dL in 90% of urines tested Multistix: 15 to 30 mg/dL Rapignost: 15 mg/dL in 90% of urines tested	More sensitive to albumin than globulins, hemoglobin, myoglobin, Bence Jones proteins, mucoproteins, or others *False positive* results owing to: • highly buffered or alkaline urine ($\geq$ pH 9): e.g., alkaline drugs, improperly preserved specimen, contamination with quaternary ammonium compounds *False negative* results owing to: • presence of protein other than albumin

TABLE 7–3.   A COMPARISON OF THE SENSITIVITY AND SPECIFICITY OF REAGENT STRIPS *Continued*

TEST	SENSITIVITY	SPECIFICITY
		• substances that induce color mask results, e.g., drugs (phenazopyridine), beet ingestion
Glucose	Chemstrip: 40 mg/dL, in 90% of urines tested Multistix: 75 to 125 mg/dL Rapignost: 45 mg/dL in 90% of urines tested	Specific for glucose Affected by high specific gravity and low temperatures *False positive* results owing to: • strong oxidizing agents, e.g., bleach • peroxide contaminants *False negative* results owing to: • ascorbic acid (≥ 50 mg/dL) • improperly stored specimens, i.e., glycolysis
Ketones	Chemstrip: 9.0 mg/dL acetoacetate and 70 mg/dL acetone, in 90% of urines tested Multistix: 5.0 to 10 mg/dL acetoacetate Rapignost: 8.0 mg/dL acetoacetate and 50 mg/dL acetone, in 90% of urines tested	Does not detect β-hydroxybutyrate *False positive* results owing to: • compounds containing free-sulfhydryl groups, e.g., MESNA, captopril, *N*-acetylcysteine • highly pigmented urines • atypical colors with phenylketones and phthaleins • large amounts of levodopa metabolites *False negative* results owing to: • improper storage, i.e., volatilization and bacterial breakdown
Bilirubin	Chemstrip: 0.5 mg/dL conjugated biliubin in 90% of urines tested Multistix: 0.4 to 0.8 mg/dL conjugated bilirubin Rapignost: 0.5 mg/dL conjugated bilirubin in 90% of urines tested	*False positive* results owing to: • drug induced color changes, e.g., phenazopyridine, indican-indoxyl sulfate • large amounts of chlorpromazine metabolites *False negative* results owing to: • ascorbic acid (≥ 25 mg/dL) • high nitrite concentrations • improper storage, i.e., oxidation or hydrolysis to nonreactive biliverdin and free bilirubin
Urobilinogen	Chemstrip: 0.4 mg/dL urobilinogen Multistix: 0.2 mg/dL urobilinogen Rapignost: 1.0 mg/dL urobilinogen	The total absence of urobilinogen cannot be determined. Reactivity increases with temperature, optimum 22–26°C *False positive* results owing to: Multistix: • any other Ehrlich-reactive substance • atypical colors owing to sulfonamides, *p*-aminobenzoic acid, *p*-aminosalicylic acid • substances that induce color mask results, e.g., drugs (phenazopyridine), beet ingestion Chemstrip and Rapignost: • substances that induce color mask results, e.g., drugs (phenazopyridine), beet ingestion *False negative* results owing to: • formalin (> 200 mg/dL), a urine preservative • improper storage, i.e., oxidation to urobilin
Ascorbic acid	Rapignost: 20 mg/dL, in 90% of urines tested	No interferences known; however, substances with similar redox potentials could cause false positive results

nuric. These terms are simply descriptive and, unlike isosthenuria, do not imply renal dysfunction.

The kidneys excrete the solutes necessary in the water that is not needed by the body. Because solute and water intake varies, so does the urine's specific gravity. Normally, the urine's specific gravity ranges from 1.002 to 1.035. Values below or above this range require further investigation, because it is physiologically impossible to produce a urine with a specific gravity equal to 1.000 or one greater than approximately 1.040. Specimens with values of approximately 1.000 should be checked by a second method; the laboratorian can also confirm that the specimen is actually urine by performing a creatinine or urea determination. In addition, the laboratorian should verify that the appropriate quality control materials have been performed and documented to ensure the functional integrity of the results obtained. Extremely high specific gravity specimens of 1.040 or more may occur because of the excretion of radiographic contrast media or mannitol. In these cases, the urine concentration can be accurately assessed by osmometry or by using the specific gravity reagent strip method.

Despite a full range of possible values, the specific gravities of the majority of random urine specimens vary between 1.015 and 1.025. During excessive sweating, dehydration, or fluid restriction, urine specific gravity values usually exceed 1.025.

PRINCIPLE. Both Miles, Inc. and Boehringer Mannheim Corporation offer a reagent strip chemistry test for specific gravity, whereas Behring Diagnostics, Inc. does not. Some disagreement surrounds the use of determining specific gravity (SG) by the reagent strip method because it does not measure the "true" or total solute content but only those solutes that are ionic (SG_{ionic}). It is only these ionic solutes, however, that reflect the renal concentrating and secreting ability of the kidneys and are therefore of diagnostic value. Because of the diversity in methods available for measuring specific gravity and for detecting and measuring solutes, it is imperative that healthcare providers are in-

formed of the test method employed in their laboratory and its principle, sensitivity, specificity, and limitations. All methods available for specific gravity determination are discussed at length in Chapter 6 and summarized in Table 6–7. For a brief summary of the reagent strip principle, refer to Table 7–1.

pH

CLINICAL SIGNIFICANCE. The kidneys play a major role in the regulation of the acid-base balance of the body, as discussed in Chapter 4. The renal system, the pulmonary system, and blood buffers provide the means for maintaining homeostasis at a pH compatible with life. Endogenous acids and bases are generated daily as a result of normal metabolism; in response, the kidneys selectively excrete acid or alkali. Normally, the urine pH varies from 4.5 to 8.0. The average individual excretes a slightly acidic urine of pH 5.0 to 6.0 because endogenous acid production predominates. During and after a meal, however, the stomach secretes acid to aid in digestion; this makes the urine less acidic, or alkaline. This observation is known as the "alkaline tide."

pH values above 8.0 or below 4.5 are physiologically impossible, are not represented on commercial reagent strips, and require investigation if obtained. Most often when the pH is greater than 8.0, the specimen has been improperly preserved and stored, resulting in the proliferation of urease-producing bacteria.

Because the kidneys constantly maintain the acid-base balance of the body, the ingestion of acids or alkali or any condition that produces acids or alkali will directly affect the urine pH. Table 7–4 lists several of the common causes of an acidic and an alkaline urine. This ability of the kidneys to manipulate the urinary pH has many applications. An acidic urine prevents the formation of alkaline renal stones (e.g., calcium carbonate or calcium phosphate) and inhibits the development of urinary tract infections. An alkaline urine prevents the precipitation of and enhances the excretion of various drugs (e.g.,

TABLE 7–4. COMMON CAUSES OF ACID AND ALKALINE URINE

ACID URINE	ALKALINE URINE
Diet	Diet
Protein diet	Vegetarian diet
Cranberry ingestion	Low-carbohydrate diet
	Citrus fruits
Sleep	
	Metabolic alkalosis
Metabolic alkalosis	Vomiting
Diabetic ketoacidosis	Gastric lavage
Starvation	
Severe diarrhea	Respiratory alkalosis
Uremia	Hyperventilation
Poisons (e.g., ethylene glycol,	
methanol)	Renal disease
	UTI—urease producing bacteria, e.g.,
Respiratory acidosis	*Proteus* sp., *Pseudomonas* sp.
Emphysema	Renal tubular acidosis (RTA)
Chronic respiratory diseases	
	Medications used to induce
Renal disease	Sodium bicarbonate
UTI—acid producing bacteria,	Potassium citrate
e.g., *Escherichia coli*	Acetazolamide
Chronic renal failure	
Medications used to induce	
Ammonium chloride	
Ascorbic acid	
Methionine	
Mandelic acid	

sulfonamide, streptomycin, salicylate) and prevents stone formation from calcium oxalate, uric acid, and cystine crystals.

The urinary pH provides valuable information for assessing and managing disease and determining the suitability of a specimen for chemical testing. Correlating the urinary pH with a patient's condition aids in the diagnosis of disease (e.g., production of an alkaline urine despite a metabolic acidosis is characteristic of renal tubular acidosis). Individuals with a history of stone formation can monitor their urinary pH and use this information to modify their diets if necessary. Highly alkaline urine of pH 8.0 to 9.0 can also interfere with chemical testing, particularly in protein determination.

METHODOLOGIES

Reagent Strip. All commercial reagent strips, regardless of the manufacturer, are based on a double-indicator system using bromthymol blue and methyl red. This indicator combination produces distinctive color changes from orange (pH 5.0) to green (pH 7.0) to blue (pH 9.0).

(7–1)

$$\text{Ind}^- + \text{H}^+ \text{ ions} \longrightarrow \text{H} - \text{Ind}$$

Indicator dyes   Reduced dye
(yellow)   (green to blue)

The range provided on the strips is from pH 5.0 to pH 9.0 in either 0.5 or 1.0 pH increments, depending on the manufacturer. No interferences with test results are known, and the results are not affected by protein concentration. However, erroneous results can occur from pH changes caused by 1) improper storage of the specimen with bacterial proliferation (a falsely increased pH); 2) contamination of the specimen container prior to collection (a falsely increased or decreased pH depending on the agent); or 3) improper reagent strip technique, causing the acid buffer from the protein test pad to contaminate the pH test area (a falsely decreased pH).

pH Meter. Although the accuracy provided by a pH meter is not usually necessary, a pH meter is an alternative method for determining the urine pH. Various pH meters are available; the manufacturer's operating instructions supplied with the instrument must be followed to ensure its proper usage and valid results. Nevertheless, the components involved in and the principle behind all pH meters are basically the same.

A pH meter consists of a silver-silver chloride indicator electrode with a pH-sensitive glass membrane connected by a salt bridge to a reference electrode (usually a calomel electrode, $Hg-Hg_2Cl_2$). When the indicator electrode is placed in urine, a difference in the H^+ activity develops across the glass membrane. This causes a change in the potential difference between the indicator and the reference electrodes. This voltage difference is registered by a voltmeter and converted to a pH reading. Because pH measurement is temperature dependent and pH decreases with increasing temperature, it is necessary that pH measurements be adjusted for the temperature of the urine when it is measured. Newer pH meters perform this temperature compensation automatically.

A pH meter is calibrated using two or three commercially available standard buffer solutions. Accurate pH measurements require that accurate standardization of the pH meter, using at least two different standards in the pH range of the test solution, is performed; that the pH-sensitive glass is adequately cleaned and maintained to prevent protein build-up or bacterial growth; and that an adjustment for the temperature of the test solution is made either manually or automatically.

pH Test Papers. Various indicator papers are available with different pH ranges and sensitivities. Micro Essentials Laboratory, Whatman, Inc., and EM Science manufacture comparable products readily available from medical product distributors. The indicator papers will not add impurities to the urine and will produce sharp color changes for

comparison to the supplied color chart of pH values.

Blood

CLINICAL SIGNIFICANCE. As discussed in Chapter 6, blood present in the urine can either result in various presentations of color or not be visually evident at all. Historically, either color and clarity or microscopic viewing was used to indicate the presence of blood in the urine. Chemical methods now provide a rapid and sensitive means for detecting blood's presence. Blood can enter the urinary tract anywhere from the glomeruli to the urethra or it can actually be a contaminant in the urine resulting from the collection procedure. Red blood cells readily lyse in alkaline or dilute urine (with a specific gravity of 1.010 or less) and release their hemoglobin. Without the current chemical means available, the presence of hemoglobin would go undetected. True hemoglobinuria—free hemoglobin directly passing the glomeruli into the ultrafiltrate—is uncommon. Most often, intact red blood cells enter the urinary tract and undergo various amounts of lysis. **Hematuria** is the term used to describe an abnormal amount of red blood cells in the urine; whereas **hemoglobinuria** indicates the urinary presence of hemoglobin.

Because even small increases in the amount of red blood cells in urine is diagnostically significant, chemical methods available detect the presence of the heme moiety. Whether red blood cells are intact or lysed, these sensitive chemical methods will detect their presence. However, other substances also contain heme groups, particularly myoglobin (MW 17,000), which readily passes the glomerular filtration barrier and is increased when muscle is damaged by trauma or disease. As a result, a positive chemical test for blood indicates the presence of red blood cells, hemoglobin, or myoglobin. Whether one of these three substances or all are present requires confirmation and differentiation. Correlation with the urine microscopic results, the appearance of the patient's plasma, and the results of plasma chemical tests may be necessary to confirm which substances are present.

Hematuria and Hemoglobinuria. A distinguishing feature between hematuria and hemoglobinuria is the clarity of the urine. Hematuria often presents with a cloudy or smoky urine specimen, whereas the urine is clear with true hemoglobinuria. The urine colors for both are similar, and color variations range from normal yellow to pink, red, or brown, depending on the amount of blood or hemoglobin present. In addition, the appearance of these specimens is affected by the urines' pH. An alkaline urine promotes red blood cell lysis and hemoglobin oxidation.

Numerous diseases of the kidneys or urinary tract, as well as trauma, drug therapy, or strenuous exercise, can result in hematuria and hemoglobinuria (Table 7–5). The detection of hematuria or hemoglobinuria is an early indicator of disease that is not always evident visually and always requires further investigation. The amount of blood present in a urine specimen has no correlation with disease severity, nor can the amount of blood alone identify the location of the bleed. In combination with a microscopic examination, however, glomerular or tubular origin can be indicated by the presence of red blood cells in casts.

As stated before, true hemoglobinuria is uncommon. Any condition resulting in intravascular hemolysis has the potential of producing hemoglobinuria. Free hemoglobin in the blood is rapidly bound by plasma haptoglobin, however. This hemoglobin-haptoglobin complex is too large to pass through the glomerular filtration barrier, so it remains in the bloodstream and is removed from the circulation by the liver and metabolized. If all available haptoglobin is bound, any additional free hemoglobin will readily pass through the glomeruli with the ultrafiltrate. As dissociated $\alpha\beta$ dimers (with a MW of approximately 38,000), hemoglobin is reabsorbed principally by the proximal renal tubules and catabolized to ferritin. The ferritin is denatured to form **hemosiderin,** a storage form of iron, that is insoluble in aqueous solutions. Hemosiderin usually appears in the urine 2 to 3 days following a hemolytic episode. It appears as yellow-brown granules in sloughed tubular cells, free-floating granules, or casts. A Prussian blue staining test (Rous test) performed on a concentrated urinary sediment aids in the visualization and identification of hemosiderin. The presence of urinary hemosiderin is intermittent and should not be solely relied on to confirm a hemolytic episode or the presence of a chronic hemolytic condition. Table 7–6 compares the urine and plasma values for

TABLE 7–5. CAUSES OF HEMATURIA, HEMOGLOBINURIA, AND MYOGLOBINURIA

Hematuria
  Renal and urinary tract disease, e.g., glomerulonephritis, pyelonephritis, cystitis, calculi, tumors
  Extrarenal disease, e.g., malignant hypertension, malaria, acute febrile episodes, appendicitis, tumors
  Trauma
  Strenuous exercise, e.g., marathon running
  Drugs, e.g., anticoagulants, cyclophosphamide
Hemoglobinuria
  Intravascular hemolysis, e.g., transfusion reactions, hemolytic anemia, paroxysmal nocturnal hemoglobinuria
  Extensive burns
  Strenuous exercise, e.g., marching, karate
  Infections, e.g., syphilis, mycoplasma
Myoglobinuria
  Skeletal or cardiac muscle injury owing to crushing injury, surgery, ischemia, burns
  Seizures
  Toxins, e.g., heroin, animal venoms
  Metabolic, e.g., alcoholic myopathy, carbon monoxide
  Polymyositis and dermatomyositis
  Severe exercise

TABLE 7–6.   COMPARISON OF SELECTED URINE AND PLASMA COMPONENTS IN MILD AND SEVERE HEMOLYTIC EPISODES

| TEST | NORMAL VALUES | INTRAVASCULAR HEMOLYSIS | |
		Mild (chronic)	Severe (acute)
Urine			
Bilirubin (conjugated)	Absent	Absent	Absent
(unconjugated)	Absent	Absent	Absent
Urobilinogen	Normal (≤ 1.0 mg/dL)	Normal to increased	Increased
Blood (hemoglobin)	Absent	Absent	Present
Hemosiderin	Absent	Absent	Present
Plasma			
Bilirubin (conjugated)	up to 0.2 mg/dL	Normal	Normal
(unconjugated)	0.8 to 1.0 mg/dL	Increased	Increased
Haptoglobin	83 to 267 mg/dL	Decreased	Absent
Free hemoglobin	1.0 to 5.0 mg/dL	Normal	Increased

Brunzel, 1990.

various analytes during chronic and acute hemolytic episodes.

Myoglobinuria. Myoglobin is a monomeric heme-containing protein involved in the transport of oxygen in muscles. When skeletal or cardiac muscle is damaged as a result of a crushing injury, vigorous physical exercise, or ischemia, myoglobin is released into the blood. Because of its small molecular size (MW 17,000), myoglobin readily passes the glomerular filtration barrier and is reabsorbed by the proximal tubules. Nontraumatic disorders such as alcohol overdose, toxin ingestion, or certain metabolic disorders can result in myoglobinuria (see Table 7–5). In fact, nontraumatic **myoglobinuria** with acute renal failure is relatively common in patients with an alcohol overdose or a history of cocaine or heroin addiction (Shihabi, 1989). Myoglobinuria may be obvious based on the patient's medical history and presenting symptoms such as a crushing injury; however, nontraumatic rhabdomyolysis (muscle damage) has vague symptoms (nausea, weakness, swollen, tender muscles) and often requires chemical analysis to diagnose.

Differentiation of Hemoglobinuria and Myoglobinuria. Myoglobin appears to be more toxic to renal tubules than hemoglobin is. The reason for this is unclear but may be related to their difference in glomerular clearance and to other factors such as hydra-

tion, hypotension, and aciduria. Differentiating between hemoglobinuria and myoglobinuria can be difficult, but it is important for diagnosis, for predicting the patient's risk for acute renal failure, and for treatment.

Visual inspection of the urine and plasma can help distinguish between hemoglobinuria and myoglobinuria, but these gross observations are of limited value. Hemoglobinuria causes either a red or brown urine, whereas myoglobinuria causes a brown urine. Hemoglobin is not cleared as rapidly from the plasma as myoglobin; therefore, with hemoglobinuria, the plasma often shows various degrees of hemolysis. In contrast, myoglobin is rapidly cleared by the glomerular filtration barrier, and the appearance of the plasma is normal.

Traditionally, the differentiation of hemoglobin and myoglobin in clinical laboratories has relied on the ammonium sulfate precipitation method. This method is based on the different solubility characteristics of hemoglobin and myoglobin when saturated with 80 percent ammonium sulfate. At this salt concentration, hemoglobin precipitates out of solution, whereas, myoglobin remains soluble in the supernatant. Only red- or brown-colored urine is tested, and an assessment is made by observing whether the urine color precipitates out of or remains in the supernate after 80 percent saturation with ammonium sulfate. Although this method is relatively easy, it is seriously flawed at detecting low levels of hemoglobinuria (less than 30 mg/dL), owing to the reliance on visual observation. At these low levels, false negative results for hemoglobin would be reported because no visible precipitation is observed (Shihabi, 1989). With the availability of protocols such as the one in the next paragraph, as well as immunoassays and high-performance liquid chromatography (HPLC) methods, the ammonium sulfate precipitation method for differentiation is no longer clinically useful.

The following method for differentiating between hemoglobin and myoglobin is based on a protocol recommended by Shihabi et al. in 1989 for the development of a "rhabdomyolysis/hemolysis profile." Normally, myoglobin excretion is less than 0.04 mg/dL; however, during extreme exercise, it can increase to 40 times the normal rate without adverse renal effects. Only urinary myoglobin concentrations exceeding 1.5 mg/dL are associated with the patient's risk of developing acute renal failure. Because the available blood reagent strip tests are very sensitive and capable of detecting approximately 0.04 mg/dL of myoglobin, urine from patients suspected of having rhabdomyolysis should be diluted 1:40 before testing for myoglobin. If the blood reagent strip test is negative on this diluted specimen, no significant rhabdomyolytic process is occurring. If the test is positive, however, the laboratorian should perform a creatine kinase (CK) determination on the patient's plasma. Because high concentrations of CK are also present in muscle tissue, a rhabdomyolytic process will cause CK values to exceed by 40 times the normal upper reference limit. If the diagnosis of hemoglobinuria versus myoglobinuria is still questionable, a plasma lactate dehydrogenase isoenzyme (LD iso) determination can be performed. Rhabdomyolysis results in an elevated LD_5 fraction, in contrast to hemolysis, in which LD_1 and LD_2 are elevated owing to their high concentration in red blood cells. Table 7-7 compares the laboratory findings that aid in the differential diagnosis of hemoglobinuria and myoglobinuria.

METHODOLOGIES

Reagent Strip Tests. The reagent strip tests available for blood detection are based on the same chemical principle: the pseudoperoxidase activity of the heme moiety. The reagent pad is impregnated with the chromogen tetramethylbenzidine and a peroxide. By the **pseudoperoxidase activity** of the heme moiety, the peroxide is reduced and the chromogen becomes oxidized, producing a color change on the reagent pad from yellow to green (Equation 7-2). Intact red blood cells are lysed on the reagent pad, releasing hemoglobin and producing a mottled green or dotted pattern.

(7-2)

$$H_2O_2 + Chromogen* \xrightarrow[\text{Mgb}]{\text{Hgb}} \begin{array}{c} \text{Oxidized} \\ \text{chromogen} \end{array} + H_2O$$

* Tetramethylbenzidine

Color charts are provided on the reagent strip container so that the laboratorian can visually assess the reagent pad for homoge-

TABLE 7-7. DIFFERENTIATION OF HEMOGLOBINURIA AND MYOGLOBINURIA

	HEMOGLOBINURIA	MYOGLOBINURIA
Urine color	Pink, red or brown	Brown (various shades)
Urine tests		
Blood by reagent strip	Positive	Positive
Plasma appearance	Hemolysis present	Normal
Plasma chemical tests		
Creatine kinase	<10 times the upper reference limit	>40 times the upper reference limit
LD* isoenzymes	LD_1 and LD_2 elevated	LD_5 elevated
Haptoglobin	Decreased	Normal

* Lactate dehydrogenase.

neous color changes resulting from hemoglobin as well as for the mottled variations resulting from intact red blood cells. Test results are reported as negative, trace, small, moderate, or large, or they are reported in the plus (1+, 2+, 3+) system.

Because intact red blood cells are not dissolved in urine, they can settle out or be removed from the urine by centrifugation. Therefore, it is important that urine specimens are well mixed and tested for blood prior to any centrifugation. Hemoglobin, on the other hand, is dissolved in the urine and will not settle out, i.e., it is detectable both in the urine before and in the supernatant after centrifugation.

Because proteins other than hemoglobin, such as myoglobin, contain the heme moiety, their presence can be detected by the blood reagent strip tests. All reagent strips, regardless of their manufacturer, are equally specific for hemoglobin and myoglobin. Other heme-containing substances, such as mitochondrial cytochromes, are present in amounts too small to be detected. See Table 7–3 for the sensitivities of the reagent strips available. To relate the sensitivity for hemoglobin to red blood cells, assuming that approximately 30 picograms of hemoglobin are contained in each red blood cell, then 10 lysed red blood cells is the equivalent of approximately 0.03 mg/dL hemoglobin (Henry, 1991).

Blood reagent strips are one of several reagent strip chemistry tests susceptible to **ascorbic acid interference.** Whenever red blood cells are observed in the microscopic examination of the urine sediment but the chemical examination is negative for blood, ascorbic acid (vitamin C) should be suspected. Ascorbic acid is a strong reducing substance that will react directly with the peroxide (H_2O_2) impregnated on the blood reagent pad and remove it from the intended reaction, thereby preventing the oxidation of the chromogen. As a result, false negative reagent strip results for blood can be obtained from specimens that contain ascorbic acid. Chemstrip reagent strips have successfully eliminated this interference by the use of an "iodate scavenger pad." On Chemstrip re-

agent strips, an iodate-impregnated mesh overlies the blood reagent pad and oxidizes any ascorbic acid before it can interfere in the chemical reaction. A different approach is taken on the reagent strips made by Behring Diagnostics, Inc. With these strips, the Rapignost blood reagent pad does not eliminate the interference; rather, the strips include an ascorbic acid test pad to detect and alert the technologist to the presence of ascorbic acid. The excretion and detection of ascorbic acid in urine, as well as a summary of the reagent strip tests affected by ascorbic acid, are discussed later in this section.

False positive results for blood can be obtained as a result of menstrual or hemorrhoidal contamination of the urine. Other causes include strong oxidizing agents such as sodium hypochlorite or hydrogen peroxide that directly oxidize the chromogen, or microbial peroxidases produced by certain bacterial strains (e.g., *Escherichia coli*) that can catalyze the reaction in the absence of the intended pseudoperoxidase, hemoglobin. Refer to Table 7–3 and the manufacturer's insert for other substances that can affect blood reagent strip results.

Leukocyte Esterase

CLINICAL SIGNIFICANCE. Significant numbers of leukocytes (white blood cells) in the urine are indicative of inflammation. The inflammation may be anywhere in the kidneys or in the lower urinary tract. Normally, few white blood cells (WBC) are found in the urine—0 to 8 per high power field or approximately 10 WBCs/μL. The number of WBCs/μL varies slightly depending on the standardized procedure used. The presence of approximately 20 WBCs/μL or more is a good indication of a pathologic process. Increased numbers of WBCs are found more often in the urine from women than from men, partly because of the greater incidence of urinary tract infections in women, but also because of the increased potential of the women's urine being contaminated with vaginal secretions.

Before the development of reagent strip tests for the detection of leukocyte esterase, the presence of WBCs was determined by the microscopic examination of the urinary sediment. Because of the multiple variations in the urine specimen itself (e.g., the time of day, the collection technique) and in the processing of urine for the microscopic examination, it has been impossible to set a reference value above which the number of WBCs present conclusively indicates disease. Instead, the presence of significant numbers of WBCs serves as a screening test indicating an inflammatory process. Because WBCs are subject to lysis, particularly in hypotonic and alkaline urine, the chemical detection of their esterases provides a means of identifying their presence even when they are no longer visible. In addition, bacteriuria, high storage temperatures, and centrifugation can result in significant cell lysis.

Increased numbers of WBCs in the urine can occur with or without **bacteriuria** (bacteria in the urine). The most commonly encountered cause of **leukocyturia,** however, is a bacterial infection involving the kidneys or urinary tract, such as pyelonephritis, cystitis, or urethritis. In these conditions, the leukocyturia is usually accompanied by bacteriuria of varying degrees. In contrast, kidney and urinary tract infections involving trichomonads, mycoses (e.g., yeast), chlamydia, mycoplasmas, viruses, and tuberculosis cause leukocyturia or **pyuria** without bacteriuria.

METHODOLOGY

Reagent Strip Tests. The reagent strip tests detect leukocyte esterases that are found in the azurophilic granules of granulocytic leukocytes. These granules are present in the cytoplasm of all granulocytes (neutrophils, eosinophils, and basophils), monocytes, and macrophages. Therefore, lymphocytes will not be detected by the reagent strip method. Several advantages of the leukocyte esterase screening test are its ability to detect the presence of intact and lysed WBCs and to provide a screening tool for the presence of WBCs that is independent of procedural variations.

All reagent strip tests for leukocyte esterase detection are based on the action of the leukocyte esterase to cleave an ester, impregnated in the reagent pad, to an aromatic compound. Immediately following hydrolysis of the ester, an azo-coupling reaction takes place between the aromatic compound produced and a diazonium salt provided on the test pad. The end result is an azo dye and a color change of the reagent pad from beige to violet (Equations 7–3 and 7–4).

(7–3)   Ester hydrolysis reaction

$$\underset{\text{(on pad)}}{\text{Ester}} \xrightarrow[\text{esterases}]{\text{leukocyte}} \underset{\text{Aromatic compound}}{\text{Ar}'}$$

(7–4)   Azo-coupling reaction

$$\underset{\substack{\text{Diazonium salt} \\ \text{(on pad)}}}{\text{Ar} - \text{N}^+ \equiv \text{N}} \quad + \quad \underset{\substack{\text{Aromatic compound} \\ \text{(from first reaction)}}}{\text{Ar}'}$$

$$\xrightarrow{\text{acid}} \underset{\text{Azodye}}{\text{Ar} - \text{N} = \text{N} - \text{Ar}'}$$

This screening test for leukocyte esterase initially detects about 10 to 25 WBCs/μL. A negative result does not rule out the presence of increased numbers of WBCs. It indicates only that the number of WBCs present is not sufficient to produce a positive response or that the WBCs present are not granulocytic leukocytes. Results for this chemical test are reported as either negative or positive. The quantitative evaluation of WBCs in the urinary sediment is part of the microscopic examination; however, lysis of these cells may have taken place. Therefore, this reagent strip test provides a means of identifying those urine specimens that require further evaluation because of an increased number of granulocytic leukocytes or their esterases.

False positive results for leukocyte esterase are most often obtained on urine specimens contaminated with vaginal discharge. Another potential source of false positive results are drugs or foodstuffs that color the urine red in an acid medium. These substances (e.g., phenazopyridine, nitrofurantoin, beets) mask the reagent pad so that its color resembles that of a positive reaction.

Highlighting the need for the laboratorian's familiarity with the limitations of each reagent strip test, substances such as significantly increased protein (500 mg/dL), glucose (3 g/dL or more) and specific gravity can reduce the sensitivity of the leukocyte esterase strip reaction and cause false negative results. Drugs such as gentamicin or cephalosporin antibiotics can also produce false negative results. In addition, strong oxidizing agents must be avoided because they interfere with the optimal reaction pH.

Nitrite

CLINICAL SIGNIFICANCE. Routine screening for urinary nitrite provides an important tool in the identification of urinary tract infections. A **urinary tract infection (UTI)** can involve the bladder (cystitis), the renal pelvis and tubules (pyelonephritis), or both. Two pathways for the development of UTIs are possible: 1) the localization of bacteria up the urethra into the bladder (ascending infection) or 2) the localization of bacteria from the bloodstream into the kidney and urinary tract. Ascending infections are by far the more prevalent type of UTIs. The microorganisms involved are usually gram-negative bacilli that are normal flora of the intestinal tract. The most common infecting microorganism is *Escherichia coli*, followed by *Proteus* species, *Enterobacter* species, and *Klebsiella* species. UTIs occur eight times more often in females than males. In addition, catheterized individuals, regardless of gender, have a high incidence of infection. The various factors involved in the incidence of UTIs are discussed under the section on UTIs in Chapter 9.

Normally, the bladder and the urine are sterile. This sterility is maintained by the constant flushing action of urine voiding. A UTI can begin, however, with urinary obstruction, bladder dysfunction, or urine stasis. Once bacteria have become established in the bladder (cystitis), ascension to the kidneys is possible but not inevitable. UTIs can be asymptomatic (asymptomatic bacteriuria) and the nitrite test provides a means of identifying patients with asymptomatic UTIs. With early intervention, the spread of infection to the kidneys and the possible development of renal failure can be prevented.

Screening the urine for nitrite and leukocyte esterase provides a means of identifying those patients with asymptomatic bacteriuria. Not all bacteria contain the enzyme (nitrate reductase) necessary to reduce nitrate to nitrite, however. Normally, nitrates are consumed in the diet (e.g., green vegetables) and excreted in the urine without nitrite formation. However, if nitrate-reducing bacteria are infecting the urinary tract and adequate bladder retention time is allowed, dietary nitrate will be converted by the bacteria to nitrite. Various factors affect nitrite formation and detection: the infecting microbe must be a nitrate-reducer; adequate time (a minimum of 4 hours) must be allowed between voids for the bacterial conversion; and adequate dietary amounts of nitrate must be consumed. In addition, nitrite detection is reduced by the subsequent conversion of nitrite to nitrogen by bacteria, and by antibiotic therapy that can inhibit normal bacterial conversion of nitrate to nitrite. Therefore, to appropriately screen for nitrite, the urine specimen of choice is the first-morning void or a specimen collected after a bladder retention of at least 4 hours. The latter requirement can be difficult in cases of a UTI in which a common presenting symptom is frequent micturition.

The screening test for urinary nitrite does not replace the traditional urine culture for the identification and quantitation of bacteria. It simply provides an indirect means of identifying the presence of nitrate-reducing bacteria in urine, rapidly and with minimal expense. In doing so, it aids in the identification of patients with asymptomatic bacteriuria who might otherwise go undiagnosed.

METHODOLOGY

The Reagent Strip Test. The reagent strip tests for nitrite are based on the same principle—the diazotization reaction of nitrite with an aromatic amine to form a diazonium salt, followed by an azo-coupling reaction (Equations 7–5 and 7–6). Both the aromatic amine for the first reaction and the aromatic compound for the second reaction are impregnated in the reagent pad. The azo-dye produced from these reactions causes a color change from white to pink.

(7–5)   Diazotization reaction

$$Ar - NH_2 \ + \ NO_2^- \xrightarrow{\text{acid}} Ar - N^+ \equiv N$$

  Aromatic amine   Nitrite   Diazonium salt
     (on pad)

(7 – 6)   Azo-coupling reaction

$$Ar - N^+ \equiv N \quad + \quad Ar'$$

Diazonium salt   Aromatic compound
(on pad)

$$\xrightarrow{\text{acid}} Ar - N = N - Ar'$$

Azodye

Results for nitrite are reported as negative or positive. Any degree of pink color is considered to be a positive result; however, there is no correlation between a positive result and the amount of the bacteria present. In fact, a negative test does not rule out the possibility of bacteriuria because of the factors previously discussed. The sensitivity of the reagent strips is such that the presence of approximately 10^5 organisms or more will produce a positive result in most cases. Table 7 – 3 shows the sensitivity and the specificity characteristics of the available reagent strips.

Substances that color the urine red in an acid medium (e.g., phenazopyridine, beets) can cause false positive nitrite results. The color induced from these substances masks the reagent pad and interferes with visual interpretation. In these cases, the microscopic examination of the urine sediment or the urine culture is the only means of identifying bacteriuria. Improper handling and storage of urine specimens can result in bacterial proliferation with nitrite formation and positive nitrite results, when in fact no in-vivo bacteriuria exists.

The presence of ascorbic acid can cause false negative nitrite results. Ascorbic acid directly reacts with the diazonium salt produced in the diazotization reaction (Equation 7 – 5) to form a colorless end-product. In this way, the azo-coupling reaction is prevented, and the reagent pad does not change color. Any factor that inhibits nitrite formation can also cause false negative results, despite bacteriuria with nitrate-reducing bacteria.

In conclusion, nitrite reagent strips provide a rapid, economical means of detecting significant bacteriuria caused by nitrate-reducing bacteria. It is a screening test only and is limited by various factors, including microorganism characteristics, dietary factors, urinary retention time, and specimen storage. Despite these disadvantages, it re-mains an important part of a routine urinalysis.

Protein

CLINICAL SIGNIFICANCE. Normal urine contains up to 150 mg (1 to 14 mg/dL) of protein each day. This protein originates both from the ultrafiltration of plasma and from the urinary tract itself. Proteins of low molecular weight (less than 40,000) readily pass through the glomerular filtration barrier and are reabsorbed. Because of their low plasma concentration, only small amounts of these proteins are seen in the urine. In contrast, albumin, a moderate-molecular-weight protein, has a high plasma concentration. This, combined with its ability — although limited — to pass through the filtration barrier, accounts for a small amount of albumin present in normal urine. Actually, less than 0.1 percent of plasma albumin enters the ultrafiltrate, and 95 percent to 99 percent of all filtered protein is reabsorbed. High-molecular-weight proteins (MW of more than 90,000) are unable to penetrate a healthy glomerular filtration barrier. The end result is that the proteins in normal urine consist of about one-third albumin and two-thirds globulins (Waller, 1989). Of the proteins that originate from the urinary tract itself, three are of particular interest: Tamm-Horsfall protein, a mucoprotein synthesized by the distal tubular cells and involved in cast formation; urokinase, a fibrinolytic enzyme secreted by tubular cells; and secretory IgA, an immunoglobulin synthesized by renal tubular epithelial cells (Waller, 1989).

The presence of an increased amount of protein in urine, termed **proteinuria,** is often the first indicator of renal disease. Early detection of protein by routine screening in a urinalysis aids in the identification, treatment, and prevention of renal disease; however, protein is not a characteristic of all renal disorders. Conditions other than renal disease can also produce an increased excretion of urine proteins. Principally, proteinuria is a result of increased amounts of protein being filtered and not reabsorbed or a reduction in the tubules' reabsorptive ability.

In the past, only the assessment of the

total urine protein concentration was available. Now, owing to technical advances, the measurement of specific proteins is possible. As a result, proteinuria can be classified into four categories: prerenal or overflow proteinuria, glomerular proteinuria, tubular proteinuria, and postrenal proteinuria. This differentiation is based on a combination of protein origination and renal dysfunction; together, they dictate the type and size of proteins observed in the urine (Table 7–8).

Overflow proteinuria results from an increased amount of plasma proteins in the blood readily passing through the glomerular filtration barrier into the urine. As soon as the level of plasma proteins returns to normal, the proteinuria will resolve. Several conditions resulting in this increased urinary excretion of low-molecular-weight plasma proteins include septicemia, with the spilling of acute-phase-reactant proteins; hemoglobinuria, following a hemolytic episode; and myoglobinuria, following muscle injury. Immunoglobulin para-proteins (kappa and lambda monoclonal light chains) are also low-molecular-weight proteins, abnormally produced in multiple myeloma and macroglobulinemia. These light chain diseases make up 12 percent of monoclonal gammopathies. Historically, the urinary presence of these immunoglobulin light chains, also known as Bence Jones proteins, was identified by the light chains' unique solubility characteristics related to temperature. If when heated a urine specimen coagulated at 40 to 60°C and redissolved at 100°C, Bence Jones proteins were present. Today, electrophoretic techniques are available to specifically identify and quantitate these light chain proteins.

Renal proteinuria may present as a glomerular pattern, a tubular pattern, or a combination—a mixed pattern. When the glomerular filtration barrier is compromised by disease, an increased amount of plasma proteins is allowed to pass into the ultrafiltrate. This condition is termed *glomerular proteinuria*. Protein reabsorption by the renal tubules is a nonselective, competitive, and threshold-limited (T_m) process. Therefore, if the capacity for protein reabsorption is exceeded, an increased amount of proteins will be excreted in the urine. As stated in Chapter 4, albumin would readily pass through the glomerular filtration barrier if not for the barrier's negative charge, which allows only a small amount of albumin to pass. Likewise, any disorder that alters the negativity of the glomerular filtration barrier will result in an increased amount of albumin freely passing into the ultrafiltrate. In addition, other moderate-molecular-weight proteins of similar charge, such as α_1-antitrypsin, α_1-acid glycoprotein, and transferrin, will also pass (Table 7–9). The glomerulus is considered to be "selective" if it is able to retard the passage of high molecular-weight proteins (MW greater than 90,000) and "nonse-

T A B L E 7 – 8.   CLASSIFICATION OF PROTEINURIA

Prerenal
   Overflow proteinuria—increase in *plasma* low-molecular-weight proteins spill into urine
   • Normal proteins, e.g., acute phase reactants, myoglobin, hemoglobin
   • Abnormal proteins, e.g., Ig light chains

Renal
   Glomerular proteinuria—defective glomerular filtration barrier
   • Selective: increase in albumin and moderate-molecular-weight proteins
   • Nonselective: increase in all proteins, including high-molecular-weight proteins
   Tubular proteinuria—defective tubular reabsorption
   • Increase in low-molecular-weight urine proteins

Postrenal
   Postrenal proteinuria—proteins produced by the urinary tract
   • Inflammation, malignancy, or injury

TABLE 7–9. PRINCIPAL PROTEINS IN GLOMERULAR PROTEINURIA

Albumin
Transferrin
α_1-antitrypsin
α_1-acid glycoprotein

lective" if discrimination is lost and high-molecular-weight proteins are allowed into the ultrafiltrate.

Glomerular proteinuria is seen in primary glomerular diseases or disorders that cause glomerular damage. It is the most common type of proteinuria encountered and also the most serious clinically. The proteinuria is usually heavy, exceeding 2.5 g/d of total protein, and can be as much as 20 g/d. Table 7–10 lists some of the conditions that can

TABLE 7–10. CAUSES OF GLOMERULAR PROTEINURIA

Primary glomerular disease
    Membranous glomerulonephritis
    Minimal change disease (lipoid nephrosis)
    Membranoproliferative glomerulonephritis
    Glomerulosclerosis, focal

Glomerular damage induced by
    Systemic disease
        Poststreptococcal glomerulonephritis
        Diabetes mellitus
        Lupus erythematosus
        Amyloidosis
        Sickle cell anemia
        Carcinoma, leukemia, lymphoma
    Infectious disease
        Malaria
        Hepatitis B
        Subacute bacterial endocarditis
    Drugs
        Penicillamine
        Lithium
        Mercury
    Transplant rejection
    Pre-eclampsia

Transitory glomerular changes
    Strenuous exercise
    Fever
    Extreme cold exposure
    Postpartum
    Postural proteinuria (orthostatic)

result in glomerular proteinuria. Glomerular proteinuria can develop into a clinical condition termed the **nephrotic syndrome.** This syndrome is characterized by proteinuria exceeding approximately 3.5 g/d, hypoalbuminemia, hyperlipidemia, lipiduria, and generalized edema. The nephrotic syndrome is a complication of numerous disorders and is discussed more fully in Chapter 9.

The detection of what seem to be minor increases in urinary albumin excretion has particular merit in patients with diabetes mellitus. Proteinuria of glomerular origin appears early in the course of diabetic nephropathy. Although the exact mechanism of proteinuria is not clearly understood, the increased glomerular permeability results from changes in the glomerular filtration barrier. The single most important factor associated with the development of glomerular proteinuria is hyperglycemia. Because glucose is capable of nonenzymatic binding with various proteins, it apparently combines with proteins of the glomerular filtration barrier, causing glomerular permeability changes and stimulating the growth of the mesangial matrix. Glomerular changes are evidenced by an increased urinary albumin excretion of 30 to 300 mg/d, compared with less than 30 mg/d excreted by a normal individual. Because rigorous treatment in the early stages of the disease can reverse these changes, sensitive chemical methods for albumin detection play an important role.

Several conditions, termed *functional proteinurias,* induce a type of mild glomerular or mixed pattern of proteinuria in the absence of renal disease. Changes in the glomerular blood flow (e.g., renal vasoconstriction) or an enhanced glomerular permeability appear to be the primary mechanisms involved. Strenuous exercise, fever, extreme cold exposure, emotional distress, congestive heart failure, and dehydration are associated with this type of proteinuria. The amount of protein excreted is usually less than 1 g/d. Functional proteinurias are transitory and resolve with time and supportive treatment.

Postural (orthostatic) proteinuria is considered to be a functional proteinuria. This condition is characterized by the urinary excretion of protein only when the individual is in an upright (orthostatic) position. A first-morning urine specimen is normal in protein content, whereas specimens collected during the day contain elevated amounts of protein. An increased renal venous pressure causing renal congestion when the patient is in the upright position is theorized as a possible mechanism resulting in glomerular changes. Although this condition is considered to be benign, persistent proteinuria may develop; evidence of glomerular abnormalities has been found by renal biopsy in a few patients (Robinson, 1961). Urinary protein excretion in postural proteinuria is usually less than 1.5 g/d. Individuals suspected of having postural proteinuria collect two urine specimens: a first-morning specimen and a second specimen collected after the patient has been in an upright position for several hours. If the first specimen is negative for protein and the second is positive, a tentative diagnosis of postural proteinuria can be made. These individuals should be monitored every 6 months and re-evaluated as necessary.

Proteinuria occurring during pregnancy is usually transient. It may be associated with toxemia, delivery, or renal infections. A wide range in the amount of protein excreted exists. Protein excretion associated with pre-eclamptic toxemia approaches 3 g/d, whereas minor increases up to 300 mg/d occur with normal pregnancies.

Tubular proteinuria is observed when normal tubular reabsorptive function is altered or impaired. When either occurs, plasma proteins normally reabsorbed, such as β_2-microglobulin, retinol-binding protein, α_2-microglobulin, or lysozyme, are found in increased concentrations in the urine. The urine total protein concentration is usually less than 2.5 g/d, with low-molecular-weight proteins predominating (Table 7–11). Although albumin is found in increased amounts, it does not approach the level found in glomerular proteinuria. In light of this, chemical testing methods that are specific for albumin (e.g., reagent strip tests) may not detect the increase in urine protein. Therefore, when tubular proteinuria is sus-

pected, a protein precipitation method sensitive to all proteins should be used, e.g., an SSA precipitation test. Originally discovered in workers exposed to cadmium dust, tubular proteinuria can result from a variety of disorders (Table 7–12). It may occur alone or in combination with glomerular proteinuria, as in chronic renal disease or renal failure, in which case the urinary proteins excreted result in a "mixed" pattern.

A condition particularly characterized by proximal tubular dysfunction is the **Fanconi syndrome.** This syndrome has the following distinctive urine findings: aminoaciduria, proteinuria, glycosuria, and phosphaturia. Associated with both inherited and acquired diseases, this syndrome of altered tubular

TABLE 7–11. PRINCIPAL PROTEINS IN TUBULAR PROTEINURIA

Albumin
β_2-microglobulin
Retinol-binding protein
α_2-microglobulin
α_1-microglobulin
Lysozyme

TABLE 7–12. COMMON CAUSES OF TUBULAR PROTEINURIA

Acute/chronic pyelonephritis
Interstitial nephritis
Renal tubular acidosis
Renal tuberculosis
Fanconi syndrome
Systemic disease
Sarcoidosis
Lupus erythematosus
Cystinosis
Galactosemia
Wilson's disease
Drugs
Aminoglycosides
Heavy metal poisoning, e.g., Cd, Pb
Sulfonamides
Penicillins
Cephalosporins
Hemolytic disorders (hemoglobin)
Muscle injury (myoglobin)
Transplant rejection
Strenuous exercise

transport mechanisms retains normal glomerular function. Heavy metal poisoning and the hereditary disease cystinosis are two common causes of the Fanconi syndrome.

Postrenal proteinuria can result from inflammation anywhere in the urinary tract, e.g., in the renal pelvis (pyelonephritis), the ureters, the bladder (cystitis), the prostate, the urethra, or the external genitalia. In addition, blood proteins that leak into the urinary tract as a result of injury and hemorrhage, or vaginal secretions contaminating the urine, can also result in proteinuria.

In summary, increased urinary protein results from 1) increased plasma proteins overflowing into the urine (prerenal); 2) renal changes—glomerular, tubular, or both; or 3) inflammation and postrenal sources. Table 7–13 compares various proteins present in normal urine with urine characteristic of renal disease—glomerular and tubular. Note the relative amount of total protein present, the size of proteins that predominate, and the dramatic difference in the percentage of protein reabsorbed.

METHODOLOGIES. Historically, qualitative or semiquantitative screening tests for urinary protein relied on protein precipitation techniques. Proteins denature upon exposure to extremes of pH or temperature; the most visible evidence of this is a decrease in their solubility. As a result, heat alone can cause protein to coagulate, and chemicals such as strong acids will induce its precipitation out of solution. Originally, the combination of heat with acetic acid was used in clinical laboratories for urinary protein detection; now, SSA at room temperature is used to detect urinary protein. All of these precipitation methods are sensitive to all proteins—i.e., both albumin and globulins are detected. Substances such as x-ray contrast media and some drugs can also produce positive results, however, necessitating the use of a second confirmatory method before reporting results.

Positive protein results should be evaluated with the urine specific gravity results. Large volumes of urine (polyuria) can give a negative protein reaction, despite significant proteinuria, if the protein present is being excessively diluted. Likewise, a trace amount of protein present in a dilute urine indicates more pathology than a trace amount in a concentrated urine. Also, an abnormally high specific gravity (greater than 1.040) is a strong indication that a radiographic contrast medium is present, which produces a delayed positive protein precipitation test (see the SSA precipitation test).

Once the presence of an increased amount of urinary protein has been established, accurate methods are available to differentiate and quantify the proteins. Electrophoresis, nephelometry, turbidimetry, and radial immunodiffusion methods are used and are discussed at length in clinical chemistry textbooks. Despite the qualitative or semiquantitative nature of the protein tests discussed here, they remain vital tools in the detection and monitoring of diseases that result in proteinuria.

Sulfosalicylic Acid (SSA) Precipitation Test. Various procedures are available for the performance of the SSA test, differing in the volume of the centrifuged urine used (3 mL vs. 11 mL) and the concentration of the SSA reagent (3.0 percent vs. 7.0 percent). Despite

TABLE 7–13.   CHARACTERIZATION OF RENAL PROTEINURIA

	NORMAL	GLOMERULAR DISEASE	TUBULAR DISEASE
Total protein (g/d)	<0.15	>2.5	<2.5
Albumin (mg/d)	50	>500	<500
β_2-microglobulin (mg/d)	0.150	0.150	20
Tubular reabsorption of filtered proteins (%)	95	3	50

Modified from Waller KV, Ward MW, et al.: Current concepts in proteinuria. Clin Chem 35:5, 1989.

these differences, the final solution concentration (urine plus reagent) is the same—0.015 g of SSA per mL of total solution.

Because particulate matter suspended in the urine can interfere with turbidity assessment, the SSA test is performed on clear supernatant urine following centrifugation. The urine supernate and reagent are added together and mixed by inversion. After a 10-minute, room-temperature incubation, the tube is inverted and evaluated. Using ordinary room light, the precipitation reaction is graded as negative, trace, 1+, 2+, 3+, 4+ according to a predetermined protocol (Table 7–14). In some institutions, the "plus" grading system is replaced with concentration values (mg/dL) corresponding to the standards used or the albumin values obtained when using reagent strips. The SSA method is sensitive to 5 to 10 mg/dL of protein, regardless of the type of protein present.

If a radiographic contrast medium is suspected because of an abnormally high specific gravity result, or if a lack of correlation exists between the SSA method and the reagent strip method, the SSA precipitate should be viewed microscopically. Drugs (e.g., penicillins) and contrast media form crystalline precipitates, whereas protein precipitates are amorphous. When the SSA result is crystalline, the protein

results obtained using the reagent strip can be reported. When the SSA precipitate is amorphous, the discrepancy between the SSA and the reagent strip method is highly indicative of the presence of urinary proteins other than albumin (e.g., globulins, Bence Jones protein), and further investigation is required (e.g., protein electrophoresis).

Although rare, false negative or decreased SSA results for protein can be obtained with extremely alkaline (pH 9.0 or greater) or highly buffered urine. The precipitating reagent (acid) is neutralized by the substances present, producing erroneous results. Because urine specimens exceeding pH 8.0 are not physiologically possible and indicate contamination or improper storage, they should not be used. However, if the urine is acidified to approximately pH 5.0 and retested using SSA, an accurate protein result can be obtained.

Reagent Strip Tests. Commercial reagent strips available for routine protein screening employ the same principle, originally described by Sorenson in 1909, and termed the **protein error of indicators.** When the pH is held constant by a buffer, certain indicator dyes will release hydrogen ions as a result of the presene of proteins (anions) and cause a color change. The reagent pad is impregnated with a buffer to maintain the test area at pH

TABLE 7–14.   SSA PRECIPITATION GRADING GUIDELINE

SSA RESULT	OBSERVATIONS	APPROXIMATE PROTEIN CONCENTRATION*
Negative	No turbidity or increase in turbidity • When the tube is viewed from the top, a circle is visible in the bottom of the test tube†	Negative
Trace	Perceptible turbidity • When the tube is viewed from the top, **a circle is NOT** visible in the test tube bottom • CAN read newsprint through mixture	Trace (5 to 20 mg/dL)
1+	Distinct turbidity WITHOUT discrete granulation • CANNOT read newsprint through mixture	30 mg/dL
2+	Turbidity with granulation; NO flocculation	100 mg/dL
3+	Turbidity with granulation AND flocculation	300 mg/dL
4+	Large clumps of precipitate or a solid mass	≥500 mg/dL

This value correlates with the reagent strip result if the protein present is albumin.
† While holding a test tube filled with a clear solution vertically, view the bottom of the tube looking through the solution from the top. A circle formed by the tube bottom is visible. As a solution increases in turbidity, this circle will no longer be evident.

3.0. If protein is present, it acts as a hydrogen receptor—accepting hydrogen ions from the pH indicator—thereby inducing a color change (Equation 7–7).

(7–7)

$$\text{Indicator dye} + \text{Protein} \xrightarrow{\text{pH } 3.0} \begin{array}{c} \text{H}^+ \text{ ions released} \\ \text{from indicator} \\ \text{(blue-green)} \end{array}$$

The intensity of the color change is directly related to the amount of protein present. Protein reagent strip results are reported as concentrations in mg/dL by matching the resultant reagent pad color to the color chart provided on the reagent strip container.

This method is more sensitive to albumin than to any other protein, and false negative results can occur if significant amounts of proteins other than albumin are present. Globulins, myoglobin, Bence Jones proteins, and mucoproteins may not be detected. Extremely alkaline (pH 9.0 or higher) or highly buffered urine can overwhelm the buffering capacity of the reagent strip to produce false positive protein results. As with the SSA method, adjusting the urine to approximately pH 5.0 and retesting using the reagent strip test can produce an accurate protein result.

In order to enhance detection of all types of proteinuria—regardless of the protein excreted—both the reagent strip method and a precipitation method should be employed. Some institutions use the SSA method to screen all specimens and then confirm any positive results using the reagent strip method. Others reverse the process, screening with the reagent strip method and confirming with the SSA method. Although initially this latter approach would appear to miss cases of proteinuria, it rarely does because the tubular reabsorption of protein is a nonselective, competitive process. Even though the increased protein present is not albumin, albumin is excreted in increased amounts as the tubules randomly reabsorb the increased amount of protein presented to them. As a result, the reagent strip detection of albumin can adequately detect most instances of proteinuria. Any discrepancy between the methods must be investigated and resolved before reporting the test results.

Sensitive Albumin Tests. Because of the need to detect even slightly increased amounts of albumin in urine that are not detectable by the routine reagent strip methods, sensitive albumin screening tests were developed. The detection and monitoring of low levels of albumin in urine aid in the identification and management of patients at risk for renal disease. Patients, particularly those with type I and type II diabetes, benefit from close monitoring of their urinary albumin concentrations. It has been shown that these patients develop low-level **albuminuria** before they present with diabetic nephropathy clinically. In addition, intervention to reduce hyperglycemia and normalize blood pressure actually reduces the progression of the disease to clinical nephropathy.

Two commercial methods are available for the rapid screening of urine for an increased amount of albumin: the Micro-Bumin-test from Miles, Inc., and Chemstrip Micral from Boehringer Mannheim Corporation. The Micro-Bumintest is based on the same principle as a reagent strip protein test—the protein error of indicators. However, it is a tablet test and able to detect 4.0 to 8.0 mg/dL of albumin. After urine and water are placed on the tablet, a positive reaction is indicated when any detectable bluish-green spot or ring becomes visible on the tablet surface. A color chart is provided for comparison; as with reagent strips, the intensity of the color produced is directly related to the amount of albumin present. This tablet test is subject to the same limitations as the reagent strip test, and although it is much more sensitive to albumin, the presence of other proteins can go undetected by this method. In other words, a negative reaction does not rule out the presence of other proteins.

The Chemstrip Micral is a unique reagent strip test employing an immunochemical reaction. Albumin in the urine binds with a soluble antibody-enzyme conjugate impregnated on the reagent strip pad. Only the albumin-conjugate immunocomplex can pass to the reaction zone of the reagent strip by a wicking action because an intermediate zone immobilizes any excess unbound conjugate. Once in the reaction zone, the enzyme (β-galactosidase) from the immunocomplex reacts with the conjugate (chlorophenolred galactoside) present to produce a red dye. Timing and technique are crucial; the manufacturer's instructions must be followed to ensure accurate test results. The Micral method is capable of detecting as little as 1.0 to 2 mg/dL (10 to 20 mg/L) of human albumin in the urine. A color chart for comparison is provided on the container, and semiquantitative results are reported from 0 to 10 mg/dL (0 to 100 mg/L). Not all positive Micral tests are evidence of abnormality because urine albumin concentrations less than 2.0 mg/dL (less than 20 mg/L) are considered to be normal. This test is specific for human albumin and will not indicate the presence of any other proteins. Table 7–15 provides a comparison of the Micral and the Micro-Bumintest methods for the detection of low levels of urinary albumin.

Glucose

CLINICAL SIGNIFICANCE. The presence of glucose in the urine is termed **glucosuria** (or **glycosuria**). Normally, all glucose that passes through the glomerular filtration barrier into the ultrafiltrate is actively reabsorbed by the proximal renal tubules. However, the tubular reabsorption of glucose is a threshold-limited process with a maximum reabsorptive capacity (T_m) averaging about 350 mg/min (the T_m for glucose differs with gender and body surface area, ranging from 250 to 360 mg/min in females and 295 to 455 mg/min in males). When the level of glucose in the blood exceeds its renal threshold level of approximately 160 to 180 mg/dL, the ultrafiltrate concentration of glucose exceeds the reabsorptive ability of the tubules and glucosuria occurs.

Glucosuria is caused by either 1) a prerenal condition, i.e., hyperglycemia, or 2) a renal condition, i.e., defective tubular absorption. Diabetes mellitus is the most common disease that results in hyperglycemia and glucosuria. This disease is characterized by ineffective glucose utilization owing to either inadequate insulin production or the production of defective insulin. As a result, patients with undiagnosed or inadequately controlled diabetes have blood glucose concentrations that exceed the renal threshold level, and glucosuria is present. The clinical presentation of diabetes mellitus is varied; often individuals are asymptomatic and initial detection results from a routine blood or urine test. Because diabetes mellitus is the seventh leading cause of death in the United States, and early intervention and treatment can prevent or delay the many long-term complications of this disease, routine screening of urine for glucose is an important part of a urinalysis.

Conditions other than diabetes mellitus can cause hyperglycemia with glucosuria. These conditions include various hormonal disorders, liver disease, pancreatic disease, central nervous system damage, and drugs (Table 7–16). The etiology, presentation, and treatment of these diseases differ; the common link is the inadequate utilization of glucose that results in glucosuria. Therefore, when a patient presents with glucosuria, further evaluation of the blood and urine is required to identify the specific disease process.

Because screening for glucose in urine and blood is routinely performed simultaneously, with abnormal findings further investigated, a brief discussion of hyperglycemia without glucosuria is necessary. Glucose freely passes through the glomerular filtration barrier; however, if this barrier is compromised because of disease, the glomerular

TABLE 7–15.   SENSITIVE ALBUMIN TESTS

	MICRAL	MICRO-BUMINTEST
Test type	Reagent strip	Tablet
Time required	5 minutes	~ 3 minutes
Principle	Immunochemical	Protein error of indicators
Sensitivity	1 to 2 mg/dL	4 to 8 mg/dL
Specificity	Albumin (human)	Albumin (any species)

TABLE 7–16. CAUSES OF GLUCOSURIA

Prerenal—hyperglycemia with glucosuria
  Diabetes mellitus
  Hormonal disorders
    Hyperthyroidism—increased thyroid hormone
    Acromegaly—increased growth hormone
    Stress, anxiety, and Cushing's disease—increased epinephrine and glucocorticoids
  Liver disease
  Pancreatic disease
  CNS damage, e.g., cerebrovascular accident
  Drugs, e.g., thiazide diuretics, steroids
Renal—defective tubular reabsorption of glucose
  Fanconi syndrome
  Cystinosis
  Heavy metal poisoning
  Genetic
  Pregnancy

filtration rate (GFR) may be decreased. In these instances, hyperglycemia can be present, but because of the decreased GFR, only limited amounts of glucose are able to pass into the ultrafiltrate. The tubules are able to reabsorb all the glucose presented to them, and glucosuria is not present. Any disease that decreases the GFR, such as renal arteriosclerosis or low cardiac output, can result in hyperglycemia without glucosuria. Figure 7–2 summarizes glucosuria mechanisms and their relationship to hyperglycemia and renal tubular function.

Sugars other than glucose can also appear in the urine, although like glucose they are normally not present. Various circumstances can result in the urinary excretion of other sugars such as galactose, fructose, lactose, maltose, or pentoses. The most significant of these is the excretion of galactose, because it signifies a disease (galactosemia) with severe and irreversible consequences. Galactosemia is a pathologic condition characterized by a congenital deficiency to metabolize galactose to glucose. The defect has several forms, all of which involve the reduction or absence of an enzyme necessary for galactose metabolism. Lactose, a disaccharide of D-galactose and D-glucose found in milk, is a principal source of dietary galactose. Infants born with these enzyme deficiencies must be recognized at birth so that milk can be eliminated from their diet. If this deficiency goes undetected, increased concentrations of galactose in the infant's blood results in the formation of galactitol and galactonate. These two intermediate products of metabolism are toxic and cause cataract formation, hepatic dysfunction, and severe mental retardation. The infant presents initially with a failure to thrive, vomiting, and diarrhea. If the condition is recognized early, galactose can be eliminated from the diet, resulting in the infant's normal growth and development. The detection of galactose and

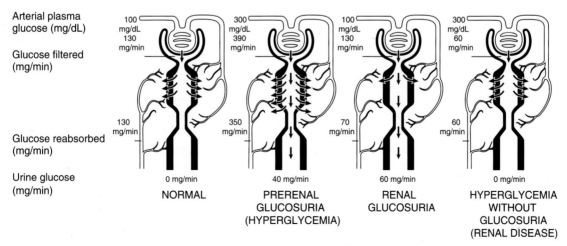

FIGURE 7–2. A schematic diagram comparing the filtration and reabsorption of glucose by the proximal tubular cells normally and in conditions of hyperglycemia and renal tubular disease.

any reducing sugar other than glucose relies on the testing of urine for reducing substances. Therefore, routine screening of urine from children less than 3 years old should include a test for reducing substances.

Lactose may be found in the urine of pregnant women or premature infants. Rarely, urine may contain fructose owing to excessive fruit or honey ingestion; pentoses (xylose and arabinose) from excessive fruit ingestion (e.g., plums, cherries) or from a rare genetic defect; or maltose and glucose together in some diabetic patients. Of the many sugars that may be present in the urine, only glucose and galactose signify pathology.

In summary, sugars are normally not excreted in the urine, and a routine urinalysis should include a screening test for them. The most common sugar encountered by far is glucose; however in children less than 2 to 3 years old, it is imperative that a screening test for any reducing sugar be performed. Other reducing substances may be found in the urine as well (e.g., homogentisic acid, ascorbic acid, salicylates). As a result, urine specimens producing positive reduction tests require further evaluation to identify the reductant present (see Copper Reduction Tests in this chapter).

METHODOLOGIES

Reagent Strip Tests. Urinary screening for glucose dates back to the Babylonians and Egyptians, who tasted urine to detect the presence of urinary sugars. Now, urinary glucose screening by a reagent strip test is a cost-effective, noninvasive means of identifying individuals with glucosuria. The glucose reagent strip was the first "dip and read" reagent strip developed by Miles, Inc., in 1950. Glucose reagent strip tests use a double sequential enzyme reaction and detect only glucose (Equations 7–8 and 7–9). Glucose oxidase impregnated on the reagent pad rapidly catalyzes the oxidation of glucose to form hydrogen peroxide (H_2O_2) and gluconic acid. The hydrogen peroxide oxidizes the chromogen on the reagent pad in the presence of peroxidase. The color change differs depending on the chromogen employed on the reagent strip.

(7–8)

$$\text{Glucose} + O_2 \xrightarrow[\text{oxidase}]{\text{glucose}} \text{Gluconic acid} + H_2O_2$$

(7–9)

$$H_2O_2 + \text{Chromogen} \xrightarrow{\text{peroxidase}} \begin{array}{c}\text{Oxidized}\\\text{chromogen}\end{array} + H_2O$$

Results are reported as negative or normal, and positive tests are assessed quantitatively in concentration units of milligrams per deciliter or grams per deciliter. Whereas virtually all glucose is reabsorbed by the renal tubules, a urinary concentration of less than 20 mg/dL is considered to be normal, and the sensitivity of glucose reagent strips is adjusted to avoid the detection of these extremely small amounts of glucose (see Table 7–3). Specific gravity and temperature can modify the sensitivity of the reagent strip for glucose. As the urine specific gravity increases or the temperature of the urine decreases (because of refrigeration), the sensitivity of the reagent strip to glucose decreases. Similarly, high concentrations of urinary ketones, *ketonuria* (40 mg/dL or more), can reduce the sensitivity of the reagent strip to low concentrations (75 to 125 mg/dL) of urinary glucose. However, ketonuria—caused by increased fat metabolism—occurs as a result of inadequate glucose utilization (in diabetes) or inadequate glucose intake (in starvation). In patients with diabetes, large amounts of glucose spill into the urine, whereas in starvation, no glucose is available to be excreted. As a result, significant ketonuria with low-level glucosuria is rarely encountered.

False positive reagent strip tests for glucose can be caused by strong oxidizing agents (e.g., sodium hypochlorite) or contaminating peroxides that directly interact with the chromogen. However, because of the specificity of the reagent strip for glucose, false negative results are more common. Ascorbic acid concentrations of 50 mg/dL or more directly reduce the hydrogen peroxide produced in the first reaction, thereby preventing the oxidation of the chromogen and causing a false negative result. Recent studies highlight the need for routine ascorbic acid detection simultaneously with glucose screening to prevent potentially dangerous false negative results for a diabetic patient (Brigden, 1992). The difference between no glucose and low levels of glucose in the urine can directly affect disease management; therefore, testing should not be compromised. Improperly stored urine specimens can also produce false negative results owing to rapid bacterial glycolysis and should be avoided.

Copper Reduction Tests. In the 19th century, the copper reduction ability of some sugars in an alkaline medium was discovered and the term "reducing sugar" was coined. Glucose, fructose, galactose, lactose, maltose, and pentoses are a few of the reducing sugars; common table sugar, sucrose, is not a reducing sugar. A sugar's reducing ability is determined by the presence of the reducing group, $\rangle C{=}O$, present in all monosaccharides. In disaccharides, the reducing group may have been used in its formation (a glycosidic linkage), in which case the resultant sugar would be nonreducing (e.g., sucrose). As a medical student, Stanley Benedict modified the original, time-consuming copper reduction test into a practical liquid test (Benedict, 1909). A tablet version of Benedict's test, the Clinitest reagent tablet (Ames, Inc., Elkhart, IN 46514), is now widely used in clinical laboratories for the detection of reducing substances.

Copper reduction tests are based on the ability of reducing substances to convert cupric sulfate to cuprous oxide, resulting in a color change from blue to green to orange. Clinitest tablets contain all the reagents necessary for this reaction: anhydrous copper sulfate, sodium hydroxide, citric acid, and sodium bicarbonate. A mixture of approximately 0.25 mL of urine (5 drops) and 0.50 mL of water (10 drops) is prepared in a test tube, to which one reagent tablet is added and allowed to stand undisturbed for 15 seconds. During this period, the mixture bubbles from the reaction of citric acid and sodium bicarbonate to form carbon dioxide. This gas blankets the reaction mixture and effectively prevents room air from participating in the chemical reaction. At the same time, the reaction is promoted by heat, generated from

the interaction of sodium hydroxide and water. After the 15-second reaction period, the tube is mixed and its color compared to the chart provided. The reaction is depicted in Equation 7–10.

(7–10)

$$CuSO_4 \underset{\text{(blue)}}{} + \frac{\text{Reducing}}{\text{substance}} \xrightarrow{\text{heat and alkali}}$$

$$\underset{\text{(yellow)}}{CuOH} + \underset{\text{(red)}}{Cu_2O} + \frac{\text{Oxidized}}{\text{substance}} + H_2O$$

Clinitest results need to be evaluated immediately; any color change occurring after 15 seconds must be ignored. If the color change is not read at 15 seconds, falsely low results may be reported if a "pass-through" phenomenon took place. The "pass-through" phenomenon occurs in the presence of high concentrations of reducing substances and is evidenced by the mixture's passing through all colors possible to orange (the highest concentration) and then back to green-brown (the low concentration). The mechanism of this phenomenon is the reoxidation of the resultant cuprous oxide to cupric oxide and other cupric complexes (green). This reoxidation can occur in the presence of extremely high concentrations of reducing substances or from the exposure of the reaction mixture to room air after the protective CO_2 gas blanket disperses. In order to observe this phenomenon *within* the 15-second reaction period, very high—physiologically impossible—glucose concentrations must be present. If a reaction mixture is not observed, however, and the 15-second time period has been exceeded, the high glucose concentrations found in diabetic patients can cause this "pass-through" phenomenon. In these instances, the color observed (after the "pass-through") no longer indicates the high glucose concentration, and falsely low results would be reported. The laboratorian's adherence to the manufacturer's procedural directions will avoid this technical error.

An alternative approach to quantifying high glucose concentrations is to perform the Clinitest method using only 2 drops of urine. Although the 5-drop method is sensitive to 250 mg/dL (0.25 g/dL) glucose, the 2-drop method requires a minimum of 350 mg/dL (0.35 g/dL) to obtain a positive result. Advantages of the 2-drop method is that it allows for glucose quantitation up to 5 g/dL and reduces the possibility of the "pass-through" effect. Semiquantitative results in grams per deciliter are obtained by comparison to the appropriate color chart, with different charts provided for the 5-drop and 2-drop methods.

Copper reduction tests are nonspecific, and many reducing substances in urine, other than sugars, can produce positive results when present in significant amounts. Table 7–17 provides a partial listing of these reducing substances. Although creatinine, ketone bodies, and uric acid are also reducing substances, the amounts present in urine, even in extreme cases, are usually insufficient to produce a positive Clinitest result. Ascorbic acid is the most commonly encountered agent producing positive copper reduction tests in the absence of glucose or causing a significant discrepancy in the results obtained with glucose reagent strip tests and the Clinitest method. Radiographic contrast media may cause false negative or decreased results. Urine of low specific gravity appears to increase the sensitivity of the Clinitest method slightly, whereas sulfonamide metabolites or methapyriline compounds interfere with it, causing decreased results.

As previously mentioned, the excretion of glucose or galactose is pathologically significant. Therefore, any urine glucose determination performed on children less than 3 years old should include a copper reduction test to screen for reducing substances formed as a result of an inherited metabolic disorder (e.g., galactosemia).

When a reducing sugar other than glucose is determined to be present, several methods are available for the separation and identification of the specific reducing sugar. Chromatographic procedures — paper or thin-layer chromatography (TLC) — predominate, with TLC requiring less time to perform. Regardless of the technique employed, each sugar is identified by comparing the unknown specimen to standards chromatographed at the same time.

Comparison of the Clinitest Method and Glucose Reagent Strip Tests. Because glucose reagent strip tests are more sensitive than the Clinitest method, it is possible to obtain a negative Clinitest result and a positive glucose reagent strip test on a urine specimen. These results would indicate a low concentration of glucose (approximately 40 to 200 mg/dL). If, on the other hand, the Clinitest result is positive and the glucose reagent strip result is negative, a reducing substance other than glucose is present. In both of these cases, it is assumed that no interfering substances are present and that all reagents and strips are functioning properly. Outdated reagent strips or tablets, as well as contaminating agents, could produce similar result combinations (Table 7–18). Because Clinitest tablets are extremely hygroscopic — they take up and retain water — it is imperative to protect them from moisture, as well as from light and heat. The tablets should be visually inspected before use to ensure their integrity.

TABLE 7–17.   REDUCING SUBSTANCES FOUND IN URINE, CAUSING POSITIVE COPPER REDUCTION TESTS

Sugars
   Monosaccharides
      Glucose
      Fructose
   Disaccharides
      Galactose
      Lactose
      Maltose
   Pentoses
      Arabinose
      Ribose
Ascorbic acid
   Vitamins or fruits
   Drug preparations (e.g., intravenous tetracycline)
Drugs and their metabolites
   Salicylates
   Penicillin
   Cephalosporins
   Nalidixic acid
   Sulfonamides
Cysteine
Homogentisic acid

TABLE 7–18. COMPARISON OF THE GLUCOSE REAGENT STRIP TEST AND CLINITEST TABLET TEST

GLUCOSE REAGENT STRIP TEST	CLINITEST TABLET TEST	POSSIBLE CAUSES OF TEST DISCREPANCY
Positive	Negative	• Reagent strip more sensitive—a low concentration of glucose present • False positive reagent strip owing to contaminants, e.g., oxidizing agents or peroxidases • Tablets defective, e.g., outdated
Negative	Positive	• **Reducing substance other than glucose present, e.g., ascorbic acid** • Reagent strip interference, e.g., high SG, low temperature • Reagent strips defective, e.g., outdated

Ketones

FORMATION. The terms ketones and ketone bodies identify three intermediate products of fatty acid metabolism: acetoacetate, β-hydroxybutyrate, and acetone (Fig. 7–3). Normally, the end-products of fatty acid metabolism are carbon dioxide and water, with no measurable ketones produced. However, when carbohydrate availability is limited, the liver must oxidize fatty acids as its main metabolic substrate. As a result, large amounts of acetyl CoA are formed, and the Krebs cycle becomes overwhelmed. In order to handle the increased acetyl CoA load, the liver mitochondria begin active ketogenesis. Large amounts of ketones are released into the blood *(ketonemia)* and provide energy to the brain, heart, skeletal muscles, and kidneys.

The amount of each ketone body in the blood can vary with the severity of the condition. However, the average distribution of ketones in both serum and urine is 78 percent β-hydroxybutyrate, 20 percent acetoacetate, and 2 percent acetone. When blood ketone concentrations exceed 70 mg/dL (the renal threshold level), renal tubular absorption is maximal and ketones are excreted in the urine (Montgomery, 1990). This condition is termed **ketonuria.** In addition, acetone that is also excreted by the lungs when the blood concentration is high causes an acetonic or fruity odor in the breath of these patients.

CLINICAL SIGNIFICANCE. Ketonemia and ketonuria result when the body mobilizes fatty acids from triglyceride stores because of the inadequate intake or availability of carbohydrates. In contrast, when excess carbohydrates are available, ketone synthesis is inhibited, causing normal blood ketone levels to be 3 mg/dL or less and causing ketone excretion in the urine of about 20 mg/d. Any condition that results in increased fat metab-

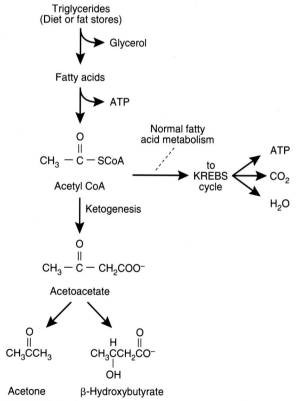

FIGURE 7–3. The formation of ketones from fatty acid metabolism.

olism can result in ketonemia and ketonuria. These conditions can be divided into three categories: 1) an inability to utilize carbohydrates; 2) an inadequate carbohydrate intake; or 3) a loss of carbohydrates. Table 7–19 provides a list of conditions that can result in significant ketone formation with subsequent ketonemia and ketonuria.

Regardless of the initiating condition, the sequence of ketone formation is the same. By far the most common clinical presentation is in the patient with uncontrolled diabetes mellitus. In these patients, carbohydrates cannot be utilized, and fat metabolism is dramatically increased. As a result, ketoacids (ketones) accumulate in the patient's plasma, causing the plasma pH and bicarbonate to decrease. In order to eliminate these ketones and the large amount of glucose present, substantial amounts of body water are excreted (diuresis). Without intervention, large amounts of electrolytes are lost in the urine and a chemical imbalance ensues, resulting in acidosis and diabetic coma. This condition is characteristically preceded by polyphagia, polydipsia, polyuria, and complaints of fatigue, nausea, and vomiting.

The detection of ketones in urine provides a valuable monitoring and management tool for type I insulin-dependent diabetic patients. Ketonuria is an early indicator of insulin deficiency, and ketoacidosis can develop slowly and progressively as a result of repeated insufficient insulin doses. In contrast, type II noninsulin-dependent diabetics rarely develop ketoacidosis (Cotran, 1989). Chapter 9 further discusses the classification of diabetes and the metabolic derangements encountered.

METHODOLOGIES. As depicted in Figure 7–3, the first ketone body formed is acetoacetate and the peripheral tissues metabolize it into β-hydroxybutyrate and acetone. None of the clinical laboratory tests for ketone detection and measurement reacts with all three ketones. Although β-hydroxybutyrate is the ketone body of greatest average concentration in ketosis, methods for its detection are indirect determinations, are difficult to perform, and are time consuming. In contrast, methods based on the nitroprusside reaction (Legal's test or Rothera's test) are rapid and can detect both acetoacetate and acetone. These tests are 15 to 20 times more sensitive to acetoacetate than they are to acetone and they do not react with β-hydroxybutyrate (Caraway, 1987).

Prior to the development of the nitroprusside test, the ferric chloride test (Gerhardt's test, 1865) was used to detect ketones. Unfortunately, many other substances most notably salicylates, can produce positive results. The search for a more specific and sensitive method for ketone detection resulted in the nitroprusside test, originally developed by Legal in 1883 and later modified by Rothera in 1908. Although it is no longer performed routinely in the clinical laboratory, the Rothera tube test is more sensitive to acetoacetate (1 to 5 mg/dL) and acetone (10 to 25 mg/dL) than the current modification available on reagent strips or tablet tests.

Reagent Strip Tests. The reagent strip tests are based on the nitroprusside reaction with sodium nitroprusside (nitroferricyanide) impregnated in the reagent pad. In an alkaline medium, acetoacetate reacts with the nitroprusside to produce a color change from beige to purple. β-hydroxybutyrate is not detected by any of the reagent strip tests; however, Chemstrip and Rapignost strips include glycine in the reagent pad to detect the presence of acetone in addition to acetoacetate. (7–11)

$$\frac{\text{Acetoacetate}}{\text{(and acetone)}} + \frac{\text{Sodium}}{\text{nitroprusside}} + \text{(Glycine)}$$

$$\xrightarrow{\text{alkaline}} \text{Purple color}$$

TABLE 7–19.   CAUSES OF KETONURIA

Inability to utilize the carbohydrates available
  Diabetes mellitus
Insufficient carbohydrate consumption
  Starvation
  Diet regimens
  Severe exercise
  Cold exposure
Loss of carbohydrates
  Frequent vomiting, e.g., pregnancy, illness
  Defective renal reabsorption, e.g., Fanconi's syndrome
  Digestive disturbances

Ketone results are reported in a variety of ways, qualitatively using the plus system (negative, 1+, 2+, 3+); as negative, small, moderate, or large; or semiquantitatively as a concentration in milligrams per deciliter (negative, 5, 15, 40, 80, 160 mg/dL). All the reagent strip tests are sensitive at 5 to 10 mg/dL of acetoacetate, with the Chemstrip and Rapignost strips also detecting acetone concentrations of 50 to 70 mg/dL.

Several agents can produce false positive reagent strip tests for ketones. Most notable are any compounds that contain free sulfhydryl groups. These include 2-mercaptoethane sulfonic acid (MESNA)—a rescue drug in the treatment of cancers; captopril —an antihypertensive drug; *N*-acetylcysteine —a treatment for acetaminophen overdose; D-penicillamine—an antibiotic; and cystine —an amino acid. Because of the increasingly widespread use of these and other agents containing free sulfhydryl groups, it is imperative not only that laboratorians be aware of these potential interferences but that they also review and confirm positive ketone results. In 1989, less than 1 percent of participating laboratories correctly reported a negative result for ketones on a College of American Pathologists' (CAP) urine survey specimen that contained only a free sulfhydryl drug (Csako, 1990).

A rapid and easy means of determining a false positive reaction owing to a free sulfhydryl-containing drug when using the reagent strip test or the tablet test (e.g., Acetest, to be discussed) is available. In high concentrations, these drugs cause the reagent strip pad to become immediately positive; however, by the appropriate read time, the color has faded dramatically or even disappeared. In contrast, the color of the reagent strip pad or reagent tablet intensifies in the presence of true ketones. Because automated reagent strip readers read the strips at a shorter interval than when the strips are read manually, many false positive results can be obtained. With lower drug concentrations, the fading of the strip or tablet color is not always evident, in which case one drop of glacial acetic acid can be added to the reagent strip pad or to the reagent tablet test.

If the purple color fades or disappears, ketones are not present. If these drugs are known or determined to be present, the detection of ketones by these methods can be very difficult (e.g., in a diabetic patient on captopril).

Highly pigmented urine can produce false positive reagent strip and tablet tests. In addition, positive or atypical colors can occur when levodopa metabolites, phenylketones, or phthaleins (e.g., bromsulphalein or phenolsulfonphthalein dyes) are present. These substances apparently react with the alkali in the test medium to produce color (Schumann, 1991).

The primary reason for false negative ketone tests is improper specimen collection and handling. Because of the rapid volatilization of acetone at room temperature and the breakdown of acetoacetate by bacteria, specimens should be tested immediately or refrigerated. Because nitroprusside is very sensitive, deterioration and subsequent nonreactivity of the reagent strips or tablets from exposure to moisture, heat, or light can cause false negative tests.

The Nitroprusside Tablet Test for Ketones (Acetest). A nitroprusside tablet test for the detection of ketones is manufactured by Miles, Inc., as the Acetest tablet test. The Acetest tablets employ the same nitroprusside reaction as the reagent strip tests. The tablets contain glycine, to allow the reaction of acetone, and lactose, which acts as a color enhancer. One advantage of this tablet test is the flexibility of specimen type—urine, serum, plasma, or whole blood can be used. One drop of the specimen is placed directly on the tablet, and after the appropriate timed interval, the tablet color is compared to the color chart provided. Positive results are evidenced by a purple color and are reported as negative, small, moderate, or large. Any pink, tan, or yellow coloration should be ignored.

Both false positive and false negative results can occur for the same reasons as those described under the section on reagent strip tests for ketones. Therefore, regardless of the nitroprusside method used, specimen and reagent integrity and the laboratorian's knowledge of potential interferences are essential to obtaining accurate results.

Bilirubin and Urobilinogen

FORMATION. Bilirubin is an intensely orange-yellow pigment that causes a characteristic coloration of plasma and urine when present in significant amounts. The principal source of bilirubin (85 percent) is hemoglobin released daily from the breakdown of senescent red blood cells in the reticuloendothelial system. Other normal sources of bilirubin are destroyed red blood cell precursors in the bone marrow or other heme-containing proteins such as myoglobin or cytochromes.

Once heme has been liberated in the peripheral tissues, it undergoes catabolism to form bilirubin. The iron is bound by transferrin and returned to the iron stores of the liver and bone marrow; the protein is returned to the amino acid pool for reutilization; and the alpha carbon from the protoporphyrin ring is expired by the lungs as carbon monoxide. This reaction sequence results in the formation of the tetrapyrrole biliverdin, which is rapidly and enzymatically reduced to bilirubin. The conversion of heme to bilirubin requires about 2 to 3 hours (Sherwin, 1989). Figure 7–4 gives a schematic representation of bilirubin formation.

Bilirubin released into the bloodstream from the peripheral tissues is water insoluble and becomes reversibly bound to albumin. This association enhances its solubility and prevents the bilirubin from crossing cell membranes into tissues where it would be toxic. While bound to albumin, bilirubin is also too large to cross the glomerular filtration barrier for urinary excretion. As the blood passes through the liver sinusoids, hepatocytes rapidly remove bilirubin from albumin in a carrier-mediated active transport process. Once within the hepatocytes, bilirubin is rapidly conjugated with glucuronic acid to produce water-soluble bilirubin monoglucuronide and diglucuronide (collectively termed conjugated bilirubin). Normally, all the conjugated bilirubin formed is excreted against a concentration gradient into the bile duct and ultimately into the

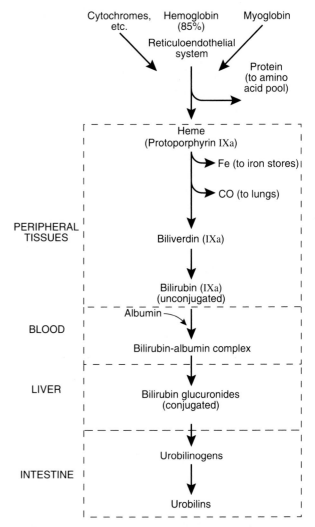

FIGURE 7–4. A schematic diagram of hemoglobin catabolism.

small intestine. Should conjugated bilirubin re-enter the systemic circulation however (e.g., because of hepatocellular disease), it can easily and rapidly be excreted by the kidneys into the urine.

Once in the intestinal tract, conjugated bilirubin is reconverted to its unconjugated form and reduced by anaerobic intestinal bacteria to form the colorless tetrapyrrole urobilinogen. A portion of this urobilinogen is subsequently reduced to stercobilinogen. Normally, about 20 percent of the urobilinogen is reabsorbed and re-enters the liver via the hepatic portal circulation; in contrast, stercobilinogen cannot be reabsorbed. Of the reabsorbed urobilinogen, the majority is re-excreted by the liver into the bile; however, 2 percent to 5 percent of the urobilinogen normally remains in the bloodstream and is carried to the kidney, where it readily passes the glomerular filtration barrier and is excreted in the urine (1 mg/dL or less). The spontaneous oxidation of urobilinogen and stercobilinogen in the large intestine results in the formation of urobilin and stercobilin. These compounds are orange-brown and account for the characteristic color of feces. Similarly, oxidation of the urobilinogen in urine to urobilin can contribute to the color observed in a urine specimen.

CLINICAL SIGNIFICANCE. Disturbances in any aspect of bilirubin formation, hepatic uptake, metabolism, storage, or excretion are possible in a variety of diseases. Depending on the dysfunction unconjugated bilirubin, conjugated bilirubin, or both may be produced in abnormally increased amounts, resulting in hyperbilirubinemia and possibly *bilirubinuria.*

In healthy individuals, only trace amounts of bilirubin (0.02 mg/dL) are excreted, and its presence is normally undetectable by the routine testing methods em-ployed. Therefore, any detectable amount of bilirubin is considered to be significant and requires further clinical investigation. Its presence indicates either the disruption of or an increase in hemoglobin catabolism. An increase in plasma bilirubin and its appearance in urine is an early indicator of liver disease and can occur before any other clinical symptoms. Its presence can be detected long before the development of **jaundice**—the yellowish pigmentation of skin, sclera, tissues, and body fluids owing to bilirubin—which appears when plasma bilirubin concentrations reach 2 to 3 mg/dL (approximately 2 to 3 times normal).

There are principally three mechanisms of altered bilirubin metabolism. They can result in an increase in urinary bilirubin, urinary urobilinogen, or both (Table 7–20 and Fig. 7–5). The first mechanism is prehepatic, indicating that the abnormality occurs before the handling of bilirubin by the liver. In other words, liver function is normal and the dysfunction is an overproduction of bilirubin from heme. This overproduction, occurs in hemolytic conditions such as hemolytic anemia, sickle cell disease, hereditary spherocytosis, and transfusion reactions, or in inef-

TABLE 7–20. CAUSES OF INCREASED URINARY BILIRUBIN AND UROBILINOGEN

CONDITION	URINARY BILIRUBIN	URINARY UROBILINOGEN

Prehepatic—increased heme degradation
  Hemolytic conditions
    Transfusion reaction
    Sickle cell disease
    Hereditary spherocytosis
  Ineffective erythropoiesis
    Thalassemia
    Pernicious anemia
	Negative	Increased

Hepatic—hepatocellular disease
  Hepatitis
  Cirrhosis
  Genetic defects
  Liver congestion
	Positive	Increased to normal

Posthepatic—obstruction
  Carcinoma
  Calculi formation
  Fibrosis
	Positive	Decreased to absent

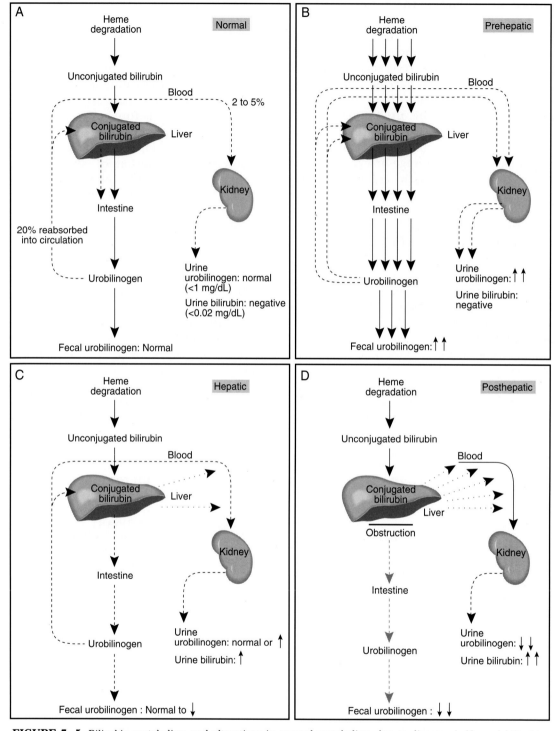

FIGURE 7–5. Bilirubin metabolism and alterations in normal metabolism due to disease. *A*, Normal bilirubin metabolism. *B*, Prehepatic alteration of bilirubin metabolism. *C*, Hepatic alteration of bilirubin metabolism. *D*, Posthepatic alteration of bilirubin metabolism.

fective erythropoietic diseases, such as thalessemia or pernicious anemia. In each of these conditions, large amounts of heme are catabolized into unconjugated bilirubin in the peripheral tissues. Because the bilirubin is unconjugated and bound to albumin, it cannot be excreted in the urine. As a result, large amounts of bilirubin are presented to the liver for conjugation and excretion into the bile. The liver has a large capacity for bilirubin conjugation; most of the unconjugated bilirubin is removed in its first pass through the liver. Because larger amounts of bilirubin are excreted into the intestine, larger amounts of urobilinogen are formed — thus, increased amounts of urobilinogen are reabsorbed into the enterohepatic circulation. As a result, the urinary bilirubin remains negative, whereas the urinary urobilinogen concentration increases above its normal value of 1 mg/dL or less.

The second mechanism of altered bilirubin metabolism is hepatic in origin and results from a variety of ongoing hepatocellular disease processes. In hepatic conditions, the ability of the liver to perform the tasks of bilirubin uptake, conjugation, and excretion are affected. The severity of the disease, and therefore the amount of bilirubin or urobilinogen found in the urine, vary. Depending on the extent of hepatocellular damage, conjugated bilirubin leaks directly back into the systemic circulation from the damaged hepatocytes. Because the bilirubin is conjugated, is readily passes through the glomerular filtration barrier and is excreted in the urine. The re-excretion of intestinally reabsorbed urobilinogen is also affected by hepatocellar damage. Because less urobilinogen may be removed from the portal circulation by the diseased liver, more urobilinogen is presented to the kidneys, and the urinary urobilinogen concentration may be increased or remain normal.

The third mechanism of altered bilirubin metabolism involves posthepatic obstructions of the bile duct or biliary tree. In these conditions, the liver functions normally; however, conjugated bilirubin presented for excretion is unable to pass into the intestine because of the obstruction. Consequently, conjugated bilirubin accumulates in the liver and eventually overflows or backs up into the systemic circulation. The conjugated bilirubin is rapidly cleared by the kidneys, resulting in bilirubinuria. At the same time, very little or no bilirubin passes into the intestine. As a result, no urobilinogen is formed and none is available for intestinal reabsorption. Because of this, the feces of patients with posthepatic obstructions are characteristically acholic (pale white) because the customary bile pigments (i.e., stercobilin, urobilin) are lacking.

BILIRUBIN METHODOLOGIES

Physical Examination. As a result of bilirubin's characteristic pigmentation, its presence is often suspected in distinctly dark yellow-brown or amber urine specimens, which are sometimes described as "beer brown." These urines when shaken will usually develop a yellow foam, indicating the presence of bilirubin. Because clinically significant increases in urinary bilirubin can be small and may not appreciably alter these physical characteristics, a chemical test for bilirubin should be included in all routine urinalyses.

Reagent Strip Tests for Bilirubin. The reagent strip tests for bilirubin are based on the coupling reaction of a diazonium salt impregnated in the reagent pad with bilirubin, in an acid medium to form an azodye — azobilirubin. This azo-coupling reaction produces a color change from light tan to beige or pink (Equation 7–12).

(7–12) Azo-coupling reaction

$$\underset{\substack{\text{glucuronide}\\\text{Aromatic compound}}}{\text{Bilirubin}} + \underset{\text{Diazonium salt}}{\text{Ar} - \text{N}^+ \equiv \text{N}}$$

$$\xrightarrow{\text{acid}} \underset{\text{Azodye (brown)}}{\text{Azobilirubin}}$$

Results are reported as negative, small, moderate, or large, or, using the plus system, negative, 1+, 2+, 3+. The reagent strip tests are sensitive to approximately 0.5 mg/dL of conjugated bilirubin. Before bilirubin detection by this method is possible, about a 25-fold increase in urinary bilirubin excretion is necessary. Various drugs that color the urine red in an acid medium, e.g, phenazopyridine, can cause false positive reactions. Other drugs, such as large amounts of chlorpromazine metabolites, can react directly with the diazonium salt to produce a false positive test.

False negative results can occur as a result of ascorbic acid (greater than or equal to 25 mg/dL) that reacts directly with the diazonium salt to form a colorless end-product; as a result, bilirubin is prevented from participating in the azo-coupling reaction. Elevated nitrite concentrations resulting from UTIs may interfere by the same mechanism described for ascorbic acid. Because bilirubin is very unstable, improper specimen storage can result in false negative bilirubin tests. Bilirubin can rapidly photo-oxidize to biliverdin or hydrolyze to free bilirubin when exposed to artificial light or sunlight. Neither of these compounds reacts appreciably with reagent strip tests; once this bilirubin conversion has taken place, false negative results will be obtained. Bilirubin's light sensitivity is temperature dependent; it is enhanced at room temperature and retarded at low or refrigerator temperatures.

Diazo Tablet Test for Bilirubin (Ictotest Method). A tablet test for the detection of bilirubin in urine is available from Miles, Inc., as the Ictotest method. This tablet test is based on the same azo-coupling reaction of bilirubin with a diazonium salt as the commercial reagent strips. A notable difference is its enhanced sensitivity to bilirubin concentrations as low as 0.05 to 0.1 mg/dL. This represents approximately a four-fold greater sensitivity to bilirubin than the reagent strip tests. Because of this sensitivity difference, it is not unusual for a urine specimen to give a positive Ictotest result for bilirubin when the reagent strip test gives a negative result. When specific requests are made for a urine bilirubin determination or when bilirubin is suspected from the physical examination and the reagent strip result is negative, the Ictotest method should be performed.

The Ictotest method is quickly and easily performed. Urine (10 drops) is added to a special absorbent pad provided. Then, one Ictotest tablet is placed atop the premoistened pad and 2 drops of water are added to the tablet and allowed to flow onto the pad. After 30 seconds, the tablet is removed and the absorbent pad is observed for the development of any purple or blue coloration, indicating a positive test. Any other coloration, such as red or pink, is considered a negative test result for bilirubin. Because the chemical principle of the Ictotest method and the reagent strip tests are similar, the tablet test is subject to the same interferences as discussed with the reagent strip tests.

UROBILINOGEN METHODOLOGIES. Urobilinogen is normally present in urine in concentrations of 1 mg/dL or less (approximately 1 Ehrlich unit) or 0.5 to 2.5 mg/d. Although both qualitative and quantitative procedures are available for urobilinogen detection, qualitative screening tests predominate. Because urobilinogen excretion is enhanced in alkaline urine, the specimen of choice for quantitation or monitoring would be a 2-hour collection following the midday meal (i.e., 2:00 to 4:00 PM). This collection would correlate with the typical "alkaline tide" observed in urinary pH following meals. Quantitative urobilinogen procedures are rarely performed, however; because the information they convey regarding liver function can be obtained by other, more specific, liver-function tests.

Urobilinogen is very labile in acid urine and is easily photo-oxidized to urobilin. Because urobilin is nonreactive in the methods employed for urobilinogen detection, urine collection and handling procedures must be followed to ensure the integrity of the specimen. Urine specimens should be fresh or appropriately preserved and at room temperature for testing (see Chapter 3).

The Watson-Schwartz test, which is used primarily for the detection of porphobilinogen, can be used to specifically identify urobilinogen. This test may be used to differentiate urobilinogen from other Ehrlich-reactive substances that can mask reagent strip test results. See the details of the Watson-Schwartz test under the Porphobilinogen section in this chapter.

The "Classic" Ehrlich's Reaction. Before the development of reagent strip tests, **Ehrlich's reaction** was used for qualitative screening for urobilinogen. It is based on the reaction of urobilinogen with p-dimethylaminobenzaldehyde (Ehrlich's reagent) in an acid medium to produce a characteristic magenta or red chromophore. Numerous substances react with Ehrlich's reagent to produce a red color and are often collectively termed "Ehrlich-reactive" substances (Table 7–21). The test is performed by mixing 1 part Ehrlich's reagent to 10 parts urine in a tube and observing the mixture for any pink color after a 5-minute incubation.

(7–13)

$$\text{Urobilinogen} + \frac{\text{Ehrlich's}}{\text{reagent}} \xrightarrow{\text{acid}} \frac{\text{Red}}{\text{chromophore}}$$

Serial dilutions (1:10, 1:20, 1:30, etc.) of urine could be made and the urine concentration semiquantitated. Any perceptible pink color is considered to be a positive test result; normal urobilinogen concentrations may be positive up to the 1:20 dilution. This tube test is no longer routinely performed for urobilinogen screening because it is time consuming, nonspecific, and costly. However, various modifications (e.g., the Watson-Schwartz and Hoesch tests) are used to screen for urinary porphobilinogen.

Reagent Strip Tests for Urobilinogen

Multistix Reagent Strips. The principles for urobilinogen reagent strip tests, including their sensitivity and specificity, differ depending on the testing product used. Ames Multistix reagent strips are based on the classic Ehrlich's reaction. The reagent pad is impregnated with Ehrlich's reagent (p-di-

TABLE 7–21. SOME EHRLICH-REACTIVE SUBSTANCES FOUND IN URINE

Urobilinogen
Porphobilinogen
Indican
5-HIAA
Drugs
Methyldopa
Chlorpromazine
Sulfonamides
p-Aminosalicyclic acid
Procaines

methylaminobenzaldehyde), a color enhancer, and an acid buffer. As urobilinogen reacts with the Ehrlich's reagent to form the red-colored chromophore, the reagent pad changes from light pink to dark pink.

(7–14) Ehrlich's reaction

$$\begin{array}{c}\text{Ehrlich's reactive} \\ \text{substance} \\ \text{Urobilinogen}\end{array} + \begin{array}{c}p\text{-dimethylamino-} \\ \text{benzaldehyde} \\ \text{Ehrlich's reagent}\end{array}$$

$$\xrightarrow{\text{acid}} \text{Red chromophore}$$

False positive results can occur owing to the presence of any Ehrlich's reactive substance. However, this reaction can be variable and should not be relied on to screen for substances other than urobilinogen, e.g., porphobilinogen (Kanis, 1973). Another problem are substances that mask the reagent pad with a drug-induced or atypical color (e.g., phenazopyridine, red beets, azo dyes). As a result, these colors interfere with the visual interpretation of the test. Formalin, a urine preservative, inhibits the reaction, whereas a high concentration of nitrites can interfere with the reaction. The reactivity of the reagent strip increases with temperature; therefore, urine specimens should be at room temperature when tested.

Chemstrip and Rapignost Reagent Strips. Chemstrip and Rapignost reagent strip tests for urobilinogen are based on an azo-coupling reaction. A diazonium salt, impregnated in the reagent pad, reacts with urobilinogen in the acid medium of the reagent strip pad (Equation 7–15). The azodye produced by the reaction causes a color change from white to pink.

(7–15) Azo-coupling reaction

$$\underset{\text{Aromatic cmp}}{\text{Urobilinogen}} + \underset{\text{Diazonium salt}}{\text{Ar} - \text{N}^+ \equiv \text{N}} \xrightarrow{\text{acid}} \underset{\text{(red)}}{\text{Azodye}}$$

Unlike Multistix strips, these reagent strip tests are specific for urobilinogen. False positive results can be caused by substances that mask the reagent pad with their own color, thereby interfering with color interpretation (e.g., phenazopyridine, red beets, azo dyes). False negative results occur because of nitrites (more than 5 mg/dL) and formalin or from improper storage of the urine specimen.

Regardless of the reagent strip used, urobilinogen results of 1 mg/dL or less are reported as such and are considered normal. Increased urobilinogen values are reported semiquantitatively in milligrams per deciliter (1 mg/dL is approximately equivalent to 1 Ehrlich unit). All reagent strip tests are sensitive to normal levels of urobilinogen in urine; see Table 7–1 for their individual sensitivity limits. Note, however that the absence of urobilinogen is unable to be determined. In other words, these tests cannot clearly or reliably indicate a decrease in or the absence of urinary urobilinogen. The absence of urobilinogen formation and therefore urinary excretion is best reflected by fecal analysis (acholic stool) or from blood profiles involving bilirubin analysis, as previously discussed for bilirubin.

It should be apparent that different results can be obtained when testing a urine with both a nonspecific reagent strip test for urobilinogen (i.e., Multistix strips) and a specific reagent strip test (i.e., Chemstrip and Rapignost strips). Urine specimens containing significant amounts of other Ehrlich-reactive substances can give higher values using Multistix reagent strips than would be obtained with Chemstrip or Rapignost reagent strips.

Porphobilinogen

CLINICAL SIGNIFICANCE. Porphobilinogen (PBG) is a porphyrin precursor and an important intermediate compound in the formation of heme (Fig. 7–6). It is formed when two molecules of δ-aminolevulinic acid (ALA) condense in a reaction catalyzed by ALA dehydratase. Subsequently, four molecules of PBG condense to form the first porphyrinogen, uroporphyrinogen. The porphyrinogens can spontaneously and irreversibly oxidize to form their respective porphyrins. Once this process has taken place, the porphyrin cannot re-enter the heme synthetic pathway; it has no biologic function and must be excreted. Normally, heme synthesis is so closely regulated that only trace amounts of the por-

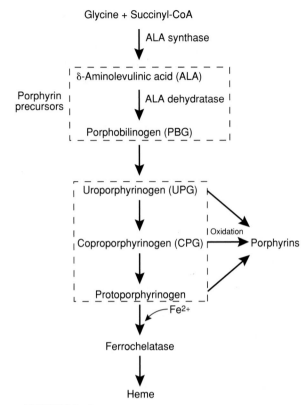

FIGURE 7–6. A schematic diagram of heme synthesis.

phyrin precursors, ALA (at less than approximately 1.4 mg/dL) and PBG (at less than approximately 0.4 mg/dL), are formed. If heme synthesis is disrupted, however, the porphyrin precursors or porphyrins will accumulate depending on the defect in the pathway. This synthesis actually occurs in all mammalian cells, although the major sites of heme production are the bone marrow and the liver. Various inherited or induced disorders are characterized by increased urinary amounts of porphyrin precursors (PBG and ALA) or porphyrins **(porphyrinuria).**

The rate-limiting step in heme synthesis is the first reaction catalyzed by ALA synthase and is subject to end-product inhibition by heme. In other words, in the presence of sufficient heme, this pathway is retarded or inhibited; however, if adequate heme is lacking, the pathway is stimulated to increase its formation. Should an enzyme required in the synthetic pathway be absent, decreased, defective, or inhibited, the compound immediately preceding that enzyme's action would accumulate. For example, in acute intermittent porphyria (AIP), the enzyme PBG deaminase is deficient, and porphobilinogen as well as ALA accumulate. In addition, because heme is not being formed to inhibit the pathway, it is stimulated even more, resulting in further overproduction of the porphyrin precursors. Because these porphyrin precursors have a low renal threshold, they are rapidly removed from the blood and appear in the urine. Increased amounts may be detected or suspected when performing a routine urinalysis.

Although both urinary screening and quantitative tests are available for porphobilinogen, no screening procedure for ALA is currently possible. The various inherited and induced disorders that result in the overproduction of porphyrin precursors or porphyrins, as well as their clinical features, diagnosis, and treatment, are discussed in Chapter 9.

METHODOLOGIES

Physical Examination. The porphyrin precursor, porphobilinogen, is colorless and nonfluorescent. In contrast, its oxidative form, porphobilin, is dark red. As a result, urine containing porphobilin may appear dark red, often described as looking like the color of port wine. A red-colored urine initially implies blood or hemoglobin, but when the test for blood is negative, porphyria should be one of several possibilities suspected. The urine may also appear normal in color initially, but upon standing the specimen may be observed to take on a pink to red color, as photooxidation of porphobilinogen takes place. Keep in mind that the visual observation of a red color is highly dependent on the urine concentration, which varies with hydration; in addition, other chromogens normally present in the urine can affect the color.

The Hoesch Test for Porphobilinogen. The Hoesch test is basically an inverse Ehrlich's reaction. In other words, the volume ratio of urine to reagent is reversed. The reaction mixture maintains a highly acidic condition and urobilinogen is prevented from reacting, except when present in extremely high concentrations, i.e., greater than 20 mg/dL. Because the Hoesch test is rapid, easy to perform, and sensitive, it is usually performed

first when screening for porphobilinogen. To perform the Hoesch test, 2 mL of modified Ehrlich's reagent (Hoesch reagent) is placed in a tube and 2 drops of urine are added. A deep pink or red color will develop instantaneously at the interface of the reagent and the urine if porphobilinogen is present. When the tube is agitated, the color is dispersed throughout the mixture. The intensity of the color relates directly to the porphobilinogen concentration; however, quantitation is not performed by this method. The Hoesch test detects porphobilinogen concentrations as low as 2 mg/dL.

Despite its sensitivity and specificity for porphobilinogen, interpretation of the Hoesch test can be difficult owing to the development of atypical colors. In order to resolve questionable results, the Hoesch test is often confirmed by the Watson-Schwartz test. False positive or questionable results can be caused by indoles or drugs (e.g., phenazopyridine). Methyldopa is also capable of producing false positive results in both tests. However, the Hoesch test requires the presence of very large amounts of these substances to give a false positive result and therefore is preferred over the Watson-Schwartz test if porphobilinogen is suspected or known to be present.

The Watson-Schwartz Test for Porphobilinogen and Urobilinogen. The Watson-Schwartz test is a modification of the original Ehrlich's reaction and is used routinely as a urine screening test for porphobilinogen. Porphobilinogen can be differentiated from urobilinogen and from other Ehrlich-reactive substances. This test is based on the different solubility characteristics of porphobilinogen and urobilinogen with regard to pH and solvent type. Essentially Ehrlich's reaction is performed but with solvents of slightly different polarity; the layer in which the red chromophore resides identifies the substance present.

To perform the qualitative Watson-Schwartz test, equal parts (approximately 2 mL each) of urine and Ehrlich's reagent are mixed in a tube. The volume is doubled by adding saturated sodium acetate (approximately 4 mL) and the solution is mixed again. A positive test will result in the development of a characteristic red or magenta color (the aldehyde chromophore) at this step.

(7–16) Modified Ehrlich's reaction

$$\text{Porpho-} + \text{Ehrlich's} + \text{Sodium}$$
$$\text{bilinogen} \quad \text{reagent} \quad \text{acetate}$$

$$\xrightarrow{\text{acid}} \text{Red chromophore}$$

(7–17)

Red chromophore + Chloroform
→ Aqueous layer (top): Porphobilinogen and others
→ Chloroform layer: Urobilinogen

(7–18)

Red chromophore + Butanol
→ Butanol layer (top): Urobilinogen and others
→ Aqueous layer: Porphobilinogen

If the mixture does not show a red color or if an orange color develops, the test is negative. Next, an extraction is performed by adding chloroform (approximately 2 to 5 mL) to the mixture, followed by vigorous shaking. The phases are allowed to separate. If the red color resides only in the aqueous phase (the top layer), porphobilinogen or another Ehrlich-reactive substance is present and a butanol extraction must be performed. If the red color resides only in the chloroform phase (the bottom layer), increased amounts

of urobilinogen are present. If color is in both phases, the aqueous layer must be re-extracted with chloroform to ensure complete extraction of the red chromophore for identification.

To perform the butanol extraction, the aqueous phase (the top layer) is transferred to another tube and an equal volume of butanol is added. The tube should be shaken vigorously and the phases allowed to separate. If the red color remains in the aqueous phase (now the bottom layer), porphobilinogen is present. If the red color is in the butanol phase (the top layer), urobilinogen or other Ehrlich-reactive substances are present. Table 7–22 provides a summary for interpreting the Watson-Schwartz test.

The Watson-Schwartz test is capable of detecting porphobilinogen concentrations greater than 0.6 mg/dL (Pierach, 1977) and therefore is more sensitive than the Hoesch test. However, other Ehrlich-reactive substances also produce a positive test, requiring butanol extraction for differentiation.

Ascorbic Acid

CLINICAL SIGNIFICANCE. Ascorbic acid, also known as vitamin C, is a water-soluble vitamin. This means that it does not require fat for absorption and that any excess vitamin ingested is immediately excreted in the urine as ascorbic acid or its metabolite— oxalic acid (oxalate). Of the oxalates present in normal urine, approximately 50 percent are derived from ascorbic acid metabolism. Ascorbic acid functions as an enzyme cofac-

T A B L E 7 – 2 2.   A TEST RESULT SUMMARY FOR THE WATSON-SCHWARTZ TEST

	PORPHOBILINOGEN	UROBILINOGEN	OTHER EHRLICH REACTIVE SUBSTANCES
Chloroform extraction			
Aqueous phase (top layer)	Red	No color*	Red
Chloroform phase (bottom layer)	No color*	Red	No color*
Butanol extraction			
Butanol phase (top layer)	No color*	Red	Red
Aqueous phase (bottom layer)	Red	No color*	No color*

* The urine mixture is usually colorless or pale yellow; the yellow color owing to urea will vary with the urine's concentration.

tor in connective tissue proteins. Humans cannot synthesize vitamin C; therefore, dietary intake of vitamin C is essential. Major dietary sources are citrus fruits and vegetables (tomatoes, green peppers, cabbage, leafy greans). Ingestion of megadoses of vitamin C is a common practice although the efficacy of these high doses in the prevention of the common cold and cancers or in the prolongation of life has not been scientifically proven. Regardless, excess daily intake can result in increased urinary excretion of ascorbic acid. Normally, without supplementation, urinary excretion averages less than 5 mg/dL of vitamin C. With supplementation, however, significant intra-individual variations in urinary vitamin C concentrations are obtained.

In a recent study, 22.8 percent of routine urine specimens tested positive for ascorbic acid (Brigden, 1991). The mean urinary concentration was 37.2 mg/dL (2120 μmol/L), with values ranging from 7.1 to 339.5 mg/dL (405 to 19,350 μmol/L). The presence of ascorbic acid has serious implications on several of the reagent strip tests used in routine urinalysis. Therefore, either routine urinalysis protocols should include a screening test for ascorbic acid, or reagent strip tests that are not subject to its interference should be used.

THE MECHANISMS OF INTERFERENCE. Ascorbic acid is a strong reducing agent owing to its ene-diol group (Fig. 7–7). As a

hydrogen donor, it readily oxidizes to dehydroascorbic acid, a colorless compound. Reagent strip tests using a diazonium salt or hydrogen peroxide are subject to ascorbic acid interference. Whether these compounds are impregnated in the reagent pad or are produced by a first reaction, they are removed, preventing the reaction intended. As a result, colorless dehydroascorbic acid is produced, no positive color change is observed, and a false negative test is obtained. Bilirubin, nitrite, glucose, and blood reagent strip tests are vulnerable to ascorbic acid interference (Table 7–23). However, owing to reagent strip variations, some brands are more sensitive than others to this interference (see the discussion of this interference under each specific test section or in Table 7–3: Reagent Strip Specificity).

The presence of ascorbic acid in urine is most often suspected when the microscopic examination reveals the presence of red blood cells but the reagent strip test for blood is negative. Ascorbic acid's effect on decreasing glucose reagent strip results is less obvious and may be suspected only when ketones are positive and glucose negative or when a discrepancy exists between the copper reduction test and the reagent strip test for glucose. Although chemical techniques are being employed to reduce ascorbic acid interference (e.g., iodate scavenger pad), it remains a source of false negative chemical tests.

METHODOLOGIES

Reagent Strip Test. Only Rapignost, manufactured by Behring Diagnostics, Inc., includes an ascorbic acid test on its reagent strips. It is based on the action of ascorbic acid to reduce a dye impregnated on the reagent pad. The reduced dye results in a distinct color change from blue to orange (Equation 7–19).

(7–19)

L-Ascorbic acid + Oxidized dye $\xrightarrow{\text{buffer}}$

Reduced dye + Dehydroascorbic acid

This reagent strip test produces positive results with ascorbic acid concentrations as low as 7.0 mg/dL (Brigden, 1991) and con-

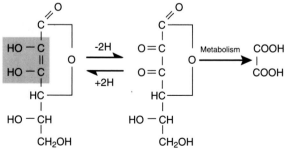

FIGURE 7–7. Ascorbic acid. The highlighted ene-diol group of ascorbic acid is responsible for its strong reducing ability (i.e., as a hydrogen donor). Normally, the principal metabolite of ascorbic acid—oxalic acid (oxalate)—accounts for approximately 50 percent of the urinary oxalate excreted daily.

TABLE 7–23.   SUMMARY OF ASCORBIC ACID INTERFERENCE WITH REAGENT STRIP TESTS

TEST AFFECTED	ASCORBIC ACID CONCENTRATION NEEDED	REACTS WITH
Blood*	≥ 9 mg/dL	H_2O_2 on reagent pad
Bilirubin	≥ 25 mg/dL	Diazonium salt on reagent pad
Nitrite	≥ 25 mg/dL	Diazonium salt produced by first reaction
Glucose	≥ 50 mg/dL	H_2O_2 produced by first reaction

* Chemstrip reagent strip tests for blood are significantly resistant to high ascorbic acid concentrations. At a hemoglobin concentration of 0.6 mg/dL, positive results were obtained despite the presence of 70 mg/dL ascorbic acid.

sistently detects 20 mg/dL of ascorbic acid in 90 percent of the urines tested. No test interferences are currently known; however, other substances with similar oxidation-reduction potentials could possibly cause false positive results. Results are reported as either negative or positive.

Another strip test for the detection and semiquantitation of ascorbic acid in foodstuffs, such as wine, fruit, and vegetable juices, is manufactured by E. Merck as the Merckoquant ascorbic acid test. These reagent strips are based on the same principle as Rapignost strips but employ phosphomolybdate. As this dye is reduced by ascorbic acid to molybdenum blue, a color change from yellow to blue is observed. The lowest level of ascorbic acid detectable is 5 mg/dL, and a possibility of interference from substances with similar reduction potential remains.

Automation in the Urinalysis Laboratory

A goal of the urinalysis laboratory is to maximize productivity and testing quality, while keeping costs and turnaround time at a minimum. Convenience and simplicity are also sought in the development of new techniques and methods. In seeking to achieve these goals, the first reagent strip tests were developed. Since then, reagent strips have dramatically changed the way in which a urinalysis has been performed. Their usage streamlined the chemical examination, significantly reduced the time required, and in-

creased the number of specimens that could be analyzed in a given time period. Since the development of reagent strips, efforts have focused on increasing the consistency in reagent strip reading (e.g., color interpretation, timing), as well as increasing the specimen throughput. This has resulted in the development of both semi-automated reflectance photometry instruments that read commercial reagent strips and a complete urinalysis workstation.

Reflectance Photometry

When light strikes a matte or unpolished surface (e.g., a reagent strip), some light is absorbed and the remaining is scattered or reflected in all directions. The scattered light is termed diffuse **reflectance.** Substances such as magnesium carbonate or barium sulfate completely reflect all incident light and, therefore, can serve as reflectance calibration standards. Reflectance measurements are performed at specific wavelengths and are expressed as percent reflectance. The percent reflectance (% R) is the ratio of the test reflectance (R_t) compared to the calibration reflectance (R_c) multiplied by the percent reflectivity of the calibration reference, which is usually 100 percent (Equation 7–20).

(7–20)

$$\% R = \frac{R_t}{R_c} \times 100$$

The relationship between concentration and reflectance is not linear, however. This necessitates a microprocessor to employ complex algorithms to change the relationship to a linear one. Because the color of the reaction on the reagent test pad dictates the wavelength of light needed for reflectance measurements, each reflectance photometer must have a means of selecting the appropriate wavelength for each test. It selects the wavelength by using either filters or a monochromatic light source (e.g., light emitting diode, or LED) of the appropriate wavelength.

Instrumentation

Currently, three manufacturers market reflectance photometers for use with their respective reagent strips: Miles, Inc.: the Ames Clinitek 200+; Boehringer Mannheim Diagnostics: the Chemstrip Urine Analyzer; and Behring Diagnostics: the Rapimat II/T. Table 7–24 compares the various features of these reagent strip readers. Each reader is specifically designed for use with its manufacturer's products; however, the basic principle of reflectance photometry employed by all of them is the same. All instruments are user friendly, with both audio and visual prompts to aid in their operation. Once the reagent strip has been appropriately placed in the instrument, the microprocessor controls the remaining aspects of testing. It mechanically moves the strip into the reflectometer, turns on the appropriate light source, records the reflectance data, calculates results, and removes the strip for disposal.

The Ames Clinitek 200+ instrument utilizes a single tungsten light source and a filter wheel to select the appropriate wavelength for each of its 10 reagent test areas. The strip is placed onto a transport platform and is automatically advanced under two read heads for timed reflectance measurements and eventually moves into a waste receptacle. The instrument's microprocessor stores the readings until they are complete, then prints them on an internal tape printout. Optional printing on report forms is also available. The reflectometer should be calibrated daily, but it does not provide a permanent copy of the calibration for record keeping. Maintenance of the reflectometer consists primarily of daily cleaning of the transport platform and the areas in contact with the reagent strips and emptying of the waste receptacle.

The Chemstrip Urine Analyzer uses six individual reflectometers to read the reagent strip reactions—two read heads, each with three light-emitting diodes (LEDs). Each reflectometer has a LED as its monochromatic light source and a phototransistor detector. The reagent strip is placed on the transport tray and is automatically taken into the instrument. Once inside, the dual read heads

TABLE 7–24. COMPARISON OF REFLECTANCE PHOTOMETER FEATURES

FEATURE	CLINITEK 200+	CHEMSTRIP URINE ANALYZER	RAPIMAT II/T
Calibration frequency	Daily	Every 2 weeks	Weekly (or every 1000 determinations)
Printout of calibration values	No	Yes	Yes
Warm-up time	2 minutes	None	Approximately 1 minute
Abnormal result flags	Preset values	User selects values	User selects values
Urine color compensation	No	Yes	Yes
Leukocyte esterase enhanced thermostatically	No	No	Yes
Specific gravity options			
Interface for external SG-meter	Yes	Yes	Yes
Reagent strip SG	Yes	Yes	No
Optional entry of microscopic results	No	Yes	Yes
Reflectance photometer light source	Tungsten	LEDs (6)	LEDs (13)
Bar code capability	No	Yes	Yes
Memory capacity	200 sample results	300 sample results	300 sample results

over each reaction pad take reflectance readings at microprocessor-controlled intervals. Urine color compensation is made possible by the use of a color reference pad on the reagent strips, and appropriate strip alignment in the instrument is ensured with a photosensor. Because stray light is a potential problem with many reflectometers so closely arranged, each reagent pad is read individually. The instrument's microprocessor stores all reflectance readings, calculates the respective concentration (correcting for urine color if necessary), and prints the results. Both the physical characteristics and microscopic results can be entered into the microprocessor for inclusion on the final printed report. Calibration of the instrument is recommended every 2 weeks, and the numerical calibration values are printed out for a permanent record. Daily maintenance involves cleaning the strip transport plate and emptying the reagent strip waste tray.

The Rapimat II/T instrument utilizes 13 separate reflectometers. Each includes a LED and a phototransistor detector aligned on a single sensor head. Ten of the reflectometers are used to evaluate the chemistry reagent strip tests, one evaluates the urine color compensation pad, one confirms the appropriate reagent strip alignment, and the last is available for future applications. The reagent strip is placed on a "paper conveyor belt" and taken into the instrument. The leukocyte esterase test pad is thermostatically warmed to enhance this enzymatic reaction. At the appropriate timed interval, the reflectance reading for each chemistry reaction is taken and the results are adjusted for urine color if necessary and stored by the microprocessor. Chemistry results can be stored or printed out; in addition, both the physical and microscopic examination results can be entered and included on the printed report. Weekly cleaning of the instrument, recommended by the manufacturer, necessitates weekly calibration. However, should 1,000 determinations take place in less than 1 week, the instrument will prompt the operator to recalibrate it.

Urinalysis Workstation

International Remote Imaging Systems, Inc. (IRIS) (Chatsworth, CA) has developed a workstation for the performance of an entire routine urinalysis, including a "slideless" microscopic examination. The approach taken in the development of this instrument was to decrease labor costs and increase productivity by automating the entire urinalysis procedure. Because uncentrifuged urine is used, it reduces both specimen handling and processing time. The microscopic examinations are standardized, increasing accuracy and precision. In addition, data entry is minimized because all entries made by the operator, as well as results obtained by the instrument, are held within its microprocessor. These can be directly printed on a multicopy form or transmitted to a laboratory computer system, saving time and potential transcription errors.

The Yellow IRIS Model 450 workstation consists of a modified Ames Clinitek-10-semi-automated reagent strip reader for performing the chemical examination; an IRIS Mass Gravity Meter for the direct determination of specific gravity; and Automated Intelligent Microscopy (AIM) technology for the microscopic examination. In addition, a microprocessor-based computer monitors each aspect of the analysis from specimen handling to result reporting.

Although the Yellow IRIS is automated, interactive operation between a laboratorian and the instrument's many data processing capabilities is needed to perform all three components of a complete urinalysis—the physical, chemical, and microscopic examinations. Before analysis, the patient identification information, collection time, and physical characteristics of a well-mixed uncentrifuged urine specimen are entered into the system using a touch screen. A nine-test Ames reagent strip is dipped into the urine and placed into the test reader of an IRIS Modified Ames Clinitek 10. This reflectance photometer measures the reflectance on each pad at two different wavelengths. This bichromatic technique allows for correction of the reflectance readings for urine color with each specimen. In addition, this reflectometer automatically calibrates the reagent strip prior to each determination.

While the chemical reagent strip results are being determined, the specific gravity determination and microscopic examination can be performed. The uncentrifuged urine specimen is poured into an entry port until the display indicates "adequate sample"—approximately 6 mL. Specimen volumes of less than 6 mL can be processed by making a dilution and entering the dilution factor into the instrument. When this is done, calculation corrections are automatically made after the completion of the specific gravity and microscopic analysis. The chemical examination must be performed first, however, on the undiluted urine specimen.

After the specimen is introduced, the Yellow IRIS performs the specific gravity determination and the microscopic examination automatically. A controlled flow of specimen is presented to the specific gravity subsystem and to the slideless microscope. The specific gravity determination uses approximately 2 mL of the urine specimen. This direct measure of urine density is temperature compensated and linear to 1.080. It is calibrated daily during the automatic self-test procedure and requires minimal maintenance to ensure that it is clean.

The patented system for microscopic examination is performed using a flow chamber that hydrodynamically orients and focuses elements in the urine specimen stream for exposure to a sophisticated video camera with high speed stroboscopic illumination. Each specimen is stained with a supravital stain before it is slowly fed at approximately 30 cm/sec (3 μL) to the camera (Lifshitz, 1990). The instrument takes approximately 500 to 1,500 pictures or frames of the unconcentrated urine stream as it passes before the camera. Approximately 530 frames correspond to one microscopic field of a concentrated urine sediment (Lifshitz, 1990). The urine stream can be evaluated using both low- and high-power magnification; the individual particles detected are ranked by size

and shape and are counted by the microprocessor. Following a low-power examination, a complex algorithm is used to determine if the specimen needs evaluation using high-power magnification. The preselected parameters that trigger a high-power examination are adjustable using either particle count limits or reagent strip chemistry abnormalities.

Following the slideless microscopic analysis, the Yellow IRIS displays in color all particles encountered ranked according to size. It tentatively identifies each entity and requires the operator to confirm their identity or edit them if necessary. Meanwhile, the instrument automatically cleans and prepares itself for the introduction of a new specimen. Results can be sent directly to a laboratory computer system and to an optional printer for hard copy chartable reports. Although as many as 45 specimens can be processed each hour, this number will vary based on the microscopic default parameters selected.

In summary, the Yellow IRIS cannot operate by itself; it requires an operator to introduce the specimen and physical characteristics and to confirm the instrument's microscopic findings. It is faster than a routine urinalysis that uses a semi-automated reagent strip reader, primarily because the urine is evaluated without centrifugation. Other advantages of the instrument include a standardized microscopic examination; limited specimen handling that reduces the laboratorian's exposure to a potential biohazard; and enhanced sensitivity and specificity because all specimens have microscopic examinations performed. Several disadvantages of the instrument include the high instrument price and the inability to identify some unusual cellular casts and crystals. Routine cleaning and maintenance schedules must be maintained to eliminate downtime for cleaning and recalibration.

References

Benedict SR: A reagent for the detection of reducing sugars. J Biol Chem 5:485, 1909.

Brigden ML, Edgell D, et al: High incidence of significant urinary ascorbic acid concentrations in a west coast population—implications for routine urinalysis. Clin Chem *38:*3, 1992.

Brunzel NA: Introduction to urinalysis. Unpublished laboratory manual, University of Minnesota Division of Medical Technology, 1990.

Caraway WT, Watts NB: Carbohydrates. *In* Tietz NW (ed.): Fundamentals of Clinical Chemistry (3rd ed.), Philadelphia, W. B. Saunders Company, 1987, p. 439.

Cotran RS, Kumar V, Robbins SL: Robbins' Pathologic Basis of Disease (4th ed.), Philadelphia, W. B. Saunders Company, 1989, p. 1002.

Csako G: Causes, consequences, and recognition of false-positive reactions for ketones. Clin Chem *36:*7, 1990.

Kanis JA: Detection of urinary porphobilinogen. Lancet *1:*1511, 1973.

Labbe RF, Lamon JM: Porphyrins and disorders of porphyrin metabolism. *In* Tietz NW (ed.): Fundamentals of Clinical Chemistry (3rd ed.), Philadelphia, W. B. Saunders Company, 1987, p. 834.

Lifshitz MS, De Cresce, R (eds.): The Instrument Report. Chicago, Applied Technology Associates, Inc., *2*(1):4, 1990.

Montgomery R, Conway TW, Spector AA: Lipid metabolism. *In* Biochemistry, a Case-Oriented Approach, St. Louis, C. V. Mosby Company, 1990, p. 455.

National Committee for Clinical Laboratory Standards. Routine urinalysis. Proposed Guideline. NCCLS Document GP16-T (ISBN 1-56238-183-0), *12*(26):5, 1992.

Pierach CA, Cardinal R et al: Comparison of the Hoesch and Watson-Schwartz tests for urinary porphobilinogen. Clin Chem *23:*1666, 1977.

Robinson RR, Glover SN, et al: Fixed and reproducible orthostatic proteinuria. Am J Pathol *39:*291, 1961.

Schumann GB, Schweitzer SC: Examination of urine. *In* Henry JB (ed.): Clinical Diagnosis and Management by Laboratory Methods (18th ed.), Philadelphia, W. B. Saunders Company, 1991, p. 409.

Sherwin JE: Liver function. *In* Kaplan LA, Pesce AJ (eds.): Clinical Chemistry, Theory, Analysis, and Correlation (2nd ed.), St. Louis, C. V. Mosby Company, 1989, p. 363.

Shihabi ZK, Hamilton RW, Hopkins MB: Myoglobinuria, hemoglobinuria, and acute renal failure. Clin Chem *35:*8, 1989.

Waller KV, Ward MW, et al: Current concepts in proteinuria. Clin Chem *35:*5, 1989.

Bibliography

Bender GT: Principles of Chemical Instrumentation, Philadelphia, W. B. Saunders Company, 1987.

Narayanan S: Principles and Applications of Laboratory Instrumentation, Chicago, ASCP Press, 1989.

Study Questions

1. **To preserve the integrity of reagent strips, it is necessary that they are**

   A. humidified adequately.

   B. stored in a refrigerator.

   C. stored in a tightly capped container.

   D. protected from the dark.

2. **Using quality control materials, reagent strip performance should be checked**

   1. at least once daily.
   2. when a new bottle of strips or tablets is opened.
   3. when a new lot number of strips or tablets is placed into use.
   4. once each shift by each laboratorian performing urinalysis testing.

      A. 1, 2, and 3 are correct.

      B. 1 and 3 are correct.

      C. 4 is correct.

      D. All are correct.

3. **Which of the following is NOT checked by quality control materials?**

   A. The technical skills of the personnel performing the test.

   B. The integrity of the specimen, i.e., that the specimen was properly collected and stored.

   C. The test protocol, i.e., that the procedure was performed according to written guidelines.

   D. The functioning of the equipment used, e.g., the refractometer, the reagent strip readers.

4. **Quality control materials used to assess the performance of reagent strips and tablet tests must**

   A. be purchased from a commercial manufacturer.

   B. yield the same results regardless of the commercial brand used.

   C. contain chemical constituents at realistic and critical detection levels.

   D. include constituents to assess both the chemical and the microscopic examinations.

5. **Which of the following is NOT a source of erroneous results when using reagent strips?**

   A. Testing a refrigerated urine specimen
   B. Timing using a clock without a second hand
   C. Allowing excess urine to remain on the reagent strip
   D. Dipping the reagent strip briefly into the urine specimen.

6. **Select the primary reason why tablet (e.g., Ictotest) and chemical tests (e.g., SSA) are generally performed.**

   A. They confirm results suspected about the specimen.
   B. They are alternative testing methods for highly concentrated urines.
   C. Their specificity differs from that of the reagent strip test.
   D. They are more sensitive to the chemical constituents in urine.

7. **In a patient with chronic renal disease in whom the kidneys can no longer adjust urine concentration, the urine specific gravity would be**

   A. 1.000.
   B. 1.010.
   C. 1.020.
   D. 1.030.

8. **Urine pH normally ranges from**

   A. 4.0 to 9.0.
   B. 4.5 to 7.0.
   C. 4.5 to 8.0
   D. 5.0 to 6.0.

9. **Urine pH can be modified by all of the following EXCEPT**

   A. diet.
   B. increased ingestion of water.
   C. ingestion of medications.
   D. urinary tract infections.

10. **The "double indicator system" employed by commercial reagent strips to determine urine pH uses which two indicator dyes?**

    A. Methyl orange and bromphenol blue
    B. Methyl red and bromthymol blue
    C. Phenol red and thymol blue
    D. Phenolphthalein and litmus

11. **All of the following can result in inaccurate urine pH measurements EXCEPT**

    A. having large amounts of protein present in the urine.
    B. double-dipping the reagent strip in the specimen.
    C. maintaining the specimen at room temperature for 4 hours.
    D. allowing excess urine to remain on the reagent strip during the timing interval.

12. **Which of the following aids in the differentiation of hemoglobinuria and hematuria?**

    A. Urine pH
    B. Urine color
    C. Leukocyte esterase test
    D. Microscopic examination

13. **Select the correct statement(s).**

    1. Myoglobin and hemoglobin are readily reabsorbed by renal tubular cells.
    2. Hemosiderin, a soluble storage form of iron, is found in aqueous solutions.
    3. When haptoglobin is saturated, free hemoglobin passes through the glomerular filtration barrier.
    4. Hemosiderin is found in the urine during a hemolytic episode.

       A. 1, 2, and 3 are correct.
       B. 1 and 3 are correct.
       C. 4 is correct.
       D. All are correct.

14. **Which statement about hemoglobin and myoglobin is true?**

    A. They both are heme-containing proteins involved in oxygen transport.
    B. Their presence is suspected when both the urine and the serum are colored red.
    C. Their presence in serum is associated with high creatine kinase values.
    D. They precipitate out of solution when the urine is 80-percent saturated with ammonium sulfate.

15. **On the reagent strip test for blood, any hemoglobin present in urine catalyzes the**

    A. oxidation of both the chromogen and the hydrogen peroxide.
    B. oxidation of the chromogen in the presence of hydrogen peroxide.
    C. reduction of the pseudoperoxidase while the chromogen undergoes a color change.
    D. reduction of the chromogen while the hydrogen peroxide becomes oxidized.

16. **Which of the following blood cells will NOT be detected by the leukocyte esterase pad because it lacks esterases?**

    A. Eosinophils
    B. Lymphocytes
    C. Monocytes
    D. Neutrophils

17. **A microscopic examination of a urine sediment revealed an average of two to five WBCs per high-power field, whereas the leukocyte esterase test by reagent strip was negative. Which of the following best accounts for this discrepancy?**

    A. The urine is contaminated with vaginal fluid.

    B. Many WBCs are lysed and their esterase has been inactivated.

    C. Ascorbic acid is interfering with the reaction on the reagent strip.

    D. The amount of esterase present is below the sensitivity of the reagent strip test.

18. **Which of the following statements describes the chemical principle involved on the leukocyte esterase pad of commercial reagent strips?**

    A. Leukocyte esterase reacts with a diazonium salt on the reagent pad to form an azodye.

    B. An ester and a diazonium salt combine to form an azodye in the presence of leukocyte esterase.

    C. An aromatic compound on the reagent pad combines with leukocyte esterase to form an azodye.

    D. Leukocyte esterase hydrolyzes an ester on the reagent pad, then an azo-coupling reaction results in the formation of an azodye.

19. **Which of the following conditions most likely account for a negative nitrite result on the reagent strip despite the presence of large amounts of bacteria?**

    1. The bacteria present did not have enough time to convert nitrate to nitrite.

    2. The bacteria present are not capable of converting nitrate to nitrite.

    3. The patient is not ingesting adequate amounts of nitrate in the diet.

    4. The urine is very dilute and the level of nitrite present is below the sensitivity of the test.

       A. 1, 2, and 3 are correct.

       B. 1 and 3 are correct.

       C. 4 is correct.

       D. All are correct.

20. **The chemical principle of the nitrite reagent pad is based on the**

    A. pseudoperoxidase activity of nitrite.

    B. diazotization of nitrite followed by an azo-coupling reaction.

    C. azo-coupling action of nitrite with a diazonium salt to form an azodye.

    D. hydrolysis of an ester by nitrite combined with an azo-coupling reaction.

21. **Which of the following can result in false positive nitrite results?**

    A. Ascorbic acid

    B. Vaginal contamination

    C. Strong reducing agents

    D. Improper specimen storage

22. **Normally, daily urine protein excretion does NOT exceed**

    A. 150 mg/d.   C. 1.5 g/d.
    B. 500 mg/d.   D. 2.5 g/d.

23. **Which of the following proteins originates in the urinary tract?**

    A. Albumin   C. β_2-microglobulin
    B. Bence Jones protein   D. Tamm-Horsfall protein

24. **Match the type of proteinuria to its description.**

    Description

    _____ A. Defective protein reabsorption in the nephrons

    _____ B. Increased urine albumin and mid- to high-molecular-weight proteins in urine

    _____ C. Increase of low-molecular-weight proteins in urine

    _____ D. Immunoglobulin light chains in the urine

    _____ E. Proteins originating from a bladder tumor

    _____ F. Protein excreted only in an orthostatic position

    _____ G. Hemoglobinuria and myoglobinuria

    _____ H. Nephrotic syndrome

    _____ I. Fanconi syndrome

    Type of Proteinuria

    1. Overflow proteinuria
    2. Glomerular proteinuria
    3. Tubular proteinuria
    4. Postrenal proteinuria

25. **Which of the following statements about Bence Jones protein is correct?**

    A. It consists of kappa and lambda light chains.
    B. It is often found in the urine of patients with multiple sclerosis.
    C. It precipitates when the urine is heated to 100°C and redissolves when cooled to 60°C.
    D. It can produce a positive reagent strip protein test and a negative sulfosalicylic acid precipitation (SSA) test.

26. **A urine specimen is tested for protein by reagent strip and by the SSA test. The reagent strip result is negative and the SSA result is 2+. Which of the following statements best explains this discrepancy?**

    A. A protein other than albumin is present in the urine.
    B. The reagent strip result is falsely negative due to the urine's pH of 8.0.
    C. A large amount of amorphous urates in the urine caused the false positive SSA result.
    D. The time interval for reading the reagent strip pad was exceeded, causing a false negative result.

27. **Which of the following best describes the chemical principle of the protein reagent strip test?**

    A. The protein reacts with an immunocomplex on the pad, which results in a color change.
    B. The protein causes a pH change on the reagent strip pad, which results in a color change.
    C. The protein accepts hydrogen ions from the indicator dye, which results in a color change.
    D. The protein causes protons to be released from a polyelectrolyte, which results in a color change.

28. **A urine specimen is tested for glucose by a reagent strip and by the Clinitest method. The reagent strip result is 100 mg/dL and the Clinitest result is 500 mg/dL. Which of the following statements would best account for this discrepancy?**

    A. The Clinitest tablets have expired or were improperly stored.
    B. A large amount of ascorbic acid is present in the specimen.
    C. A strong oxidizing agent (e.g., bleach) is contaminating the specimen.
    D. The reagent strip is exhibiting the "pass-through" phenomenon, which results in a falsely low value.

29. **Which of the following substances if present in the urine will result in a negative Clinitest?**

    A. Fructose
    B. Lactose
    C. Galactose
    D. Sucrose

30. **The glucose reagent strip test is more sensitive and specific for glucose than the Clinitest method because it detects**

    A. other reducing substances and higher concentrations of glucose.
    B. no other substances and higher concentrations of glucose.
    C. other reducing substances and lower concentrations of glucose.
    D. no other substances and lower concentrations of glucose.

31. **Which of the following statements about glucose is false?**

    A. Glucose readily passes the glomerular filtration barrier.
    B. Glucose is passively reabsorbed in the proximal tubule.
    C. Glucosuria occurs when plasma glucose levels exceed 160 to 180 mg/dL.
    D. High plasma glucose concentrations are associated with damage to the glomerular filtration barrier.

32. The "pass-through" phenomenon observed with the Clinitest method when large amounts of glucose are present in the urine is due to

    A. the "carmelization" of the sugar present.

    B. the reduction of copper sulfate to green-brown cupric complexes.

    C. the depletion of the substrate, i.e., not enough copper sulfate present initially.

    D. the re-oxidation of the cuprous oxide formed to cupric oxide and other cupric complexes.

33. The glucose specificity of the "double sequential enzyme reaction" employed on reagent strip tests is due to the use of

    A. gluconic acid.

    B. glucose oxidase.

    C. hydrogen peroxide.

    D. peroxidase.

34. Which of the following ketones are NOT detected by the reagent strip or tablet test?

    A. Acetone

    B. Acetoacetate

    C. Acetone and acetoacetate

    D. β-hydroxybutyrate

35. Which of the following can cause false positive ketone results?

    A. A large amount of ascorbic acid in urine

    B. Improper storage of the urine specimen

    C. Drugs containing free sulfhydryl groups

    D. A large amount of glucose, i.e., glucosuria

36. Which of the following will NOT cause ketonemia and ketonuria?

    A. The inability to utilize carbohydrates.

    B. An inadequate intake of carbohydrates.

    C. An increased metabolism of carbohydrates.

    D. The excessive loss of carbohydrates.

37. The ketone reagent strip and tablet tests are based on the reactivity of ketones with

    A. ferric chloride.

    B. ferric nitrate.

    C. nitroglycerin.

    D. nitroprusside.

38. Which of the following statements about bilirubin is true?

    A. Conjugated bilirubin is water insoluble.
    B. Bilirubin is a degradation product of heme catabolism.
    C. Unconjugated bilirubin readily passes through the glomerular filtration barrier.
    D. The liver conjugates bilirubin with albumin to form conjugated bilirubin.

39. The bilirubin reagent strip and tablet tests are based on

    A. Ehrlich's aldehyde reaction.
    B. The oxidation of bilirubin to biliverdin.
    C. The reduction of bilirubin to azobilirubin.
    D. The coupling of bilirubin with a diazonium salt.

40. Which of the following are characteristic urine findings from a patient with hemolytic jaundice?

    A. A positive test for bilirubin and an increased amount of urobilinogen
    B. A positive test for bilirubin and a decreased amount of urobilinogen
    C. A negative test for bilirubin and an increased amount of urobilinogen
    D. A negative test for bilirubin and a decreased amount of urobilinogen

41. Which of the following results are characteristic urine findings from a patient with an obstruction of the bile duct?

    A. A positive test for bilirubin and an increased amount of urobilinogen
    B. A positive test for bilirubin and a decreased amount of urobilinogen
    C. A negative test for bilirubin and an increased amount of urobilinogen
    D. A negative test for bilirubin and a decreased amount of urobilinogen

42. Which of the following conditions can result in false positive bilirubin results?

    A. Elevated concentrations of nitrite
    B. Improper storage of the specimen
    C. Ingestion of ascorbic acid
    D. Ingestion of certain medications

43. Urobilinogen is formed from the

    A. conjugation of bilirubin in the liver.
    B. reduction of conjugated bilirubin in bile.
    C. reduction of bilirubin by intestinal bacteria.
    D. oxidation of urobilin by anaerobic intestinal bacteria.

44. Which of the following statements about urobilinogen is true?

    A. Urobilinogen is not normally present in urine.
    B. Urobilinogen excretion is usually decreased following a meal.
    C. Urobilinogen excretion is an indicator of renal function.
    D. Urobilinogen is labile and will readily photo-oxidize to urobilin.

45. The classic Ehrlich's reaction is based on the reaction of urobilinogen with

A. diazotized dichloroaniline.

B. *p*-aminobenzoic acid.

C. *p*-dichlorobenzene diazonium salt.

D. *p*-dimethylaminobenzaldehyde.

46. Which of the following chemical principles is the most specific for the detection of urobilinogen?

A. The azo-coupling reaction

B. Ehrlich's reaction

C. The Hoesch test

D. The Watson-Schwartz test

47. Which of the following statements about porphobilinogen is true?

A. Porphobilinogen is red and fluoresces.

B. Normally, only trace amounts of porphobilinogen are formed.

C. Porphobilinogen is an intermediate product in bilirubin formation.

D. Porphobilinogen production is the rate-limiting step in heme synthesis.

48. A Watson-Schwartz test is performed on a urine specimen. The following results are seen:
Chloroform tube: red color in the bottom layer
Butanol tube: red color in the top layer
These results indicate the presence of

A. Urobilinogen

B. Porphobilinogen

C. Urobilinogen and other Ehrlich-reactive substances

D. Porphobilinogen and other Ehrlich-reactive substances

49. Which of the following features is/are different when comparing the Hoesch and Watson-Schwartz tests?

1. The pH of the reaction mixture.

2. The concentration of the Ehrlich's reagent used.

3. The volume ratio of urine to Ehrlich's reagent in the reaction mixture.

4. The sensitivity and specificity for porphobilinogen and urobilinogen.

A. 1, 2, and 3 are correct.

B. 1 and 3 are correct.

C. 4 is correct.

D. All are correct.

50. **Which of the following reagent strip tests can be affected by ascorbic acid, resulting in falsely low or false negative results?**

   1. Blood
   2. Bilirubin
   3. Glucose
   4. Nitrite
      A. 1, 2, and 3 are correct.
      B. 1 and 3 are correct.
      C. 4 is correct.
      D. All are correct.

51. **Which of the following best describes the mechanism of ascorbic acid interference?**

   A. Ascorbic acid inhibits the oxidation of the chromogen.
   B. Ascorbic acid inactivates a reactant, promoting color development.
   C. Ascorbic acid removes a reactant from the intended reaction sequence.
   D. Ascorbic acid interacts with the reactants, producing a color that masks the results.

52. **Which of the following statements about reflectance photometry is true?**

   A. Reflectance photometry measures absorbed light.
   B. The color of the reaction dictates the intensity of light used.
   C. The relationship between reflectance and concentration is linear.
   D. Reflectance measurements are performed at specific wavelengths.

Microscopic Examination of Urine Sediment

LEARNING OBJECTIVES

After studying this chapter, the student should be able to

1. Discuss the importance of standardizing the microscopic examination of urine and describe how this standardization is achieved in the clinical laboratory.

2. Describe microscopic and staining techniques used to enhance the visualization of the formed elements in urinary sediment.

3. Describe the microscopic appearance and clinical significance of erythrocytes and leukocytes in urine and correlate their presence with the physical and chemical examination of urine.

4. Describe the microscopic characteristics and location of each type of epithelium found in the urinary tract, i.e., squamous, transitional, and renal tubular epithelium (proximal, distal, and collecting duct).

5. Summarize briefly the clinical significance of increased sloughing of the urinary tract epithelium.

6. Describe the formation, composition, and clinical significance of urinary cast formation.

7. State the categories into which casts are classified; discuss the clinical circumstances that result in the formation of each cast type; and correlate the presence of casts with the physical and chemical examination of urine.

8. Describe the development of urinary crystals, including at least three factors that influence their formation.

9. Describe the characteristic form of each major type of urinary crystal; categorize each crystal type as being found in acid, neutral, or alkaline urine; and discuss the clinical significance of each crystal type.

10. Identify the following formed elements found in urine sediment or vaginal secretions and discuss their clinical significance:
    - bacteria
    - clue cells
    - fat
    - fecal contaminants
    - fibers
    - hemosiderin
    - mucus threads
    - parasites
    - spermatozoa
    - starch
    - trichomonads
    - yeast

casts: cylindrical bodies that form in the lumen of the renal tubules. Their core matrix is principally made up of Tamm-Horsfall mucoprotein, although other plasma proteins can be incorporated. Because casts are formed in the tubular lumen, any chemical or formed element present, e.g., cells, fat, and bacteria, can also be incorporated into its matrix. When excreted in the urine, casts are enumerated and classified by the type of inclusions present.

clue cells: squamous epithelial cells with large numbers of bacteria adhering to them. They appear soft and finely granular with indistinct or "shaggy" cell borders. To be considered a clue cell, the bacteria do not need to cover the entire cell, but the bacterial organisms must extend beyond the cell's cytoplasmic borders. Clue cells are characteristic of bacterial vaginosis, a synergistic infection involving *Gardnerella vaginalis* and anaerobic bacteria.

collecting duct cells: cuboidal or polygonal cells approximately 12 to 20 μm in diameter with a large, centrally located dense nucleus. These cells form the lining of the collecting tubules and become larger and more columnar as they approach the renal calyces.

crystals: entities formed by the solidification of urinary solutes. These urinary solutes can be made of a single element, a compound, or a mixture and are arranged in a regular repeating pattern throughout the crystalline structure.

cytocentrifugation: a specialized centrifuge procedure used to produce a monolayer of the cellular constituents in various body fluids on a microscope slide. The slides are fixed and stained, providing a permanent preparation for cytologic studies.

distal convoluted tubular cells: oval to round cells approximately 14 to 25 μm in diameter with a small, central to slightly eccentric nucleus and a dense chromatin pattern. These cells form the lining of the distal convoluted tubules.

KOH preparation: a preparation technique used to enhance the viewing of fungal elements. Secretions obtained using a sterile swab are suspended in saline. A drop of this suspension is placed on a microscope slide, followed by a drop of 10 percent KOH (potassium hydroxide). The slide is warmed and viewed microscopically. KOH destroys most formed elements with the exception of bacteria and fungal elements.

lipiduria: the presence of lipids in the urine.

maltese cross pattern: a design that appears as an orb divided into four quadrants by a bright maltese-style cross. When the microscopist uses polarizing microscopy, cholesterol droplets exhibit this characteristic pattern, which aids in their identification. Other substances, such as starch granules, can show a similar pattern.

oval fat bodies: renal tubular epithelial cells or macrophages with inclusions of fat or lipids. Often these cells are engorged such that specific cellular identification is impossible.

proximal convoluted tubular cells: large (approximately 20 to 60 μm in diameter), oblong or cigar-shaped cells with a small, often eccentric, nucleus (or they can be multinucleated) and a dense chromatin pattern; these cells form the lining of the proximal tubules.

Prussian blue reaction (also called the **Rous test**): a chemical reaction used to identify the presence of iron. Iron-containing granules, e.g., hemosiderin, stain a characteristic blue color when mixed with a freshly prepared solution of potassium ferricyanide-HCl.

squamous epithelial cells: large (approximately 40 to 60 μm in diameter), thin, flagstone-shaped cells with a small, condensed, centrally located nucleus (or they can be anucleated) that form the lining of the urethra in the female and the distal urethra in the male.

Tamm-Horsfall protein: a mucoprotein produced and secreted only by renal tubular cells, particularly those of the thick ascending loops of Henle and the distal and collecting tubules.

transitional (urothelial) epithelial cells: round or pear-shaped cells with an oval to round nucleus and abundant cytoplasm. They form the lining of the renal calyces, renal pelves, ureters, and bladder. These cells vary considerably in size, ranging from 20 to 40 μm in diameter depending on their location in the three principal layers of this epithelium, i.e., the superficial layer, the intermediate layers, and the basal layer.

The standardized quantitative microscopic examination of urinary sediment made its clinical laboratory debut in 1926. At that time, Thomas Addis developed a procedure to quantitate formed elements in a 12-hour overnight urine collection. The purpose of this test, the Addis count, was to follow the progress of renal diseases, particularly acute glomerulonephritis. Increased numbers of red blood cells, white blood cells, or casts in the urine indicated disease progression. A disease process was indicated when one or more of the following cell changes occurred: the number of red blood cells exceeded 500,000; the number of white blood cells exceeded 2,000,000; or the number of casts exceeded 5,000. Because other, primarily chemical, methods are currently available to monitor the progression of renal disease, the Addis count is no longer routinely performed, despite its ability to accurately detect changes in the excretion of urinary formed elements. The microscopic examination of urine sediment now plays an important role in monitoring renal disease progression and in the initial diagnosis of renal disease.

Standardization of Sediment Preparation

Commercial Systems

Ensuring the accuracy and precision of the urine microscopic examination requires standardization. This demands the laboratorian's adherence to an established laboratory protocol for the preparation of the urine sediment, including using the same supplies, step sequence, timing intervals, and equipment. All testing aspects must be followed consistently by all personnel to ensure comparable results. To achieve this consistency, several commercial urinalysis systems are available (Table 8-1). Each system seeks to consistently 1) produce the same concentration of urine or sediment volume; 2) present the same volume of sediment for microscopic examination; and 3) control microscopic vari-

ables such as the focal planes and the optical properties of the slides. All of these systems surpass the outdated practice of using a drop of urine on a glass slide and covering it with a coverslip. In addition, these commercial systems are cost competitive, easy to adapt to, and necessary to ensure reproducible and accurate results.

Each commercial system features a disposable plastic centrifuge tube with gradations for consistent urine volume measurement. The tubes are clear, allowing the assessment of the urine's macroscopic characteristics, and conical, facilitating sediment formation during centrifugation. Each commercial system's centrifuge tube is unique. The UriSystem tube is designed such that after centrifugation, it is decanted completely with a quick smooth motion and it consistently retains 0.4 mL of urine for sediment resuspension. The KOVA System utilizes a specially designed pipette, fitted for the respective diameter and shape of its centrifuge tube, to retain 1 mL of urine during decanting, in which to resuspend the sediment. The Count-10 System offers several options to retain 0.8 mL for sediment resuspension. All of the commercial systems provide tight-fitting plastic caps to eliminate spillage and aerosol formation during centrifugation.

A laboratory need not purchase all aspects of a commercial system to obtain a standardized urine sediment for microscopic analysis. An established protocol could use washable glass centrifuge tubes to prepare the sediment. After centrifugation, according to procedural guidelines, a specific volume of urine is retained and the sediment resuspended. The cost to purchase and then routinely clean reusable centrifuge tubes usually makes this technique very costly and undesirable, however.

Specimen Volume

The volume of urine recommended for a urinalysis is 12 mL; however, volumes ranging from 10 to 15 mL have been used. This volume from a well-mixed specimen contains a representative sampling of the formed ele-

TABLE 8–1.   A COMPARISON OF STANDARDIZED URINALYSIS SYSTEMS

FEATURES	COUNT-10 SYSTEM (V-TECH, INC.)	KOVA SYSTEM (ICL SCIENTIFIC)	URISYSTEM (FISHER SCIENTIFIC)
Initial volume of urine used	12 mL	12 mL	12 mL
Final urine volume with sediment	0.8 mL	1.0 mL	0.4 mL
Sediment concentration	15:1	12:1	30:1
Volume of sediment used	6 μL	6 μL	16 μL
Area for viewing	36 mm^2	32 mm^2	90 mm^2
Number of 100× fields*	11	10	28
Number of 400× fields*	183	163	459
Coverslip type	Acrylic	Acrylic	Glass
Number of specimens per slide	10	4, 10	4

* *Calculated using a "field of view" diameter for high power (400×) of 0.5 mm and for low power (100×) of 2 mm. The number of fields possible is equal to the area for viewing divided by the area per low- (or high-) power field. Note that the field of view diameter is determined by the lens system of the microscope.*

ments. This amount of urine is not always available, especially from pediatric patients. In these instances, the volume of urine may be reduced to 6 mL, and all numerical counts from the sediment exam must be doubled. In some facilities, when less than 3 mL of urine is available for testing, the urine is microscopically examined, without the sediment's being concentrated. Whenever the actual volume used to prepare the sediment for the microscopic examination is less than that routinely required, a notation must accompany the specimen report. The decision to accept specimens with volumes less than 12 mL for a urinalysis, as well as the choice of protocol, is determined by each individual laboratory.

Centrifugation

It is recommended that covered urine specimens be centrifuged at 400 to 450 g for 5 minutes. This 5-minute centrifugation time must be adhered to with all specimens to ensure uniformity. The speed is given here in relative centrifugal force (RCF) (g) because this term is independent of the centrifuge used and the size of its rotor. The speed in revolutions per minute (RPM) required to obtain 400 to 450 g will vary in different centrifuges. Nomograms provided by the centrifuge manufacturer can be used to determine the RPMs necessary, or Equation 8–1 can be used:

(8–1)

$$RCF(g) = 1.118 \times 10^{-5} \times \text{radius in cm} \times RPM^2$$

In this equation, the radius in centimeters refers to the length of the rotor from its center to the outermost point of the cup or trunnion when the rotor is in its horizontal position.

A centrifugation speed of 450 g allows for optimal sediment concentration without the disruption of fragile formed elements such as cellular casts. In addition, the centrifuge brake should not be used because it can prematurely resuspend the sediment, resulting in erroneously decreased numbers of formed elements present in the concentrated sediment. In many laboratories, centrifuges are used by multiple personnel for performing numerous and varied procedures. If the centrifuge settings, including the brake setting, are not checked when the laboratorian is preparing the urine sediments, the established procedural guidelines are not followed and the resultant sediments may show dramatic reductions in their formed elements because of this processing change. Using a control material for the microscopic examination or performing duplicate testing with another laboratory will detect this often subtle but crucial change in sediment preparation.

Sediment Concentration

Following centrifugation, the covered urine specimens should be carefully removed and all specimens equally concentrated. When using standardized commercial systems, the combination of the plastic centrifuge tube and its corresponding pipette accomplishes this task through the consistent retention of a specific volume of urine. Different brands of centrifuge tubes and pipettes should not be intermixed. Using products of different brands can result in changes in the volume of urine retained and therefore changes in the actual sediment concentration. Table 8–1 shows how commercial systems vary in the sediment concentration produced, ranging from a 12:1 to 30:1 concentration. Manual techniques traditionally strive toward a 12:1 concentration with supernatant urine removed, either by using a disposable pipette or by decanting the urine until 1 mL of urine is retained for sediment resuspension.

Volume of Sediment Viewed

A standardized slide should be used for the microscopic examination of the urine sediment. Its use ensures that the same volume of sediment is presented for viewing each time. These standard slides are made of molded plastic with a built-in coverslip of consistent optical quality (or a glass coverslip, if the UriSystem is used). With a disposable transfer pipette, urine sediment is presented to the chamber, and the chamber fills by capillary action. This technique allows for the uniform distribution of the sediment's formed elements throughout the viewing area of the slide.

Glass microscope slides and coverslips are not recommended because they do not yield standardized, reproducible results (NCCLS, 1992). If they must be used, however, the laboratorian should always pipette an exact amount (e.g., 20 μL) of the resuspended sediment onto the glass slide using an automatic pipette. The volume of sediment selected will depend on the size of the cov-

erslip used and should be established in the laboratory protocol. Ideally, the sediment volume should just fill the area beneath the coverslip without excess. Bubbles and uneven distribution of the sediment components can result from application of the coverslip (e.g., heavier components such as casts will be more concentrated near the coverslip edges). If the microscopic examination shows the distribution of formed elements to be particularly uneven, a new suspension of the sediment should be prepared for viewing. Because all the commercial systems have been proven to be far superior to the "drop on a slide" method, this technique should no longer be used for the microscopic examination of urine (Schumann, 1986).

Routinely, formed elements are enumerated at either low power or high power, never both. High-power magnification is often used to differentiate a component. For example, to identify the cell type in a cellular cast, high power is used; however, the number of casts reported would be an average of the number of these casts viewed per low-power field. The average number of formed elements found in 10 low-power fields or 10 high-power fields is always reported.

When the laboratorian is performing a standard microscopic examination, the volume of sediment viewed in each microscopic field of view, using low-power or high-power magnification, is determined by two factors: the optical lenses used by the microscope for magnification and the standardized slide system used. These variations account for the differences seen in reference ranges for microscopic formed elements; they also prevent the comparison of microscopic results obtained in laboratories using different microscopes and commercial slides. However, if each laboratory would relate the number of formed elements found in the microscopic exam to the volume of urine tested instead of per low- or high-power field, interlaboratory result comparisons would be possible.

To convert the number of formed elements observed per low- or high-power field to the number present per milliliter of urine tested, a few calculations are necessary

T A B L E 8 – 2.   CONVERSION OF THE NUMBER OF FORMED ELEMENTS PRESENT IN A MICROSCOPIC FIELD TO THE NUMBER OF FORMED ELEMENTS PRESENT IN A VOLUME OF URINE

1. Calculate the areas of the low-power and the high-power fields of view for your microscope using the formula: Area $= \pi r^2$.

   For example:
   Diameter of high-power field view $= 0.5$ mm
   Radius of high-power field view $= 0.25$ mm
   Area of high-power field view $= 0.196$ mm^2

2. Calculate the maximum number of low-power and high-power fields possible using your microscope and the standardized microscope slides (see manufacturer's information or Table 8–1) in use as follows:

$$\frac{\text{Total coverslip area for viewing}}{\text{Area per high-power field (or low-power field)}} = \text{Number of view fields possible}$$

   For example, using a KOVA slide and the microscope lens given in step 1 above:

$$\frac{32 \text{ mm}^2}{0.196 \text{ mm}^2} = 163 \text{ fields of view possible using high power}$$

3. Calculate the field conversion factor, which is the number of microscope fields per milliliter of urine tested, as follows:

$$\frac{\text{Number of view fields possible}}{\text{Volume of sediment} \underset{\times}{} \text{Concentration}} = \frac{\text{Number of view fields}}{1 \text{ mL of urine tested}}$$
$$\text{viewed (mL)} \quad \text{factor}$$

   For example, using the KOVA system specimen preparation and a KOVA slide:

$$\frac{163 \text{ high-power fields of view possible}}{0.006 \text{ mL sediment} \times 12} = Approximately \ \frac{2200 \text{ high-power fields}}{mL \text{ urine}} = Field \ conversion \ factor$$

4. Convert the number of formed elements observed per high-power field (or low-power field) to the number present per milliliter of urine by multiplying the number observed per view field by the appropriate field conversion factor.

   For example, 2 RBCs are observed per high-power field. Therefore:

$$\frac{2 \text{ RBCs}}{\text{High power field}} \times \frac{2200 \text{ high-power fields}}{mL \text{ urine}} = \frac{4400 \text{ RBCs}}{mL \text{ urine}}$$

(Table 8–2). First, the area of the field of view for both the low- and high-power fields must be determined. This calculation uses the diameter for the field of view (obtained from the manufacturer's information supplied with the objective lens system of the microscope) and the formula for the area of a circle (area $= \pi r^2$). Because a standardized commercial microscope slide presents the same volume of sediment in a known viewing area (see Table 8–1) and the area viewed in each microscopic field is known, the "field conversion factors" remain constant. Once the field conversion factors for a particular microscope and the standardized microscope slide system used are determined, obtaining the

number of formed elements per milliliter of urine requires only a single multiplication step. Table 8–2 outlines these calculations and includes an example.

Enhancing Urine Sediment Visualization

The visualization of urine sediment components can be difficult when using brightfield microscopy because the refractive index of the urine and of many of the urine's components are similar and lack sufficient contrast for optimal viewing. Staining, which changes the refractive index of formed elements, can make components more visible. Changing the type of microscopy used can also facilitate the visualization of low-refractility components or can confirm the identity of suspected substances (e.g., fat). Hyaline casts, mucus threads, and bacteria are extremely difficult to see using brightfield microscopy and often require the use of stains or a change in microscopy to be observed. These techniques facilitate the observation of the fine detail necessary for specific identification (e.g., distinguishing a white blood cell from a renal tubular cell). They also help to differentiate "look-alike" entities, such as an uncommon form of calcium oxalate crystal that resembles red blood cells, or to distinguish between mucus threads and hyaline casts. Table 8–3 summarizes the visualization techniques discussed in this chapter.

Staining Techniques

Supravital Stains

Numerous stains have been used to enhance the visualization of urine sediment; generally, each institution has a stain that it uses most often. The most commonly used stain is a supravital stain consisting of crystal-violet and safranin, also known as the Sternheimer-Malbin stain (Fig. 8–1). This stain facilitates formed element identification by allowing more detailed images of the internal structure, particularly of white blood cells, epithelial cells, and casts. Other formed elements (e.g., red blood cells, mucus) stain characteristically; these reactions are noted on the package inserts provided with commercially prepared stains. Although the Sternheimer-Malbin stain is available commercially, it can also be readily prepared by the laboratory if desired (Sternheimer, 1951). One disadvantage is that in strongly alkaline urines, this stain will precipitate, thereby inhibiting the microscopic visualization of formed elements.

Another good supravital stain for urine sediment is a 0.5 percent solution of toluidine blue (Figs. 8–2 and 8–3). It is a metachromatic dye that stains various cell components differently; hence, the differentiation between the nucleus and the cytoplasm becomes more apparent. The toluidine blue stain enhances the specific identification of cells and aids in distinguishing cells of similar size, such as leukocytes and renal collecting duct cells.

TABLE 8–3. VISUALIZATION TECHNIQUES TO ASSIST IN THE MICROSCOPIC EXAMINATION OF URINE SEDIMENT

TECHNIQUE	FEATURES
Staining Techniques	
Supravital stains	
Sternheimer-Malbin	Characteristically stains cellular structures and other formed elements
0.5% toluidine blue	Enhances the nuclear detail of cells
Acetic acid	Accentuates the nuclei of leukocytes
Fat stains—Sudan III and Oil Red O	Confirms the presence of triglyceride and neutral fats by characteristically staining them orange to red
Gram stain	Identifies bacteria; differentiates them as gram-negative or gram-positive
Prussian blue reaction	Identifies hemosiderin, free-floating or in epithelial cells
Hansel stain	Enhances the identification of eosinophils
Microscopic Techniques	
Phase contrast microscopy	Enhances the imaging of translucent or low-refractile formed elements
Interference contrast microscopy	Enhances the imaging of formed elements by producing 3-dimensional images
Polarizing microscopy	Confirms the presence of cholesterol droplets by their characteristic maltese cross formation; aids in the identification of crystals

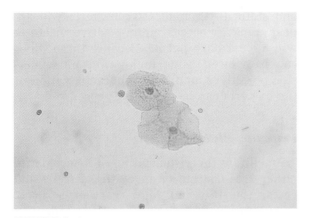

FIGURE 8–1. Two squamous epithelial cells stained using Sternheimer-Malbin stain. Brightfield microscopy at a magnification of 100×.

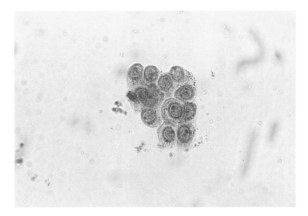

FIGURE 8–2. Fragment of renal collecting duct epithelial cells stained with 0.5% toluidine blue. Brightfield microscopy at a magnification of 400×.

Acetic Acid

Although acetic acid is not actually a stain, it can be helpful in identifying white blood cells. White blood cells can appear small, especially in hypertonic urine, with their nuclei and granulation not readily apparent. By adding 1 to 2 drops of a 2 percent solution of acetic acid to a few drops of urine sediment, the nuclear pattern of white blood cells and epithelial cells is accentuated, whereas red blood cells lyse.

Fat or Lipid Stains

Sudan III or Oil Red O is often used to confirm the presence of neutral fat or triglyceride suspected during the microscopic examination (Fig. 8–4). Fats or lipids stain orange or red and may be found free-floating as droplets or globules; within renal cells or histiocytes, aptly termed oval fat bodies; or within the matrix of casts, as either globules or oval fat bodies. It is important to note that only neutral fats (e.g., triglyceride) will stain. Cholesterol and cholesterol esters do not stain and are confirmed with polarizing microscopy. The distinction between triglyceride and cholesterol is primarily academic because the renal disease implications are the same regardless of the identity of the fat. The urinalysis laboratory can use either fat stains or polarizing microscopy to confirm the presence of fat; the confirmation method

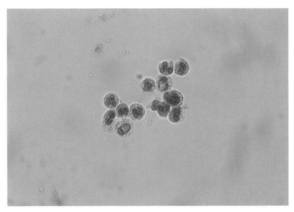

FIGURE 8–3. Leukocytes stained with 0.5% toluidine blue. Brightfield microscopy at a magnification of 400×.

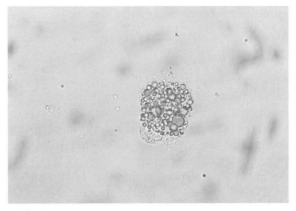

FIGURE 8–4. Oval fat body stained with Sudan III stain. Note the characteristic orange-red coloration of neutral fat globules. Brightfield microscopy at a magnification of 400×.

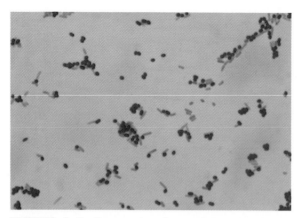

FIGURE 8–5. Gram stain of gram-negative rods and gram-positive cocci. Brightfield microscopy at a magnification of 1000×.

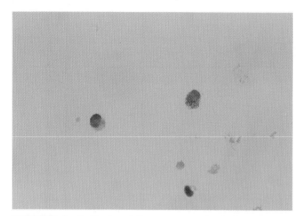

FIGURE 8–6. Eosinophil in urine stained with Hansel stain. Cytospin, 400×.

selected is usually determined by cost, personnel preference, and convenience.

Gram Stain

Although Gram stain is primarily used in the microbiology laboratory, it may at times be used in the urinalysis laboratory. Gram stain provides a means of positively identifying bacteria in the urine and differentiating them as gram-negative or gram-positive (Fig. 8–5). To perform a Gram stain, the laboratorian must first obtain a dry preparation of the urine sediment on a microscope slide, e.g., by smearing or cytocentrifugation. As in the microbiology laboratory, the slide is heat-fixed and stained. Gram-negative bacteria will appear pink, whereas gram-positive bacteria will appear dark purple. Because these slides can be viewed using high-power oil immersion objectives, additional characterization of the bacteria can be made (e.g., cocci, rods).

Prussian Blue Reaction

To facilitate the visualization of hemosiderin, either free-floating or in epithelial cells and casts, the Prussian blue reaction is used. First described by Rous in 1918 to identify urinary siderosis, the Prussian blue reaction stains the iron of hemosiderin granules a characteristic blue color (Rous, 1918). See the section on hemosiderin later in this chapter for more discussion of this reaction and its use.

Hansel Stain

Hansel stain (methylene blue and eosin-Y in methanol, Lide Labs, Inc.) is used in the urinalysis laboratory to specifically identify eosinophils in the urine (Fig. 8–6). Whereas Wright stain or Giemsa stain will also distinguish eosinophils, Hansel stain is preferred (Nolan, 1986). Patients with acute interstitial nephritis owing to hypersensitivity to a medication such as a penicillin derivative may have increased numbers of eosinophils in the urine sediment. Identification of this renal disease is very important because it is one of the few renal diseases that has a quick and effective treatment: the cessation of administration of the drug. Failure to do so can result in permanent renal damage.

Microscopy Techniques

Phase Contrast Microscopy

As described in Chapter 1, phase contrast microscopy converts variations in refractive index into variations in contrast and is ideally suited for viewing urinary sediment (Fig. 8–7). Phase contrast microscopy permits more detailed visualization of translucent or low-refractile components and living cells than is possible with brightfield microscopy. This technique enables traditionally difficult-to-view formed elements—hyaline casts and mucus threads—to be readily identified. In addition, microscopic examinations are generally performed faster, a direct reflection of the increased visualization afforded using phase contrast microscopy.

Polarizing Microscopy

In the urinalysis laboratory, polarizing microscopy is most often used to confirm the presence of fat, specifically cholesterol. Cholesterol is birefringent, and like its counterpart triglyceride, it can be found as free-floating droplets or in cells (oval fat bodies) and casts. In droplet form, cholesterol produces a characteristic **maltese cross pattern** with polarized light (Fig. 8–8*A*). These droplets appear as orbs against a black background divided into four quadrants by a bright maltese-style cross. If a first-order red compensator plate is used, opposing quadrants in the orb will be yellow or blue depending on their orientation, and the background is red-violet (Fig. 8–8*B*). Starch granules also show a similar maltese cross pattern; however, when the laboratorian uses brightfield microscopy, starch granules are readily distinguished from cholesterol by their characteristic dimple, variation in size and shape, and difference in refractility. Be-

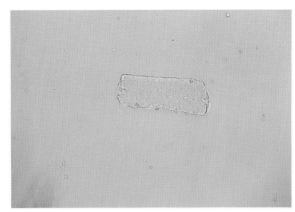

A

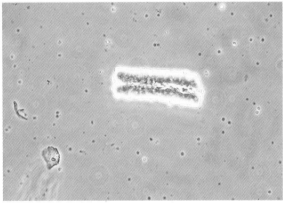

B

FIGURE 8–7. Waxy cast. *A,* Brightfield microscopy at a magnification of 100X. *B,* Phase contrast microscopy at a magnification of 100X. Note the central fissure and increased detail revealed using phase contrast microscopy.

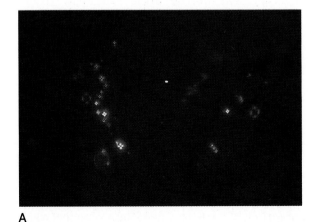

A

B

FIGURE 8–8. *A,* Cholesterol droplets displaying their characteristic maltese cross pattern using polarized microscopy at a magnification of 400X. *B,* Polarizing microscopy with a first-order red compensator plate at a magnification of 400X.

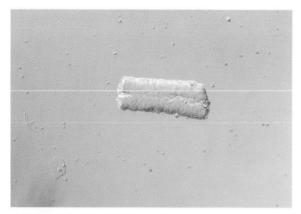

FIGURE 8–9. Three-dimensional image of the waxy cast in Figure 8–7 using differential interference contrast (Nomarski) microscopy at a magnification of 100×. Compare images obtained in these two figures.

cause fatty acids and triglyceride are not anisotropic, they are not identified by polarizing microscopy.

When the laboratorian is performing urine sediment examinations, polarizing microscopy can also be helpful in the differentiation of crystals from cells (e.g., red blood cells from an uncommon form of calcium oxalate; see Fig. 8–57 later in this chapter); waxy casts from fibers (see Fig. 8–93 later in this chapter); or amorphous material from some coccoid bacteria.

Interference Contrast Microscopy

Two types of interference microscopy are discussed in Chapter 1. Both differential interference contrast (Nomarski) microscopy and modulation contrast (Hoffman) microscopy provide detailed 3-dimensional images of high contrast and resolution (Fig. 8–9). Although their use is ideally suited for the microscopic examination of the formed elements found in urine sediment, their increased cost often cannot be justified by the traditional urinalysis laboratory. With experience, however, these microscopic techniques are easy to use and less time-consuming than brightfield microscopy because of the enhanced specimen imaging. In addition, once a brightfield microscope has been modified for modulation contrast microscopy, it can easily be used for brightfield, polarizing, and other techniques by simply removing the specialized slit aperture from the light path.

Cytocentrifugation and Cytodiagnostic Urinalysis

Cytocentrifugation

Cytocentrifugation is used to produce permanent microscope slides of urine sediment. Because a monolayer of sediment components is desired, the amount or volume of urine sediment needed to prepare the slide will vary and requires an initial microscopic examination. The appropriate amount of a concentrated urine sediment is added to a specially designed cartridge fitted with a microscope slide that is placed in a cytocentrifuge (e.g., Cytospin, Shandon Southern Instruments). After cytocentrifugation, a dry circular monolayer of sediment components remains on the slide. The slide is permanently fixed using an appropriate fixative and is stained. For cytology studies, Papanicolaou stain is preferred; however, if Papanicolaou stain is not available or time is a factor, Wright stain can be used. The end result is a monolayer of formed elements with their structural details greatly enhanced by staining. This enables the quantitation and differentiation of white blood cells and epithelial cells present in the urine sediment. If desired, these slides can also be viewed using high-power oil immersion objectives and can be retained permanently in the laboratory for later reference or review.

Cytodiagnostic Urinalysis

Thomas Addis established the value of identifying increased numbers of urine cellular elements as evidence of disease progression in 1926. Today, the ability to perform urinary differential cell counts enables the identification of and the discrimination between renal diseases. Although a cytodiagnostic urinalysis need not be performed on all urine specimens, it plays an important role in the early detection of renal allograft rejection and in the differential diagnosis of renal disease. Cytodiagnostic urinalysis involves making a 10:1 concentration of a first morning urine, followed by cytocentrifugation of the urine sediment and Papanicolaou staining (Schumann, 1986). Although cytodiagnostic urinalysis requires more time to perform, it is uniquely valuable in the identification of blood cell types, cellular fragments, epithelial cells (both atypical and neoplastic), cellular inclusions (both viral and nonviral), and cellular casts.

Formed Elements in Urinary Sediment

A wide range of formed elements may be encountered in the microscopic examination of urine sediment. These formed components may originate from any part of the urinary tract, from the glomerulus to the urethra, or may result from contamination (e.g., menstrual blood, spermatozoa, fibers, starch). Many components are cellular, such as blood cells and epithelial cells; others are chemical, such as the variety of crystalline and amorphous substances that may be present in the sediment. **Casts** — cylindrical bodies with a Tamm-Horsfall protein matrix — actually form in the lumen of the renal tubules and are flushed into the urine. Opportunists such as bacteria, yeast, and trichomonads may also be encountered in the urinary sediment. Not all of these formed elements indicate a pathologic process. The presence of large amounts of "abnormal" components has diagnostic significance, however.

Identifying and enumerating the components found in urine sediment provide a means of monitoring disease progression or resolution. Determining at what point the amount of each element present indicates a pathologic process requires familiarity with

TABLE 8–4.   A REFERENCE RANGE FOR MICROSCOPIC EXAMINATION*

COMPONENT	NUMBER	MAGNIFICATION
Red blood cells	0 to 3	Per high-power field
White blood cells	0 to 8	Per high-power field
Casts	0 to 2 hyaline	Per low-power field
Epithelial cells		
Squamous	Few	Per low-power field
Transitional	Few	Per high-power field
Renal	Few	Per high-power field
Bacteria and yeast	Negative	Per high-power field

* *Using the UriSystem.*

the expected normal or reference range for each component (Table 8–4). Normally, a few red blood cells, white blood cells, epithelial cells, and hyaline casts may be observed in the urine sediment from normal, healthy individuals. Their actual numeric value varies and depends on the standardized slide system used for the microscopic examination (Mahon, 1990). Because changes occur in unpreserved urine, factors such as the type of urine collection and how the specimen has been stored can have an impact on the formed elements observed during the microscopic examination.

This section discusses in detail the variety of formed elements possible in urine sediment. The origin of each component and its clinical significance, the possible variations in shape and composition, and techniques used to facilitate differential identification are also presented.

Blood Cells

Red Blood Cells

MICROSCOPIC APPEARANCE. Because of their small size, approximately 8 μm in diameter and 3 μm in depth, red blood cells in urine are observed using high-power magnification. Red blood cells have no nucleus; they normally appear as smooth biconcave discs; and they are moderately refractile. Red blood cells may present for view from any angle;

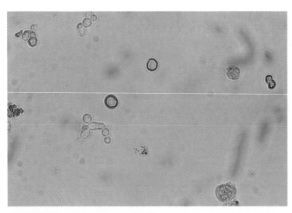

FIGURE 8–10. Three red blood cells—two viewed from above appear as biconcave discs, and one viewed from the side appears hourglass-shaped. Also present are budding yeast and several white blood cells. Brightfield microscopy, sedistain, at a magnification of 400X.

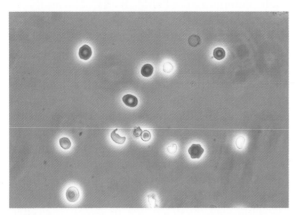

FIGURE 8–11. Dysmorphic, and crenated red blood cells. A single ghost red blood cell is located at top of view. Phase contrast microscopy at a magnification of 400X.

they can have an hourglass shape if viewed from the side or appear as discs with a central pallor if viewed from above (Fig. 8–10). When present in hypertonic urine, red blood cells become smaller as water is lost from the cell by osmosis, and they become crenated. As they crenate, erythrocytes lose their biconcave disc shape and become spheres covered with spicules or crenations. Because of these membrane changes, these crenated cells appear rough microscopically as compared with normal erythrocytes. In hypotonic urine, erythrocytes swell and release their hemoglobin to become ghost cells: intact cells without hemoglobin. These empty cells, outlined by their membranes, appear as colorless, empty circles. Because their hemo-

globin has been lost, ghost cells are extremely difficult to see using brightfield microscopy; however, they are readily visible with phase contrast or interference contrast microscopy (Fig. 8–11). Alkaline urine promotes red blood cell lysis and disintegration, resulting in ghost cells and erythrocyte remnants. All of the red blood cell shapes described—normal biconcave discs, crenated cells, and ghost cells—may be found in the same urine sediment.

Dysmorphic or distorted erythrocytes may also be observed (see Fig. 8–11). Although occasionally these cells are present along with normal erythrocytes in the urine of healthy individuals, their increased numbers are directly related to glomerular damage (Fairley, 1982). Sickle cells have also been observed in the urine sediment of patients suffering from sickle cell disease.

Normally, red blood cells are found in the urine of healthy individuals and do not exceed 0 to 3 per high-power field or 3 to 12 per microliter of urine sediment (Schumann, 1991). Semiquantitation is made by observing 10 representative high-power fields and averaging the number of erythrocytes seen in each. Although red blood cells are nonmotile, they are capable of passing through pores only 0.5 μm (500 nm) in diameter as foot processes (Bessis, 1973). In addition, during inflammation, red blood cells can be transported out of capillaries by the same mechanism as inert, insoluble substances (Bessis, 1973). All red blood cells in urine originate from the vascular system. The integrity of the normal vascular barrier in the kidneys or urinary tract can be damaged by injury or disease, causing leakage of red blood cells into any part of the urinary tract. Increased numbers of red blood cells along with red blood cell casts are indicative of a renal bleed, either glomerular or tubular in origin. These urines also have significant proteinuria. When an increased number of red blood cells is present without casts or proteinuria, the bleed is occurring below the kidney or may be due to contamination (e.g., menstrual or hemorrhoidal).

CORRELATION WITH PHYSICAL AND CHEMICAL EXAMINATIONS. Red blood cells observed during the microscopic examination should be correlated with both the physical and chemical examinations. Macroscopically, the urine sediment may also indicate the presence of red blood cells, i.e., red color in the sediment button. Sometimes specimens have a positive chemical test for blood, but the microscopic examination reveals no red blood cells. This can be accounted for by the fact that red blood cells readily lyse and disintegrate in hypotonic or alkaline urine. This lysis can even occur within the urinary tract, anywhere from the tubules to the bladder. As a result, the laboratorian may encounter urine specimens that contain only hemoglobin from red blood cells that are no longer intact or microscopically visible. One must also be alert to other substances that can produce a false positive chemical test for blood, such as myoglobin, microbial peroxidases, and strong oxidizing agents (see Chapter 7).

In specimens in which red blood cells are found microscopically but the chemical screen for blood is negative, ascorbic acid interference should be suspected. If this substance is ruled out, it is possible that the formed elements are not red blood cells but yeast or an unusual form of calcium oxalate crystals (see Fig. 8–57). In these cases, the formed elements' identity must be confirmed by an alternative technique (e.g., staining, polarizing microscopy).

In most cases of hematuria, even though hemoglobin is a protein, it does not contribute to the protein result obtained by the chemical reagent strip. Hemoglobin must be present in the urine in an amount exceeding 10 mg/dL before it is detected by the current chemical reagent strip tests for protein. However, this level of hemoglobin will produce a trace result by sulfosalicylic acid precipitation. In other words, if the chemical reagent strip test for blood reads less than large (3+), hemoglobin is not affecting the protein result; if the blood result is greater than or equal to large (3+), hemoglobin may or may not be contributing to the protein result obtained by the chemical reagent strip tests.

LOOK-ALIKES. Other components in urine sediment such as yeast, a form of calcium oxalate crystals, oil droplets, or air bubbles can resemble red blood cells. Even white blood cells can be difficult to distinguish from red blood cells in a hypertonic urine specimen. In this case, using acetic acid or toluidine blue stain to accentuate the nuclei of the white blood cells is advantageous. The techniques described earlier in this chapter are useful for the differentiation of these formed elements. A Sternheimer-Malbin stain characteristically colors red blood cells, whereas neither yeast nor calcium oxalate crystals stain. The laboratorian can also use polarizing microscopy to identify calcium oxalate crystals or use acetic acid, which lyses red blood cells but does not eliminate yeast or calcium oxalate crystals.

Yeast varies in size; tends to be spherical or ovoid, rather than biconcave; and often exhibits budding. Each of these characteristics helps to differentiate yeast from red blood cells.

Bubbles or oils in droplet form contaminating the urine sediment can be distinguished from red blood cells because of their variation in size, uniformity in appearance, and high refractility. Although these characteristics may be evident to an experienced microscopist, they may not be as obvious to a novice.

CLINICAL SIGNIFICANCE. Numerous conditions can result in hematuria, i.e., the presence of increased red blood cells in the urine. Smoking has been associated with hematuria, as has normal exercise (Freni, 1977). The conditions resulting in hematuria are outlined in Table 7–5 and include various renal diseases such as glomerulonephritis, pyelonephritis, cystitis, calculi, tumors, and trauma. Anticoagulant drugs and drugs that induce a toxic reaction, such as sulfonamides, can also cause increased numbers of red blood cells in the urine sediment. Therefore, any condition that results in inflammation or compromises the integrity of the vascular system throughout the urinary tract can result in hematuria. In addition, specimens contaminated with vaginal secretions or hemorrhoidal blood will also falsely imply hematuria.

Leukocytes (White Blood Cells)

NEUTROPHILS

Microscopic Appearance. Neutrophils, the most common granulocytic leukocytes found in urine, are approximately 10 to 14 μm in diameter—larger than erythrocytes, but similar in size to the small epithelial cells lining the renal tubular collecting ducts. They are spherical cells with characteristic cytoplasmic granules and lobed or segmented nuclei (Fig. 8–12). Unstained, they have a grayish hue and appear grainy. Neutrophils may occur singly or aggregated in clumps; clumping, which often occurs in acute inflammatory conditions, makes their enumeration difficult (Fig. 8–13).

In fresh urine specimens, the characteristic features of neutrophils are often readily apparent by brightfield microscopy; however, as the neutrophils age and begin to disintegrate, their lobed nuclei fuse, and their characteristic features eventually resemble those of a mononuclear cell. This can make neutrophils extremely difficult to distinguish from renal tubular collecting duct cells. Hypotonic urine causes white blood cells to swell and become spherical balls that lyse as rapidly as 50 percent in 2 to 3 hours at room temperature. In these large swollen cells, the brownian movement of the refractile cytoplasmic granules is often evident, giving the descriptive name "glitter cells" to these edemic leukocytes. In hypertonic urine, leukocytes become smaller as water is lost osmotically from the cells; however, leukocytes do not crenate.

In addition to the fusion of the neutrophils' lobed nuclei, evidence of their and other leukocytes' disintegration is indicated by the formation of blebs (Fig. 8–14). These vacuoles develop within the cell periphery or on their outer membranes; they appear to be empty or may contain a few small granules. As these changes continue, the blebs or vacuoles can detach and become free-floating in the urine. They may also develop and remain within the cell, pushing the cytoplasm to one side and giving rise to large pale areas intercellularly. Another degenerative change is

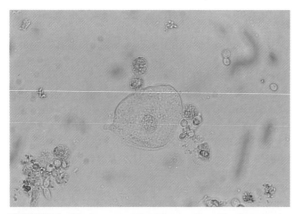

FIGURE 8–12. Several white blood cells with characteristic cytoplasmic granules and lobed nuclei surrounding a squamous epithelial cell. Budding yeast cells are also present. Brightfield microscopy, sedistain, at a magnification of 400X.

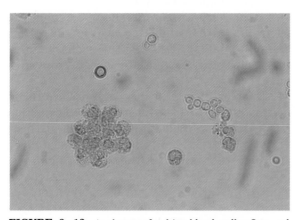

FIGURE 8–13. A clump of white blood cells. One red blood cell and budding yeast are also present. Brightfield microscopy, sedistain, at a magnification of 400X.

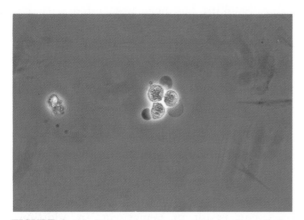

FIGURE 8–14. Disintegrating white blood cells with the formation of blebs. Phase contrast microscopy at a magnification of 400X.

the development of numerous finger- or worm-like projections protruding from their surfaces (Fig. 8–15). These long filaments, termed myelin forms, are breakdown products of the cells' membrane. As these cells die, additional vacuolization, rupturing, or pseudopod formation may be observed.

Normally, leukocytes are observed in the urine of healthy individuals. Semiquantitation is made by observing 10 representative high-power fields and averaging the number of leukocytes found in each. Values range from 0 to 8 cells per high-power field or approximately 10 cells per microliter of urine sediment using a standardized microscope slide. These normal values are not surprising because leukocytes are a normal component in the secretions of both the male and female genital tracts. Any clumping of leukocytes evident during the microscopic examination is reported, because leukocyte enumeration is directly affected. Because leukocytes are motile, they are capable of entering the urinary tract at any point. In response to an inflammatory process, leukocytes move through the tissues in an ameboid fashion (chemotaxis). Although they are spherical within the blood stream or in the urine, the cytoplasm and nucleus of leukocytes are readily deformable, allowing them to leave the peritubular capillaries and migrate through the renal interstitium.

If the microscopic examination reveals white blood cell casts, cellular casts, or granular casts in the sediment, the leukocytes are believed to be of renal origin and indicate an upper urinary tract infection. The chemical reagent strip test for protein should also reveal increased amounts of urine protein. In contrast, a lower urinary tract infection, one that is localized below the kidney, presents with increased leukocytes but without increased numbers of casts and only small amounts of protein, if any.

Correlation with the Physical and Microscopic Examinations. When leukocytes are present in the urine in increased numbers, the urine may be cloudy; depending on the extent of the infection, the urine can have a strong, foul odor. A macroscopic examination

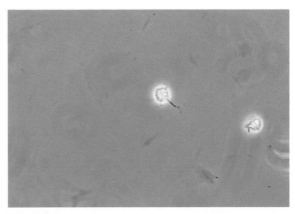

FIGURE 8–15. Formation of myelin filaments in disintegrating white blood cells. Phase contrast microscopy at a magnification of 400×.

of the sediment button may show a large amount of gray-white material: the concentrated leukocytes. Because leukocytes readily lyse in urine, discrepancies may occur between the number of cells seen microscopically and the results obtained with the leukocyte esterase chemical screening test. A positive chemical screening test for leukocyte esterase, despite few or no white blood cells evident microscopically, can result from cellular lysis and disintegration. Also, different leukocytes contain varying amounts of granules and therefore differing amounts of leukocyte esterase; some cells, such as lymphocytes, contain no leukocyte esterase. If increased numbers of leukocytes appear in the urine, but the leukocyte esterase screening test is negative, the microscopist must ensure that the cells are granulocytic leukocytes and that the reagent strips are functioning properly. Although the leukocyte esterase screening test usually detects 10 to 25 white blood cells/μL, the amount of esterase present may be insufficient to produce a positive response.

Look-alikes. As mentioned earlier, some renal tubular epithelial cells and at times even red blood cells can be difficult to distinguish from leukocytes. A 2 percent acetic acid solution or, better yet, a 0.5 percent toluidine blue solution will reveal the nuclear details of the cells present and allow the

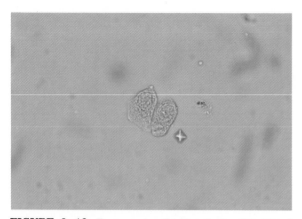

FIGURE 8-16. Two renal collecting duct cells stained with 0.5% toluidine blue. Note their polygonal shape and the nuclear detail distinguishing them from leukocytes. Brightfield microscopy at a magnification of 400×.

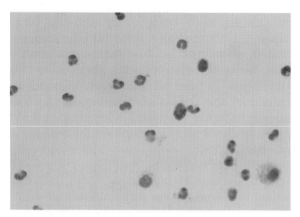

FIGURE 8-17. Eosinophil in urine, stained with Hansel stain. Brightfield microscopy, cytospin, at a magnification of 400×.

cells' positive identification. The large, dense nuclei of collecting duct cells and their polygonal shape help to distinguish collecting duct cells from spherical white blood cells, which have characteristic cytoplasmic granulation (Fig. 8-16). Staining with Sternheimer-Malbin stain or toluidine blue, or using contrast interference microscopy, can also produce more detailed cellular images for specific identification.

Clinical Significance. An increased amount of leukocytes in the urine is termed leukocyturia. Almost all renal diseases and inflammatory conditions of the urinary tract present with increased numbers of leukocytes, particularly neutrophils, in the urine.

Both bacterial and nonbacterial causes of inflammation result in leukocyturia. Bacterial infections include pyelonephritis, cystitis, urethritis, and prostatitis; nonbacterial infections include nephritis, glomerulonephritis, chlamydia, mycoplasmosis, tuberculosis, trichomonads, and mycoses. The latter two microbes, trichomonads and mycoses, often appear as a vaginal contaminant in the urine from women. Although these organisms can infect the urinary tract, it is rare—their presence usually indicates a vaginal infection. Their presence in the urine from a male, however, indicates a urinary tract infection.

EOSINOPHILS. In a routine microscopic examination of unstained urine sediment, the discrimination of eosinophils from neutrophils is often impossible despite their bilobed nuclei and slightly larger size. When specifically requested, urine specimens for eosinophil detection should be cytocentrifuged and stained using Hansel stain. This stain is considered superior to Wright stain in detecting eosinophils in urine (Corwin, 1989) (Fig. 8-17). Acute interstitial nephritis (AIN) and, occasionally, chronic urinary tract infections (UTIs) present with eosinophiluria. The presence of eosinophil casts is diagnostic of AIN. Overall, eosinophiluria is a good predictor of AIN associated with drug hypersensitivity, particularly hypersensitivity to penicillin and its derivatives. Untreated AIN can lead to permanent renal damage; however, if detected early, simply ceasing administration of the drug can result in the return of normal renal function. In cases of acute allograft rejection, the presence of large numbers of eosinophils in a kidney biopsy specimen is considered a poor prognostic indicator (Weir, 1986).

LYMPHOCYTES. Although lymphocytes are normally present in the urine, these leukocytes are usually not recognized because of their small numbers. When supravital stains are used or a cytodiagnostic urinalysis using Wright or Papanicolaou stain is performed, they are more readily apparent and identified (Fig. 8-18). Most prevalent in the urine are small lymphocytes, approximately 6 to 9 μm in diameter. They have a single round to slightly oval nucleus and scant clear cytoplasm that usually extends out from one side of the cell. Lymphocytes are present in inflammatory conditions such as acute pyelonephritis; however, because neutrophils predominate, lymphocytes are often not recognized. In contrast, patients experiencing renal transplant rejection will also have leukocyturia; however, lymphocytes predominate. Because lymphocytes do not contain leukocyte esterases, they will not produce a positive screening test by reagent strip tests, regardless of the number of lymphocytes present in the urine.

MONOCYTES AND MACROPHAGES (HISTIOCYTES). Both monocytes and macrophages may be seen in urine sediment. They are actively phagocytic cells, capable of phagocytizing bacteria, viruses, antigen-antibody complexes, red blood cells, and both organic and inorganic substances (e.g., fat, hemosiderin). The primary functions of these cells are to defend against microorganisms, to remove dead or dying cells and cellular debris, and to interact immunologically with lymphoid cells. Renal tubulointerstitial diseases resulting from infections or immune reactions will draw monocytes and macrophages to the site of inflammation by chemotaxis — i.e., their directional movement is a response to a chemoattractant stimulus.

Monocytes can range in diameter from 20 to 40 μm. They have a single large nucleus that is round to oval and often indented. The cytoplasm can be abundant and contains azurophilic granules. Because monocytes are actively phagocytic cells, large vacuoles often containing debris or organisms can be identified within them (Fig. 8–19).

Macrophages are derived from monocytes; when they reside in interstitial tissues, they are often called histiocytes. Although they average 30 to 40 μm in diameter, they can be as small as 10 μm or as large as 100 μm in diameter. When they are small, their oval nuclei and azurophilic granules make them difficult to distinguish from neutrophils. Because macrophages transform from monocytes, they are often encountered with irregular, kidney-shaped nuclei and abundant cytoplasm. They are actively phagocytic, so their cytoplasm is often vacu-

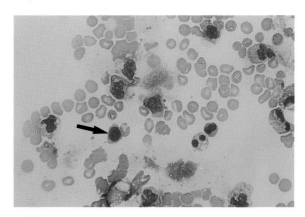

FIGURE 8–18. Lymphocyte *(arrow)* in urine sediment. Brightfield microscopy, cytospin, at a magnification of 400×.

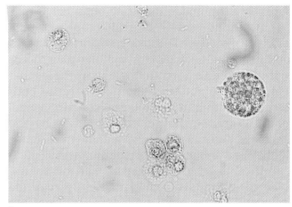

A

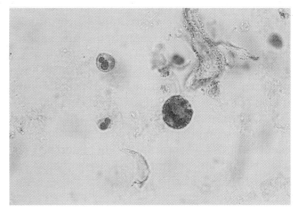

B

FIGURE 8–19. Macrophages and several white blood cells. *A,* Brightfield microscopy at a magnification of 400×. *B,* Brightfield microscopy, sedistain, at a magnification of 400×.

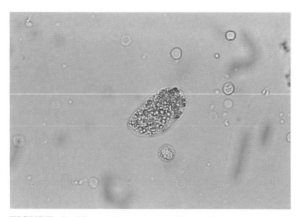

FIGURE 8–20. Oval fat body. The cell has numerous highly refractile fat globules and other inclusions. Bright-field microscopy at a magnification of 400X.

olated. Owing to their variable size and appearance, macrophages can be difficult to identify in an unstained urine sediment.

Both monocytes and macrophages are more easily identified using supravital stains on the urine sediment or making a cytocentrifuged preparation followed by Wright or Papanicolaou stain. In addition, because both monocytes and macrophages contain azurophilic granules, they can be detected by the chemical screening test for leukocyte esterase if they are present in sufficient numbers.

In a microscopic examination of an unstained urine sediment, monocytes can be misidentified as renal tubular cells. They are of similar size, and both are mononucleated. Renal tubular epithelial cells tend to have distinct cellular borders and dense nuclei compared to either monocytes or macrophages, however.

When monocytes or macrophages have ingested lipoproteins and fats, these globular inclusions are distinctly refractile (Fig. 8–20). Called oval fat bodies, they are impossible to distinguish from renal tubular cells that can also absorb fats. The microscopist can use either polarizing microscopy or fat stains to confirm the identity of these cellular inclusions.

Epithelial Cells

The laboratorian will encounter various types of epithelial cells in urine sediment.

Some epithelial cells result from the normal cell turnover of aging cells, whereas others represent epithelial damage and sloughing owing to inflammatory processes or renal disease. Familiarity with the type of epithelium found in each portion of the kidney and the urinary tract helps the laboratorian localize the origin of the cells found in the urine sediment. In addition, the presence of large amounts of some cell types can indicate an improperly collected specimen, whereas increased numbers of others indicate a severe pathologic process. Whenever epithelial cells are encountered with abnormal characteristics, such as unusual size, shape, inclusions, or nuclear chromatin pattern, further cytology studies are necessary. These cells may indicate neoplasia in the genitourinary tract. Essentially three types of epithelial cells are found in the urine sediment: squamous, transitional (urothelial), and renal tubular epithelial cells (Table 8–5). By far the most common epithelial cells found in the urine are squamous epithelial cells.

Renal epithelial cells include several distinctively different cell types, each deriving from a different part of the renal tubule (i.e., collecting duct cell, proximal convoluted tubular cell, distal convoluted tubular cell). The type of cell encountered will depend on the location of the disease process that is causing the epithelium to be injured and sloughed. Although the identification of some epithelial cells can be difficult in wet preparations, techniques are available to facilitate the cells' proper identification. Each laboratory should have a policy that addresses urine sediments with unusual or abnormal cellularity, such as atypical cells or cellular fragments. This policy may simply involve forwarding the specimen to the cytology department for analysis or performing a cytodiagnostic urinalysis. Because both the presence of certain types of epithelial cells and the number of epithelial cells present can be clinically significant, it is important that the microscopist use the techniques available to ensure the proper identification and reporting of epithelial cells.

During the microscopic examination, squamous epithelial cells are readily observed using low-power magnification owing

TABLE 8–5.   A COMPARISON OF EPITHELIAL CELLS FROM THE URINARY TRACT

CELL TYPE	SIZE (DIAMETER)	SHAPE	NUCLEUS
Squamous epithelial cells	40 to 60 μm	Thin, flagstone-shaped, with distinct edges. These cells have a large amount of cytoplasm with fine granulation that increases with degeneration.	Small (approximately 8 μm), centrally located, can be anucleated.
Transitional (urothelial) epithelial cells	20 to 40 μm	Variable, depending on the cell layer sloughed. *Superficial layer* cells are larger, round or pear-shaped; *intermediate layer* cells are smaller and rounder; *deep basal layer* cells are small and can be elongated or columnar-like. The cell edges are distinct and the cell appears "firm."	Small (8 to 14 μm), centrally located, oval to round with variable density in the chromatin pattern.
Renal tubular epithelial cells Collecting duct cells	12 to 20 μm	Variable. Polygonal or cuboidal from small ducts; columnar from larger ducts. Relatively smooth cytoplasm.	Large, moderately dense, round nucleus that takes up approximately two-thirds of the cytoplasm. In columnar cells, the nucleus is usually slightly eccentric.
Distal convoluted tubular cells	14 to 25 μm	Oval to round with grainy cytoplasm.	Small, round, dense nucleus; centered or slightly eccentric.
Proximal convoluted tubular cells	20 to 60 μm	Oblong or cigar-shaped. These cells have a large amount of grainy cytoplasm. The cell edges are not sharply defined. They can resemble casts.	Small, round, dense nucleus; eccentric; can be multinucleated.

to their large size. In contrast, both transitional and renal epithelial cells are assessed using high-power magnification. After observing their presence in 10 representative fields of view at the appropriate magnification, the microscopist reports each type of epithelial cell encountered as few, moderate, or many.

Squamous Epithelial Cells

Squamous epithelial cells are the most common and largest epithelial cells found in the urine (Fig. 8–21). They line the entire urethra in the female, but only the distal portion of the urethra in the male. Routinely, the superficial layers of the squamous epithelium are desquamated and replaced by new, underlying epithelium. In women, large numbers of squamous epithelial cells in the urine sediment often represent vaginal or perineal contamination; in uncircumcised men, their

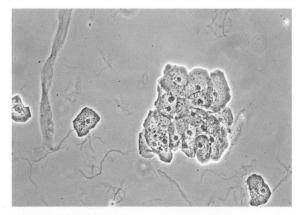

FIGURE 8–21. Squamous epithelial cells—one large clump and several individual cells. Note their large, thin, flagstone-shaped appearance, centrally located nuclei, and stippled cytoplasm (stippling increases with cellular degeneration). A few ribbon-like mucus threads are also present. Phase contrast microscopy at a magnification of 100X.

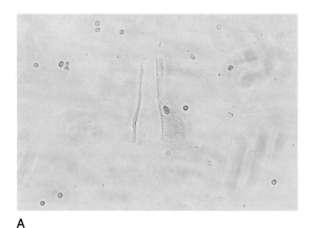

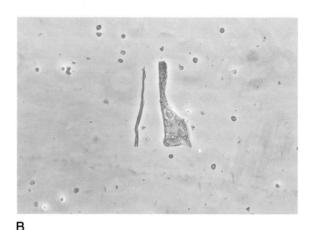

A   B

FIGURE 8-22. Two squamous epithelial cells. The cell on the left is presenting a side view, demonstrating how flat these cells are. The upper edge of the cell on the right is curled, producing an unusual form. *A*, Brightfield microscopy, sedistain, at a magnification of 200×. *B*, Phase contrast microscopy at a magnification of 200×.

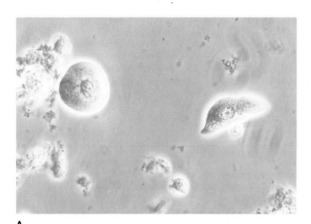

A

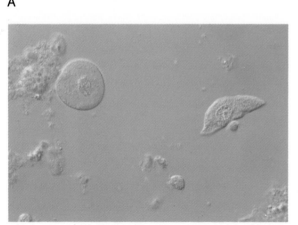

B

FIGURE 8-23. Two transitional (urothelial) epithelial cells. *A*, Phase contrast microscopy at a magnification of 400×. *B*, Interference contrast microscopy at a magnification of 400×.

presence also suggests specimen contamination. Squamous epithelial cells are large (40 to 60 μm), thin, flagstone-shaped cells with distinct edges that can appear in clumps. They have a small, condensed, centrally located nucleus about the size of an erythrocyte, or they can be anucleated. Their large amount of cytoplasm is often stippled with fine granulation (keratohyalin granules), which increases as the cell further degenerates. Squamous epithelial cells can be observed in unusual conformations, because their edges can fold over or curl (Fig. 8-22).

Easily identified using low-power magnification, squamous cells are the only epithelial cells assessed using this magnification. Squamous epithelial cells in urine specimens rarely have diagnostic significance and usually indicate specimen contamination.

Transitional (Urothelial) Epithelial Cells

The renal calyces, renal pelves, ureters, and bladder are lined with several layers of transitional epithelium (Fig. 8-23). In the male, this type of epithelium also lines the urethra except for the distal portion, whereas in the female, transitional epithelium ceases at the base of the bladder. **Transitional (urothelial) epithelial cells** are considerably variable in size. This size variation relates directly to their location in the three principal layers of the transitional epithelium. The cells in the uppermost or superficial layer are large (30 to 40 μm), flattened cells. Cells from the intermediate layers are smaller and rounder (20 to 30 μm), whereas those from the single basal layer tend to be elongated or columnar.

A few transitional epithelial cells are present in the urine sediment from normal healthy individuals and represent the routine sloughing of old epithelium. In urine sediments, the most prevalent form of the transitional cells is the superficial type—round or pear-shaped, with a dense oval to round nucleus and abundant cytoplasm (Fig. 8–24). The nucleus is about the size of a red or white blood cell, and the peripheral borders of both the nucleus and the cell membrane are distinctly outlined.

In cases of a UTI, increased numbers of transitional epithelial cells are often present in the urine. At times clusters or sheets of transitional epithelium will be encountered following urinary catheterization or other types of instrumentation procedures. However, if these cell sheets are seen without these procedures, they indicate a pathologic process that requires further investigation, e.g., transitional cell carcinoma.

Renal Tubular Epithelial Cells

As described in Chapter 4, each portion of a renal tubule is lined with a single layer of a characteristically different epithelium. A few renal tubular cells appear in urine from normal healthy individuals and represent the routine replacement of aging or old epithelium in the renal tubules. Newborn infants have more renal tubular cells in their urine than do older children or adults.

In routine microscopic examinations of urine, two types of renal epithelial cells are enumerated and reported—convoluted tubular cells and collecting duct cells.

CONVOLUTED RENAL TUBULAR CELLS. Because the cytoplasm of convoluted tubular cells is coarsely granular and their nuclei are not readily visible when using brightfield or phase contrast microscopy, these cells can resemble granular casts. Staining the urine sediment greatly enhances visualization of the nuclei and the cells' correct identification. Cytocentrifugation followed with Pa-

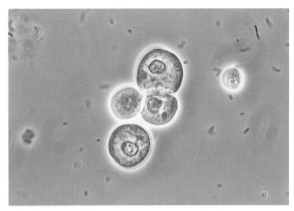

FIGURE 8–24. Four transitional (urothelial) epithelial cells. Phase contrast microscopy at a magnification of 400×.

panicolaou's staining of the urine sediment can also be used to specifically identify these cells.

Differentiating between proximal convoluted tubular cells and distal convoluted tubular cells is difficult and is based primarily on size and shape. Usually differentiation between proximal and distal convoluted tubular cells is not necessary, however, and these cells are collectively reported as "convoluted" renal tubular cells.

Proximal convoluted tubular cells are relatively large (20 to 60 μm in diameter) with granular cytoplasm. They are oblong or cigar-shaped (Fig. 8–25A and B), a characteristic that makes them resemble small granular casts. They have a small, often eccentric, nucleus with a dense chromatin pattern and can be multinucleated.

Distal convoluted tubular cells (approximately 14 to 25 μm in diameter) are round to oval and are smaller than cells of the proximal tubule (Fig. 8–25C). They have a small dense nucleus that is usually eccentric and have a granular cytoplasm, much like that of proximal tubular cells.

Both proximal and distal convoluted tubular cells are found in the urine as a result of acute ischemic or toxic renal tubular disease (e.g., acute tubular necrosis) from heavy metals or drug (aminoglycosides) toxicity.

COLLECTING DUCT CELLS. Collecting duct cells range from 12 to 20 μm in diameter and are cuboidal, polygonal, or columnar

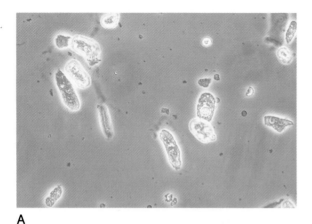

A

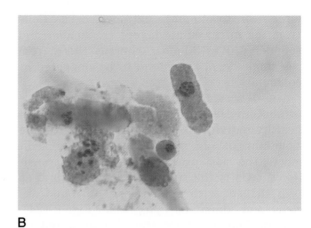

B

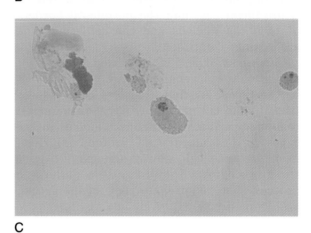

C

FIGURE 8–25. Convoluted tubular epithelial cells. *A,* Numerous proximal convoluted tubular cells. Note the similarity in shape to granular casts and that their nuclei are not readily apparent in many cells. Phase contrast microscopy at a magnification of 200×. *B,* Sediment stained with 0.5% toluidine blue. A large cast-like proximal tubular cell and a smaller round distal tubular cell are present with two hyaline casts and other debris. Brightfield microscopy at a magnification of 400×. *C,* A single proximal tubular cell stained with 0.5% toluidine blue. Note the indistinct cell margins, granular cytoplasm, and small eccentric nucleus. Brightfield microscopy at a magnification of 200×.

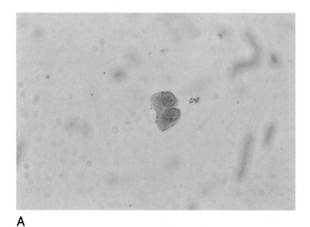

A

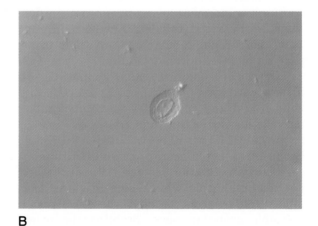

B

FIGURE 8–26. Renal collecting duct epithelial cells. *A,* Two cells with an intact edge. Brightfield microscopy, toluidine blue stain, at a magnification of 400×. *B,* A single cell. Interference contrast microscopy at a magnification of 400×.

(Fig. 8-26). They are never round. The microscopist must always look for a corner or straight edge on the cell before identifying it. Macrophages or monocytes are round or spherical and are sometimes misidentified as collecting duct cells. Collecting duct cells have a single large, moderately dense nucleus that takes up approximately two-thirds of its relatively smooth cytoplasm. Collecting duct cells become larger and more columnar as they reach the renal calyces. Urine sediments can contain increased numbers of collecting duct cells in all types of renal diseases, including nephritis, acute tubular necrosis, kidney transplant rejection, and salicylate poisoning.

In contrast to proximal and distal convoluted tubular cells, collecting duct cells may be observed as fragments of undisrupted tubular epithelium (Fig. 8-27; see Fig. 8-2). To be identified as a fragment, at least three cells must be sloughed together with a bordering edge intact. Their presence reveals severe tubular injury, as well as damage to the epithelial basement membrane. Indicating ischemic necrosis of the tubular epithelium, collecting duct fragments can be found following trauma, shock, or sepsis. In addition to these renal cell fragments, pathologic casts (e.g., granular, waxy, renal tubular cell) and increased numbers of blood cells are usually present.

RENAL TUBULAR CELLS WITH ABSORBED FAT. Renal tubular cells that are engorged with absorbed fats from the tubular lumen or degenerating their own intracellular lipids are called **oval fat bodies.** With the microscopic examination of the urine sediment, the microscopist can observe great variations in the oval fat bodies. Some cells may present with many large, highly refractile droplets; others present with only a small number of apparently glistening granules. Because oval fat bodies are often indicative of glomerular dysfunction with renal tubular cell death and the leakage of plasma components into the urine, they are always accompanied by increased amounts of urinary protein and cast formation. Oval fat bodies are positively identified using polarizing microscopy or fat stains such as Sudan III or Oil

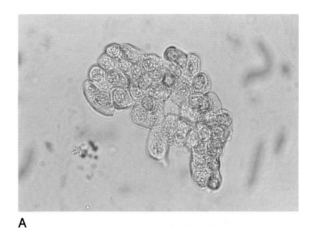

A

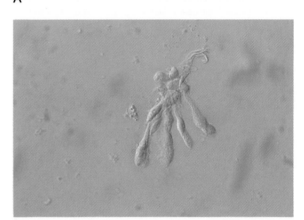

B

FIGURE 8-27. *A,* Fragment of renal collecting duct epithelial cells. Brightfield microscopy at a magnification of 400×. *B,* Fragment of renal collecting duct epithelial cells in "spindle" form, indicative of regeneration of the tubular epithelium after injury. Interference contrast microscopy at a magnification of 400×.

Red O. For more discussion on fat identification in urine, see the subsection on fats under the miscellaneous formed elements section later in this chapter.

Casts

Formation and General Characteristics

Unique to the kidney, urinary casts are formed in the distal and collecting tubules with a core matrix of **Tamm-Horsfall protein.** This mucoprotein is secreted *only* by renal tubular cells, particularly those of the distal and collecting tubules. As the tubular lumen contents become concentrated, Tamm-Horsfall protein forms fibrils that attach it to

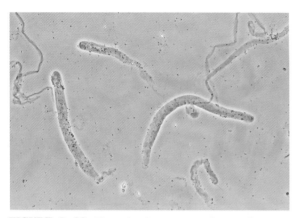

FIGURE 8–28. Three hyaline casts and several mucus threads. Phase contrast microscopy at a magnification of 100×.

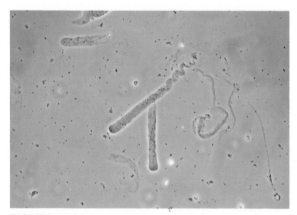

FIGURE 8–29. Three hyaline casts. The one with a tapered end is frequently called a cylindroid. Phase contrast microscopy at a magnification of 100×.

the lumen cells, holding it temporarily in place while it enmeshes any substances present into its matrix. Any urinary component, whether chemical or a formed element, can be found incorporated into a cast. Eventually, the formed cast detaches from the tubular epithelial cells and is flushed through the remaining portions of the nephron and eventually into the urine.

Because casts are formed within the tubules, they are cylindrical and microscopically always appear thicker in the middle than along their edges (Fig. 8–28). They have essentially parallel sides with ends that can be rounded or straight (abrupt). The shape and size of urinary casts can be extremely variable depending on the diameter and shape of the tubule in which they were formed. The narrower the tubular lumen, the narrower the resulting cast. Sometimes the microscopist will encounter casts that appear to be well formed at one end, yet are tapered or have a tail at the other end (Fig. 8–29). These casts, often called cylindroids, result from cast formation in a portion of the tubules where the lumen width differs (naturally or from disease), from incomplete cast formation, or from cast disintegration. Because they have the same clinical significance as completely formed casts, cylindroids are not enumerated separately.

Very wide or broad casts may be encountered (Fig. 8–30) during the microscopic ex-

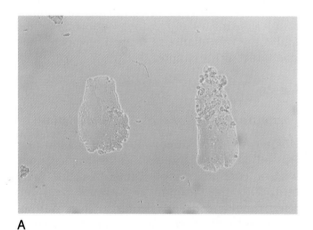

A

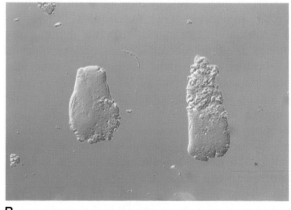

B

FIGURE 8–30. Two broad, granular to waxy casts. *A,* Brightfield microscopy at a magnification of 100×. *B,* Interference contrast microscopy at a magnification of 100×.

amination of the urine sediment. These casts reflect extremely dilated tubules or the wide collecting ducts in which they were formed. Because collecting ducts serve several nephrons, cast formation within them indicates pronounced urinary stasis and renal disease. If a cast forms in a distal tubule and when released for excretion encounters another cast being formed or a tubular obstruction, the first (narrower) cast can be compressed to form a cast that appears convoluted (Fig. 8–31). Casts can be short and stubby, long and thin, or any combination. They may be straight, curved, or convoluted. Because casts may be retained in the tubule for varying lengths of time, the substances enmeshed in its matrix can disintegrate. In addition, the cast matrix itself can undergo changes that become apparent microscopically, e.g., transition from a granular to waxy cast (See Figs. 8–30 and 8–44). Some casts are fragile and easily broken into chunks if the urine sediment is mixed too vigorously during its resuspension (Fig. 8–32). In addition, hypotonic and alkaline urine promotes the disintegration of casts in the urine sediment.

Numerous factors such as an acid pH, increased solute concentration, urinary stasis, and increased plasma proteins enhance cast formation. In an acidic environment, precipitation of solutes and gelation of protein are enhanced. Similarly, high solute concentrations facilitate the precipitation of solute crystals out of solution. Because acidification and concentration of the urine ultrafiltrate occur in the distal and collecting tubules, these tubules are the sites of most cast formation. Urinary stasis may occur because of obstruction from disease processes or congenital abnormalities. This stasis promotes the accumulation and concentration of ultrafiltrate components; hence, cast formation. In conditions that cause increased amounts of plasma proteins (e.g., albumin, globulins, hemoglobin, myoglobin) in the lumen ultrafiltrate, cast formation is greatly enhanced. These proteins become incorporated into the Tamm-Horsfall matrix along with any cells and cellular or granular debris that happens to be present.

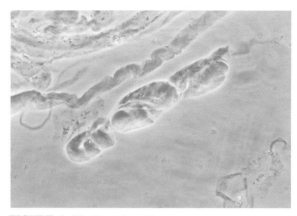

FIGURE 8–31. Convoluted hyaline cast, formed initially in a tubule and later compressed in a tubule of larger diameter. Phase contrast microscopy at a magnification of 200×.

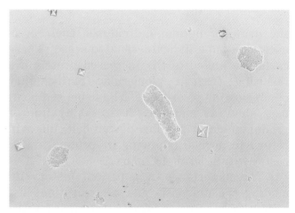

FIGURE 8–32. One intact finely granular cast and two broken pieces of a cast. Brightfield microscopy at a magnification of 100×.

Clinical Significance

A few hyaline or granular casts may be present in the urine sediment from normal, healthy individuals. Casts reflect the status of the renal tubules; therefore, with renal disease, increased numbers of casts are found in the urine sediment (Fig. 8–33). The number of casts reflects the extent of tubular involvement and the severity of the disease. Both the type of casts and their numbers provide valuable information to the clinician, because some casts are characteristic of specific renal diseases (e.g., eosinophil casts). One exception needs to be noted. Following strenuous exercise (athletic pseudonephritis), increased numbers of casts can be found in

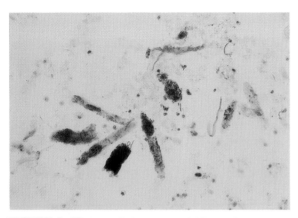

FIGURE 8–33. A single low-power field revealing several casts of various types—cellular, granular, and mixed. Brightfield microscopy, sedistain, at a magnification of 100×.

TABLE 8–6 CLASSIFICATION OF URINARY CASTS

Homogeneous matrix
  Hyaline
  Waxy
Cellular inclusions
  Red blood cells
  Leukocytes
  Renal tubular epithelial cells
  Mixed cells
  Bacteria
Other inclusions
  Granular
  Fat globules—cholesterol, triglycerides
  Hemosiderin granules
  Crystals
Pigmented
  Bilirubin
  Hemoglobin
  Myoglobin
Size
  Broad

the urine of normal individuals; their presence does not indicate renal disease. These casts are linked to the increased proteinuria resulting from a glomerular permeability change owing to exercise. The urine sediment may show as many as 30 to 50 hyaline or granulaar casts per low-power field but will return to normal (showing no proteinuria or casts) within 24 to 48 hours.

The importance of a patient history including the diagnosis and a medications list cannot be overemphasized. It facilitates the examination of the urinary sediment by providing information that can often support or account for the numbers and types of formed elements observed. Both physical exercise and emotional stress can affect the number of formed elements observed in the urine sediment. A careful patient history can prevent misdiagnosing or overdiagnosing renal dysfunction.

Classification of Casts

Casts are classified microscopically based on the composition of their matrix and the type of substances or cells enmeshed within them (Table 8–6). Because any substance is capable of being incorporated into a cast, Table 8–6 could be expanded to include all possible inclusions; those that are listed represent the most commonly encountered casts. Keep in

mind that casts can contain more than one formed element or can be of two matrix types. Mixed cellular casts are often reported as such with a description of the entities involved: e.g., cellular cast—leukocytes and renal tubular cells. When a cast of two matrix types—half granular and half waxy—is encountered, the cast is identified using the term that has the most clinical significance. In this example, the cast should be enumerated and reported as a waxy cast.

HOMOGENEOUS MATRIX COMPOSITION

Hyaline Casts. Hyaline casts, composed primarily of a homogeneous Tamm-Horsfall protein matrix, are the most commonly observed casts in the urine sediment (Fig. 8–34*A*). This protein matrix affords the hyaline casts a low refractive index similar to urine and makes them very difficult to visualize using brightfield microscopy. They appear colorless in unstained urine sediment, with rounded ends and in various shapes and sizes. When phase or interference contrast microscopy is used, their fibrillar protein matrix is more apparent and often includes some fine granulation (Fig. 8–34*B*).

In healthy individuals, 0 to 2 hyaline casts per low-power field are considered to be normal. Increased numbers of hyaline casts can be found following extreme physiologic conditions such as strenuous exercise, dehydration, fever, or emotional stress. They also accompany pathologic casts in renal diseases and cases of congestive heart failure.

If brightfield microscopy is used, staining the sediment will greatly enhance the visualization of hyaline casts, as well as aid the microscopist in differentiating them from mucus threads that may also be present. Hyaline casts become pink with Sternheimer-Malbin stain and their edges become more clearly defined. With phase or interference contrast microscopy, hyaline casts are readily identified by the homogeneity of their matrix and their characteristic shape. Occasionally, the microscopist encounters a lone hyaline cast with a single epithelial or blood cell in its matrix or a cylindroid, a hyaline cast with a tail at one end. Both of these casts are enumerated as hyaline casts and have no diagnostic significance.

Waxy Casts. Named thus because of their waxy appearance, these casts have a high refractive index and are readily visible using brightfield microscopy. Waxy casts appear homogeneous, with their edges well defined, and often have sharp, blunt, or uneven ends. Cracks or fissures from their lateral margins or along their axes are often present and are characteristic of these casts (Fig. 8–35). In

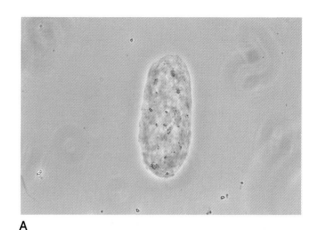

A

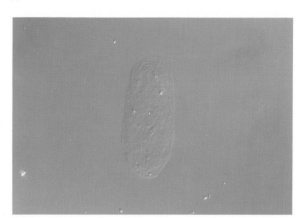

B

FIGURE 8–34. Hyaline cast. *A,* Note the appearance of the fibrillar protein matrix and the presence of fine granulation when using phase contrast microscopy at a magnification of 400X. *B,* Interference contrast microscopy at a magnification of 400X.

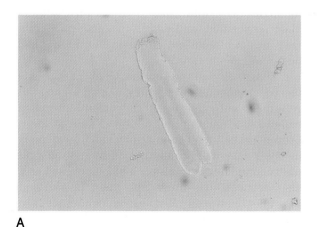

A

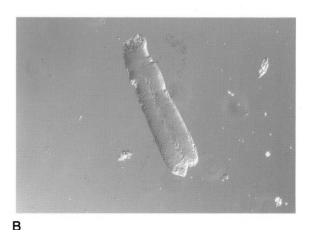

B

FIGURE 8–35. Waxy cast. *A,* Brightfield microscopy at a magnification of 100X. *B,* Interference contrast microscopy at a magnification of 100X.

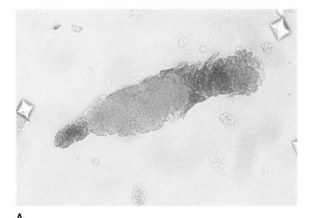

A

B

FIGURE 8–36. Cast, part granular and part waxy. Note the difference in cast diameter at one end compared to the other. This indicates initial cast formation in a narrow tubular lumen followed by stasis in a tubule with a wider lumen and further cast formation. *A*, Brightfield microscopy, sedistain, at a magnification of 200×. *B*, Interference contrast microscopy at a magnification of 200×.

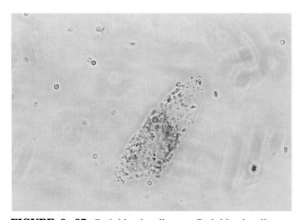

FIGURE 8–37. Red blood cell cast. Red blood cells are embedded in the cast matrix, as are granules, possibly from red blood cell degeneration. Note the free-floating red blood cells also in the sediment. Brightfield microscopy, sedistain, at a magnification of 200×.

unstained urine sediment, they are colorless, gray, or yellow; with Sternheimer-Malbin stain, they become darker pink than hyaline casts and have a diffuse, cut-glass appearance.

Waxy casts imply tubular obstruction with prolonged stasis and are often called renal failure casts. They are believed to represent an advanced stage of hyaline or granular casts (Fig. 8–36). In other words, waxy casts can form as hyaline or granular casts degrade during urinary stasis. They are often broad, indicating their formation in dilated tubules or collecting ducts. Waxy casts are most frequently found in patients with chronic renal failure. They may also be encountered in patients undergoing renal allograft rejection, with malignant hypertension, and in other acute renal diseases (e.g., acute glomerulonephritis, nephrotic syndrome).

CELLULAR INCLUSION CASTS

Red Blood Cell (Erythrocyte) Casts. The microscopic appearance of red blood cell casts varies. Some casts are packed with red blood cells; others may present principally as a hyaline cast with several clearly defined red blood cells embedded in its matrix (Figs. 8–37 and 8–38). In either case, the red blood cells must be unmistakably identified in at least a portion of the cast before it is called a red blood cell cast. In unstained urine sediments, the erythrocytes within the cast matrix cause them to be characteristically yellow or red-brown. The latter color indicates the degeneration of the erythrocytes with hemoglobin oxidation. In Sternheimer-Malbin–stained sediments, intact red cells may appear colorless or lavender in a pink homogeneous matrix.

If urinary stasis is sufficient in the affected nephrons, erythrocyte casts can degenerate into pigmented, granular casts called blood casts (Fig. 8–39). These golden-brown casts have no distinct red blood cells in their matrix because they have lysed and undergone degeneration. This process will also occur if the urine specimen is old and improperly stored. Red blood cell casts are extremely fragile, and overly vigorous resuspension of the urine sediment can result in their being broken into pieces. Microscopically, chunks of casts would be present and may be difficult to identify.

Phase and interference contrast microscopy aid in the identification of red blood cell casts by enhancing the detail of the cells trapped within the cast matrix. Because free-floating red blood cells are also present, the optical sectioning ability of these techniques enables better visualization to ensure that cells are actually within the cast matrix and not simply superimposed on its surface.

Erythrocyte casts are diagnostic of intrinsic renal disease. Their red blood cells are most often of glomerular origin (e.g., glomerulonephritis) but can also result from tubular damage (e.g., acute interstitial nephritis). When red blood cells are able to pass into the tubular ultrafiltrate, so do plasma proteins; therefore, varying degrees of proteinuria will also be present. The detection and monitoring of red blood cell casts in urine sediment provide a means of evaluating a patient's response to treatment. Occasionally, a red blood cell cast will be observed in the urine of a healthy individual. This finding usually follows strenuous exercise (i.e., athletic pseudonephritis), particularly after participation in contact sports such as football, basketball, or boxing. As with the other urine findings associated with this condition, the urine sediment will return to normal within 24 to 48 hours.

Leukocyte Casts. Leukocyte casts consist of white blood cells embedded in a hyaline cast matrix (Fig. 8–40). Because of the refractility of the cells within them, leukocyte casts can be viewed using brightfield microscopy. When the characteristic multilobed nuclei and granular cytoplasm of these cells are readily apparent, these casts are easy to identify. However, when these characteristics are not evident because of cellular degeneration, the use of supravital stains or contrast microscopy is necessary to differentiate them from renal epithelial cells. The presence of increased numbers of white blood cells, either free-floating or in clumps, would also suggest strongly that the cells in these casts are leukocytes.

The presence of leukocyte casts indicates renal inflammation or infection and requires

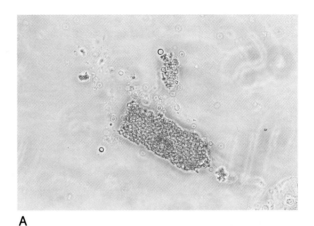

A

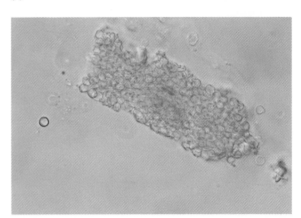

B

FIGURE 8–38. Red blood cell cast. This cast is packed with intact red blood cells. *A*, Brightfield microscopy at a magnification of 200X. *B*, Interference contrast microscopy at a magnification of 400X.

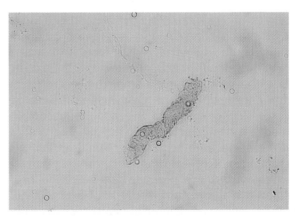

FIGURE 8–39. Blood cast. A pigmented and granular cast originating from hemoglobin and red blood cell degeneration. Note the free-floating red blood cells. Brightfield microscopy at a magnification of 200X.

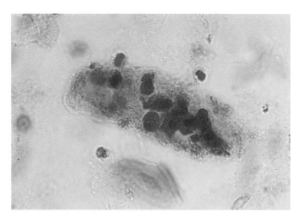

FIGURE 8-40. White blood cell cast. Brightfield microscopy, sedistain, at a magnification of 400×.

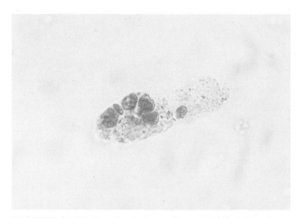

FIGURE 8-41. Renal tubular cell cast. Brightfield microscopy, sedistain, at a magnification of 400×.

further clinical investigation. The origin of the leukocytes, either glomerular or tubular, can be difficult to determine. If glomerular (e.g., glomerulonephritis), red blood cell casts will also be present and in greater numbers than leukocyte casts. With tubular diseases (e.g., pyelonephritis), leukocytes migrating into the tubular lumen from the interstitium are enmeshed in the cast matrix. In these cases, leukocyte casts are usually accompanied by bacteriuria and varying degrees of proteinuria and hematuria. Renal infections from agents other than bacteria (e.g., cytomegalovirus) are possible and must be considered when bacteriuria is not observed and when negative bacterial cultures are obtained.

Renal Tubular Epithelial Cell Casts. Renal tubular epithelial cells can become incorpo-

rated into the Tamm-Horsfall protein matrix in the same fashion as other cellular entities. These casts have a high refractive index and are readily visible using brightfield microscopy. When their characteristic large central nuclei and shape are apparent, they are easily identified (Fig. 8-41). However, as renal tubular epithelial cells become damaged, they undergo degenerative changes that can make their identification difficult. Individual renal tubular epithelial cells may be found randomly arranged within a cast or they may appear aligned as fragments of the tubular lining removed intact from the tubule. These latter casts indicate that a portion of a nephron has been severely damaged, with the tubular basement membrane stripped of its epithelium.

Because of their size similarity with white blood cells, degenerating renal tubular cells may need enhanced visualization to be differentiated and specifically identified. This can be achieved with the use of supravital stains or microscopy techniques, e.g., phase contrast or interference contrast microscopy. The presence of degenerating tubular cell casts in the urine sediment indicates intrinsic renal tubular disease. Renal tubular cell casts will be accompanied by proteinuria and often granular casts.

Mixed Cell Casts. It is not unusual to find casts that have incorporated in their matrix more than one type of cell, such as renal epithelial cells and leukocytes or erythrocytes and leukocytes. Any combination is possible. These casts are often enumerated and reported as cellular casts, with their composition provided in the report.

Bacterial Casts. Because it is difficult to visualize these small organisms within the cast matrix, these casts are often not identified as being bacterial casts. Bacterial casts are diagnostic of pyelonephritis. Because these casts usually include leukocytes, they are often reported as leukocyte casts. They are actually mixed casts. Using brightfield microscopy and staining with supravital stains or Gram stain, the microscopist's careful scrutiny of the matrix between leukocytes can often reveal embedded bacteria. Contrast interference microscopy allows better visualization of bacteria within casts because of its optical sectioning ability. Occasionally, casts that consist of bacteria without leukocytes incorporated in the protein matrix have been observed.

CASTS WITH INCLUSIONS

Granular Casts. Granular casts come in a variety of granular textures. They range from small, fine granules dispersed throughout the cast matrix to large, coarse granules (Figs. 8–42 and 8–43). Composed primarily of Tamm-Horsfall protein, cast granulation is not clinically significant. Easily viewed with brightfield microscopy because of their high refractive index, granular casts often appear colorless to shades of yellow. Granular casts can appear in all shapes and sizes, with broad granular casts considered to be an indicator of a poor prognosis.

Several mechanisms account for the granular casts observed in the urine sediment. The granules in finely granular casts have been identified as the by-products of protein metabolism, in part lysosomal, that are excreted by renal tubular epithelial cells (Haber, 1991). This mechanism accounts for the appearance of granular casts in the urine of normal, healthy individuals. A variation of this mechanism is believed to account for some casts characterized by large coarse granulation, particularly when there are no accompanying cellular casts. In these cases, as tubular cells degenerate, their intracellular components are released into the tubular lumen and become enmeshed in a cast. Other coarsely granular casts result from the degeneration of cellular casts. These casts often contain identifiable cellular remnants. In patients with intrinsic renal disease, these coarsely granular casts are usually accompanied by cellular casts. Further degeneration of granular casts into waxy casts can occur during urinary stasis (Fig. 8–44).

Urine sediment from normal healthy individuals may have an occasional finely granular cast. These casts are not as common as hyaline casts, but their numbers can increase following exercise. Patients with various types of renal disease can present with varying amounts of granular casts, both coarse and fine.

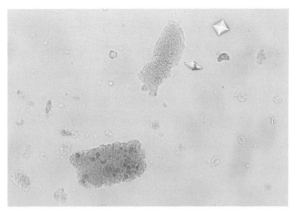

FIGURE 8–42. Two granular casts, one finely granular, the other with coarsely granular inclusions. Brightfield microscopy, sedistain, at a magnification of 200×.

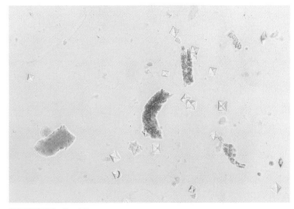

FIGURE 8–43. Finely granular and coarsely granular casts. Brightfield microscopy, sedistain, at a magnification of 100×.

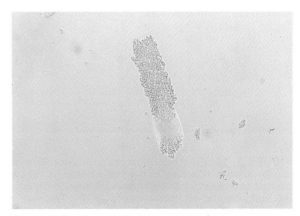

FIGURE 8–44. Coarsely granular and waxy cast. Brightfield microscopy at a magnification of 100×.

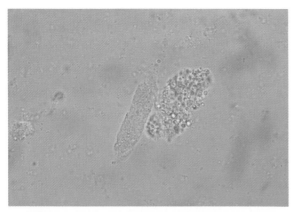

FIGURE 8–45. A fatty cast and a finely granular cast. Note the characteristic orange-red staining of the globules of neutral fat and their refractility. Brightfield microscopy, Sudan III stain, at a magnification of 400×.

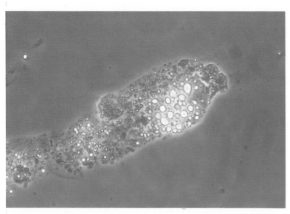

A

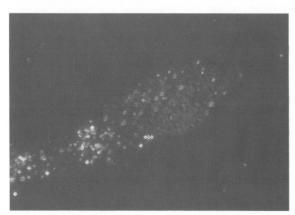

B

FIGURE 8–46. Fatty cast. Note the high refractility of the fat globule inclusions in the cast's matrix. *A,* Phase contrast microscopy at a magnification of 400×. *B,* Polarizing microscopy at a magnification of 400×. The highly refractile fat globules apparent in *A* do not exhibit a maltese cross pattern, identifying them as neutral fat; those with a maltese cross pattern are cholesterol.

Fatty Casts. Fatty casts contain free fat globules, oval fat bodies, or both, and their matrix can be either hyaline or granular. Within the cast, fat globules can vary in size and are highly refractile (Figs. 8–45 and 8–46). Oval fat bodies in casts are identified by their intact cellular membranes. Because oval fat bodies indicate renal tubular cell death, the presence of oval fat bodies in fatty casts indicates significant renal pathology. Cells other than oval fat bodies may also be present within the fatty cast matrix.

In unstained urine sediment using brightfield microscopy, lipid globules appear light yellow or brown. If fat stains such as Sudan III or Oil Red O are used, the triglycerides and neutral fat globules within the cast will stain characteristically orange or red (see Fig. 8–45), whereas cholesterol and its esters will not. In contrast, polarized microscopy will identify cholesterol and its esters by their characteristic birefringence; these globules will form a maltese cross pattern (see Fig. 8–46B). Lipids will not take up Sternheimer-Malbin stain, although the protein matrix of the cast will.

Fatty casts are accompanied by significant proteinuria and may be found in numerous renal diseases, particularly during a manifestation of nephrotic syndrome. In addition, a severe crush injury with disruption of body fat can result in fatty casts in the urine sediment.

Other Inclusion Casts. Because during cast formation any substance present in the tubular lumen can be incorporated into the Tamm-Horsfall protein matrix, both hemosiderin granules and crystals have been found in casts. Because crystals can aggregate along mucus threads to simulate a cast form, it is important to visualize that the hyaline matrix actually encases the crystals. Sulfonamide and calcium oxalate are the most commonly encountered crystal casts (Fig. 8–47). Because the presence of crystal casts indicates their precipitation within the tubules, with irritation to the tubular epithelium and possible obstruction, varying amounts of hematuria often accompany them in the urine sediment.

PIGMENTED CASTS. Pigmented casts, usually of a hyaline matrix with distinct coloration, are characterized by the pigment incorporated within the casts (Fig. 8–48). Hemoglobin, myoglobin, or bilirubin (bile) casts can be encountered in the urine sediment. Hemoglobin casts appear yellow to brown and are accompanied by hematuria. Because myoglobin casts are similar in appearance to hemoglobin casts, differentiation requires a patient history with a possible diagnosis of rhabdomyolysis or confirmation that myoglobin is present. Bilirubin characteristically colors all urine sediment constituents a yellow- or golden-brown (Fig. 8–49). Likewise, bilirubin casts have a homogeneous matrix of this coloration. In contrast, urobilin, which can impart a similar orange-brown color to urine, will not color the sediment's formed elements. Highly pigmented drugs, such as phenazopyridine, can also result in characteristically colored casts and sediment elements.

SIZE

Broad Casts. Broad casts indicate cast formation in dilated convoluted tubules or in the collecting ducts (Fig. 8–50). Because several nephrons empty into a single collecting duct, cast formation here indicates significant urinary stasis, owing to either obstruction or disease. The presence of many broad casts in the urine sediment indicates a poor prognosis. Broad casts may be of any type; however, when a significant amount of urinary stasis is involved, they principally present as granular or waxy (see Fig. 8–30). In chronic renal diseases in which nephrons have sustained previous damage, broad hyaline casts may be encountered. These casts form as a result of continued proteinuria and other factors that enhance their formation.

Correlation with the Physical and Chemical Examinations

When significant numbers of casts, particularly pathologic casts, are identified in the urine sediment, correlation with the physical and chemical examinations must be made. Increased numbers or abnormal casts must be

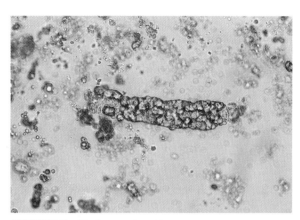

FIGURE 8–47. Cast with sulfamethoxazole crystal inclusions. Brightfield microscopy at a magnification of 200×.

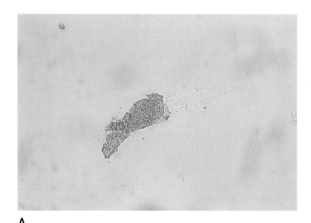

A

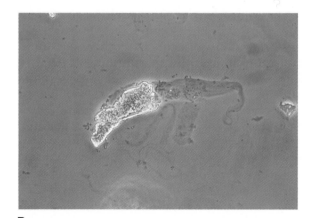

B

FIGURE 8–48. Pigmented granular cast. *A*, Brightfield microscopy at a magnification of 200×. *B*, Phase contrast microscopy at a magnification of 200×. Note the enhanced visualization of low-refractile components such as hyaline matrix and mucus with phase contrast microscopy.

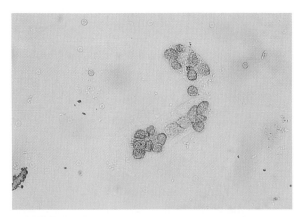

FIGURE 8-49. Bile-stained cellular cast. Brightfield microscopy at a magnification of 200X.

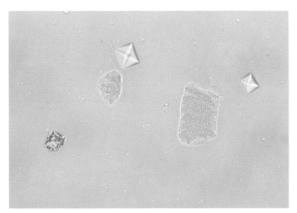

FIGURE 8-50. Broad cast and a broken cast remnant. Brightfield microscopy at a magnification of 200X.

accompanied by proteinuria, although the degree of proteinuria can vary. In contrast, proteinuria may occur without cast formation. If red blood cell casts are identified, the chemical test for blood should also be positive or its negativity accounted for before these casts are reported. Leukocyte casts may or may not be associated with a positive leukocyte esterase test depending on the type and numbers of leukocytes present. Leukocyte casts are often accompanied by bacteriuria, the most common etiologic agent of UTIs. In these cases, the nitrite test may also be positive. Bile-pigmented casts should be accompanied by a positive chemical test for bilirubin; similarly, hemoglobin- or myoglobin-pigmented casts should be accompanied by a positive chemical test for blood.

Look-alikes

To the novice microscopist, there are several formed elements in the urine sediment that can be confused with casts. Mucus threads can be mistaken for hyaline casts (see Fig. 8–75). Although they have a similar low refractive index, they are ribbon-like and their ends are not rounded, but serrated. They are irregular, whereas hyaline casts are more formed.

Various fibers, such as cotton threads or diaper fibers, may resemble waxy casts (see Figs. 8–92 and 8–93). Several distinguishing characteristics allow for their differentiation. Fibers tend to be flatter in the middle and thicker at their margins, whereas casts are cylinders, thicker in the center and thinner at their edges microscopically. In addition, fibers are more refractile than casts. Using polarizing microscopy, fibers will polarize light, whereas waxy casts will not (see Fig. 8–93). Lastly, fibers may contaminate the urine at any time, whereas casts, particularly waxy casts, must be accompanied by proteinuria. Other entities, such as squamous epithelial cells folded into a tubular shape or scratches on the coverslip surface, can also be misidentified as casts. With practice, the proper identification of these components is not difficult.

Crystals such as amorphous urates and phosphates can aggregate to simulate a cast. With polarizing microscopy, their birefringence identifies them as crystalline entities; also, the lack of a distinct matrix differentiates them from true casts.

Crystals

Crystals result from the precipitation of urinary solutes out of solution. They are normally not present in freshly voided urine, but can form as urine is stored. Most crystals are not clinically significant and can be distracting when the laboratorian is performing the microscopic examination. In addition, they can make the visualization of important formed elements difficult, especially when they are present in large numbers. Some crystals are indicative of a pathologic process; therefore, it is important that they are correctly identified and reported. Crystals are identified based on their microscopic appearance and the pH at which they are present, i.e., their solubility. It is the urinary pH that provides the information necessary to positively identify several look-alike crystals (e.g., amorphous urates from phosphates and ammonium biurate from sulfonamide).

Contributing Factors

Several factors influence crystal formation, including 1) the concentration of the solute in the urine; 2) the urinary pH; and 3) the flow of the urine through the tubules. As the glomerular ultrafiltrate passes through the tubules, the solutes in the lumen fluid are concentrated. If an increased amount of a solute is present because of dehydration, dietary excess, or medications, the ultrafiltrate can become supersaturated. This can result in the solute's precipitating into its characteristic crystalline form. Because solutes differ in their solubility, this characteristic provides a means of identifying and differentiating them. For example, inorganic salts such as oxalate, phosphate, calcium, ammonium, and magnesium are less soluble in neutral or alkaline urine. As a result, when the urine pH becomes neutral or alkaline, these solutes can precipitate out in their crystalline form. In contrast, organic solutes such as uric acid, bilirubin, and cystine are less soluble in acidic conditions and can form crystals in acidic urine. All clinically significant crystals are found in acidic urine (e.g., cystine, tyrosine, leucine), including those of iatrogenic origin (e.g., sulfonamide, ampicillin).

Crystal formation, like cast formation, is enhanced when urine flow through the renal tubules is retarded. This flow reduction allows time for the maximum concentration of the solutes in the ultrafiltrate. At the same time, the tubules are affecting pH changes in the ultrafiltrate. When the pH becomes optimal for a supersaturated solute, crystals form.

Although these factors account for crystal formation in the renal tubules, they are also involved in the development of crystals during urine storage. The solute concentration, the pH, the time allowed for formation, and the temperature all play a role in crystal formation. When these conditions are optimized, the chemicals in the urine can exceed their solubility levels and precipitate in their uniquely characteristic crystalline or amorphous forms.

In the following section, both normal and abnormal crystals are discussed and categorized according to the pH at which they form. Normal crystals are routinely reported as few, moderate, or many using high-power magnification, whereas abnormal crystals are quantitated under low-power magnification and are always confirmed before reporting. Table 8–7 summarizes the characteristics of normal and abnormal crystals of urinary solutes and their clinical significance.

Acidic Urine

AMORPHOUS URATES. Amorphous or noncrystalline forms result from the urate salts of sodium, potassium, magnesium, and calcium. Microscopically, they appear as small, yellow-brown granules (Fig. 8–51) very much like sand, and they can interfere with the visualization of other formed elements present in the urine sediment. Because refrigeration enhances the precipitation of amorphous urates, performance of the microscopic examination on fresh urine specimens often avoids the formation of amorphous urates. The urinary pigment uroerythrin readily deposits on the surfaces of urate crystals, imparting to them a characteristic pink-orange color. This coloration is apparent macroscopically during the physical examination. Often referred to as "brick dust," urate crystals indicate that the urine is acidic.

Amorphous urates are present in acidic (or neutral) urine specimens. They can be identified by observing their solubility in alkali or their dissolution when heated to approximately 60°C. If concentrated acetic acid is added and time is allowed, amorphous urates will convert to uric acid crystals. Amorphous urates have no clinical significance and are distinguished from amorphous

T A B L E 8 – 7.   CRYSTAL CHARACTERISTICS OF URINARY SOLUTES

CHEMICAL	pH	MICROSCOPIC APPEARANCE	SOLUBILITY CHARACTERISTICS	CLINICAL SIGNIFICANCE AND COMMENTS
Ammonium biurate	Alkaline (or neutral)	Spheres with striations or spicules; "thorny apple"; dark yellow-brown	Soluble in acetic acid; soluble at ~60°C; converts to uric acid with concentrated HCl	Rare in fresh urine; common and normal in old specimens
Amorphous phosphates	Alkaline (or neutral)	Amorphous, granular, colorless	Soluble in acid; *insoluble* at ~60°C	Normal; common; macroscopic appearance—white precipitate
Amorphous urates	Acid (or neutral)	Amorphous, granular, colorless to yellow-brown	Soluble in alkali; soluble at ~60°C; converts to uric acid with concentrated HCl	Normal; common; macroscopic appearance—orange-pink precipitate ("brick dust")
Ampicillin	Acid	Long, thin needles or prisms; colorless		High-dose antibiotic therapy; rare
Bilirubin	Acid	Fine needles or granules that form clusters; yellow-brown	Soluble in alkali; soluble in strong acid	Bilirubinuria; often forms during storage
Calcium carbonate	Alkaline (or neutral)	Small, granular spheres or dumbbells; colorless	With acetic acid produces CO_2 gas (effervescence)	Normal; rare
Calcium oxalate	Acid or neutral	Dihydrate—octahedral or "envelope" form; colorless Monohydrate—ovoid or dumbbell; colorless	Soluble in dilute HCl	Normal; common; also found with ethylene glycol ingestion
Calcium phosphate	Alkaline (or neutral)	Dicalcium—thin prisms in rosette or stellar pattern; prisms have one tapered end; colorless Monocalcium— irregular granular plates; colorless	Soluble in dilute acid	Normal
Cholesterol	Acid	Flat, rectangular plates with notched corners; colorless	Soluble in chloroform and ether	Lipiduria; rare; found with other forms of urinary fat
Cystine	Acid	Hexagonal plates, often layered; colorless	Soluble in alkali	Amino acid disorder—cystinosis or cystinuria; rare; resembles uric acid crystals
Leucine	Acid	Spheres with concentric circles or radial striations; dark yellow to brown	Soluble in alkali	Liver disease; aminoaciduria; rare; accompanies tyrosine
Radiographic contrast media (diatrizoate meglumine)	Acid	Two forms: long pointed needles or flat, elongated rectangular plates; colorless		Radiographic procedures; can resemble cholesterol; high specific gravity (>1.040)

TABLE 8-7.   CRYSTAL CHARACTERISTICS OF URINARY SOLUTES *Continued*

CHEMICAL	pH	MICROSCOPIC APPEARANCE	SOLUBILITY CHARACTERISTICS	CLINICAL SIGNIFICANCE AND COMMENTS
Sodium urate	Acid	Slender prisms; light yellow	Soluble in alkali; soluble at ~60°C	Normal
Sulfonamides	Acid	Yellow-brown; form varies with drug; may appear as spheres with striations, sheaves of wheat with eccentric binding, fan forms, or dense globules		Antibiotic therapy; rare
Triple phosphate (ammonium, magnesium)	Alkaline (or neutral)	Prisms with three to six sides ("coffin lids") or flat, feathery, fern-leaf form; colorless	Soluble in acetic acid	Normal
Tyrosine	Acid	Fine, delicate needles in clusters or sheaves; colorless to yellow	Soluble in alkali	Liver disease; aminoaciduria; rare
Uric acid	Acid	Pleomorphic; often flat, diamond- or lemon-shaped; may layer or form rosettes; color varies with thickness —colorless to yellow to brown	Soluble in alkali	Normal; found with chemotherapy and gout

phosphates on the basis of the urine pH, their macroscopic appearance, and their solubility characteristics.

URIC ACID. Uric acid crystals occur in several forms; the most common form is the diamond shape (Fig. 8-52). The crystals may be cube-shaped or cluster together to form rosettes (Fig. 8-53) and often show layers or laminations on their surfaces (Fig. 8-54). Although they present most often in various forms with four sides, they occasionally have six sides and may require differentiation from cystine crystals. Uric acid crystals are yellow to orange-brown, with the intensity of the color varying directly with the thickness of the crystal. As a result, thin crystals may appear colorless. Using polarizing microscopy, uric acid crystals exhibit birefringence and produce a variety of interference colors (see Figs. 8-52B and 8-53B).

Uric acid crystals are present at a low urinary pH, approximately 5.0 to 5.5, and are readily dissolved at an alkaline pH. They can appear in the urine from normal healthy individuals; however, two pathologic conditions that often show large numbers of uric acid crystals are gout and conditions of increased purine metabolism (e.g., cytotoxic drugs).

SODIUM URATE. Sodium urate crystals, a distinct form of uric acid, appear as light-yellow slender prisms (Fig. 8-55). They may be present singly or in small clusters and their ends are not pointed. Sodium urate crystals are present in an acid pH and dissolve at 60°C. They have no clinical significance and are usually reported as "urate crystals."

CALCIUM OXALATE. The most common shape of calcium oxalate crystals is its octa-

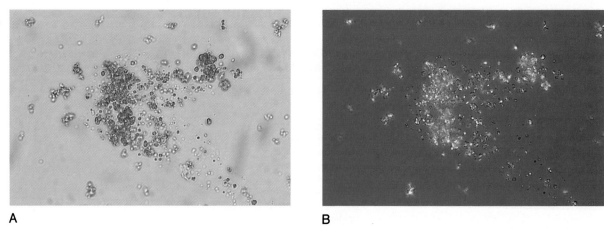

A   B

FIGURE 8-51. Amorphous urates. *A,* Brightfield microscopy at a magnification of 400×. *B,* Polarizing microscopy with first-order red compensator at a magnification of 400×.

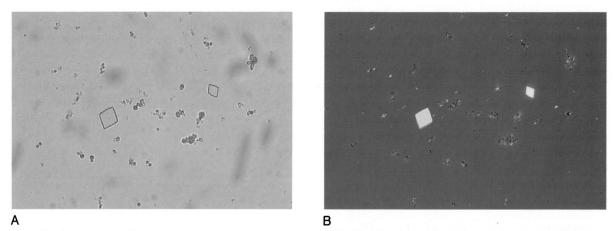

A   B

FIGURE 8-52. Amorphous urates and two uric acid crystals. *A,* Brightfield microscopy at a magnification of 400×. *B,* Polarizing microscopy with first-order red compensator at a magnification of 400×.

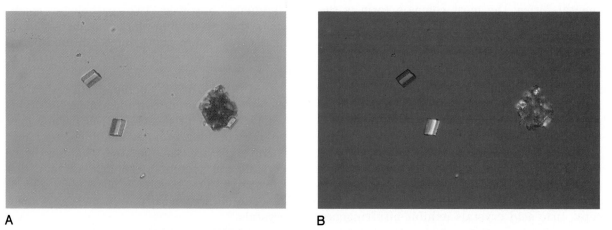

A   B

FIGURE 8-53. Uric acid crystals. *A,* A typical rosette form and two unusual cube forms. Brightfield microscopy at a magnification of 200×. *B,* Polarizing microscopy with first-order red compensator at a magnification of 200×.

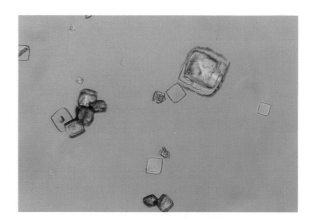

FIGURE 8–54. Uric acid crystals. These crystals can layer or laminate on top of one another. Brightfield microscopy at a magnification of 100X.

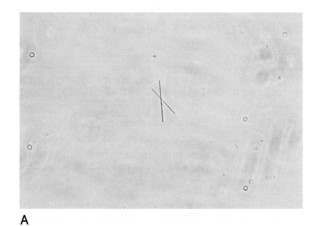

A

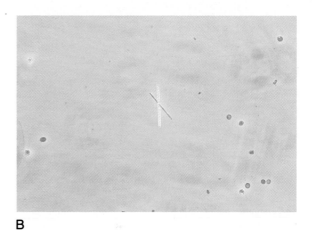

B

FIGURE 8–55. Sodium urate crystals. *A*, Brightfield microscopy at a magnification of 200X. *B*, Phase contrast microscopy at a magnification of 200X. The birefringence of these crystals is evident.

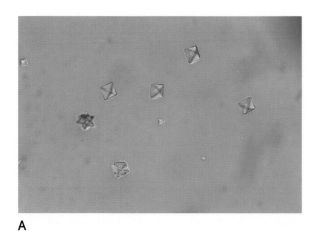

A

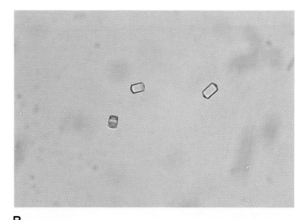

B

FIGURE 8–56. Calcium oxalate crystals. *A*, Octahedral (envelope) form of dihydrate crystals and a rosette form. Brightfield microscopy at a magnification of 200X. *B*, Atypical barrel form. Brightfield microscopy at a magnification of 400X.

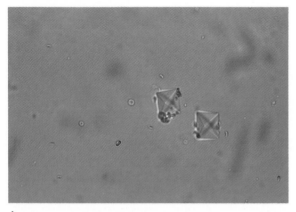

A

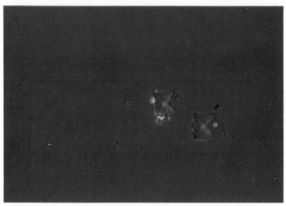

B

FIGURE 8–57. Calcium oxalate crystals. Small ovoid monohydrate crystals that resemble erythrocytes, and two large typical envelope forms of dihydrate crystals. *A,* Brightfield microscopy at a magnification of 400X. *B,* Polarizing microscopy with first-order red compensator at a magnification of 400X. The birefringence of these small ovoid crystals helps distinguish them from erythrocytes.

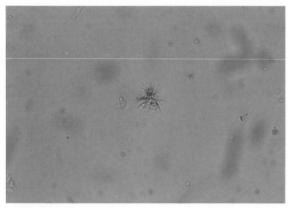

FIGURE 8–58. Bilirubin crystal. Brightfield microscopy at a magnification of 400X.

hedral or envelope form (Fig. 8–56). This dihydrate form of calcium oxalate represents two pyramids joined at their bases. When viewed from one end, they appear as squares scribed with lines that intersect in the center. In contrast, calcium oxalate monohydrate crystals are small and ovoid or dumbbell-shaped (Fig. 8–57). This rare monohydrate form resembles red blood cells and often requires differentiation using polarizing microscopy to demonstrate the birefringence of these crystals (see Fig. 8–57B).

Calcium oxalate crystals are colorless and can vary dramatically in size. Usually they are small and require high-power magnification for identification. On occasion, they may be large enough to identify using low-power magnification. Calcium oxalate crystals may cluster together and can stick to mucus threads. When this occurs, they can be mistaken for crystal casts.

Present in both acidic and neutral urine specimens, calcium oxalate crystals are often found in the urine from normal healthy individuals. The urinary calcium oxalate concentration can be increased in normal individuals through the ingestion of foods high in oxalates, such as tomatoes, asparagus, spinach, rhubarb, and oranges. Approximately 50 percent of the oxalate in urine is derived from oxalic acid, the principal metabolite of ascorbic acid (vitamin C) (see Fig. 7–7). When the body stores are saturated, the body excretes excess ascorbate and its metabolite. Once in the urine, oxalic acid combines with calcium to form calcium oxalate, resulting in increased amounts of urinary oxalate. Increased numbers of calcium oxalate crystals are also induced in pathologic conditions such as following ingestion of ethylene glycol (antifreeze) or in severe chronic renal disease.

BILIRUBIN. The amount of bilirubin in the urine can be large enough to exceed its solubility and result in the formation of bilirubin crystals (Fig. 8–58). Bilirubin crystals can take various forms, as fine needles, granules, or even plates. Always characteristically yellow-brown, they indicate the presence of large amounts of bilirubin in the urine. Frequently present in patients with liver disease, bilirubin crystals are confirmed by correlation with the chemical examination. In other words, bilirubin crystals are present only if the chemical screen for bilirubin is positive.

Bilirubin crystals are present in acid urine. They will dissolve in alkali or when strong acids are added. They are classified as abnormal crystals because bilirubinuria indicates a metabolic disease. However, because these crystals usually form in the urine following excretion, they are often not specifically reported. This information is provided on the urinalysis report in the form of the chemical examination's bilirubin result.

CYSTINE. Cystine crystals appear as colorless, six-sided (hexagonal) plates (Fig. 8–59). Their sides are not always even and they are often laminated or layered. These clear, refractile crystals tend to clump, and their shape may alter if the wet preparation is allowed to dehydrate on the microscope slide.

Present primarily in acid urine, cystine crystals are clinically significant and indicate disease, either congenital cystinosis or cystinuria. These crystals tend to deposit within the tubules as calculi, resulting in renal damage; therefore, it is important to properly identify them. Thin, hexagonal uric acid crystals can resemble cystine; the laboratorian must perform confirmatory tests before reporting cystine crystals. The chemical confirmatory test for cystine is based on the cyanide-nitroprusside reaction. Sodium cyanide reduces cystine to cysteine, and the free sulfhydryl groups subsequently react with nitroprusside to form a characteristic purple color.

Cystine crystals are present in urine with a pH of less than 8.0. They dissolve in alkali and hydrochloric acid (pH of less than 2). Because cystine crystals indicate a disease process, they are considered to be abnormal. Hence, they are quantitated and reported as the average number observed in 10 low-power fields.

TYROSINE AND LEUCINE. Tyrosine crystals appear as fine, delicate needles that are colorless or yellow (Fig. 8–60). They frequently aggregate together to form clusters or sheaves, but also appear singly or in small groups.

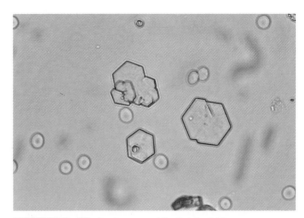

FIGURE 8–59. Cystine crystals. Brightfield microscopy at a magnification of 400X.

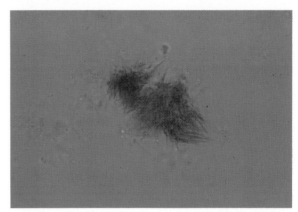

FIGURE 8–60. Tyrosine crystals. Brightfield microscopy at a magnification of 400X.

Leucine crystals are highly refractile, yellow to brown spheres. They have concentric circles or radial striations on their surface and can resemble fat globules. Unlike fat, they do not stain with fat stains or produce a maltese cross pattern with polarized light.

Both tyrosine and leucine crystals are present in acid urine and can be dissolved in alkali. Although both are rarely encountered in the urinalysis laboratory, tyrosine is found more often in the urine because it is less soluble than leucine. Sometimes leucine crystals can be forced out of solution by the addition of alcohol in tyrosine-containing urines.

These amino acid crystals are abnormal and are encountered in the urine as a result of overflow aminoaciduria. In other words,

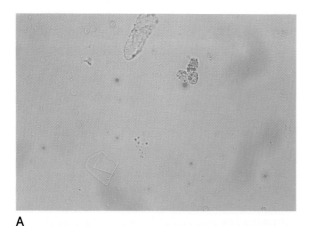

A

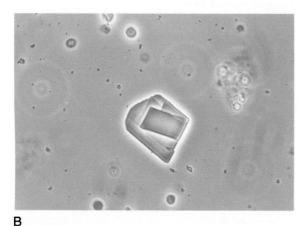

B

FIGURE 8–61. *A*, View of urine sediment with a cholesterol crystal, free-floating fat, and oval fat bodies. Brightfield microscopy at a magnification of 200X. *B*, Cholesterol crystal. Phase contrast microscopy at a magnification of 400X.

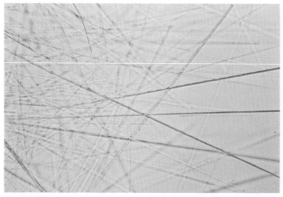

FIGURE 8–62. Ampicillin crystals. Brightfield microscopy at a magnification of 400X. (Courtesy of Patrick C. Ward, M.D.)

the concentration of these amino acids in the blood is high (aminoacidemia), resulting in their increased renal excretion. Although they are occasionally observed in patients with severe liver disease, they are usually present because of rare inherited metabolic disorders. These abnormal crystals are confirmed, preferably by chromatographic methods, before they are reported.

CHOLESTEROL. Cholesterol crystals appear as clear, flat, rectangular plates with notched corners (Fig. 8–61). They are present in acid urine and, because of their organic composition, are soluble in chloroform and ether.

Rarely observed in urine sediment, cholesterol crystals indicate large amounts of urinary cholesterol and ideal conditions promoting supersaturation and precipitation. These crystals are always accompanied by large amounts of protein and other evidence of fats, such as free-floating droplets, fatty casts, or oval fat bodies. Cholesterol crystals may be seen in nephrotic syndrome and in conditions resulting in chyluria—the rupture of lymphatic vessels into the renal tubules as a result of tumors, filariasis, etc.

Diatrizoate meglumine, an intravenous radiopaque contrast medium, forms crystals that are morphologically similar to and need to be differentiated from cholesterol crystals (see Fig. 8–66). Differentiation is achieved by correlating with the urine's chemical examination results. For example, diatrizoate meglumine crystals produce an abnormally high urinary specific gravity (i.e., greater than 1.040), and they are not associated with proteinuria or lipiduria; in contrast, cholesterol crystals are found in urine with a normal specific gravity and must be accompanied by proteinuria and lipiduria.

Although cholesterol crystals are abnormal, their formation most often occurs during urine specimen storage. Therefore, in some institutions these crystals may not be reported. Instead, lipiduria or chyluria is documented in the urinalysis report as oval fat bodies, free-floating fat, and fatty casts.

MEDICATIONS. Numerous medications are excreted by the kidneys; high urinary concentrations can result in their precipitation out of solution. These crystals are often termed iatrogenic; in other words, they result from the actions of a physician through the prescribing of a drug. Proper identification and reporting of these drug crystals are important because the crystals' presence can indicate the potential for renal damage owing to their formation within the tubules. Two commonly used antibiotics, sulfonamides and ampicillin, will be discussed in this section; other medications can form unique crystalline forms that may require further investigation for proper identification.

Ampicillin. Ampicillin crystals appear as long, colorless, thin prisms or needles (Fig. 8–62). The individual needles may aggregate into small groupings or, with refrigeration, into large clusters. Present in acid urine, ampicillin crystals indicate large doses of ampicillin and are rarely observed.

Sulfonamides. Sulfonamides appear in various forms and differ with the particular form of the drug prescribed. When initially manufactured, sulfonamide preparations were relatively insoluble and resulted in renal damage because of their crystal formation in renal tubules. Currently, these drugs have been modified and their solubility is no longer a problem. As a result, sulfonamide crystals are not found as often in urinary sediment, and renal damage because of them is uncommon.

Sulfadiazine drug crystals usually appear yellow to brown and as bundles of needles that resemble sheaves of wheat (Fig. 8–63). The constriction of the bundle may be centrally located or extremely eccentric, resulting in a fan formation. Sulfamethoxazole (e.g., Bactrim, Septra) is more commonly seen and appears as brown rosettes or spheres with irregular radial striations (Fig. 8–64). All sulfonamide crystals are highly refractile and birefringent.

Sulfonamide crystals are present in acidic urine and should be confirmed chemically before they are reported. The diazotization of sulfanilamide followed by an azo-coupling reaction is the preferred method to confirm their presence. They closely resemble ammonium biurate crystals but can be differentiated from them on the basis of their pH

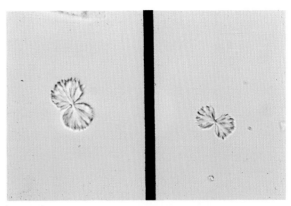

FIGURE 8–63. Sulfadiazine crystals. Brightfield microscopy at a magnification of 400×. (Courtesy of Patrick C. Ward, M.D.)

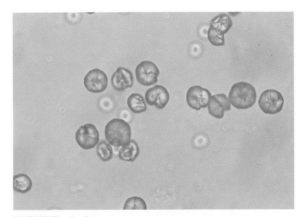

FIGURE 8–64. Sulfamethoxazole (Bactrim) crystals. Brightfield microscopy at a magnification of 400×.

and solubility and the chemical confirmatory test. A list of the patient's current and past medications can also be of value in confirming the identity of these urinary crystals.

RADIOGRAPHIC CONTRAST MEDIA. Diatrizoate salts are used as an intravenous radiographic contrast medium in x-ray procedures. They are water-soluble derivatives of triiodobenzene and are available in many preparations of the meglumine or sodium salts or in mixtures of the two. They are known by numerous product names such as Hypaque, Renografin, Cystografin, and Renovist. Because of their water solubility, they are readily excreted in the urine.

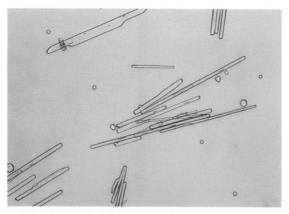

FIGURE 8–65. Radiographic contrast medium, diatrizoate meglumine (Renografin). The crystals appear in needle forms. Brightfield microscopy at a magnification of 100×.

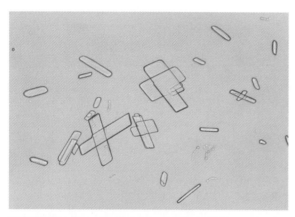

FIGURE 8–66. Radiographic contrast medium, diatrizoate meglumine (Renografin). The crystals appear as plates. Brightfield microscopy at a magnification of 100×. Compare and contrast with cholesterol crystals in Figure 8–61.

Crystals of radiographic contrast media may appear as colorless, long, pointed needles that occur singly or clustered in sheaves (Fig. 8–65) or as flat, elongated rectangular plates (Fig. 8–66). The latter form is distinguished from cholesterol crystals by the large numbers usually present, the high urine specific gravity (greater than 1.040) that accompanies them, and the lack of significant proteinuria and lipiduria.

Diatrizoate crystals appear in acidic urine and may be present up to 4 hours following the injection of the contrast medium into the patient. Besides significantly elevating the urine specific gravity, they can cause a false positive sulfosalicylic acid precipitation test for protein. A microscopic examination of the precipitate formed in this test identifies it as a crystalline substance and not protein. With interference contrast and polarizing microscopy, diatrizoate crystals produce a variety of interference colors (Fig. 8–67).

Alkaline Urine

AMORPHOUS PHOSPHATE. Amorphous phosphates are found in alkaline and neutral urine and are microscopically indistinguishable from amorphous urates. This noncrystalline form of phosphates resembles fine colorless grains of sand in the sediment (Fig. 8–68). Amorphous phosphates are differentiated from amorphous urates based on the urine pH, on their solubility characteristics,

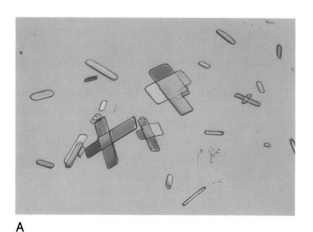

A

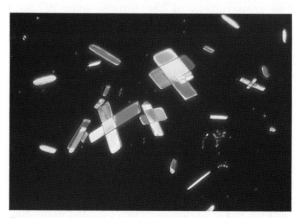

B

FIGURE 8–67. Radiographic contrast medium. *A,* Interference contrast microscopy at a magnification of 100×. *B,* Polarizing microscopy at a magnification of 100×.

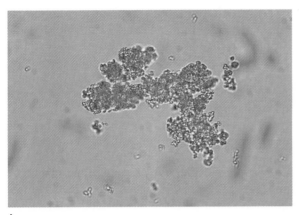

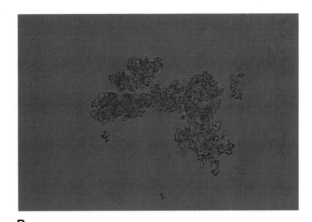

A   B

FIGURE 8–68. Amorphous phosphates. *A,* Brightfield microscopy at a magnification of 400X. *B,* Polarizing microscopy with first-order red compensator at a magnification of 400X.

and to a lesser degree on their macroscopic appearance. Large amounts of amorphous phosphates cause a urine specimen to appear cloudy; the precipitate is white, in contrast to the pink-orange color of amorphous urates. Unlike urates, they are soluble in acid and will not dissolve when heated to approximately 60°C.

Like amorphous urates, amorphous phosphates have no clinical significance and can make the microscopic examination difficult when present in large numbers. Because refrigeration enhances their deposition, specimens maintained at room temperature and analyzed within 2 hours of collection will minimize amorphous phosphate formation.

TRIPLE PHOSPHATE (AMMONIUM-MAGNESIUM PHOSPHATE). Triple phosphate crystals are colorless and appear in several different forms. The most common and characteristic form are three- to six-sided prisms, the latter described as "coffin lids" (Fig. 8–69). Not all crystals are perfectly formed, and their size can vary greatly. A feathery form that resembles a fern leaf may also be observed, although less frequently.

Present in alkaline (or neutral) urine specimens, triple phosphate crystals can be present in the urine of normal healthy individuals. They have little clinical significance, but are often present in the formation of renal calculi and are associated with UTIs characterized by an alkaline pH.

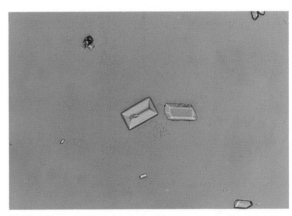

FIGURE 8–69. Triple phosphate crystals. Typical "coffin lid" form. Brightfield microscopy at a magnification of 100X.

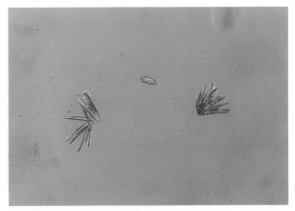

FIGURE 8–70. Calcium phosphate crystals. Prisms are arranged singly and in rosette forms. Brightfield microscopy at a magnification of 100X.

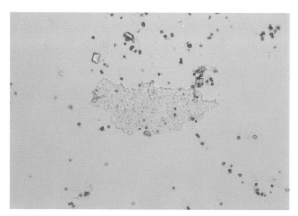

FIGURE 8–71. Calcium phosphate sheet or plate. Brightfield microscopy at a magnification of 100X.

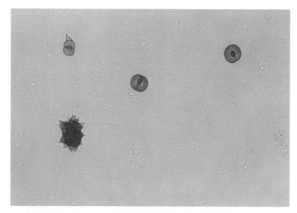

FIGURE 8–72. Ammonium biurate crystals. Spheres and a "thorny apple" form. Brightfield microscopy at a magnification of 200X.

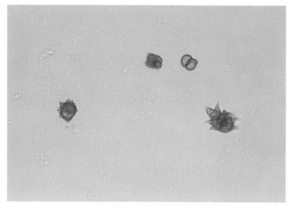

FIGURE 8–73. Ammonium biurate crystals. Several "thorny apple" forms. Brightfield microscopy, 200X.

CALCIUM PHOSPHATE. Calcium phosphate crystals may be present in two distinct forms, as dicalcium phosphate or as calcium phosphate. Dicalcium phosphate crystals, sometimes called stellar phosphates, appear as colorless, thin prisms arranged in a rosette or star-shaped pattern (Fig. 8–70). These prisms tend to have one tapered or pointed end, whereas the other appears squared off. In contrast, calcium phosphate crystals appear microscopically as irregular, granular sheets or plates (Fig. 8–71). They can be quite large and may be noticed floating on the top of a urine specimen. These colorless crystalline plates often resemble degenerated squamous epithelial cells.

Most often encountered in alkaline urine specimens, calcium phosphate crystals have no clinical significance.

AMMONIUM BIURATE. Ammonium biurate crystals appear as yellow-brown spheres with striations on the surface (Fig. 8–72). Irregular projections or spicules may also be present, giving these crystals a "thorny apple" appearance (Fig. 8–73).

Present primarily in alkaline or neutral urine, ammonium biurate crystals are not clinically significant unless found in fresh urine specimens—an extremely rare occurrence. These crystals are encountered almost exclusively in old urine specimens that have been stored for a long period of time. Therefore, if encountered in a specimen, the specimen's integrity is suspect and requires investigation to ensure proper collection and storage.

Ammonium biurate crystals dissolve in acetic acid or upon heating to approximately 60°C. Like amorphous urates, they can also be converted to uric acid crystals through the addition of concentrated hydrochloric or acetic acid. Ammonium biurate crystals can resemble some forms of sulfonamide crystals. On the basis of urinary pH, a sulfonamide confirmatory test, or the crystals' solubility characteristics, differentiation between ammonium biurate and sulfonamide crystals can be made.

CALCIUM CARBONATE. Calcium carbonate crystals appear as very small, colorless granular crystals (Fig. 8–74A). Slightly larger than amorphous material, these crystals are sometimes misidentified as bacteria because of their size and occasional rod shape. The crystals' birefringence with polarized light differentiates them from true bacteria. Calcium carbonate crystals are usually found in pairs, giving them a dumbbell shape. They may also be encountered as aggregate masses that are difficult to distinguish from amorphous material (Fig. 8–74B).

Present primarily in alkaline urine, calcium carbonate crystals are not frequently found in the urine sediment. Although they have no clinical significance, calcium carbonate crystals can be positively identified through the production of carbon dioxide gas (effervescence) with the addition of acetic acid to the sediment.

Miscellaneous Formed Elements

Mucus Threads

Mucus, a fibrillar protein, is commonly observed in urine sediment and has no clinical significance. In unstained urine sediment with brightfield microscopy, mucus can be difficult to observe because of its low refractive index. However, when the microscopist uses phase contrast or interference contrast microscopy, mucus threads are readily identified by their delicate, ribbonlike strands and irregular or serrated ends (Fig. 8–75). Mucus strands appear wavy and can take various forms as they surround other sediment elements. They may also be present as distinct strands or as a clumped mass.

Because some mucus has been shown immunohistochemically to contain Tamm-Horsfall protein, and because this protein is solely produced by the renal tubular epithelium, some mucus found in urine is at least partially derived from the renal tubules (Haber, 1991). The genitourinary tract, particularly the vaginal epithelium, is also a source of the mucus frequently observed in the urine sediments from women.

Mucus threads can be misidentified as hyaline casts because of their similar low refractive index and fibrillar protein structure.

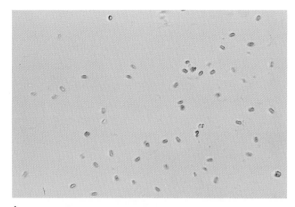

A

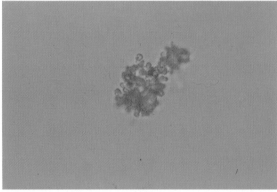

B

FIGURE 8–74. Calcium carbonate. *A,* Numerous single crystals. Brightfield microscopy at a magnification of 400X. *B,* Aggregate of calcium carbonate crystals. Brightfield microscopy at a magnification of 400X.

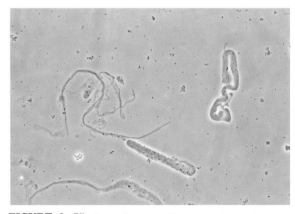

FIGURE 8–75. Several mucus threads and two hyaline casts. Phase contrast microscopy at a magnification of 100X.

The cylindrical composition of casts and their rounded ends aid in their differentiation from mucus.

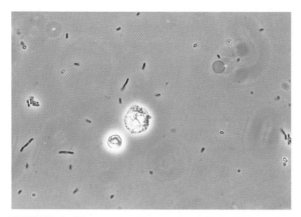

FIGURE 8–76. Urine sediment with bacteria (rods), two erythrocytes, and a leukocyte. Phase contrast microscopy at a magnification of 400×.

Bacteria

Observing bacteria in the urine sediment requires high-power magnification (Fig. 8–76). Both rod-shaped (bacilli) and coccoid forms may be identified, although the most commonly encountered are gram-negative rods. These microorganisms vary in size from long, thin rods to short, plump rods. They can appear singly or in chains depending on the species present. In wet preparations, their motility often distinguishes bacteria from amorphous substances that may also be present. Because the vagina and gastrointestinal tract normally contain bacteria, the presence of bacteria in urine frequently reflects contamination from these sources.

Bacteria are reported as few, moderate, or many per high-power field. Because urine from normal healthy individuals is sterile, the presence of bacteria in the urine sediment implies either a UTI or urine contamination. Bacteria most often ascend the urethra to cause a UTI. They can also be present owing to a fistular connection between the urinary tract and the bowel. In addition, contaminating bacteria can rapidly multiply in improperly stored urine. Therefore, this finding has clinical significance only if the urine specimen has been properly collected and stored.

For a urine sediment in which the identification of bacteria is difficult, a cytospin preparation followed by Gram staining could be performed. During UTIs, bacteriuria is usually accompanied by leukocytes in the urine sediment. When significant bacteriuria is present without leukocytes, the specimen collection and handling should be investigated.

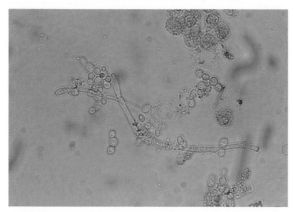

FIGURE 8–77. Budding yeast and pseudohyphae. Leukocytes are also present singly and as a clump. Brightfield microscopy at a magnification of 400×.

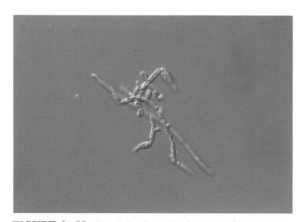

FIGURE 8–78. Pseudohyphae development due to yeast. Interference contrast microscopy at a magnification of 400×.

Yeast

Yeasts are ovoid, colorless cells that can closely resemble red blood cells (Fig. 8–77). More refractile than erythrocytes, they often present with characteristic budding forms and pseudohyphae (Fig. 8–78). Yeast can vary in size, with some species being quite large. Yeasts do not dissolve in acid and do not stain with supravital stains, two characteristics that aid in differentiating them from erythrocytes.

Yeast in the urine sediment most often represents a vaginal infection, with its subsequent contamination of the urine collection. However, because yeasts are ubiquitous—in the air and on skin—their presence could also indicate contamination from these sources. Although infrequent, primary UTIs resulting from yeasts are also possible. Hence, the health care provider must correlate the finding of the yeast with the patient's clinical picture to determine if an actual infection, whether vaginal or urethral, is present. Certain conditions, such as pregnancy, oral contraceptives, and diabetes mellitus, enhance the development of a yeast infection.

The most commonly encountered yeast in urine sediment is *Candida albicans*. Its characteristic budding and development of pseudohyphae make it readily identifiable as yeast. Another species found less frequently is *Candida glabrata*, formerly called *Torulopsis glabrata*. This species does not form pseudohyphae, and these yeast cells are often found phagocytized within white blood cells (Fig. 8–79). In immunosuppressed patients, systemic *Candida* infections are common; for some unknown reason, they have a predilection for the kidneys. During the microscopic examination, only the presence of yeast can be determined; to identify the species present requires fungal culture.

A **KOH preparation** is often used to detect yeast, hyphae, and other fungal cells in vaginal secretions. A swab of the vaginal mucosa and cervix is obtained by the physician and transported to the laboratory. The swab is placed into approximately 0.5 mL of normal saline and is mixed well to suspend the vaginal secretions in the solution. A drop of the suspension is placed on a microscope slide followed by a drop of potassium hydroxide (KOH, 10 percent) and a coverslip. The slide is warmed using a flame or a light source and is then observed microscopically

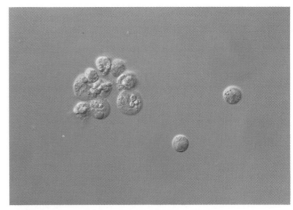

FIGURE 8–79. Leukocytes with intracellular yeast. Interference contrast microscopy at a magnification of 400X.

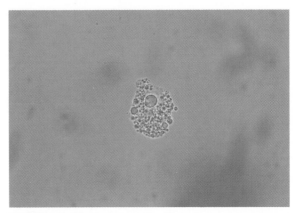

FIGURE 8–80. Oval fat body. Note the size variation of the fat globules. Brightfield microscopy at a magnification of 400X.

under both low- and high-power magnification. Using a KOH preparation enhances the visualization of fungal elements by destroying most other formed elements, with the exception of bacteria. A plain wet mount of the suspension is also observed for the presence of trichomonads and clue cells.

Fat

Fats or lipids are found in urine sediment in three forms: as free-floating fat globules, within oval fat bodies, or within a cast matrix—either as fat globules or entrapped oval fat bodies. During the microscopic examination, a distinguishing feature of lipids is their high refractility. Using brightfield microscopy, these highly refractive globules

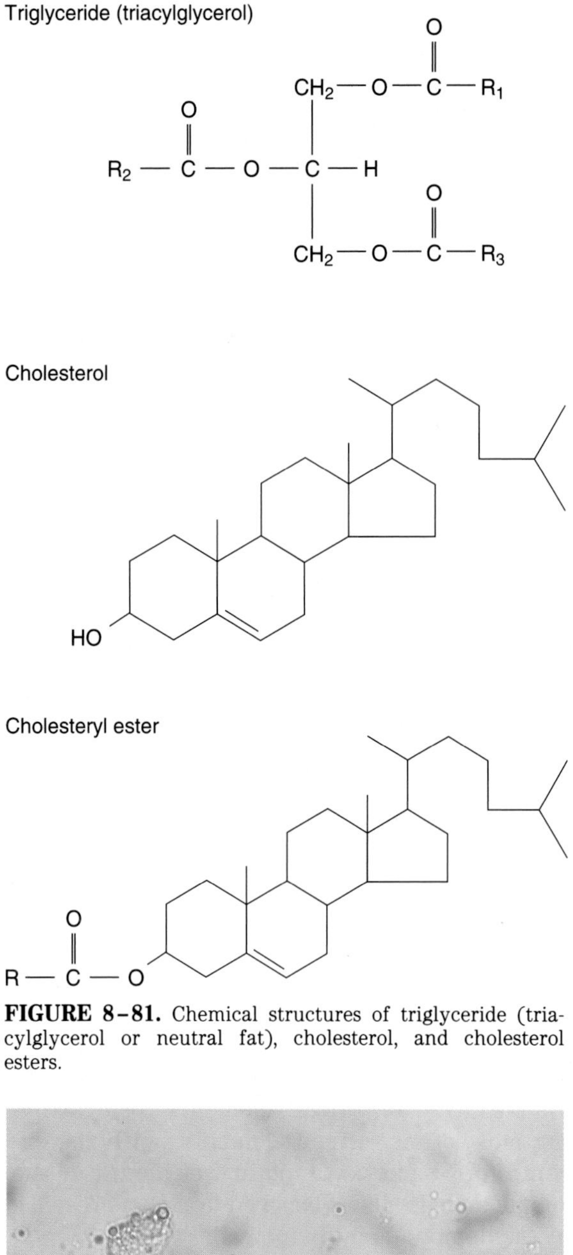

Triglyceride (triacylglycerol)

Cholesterol

Cholesteryl ester

FIGURE 8–81. Chemical structures of triglyceride (triacylglycerol or neutral fat), cholesterol, and cholesterol esters.

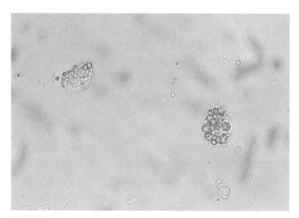

FIGURE 8–82. Two oval fat bodies stained with Sudan III stain. Note the characteristic orange-red staining of neutral fat globules. Brightfield microscopy at a magnification of 400X.

are spherical; they vary in size; and they appear light yellow or brown (Fig. 8–80).

The type of fat present can vary, and often both triglycerides and cholesterol can be demonstrated (Fig. 8–81). Triglyceride, also called neutral fat, is composed of a glycerol backbone with three fatty acids esterified to it. Adding either a Sudan III or an Oil Red O stain to the urine sediment will cause triglycerides to become characteristically orange or red (Fig. 8–82). In contrast, cholesterol and cholesterol esters do not stain and are identified by their characteristic birefringence. When polarizing microscopy is used, these cholesterol globules produce a distinctive maltese cross pattern, i.e., an orb that appears divided into four quadrants by a bright maltese-style cross (Fig. 8–83). In rare instances, cholesterol is present in a crystalline form in the urine sediment. See the crystal section of this chapter for more discussion of these unique cholesterol crystals.

Lipiduria is always clinically significant, although its presence does not pinpoint a specific diagnosis. It is present with a variety of renal diseases and may occur following severe crush injuries. It is most often encountered with nephrotic syndrome along with severe proteinuria, hypoproteinemia, hyperlipidemia, and edema. Because nephrotic syndrome can occur with glomerular, tubular, or interstitial renal diseases, as well as with metabolic diseases such as diabetes mellitus, lipids are often encountered in the urine sediment. Monitoring the presence of lipiduria can aid in following the progression or resolution of these disease processes.

Because other entities can resemble fat in urine sediment, it is important to be able to distinguish these look-alike substances. Starch granules form a similar maltese pattern with polarizing microscopy; however, they are easily distinguished from fat globules using brightfield microscopy; i.e., starch is not highly refractile, it tends to have a central dimple, and it is not spherical. The variation in size demonstrated by fat globules aids in differentiating them from erythrocytes. In addition, erythrocytes will not stain with fat dyes and are not birefringent. When using a Sternheimer-Malbin stain, lipids retain their high refractility and light yellow to brown color whether free-floating, held intracellularly, or enmeshed within a cast matrix.

Oils and creams from lubricants and lotions can also contaminate the urine. They may be introduced during the specimen collection from vaginal creams or from catheter lubricants, or during the microscopic examination from immersion oil left on an objective lens. Regardless of their source, oils and creams are identified by their homogeneity, their lack of structure, and their large droplets that often coalesce.

Hemosiderin

Hemosiderin is a form of iron resulting from ferritin denaturation. These insoluble granules can become large enough to be observed microscopically in the urine sediment, especially after they have been stained to a Prussian blue color. Unstained, hemosiderin granules appear as coarse yellow-brown granules and are often difficult to distinguish from amorphous crystalline material in the sediment (Fig. 8-84*A*).

Hemosiderin granules are found in the urine sediment 2 to 3 days following a severe hemolytic episode (e.g., transfusion reaction, paroxysmal nocturnal hemoglobinuria). In these cases, plasma haptoglobin is saturated with hemoglobin, and any remaining free hemoglobin is able to pass through the glomerular filtration barrier to be absorbed by the renal tubular epithelium. The tubular cells metabolize the hemoglobin to ferritin and subsequently denature it to form hemosiderin. Hemoglobin is toxic to cells and as these cells degenerate, hemosiderin granules appear in the urine. Hemosiderin granules may be found free-floating or within macrophages, casts, or tubular epithelial cells.

The **Prussian blue reaction,** also known as the Rous test, is used to identify hemosiderin in the urine sediment and in tissues. A concentrated urine sediment is examined for the presence of coarse yellow-brown hemosiderin granules, free-floating or within casts or tubular epithelial cells. The urine sediment

FIGURE 8-83. Cholesterol droplets demonstrating the characteristic maltese cross pattern. Polarizing microscopy with first-order red compensator at a magnification of 400X.

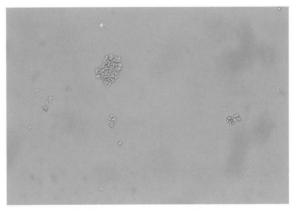

A

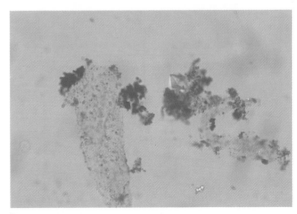

B

FIGURE 8-84. *A,* Hemosiderin granules floating free in urine sediment. Brightfield microscopy at a magnification of 400X. *B,* Hemosiderin granules after staining with Prussian blue. Brightfield microscopy at a magnification of 400X.

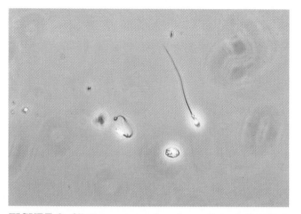

FIGURE 8–85. Spermatozoa in urine sediment. One typical and two atypical forms. Phase contrast microscopy at a magnification of 400×.

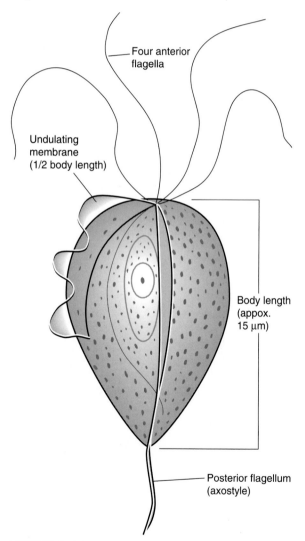

FIGURE 8–86. Schematic diagram of *Trichomonas vaginalis.*

is resuspended in a freshly prepared solution of potassium ferricyanide–HCl and allowed to stand at room temperature for 10 minutes. After centrifugation and discarding of the supernatant, the sediment is re-examined for the presence of coarse blue granules. In this preparation, hemosiderin iron causes the granules to stain Prussian blue (Fig. 8–84*B*). Because the reaction can be delayed, negative sediments are examined a second time after 30 minutes (Schumann, 1991).

Spermatozoa

Spermatozoa may be present in the urine sediment from both males and females. They have oval heads approximately 3.0 to 5.0 μm long and thin, thread-like tails about 40 to 60 μm in length (Fig. 8–85). A variety of forms may be encountered, and at times they may be found clumped in the sediment. Spermatozoa morphology is discussed further in the chapter on seminal fluid analysis.

Because urine is not a viable medium for spermatozoa, the presence of motile sperm indicates recent intercourse or ejaculation. In women, spermatozoa are usually considered a vaginal contaminant; in men, they result from either nocturnal emission or ejaculation. Spermatozoa in the urine sediment have no clinical significance.

Vaginal Contaminants

TRICHOMONAS VAGINALIS. Trichomonads, protozoan flagellates, may be observed in the urine sediment. Trichomonads appear as turnip-shaped flagellates; their unicellular bodies average 15 μm in length, although organisms as small as 5 μm and as large as 30 μm are possible. They have three to four anterior flagella and a single posterior flagellum, with an undulating membrane that extends halfway down the length of the organism (Fig. 8–86). They are mobile in wet preparations, and their characteristic flitting or jerky motion assists in identifying them. Trichomonads are similar in size to both leukocytes and renal tubular cells, and their motility, flagella, and undulating membranes help to differentiate them (Fig. 8–87).

Trichomonas vaginalis is the most common cause of parasitic gynecologic infections in women. Transmitted sexually, trichomonads most frequently represent an infection of the vagina and vulva, with their presence in the urine often indicating its contamination with vaginal secretions. In men, trichomonad infections of the urethra are usually asymptomatic. In either case, when observed in urine sediment, trichomonads are not quantitated but are simply reported as present.

Supravital staining does not appreciably enhance trichomonad identification. Both phase contrast and interference contrast microscopy permit enhanced imaging, however, as well as visualization of the trichomonads' flagella and undulating membranes. Because their characteristic motility provides the best means of positively identifying trichomonads, fresh urine specimens are desired.

CLUE CELLS AND *GARDNERELLA VAGINALIS*. *Gardnerella vaginalis* is a small gram-negative rod, often the agent of vaginitis when other organisms such as yeast or trichomonads are not present. This type of bacterial vaginosis is apparently synergistic, involving both *G. vaginalis* and anaerobic bacteria. Infections with these organisms result in the sloughing of vaginal squamous epithelial cells with large numbers of bacteria adhered to them (Fig. 8–88). The presence of these organisms causes the epithelial cells to appear soft and finely granular with indistinct cell borders, often described as having shaggy edges. Because of the large numbers of organisms adhering to the cell, its nucleus may not be visible. These characteristic squamous epithelial cells are called **clue cells.** To be considered a clue cell, the bacteria do not need to cover the entire cell; however, the bacterial organisms must extend beyond the cell's cytoplasmic borders. Often intracellular keratohyalin granules are misidentified as bacteria adhering to squamous epithelial cells. These granules vary in size and are usually larger and more refractile than bacteria.

Although clue cells are not often present in a urine specimen, they are readily recovered from a vaginal swab. The physician collects a swab of the vaginal mucosa, which is

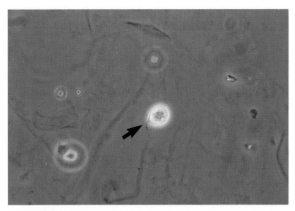

FIGURE 8–87. A trichomonad in urine sediment. Due to their rapid flitting motion, only one of the flagella is visible in this view *(arrow)*. Mucus, white blood cells, and other trichomonads are present but not in focus at this focal plane. Phase contrast microscopy at a magnification of 400×.

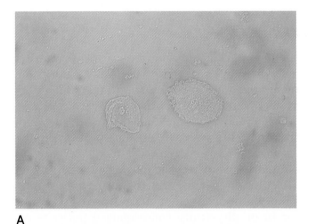

A

B

FIGURE 8–88. The slightly larger squamous epithelial cell with indistinct, shaggy cytoplasmic edges is a "clue cell." The cell with well-defined cytoplasmic edges is a normal squamous epithelial cell. *A,* Brightfield microscopy at a magnification of 200×. *B,* Phase contrast microscopy at a magnification of 200×.

then transported to the laboratory. The swab is placed into approximately 0.5 mL of normal saline and agitated to suspend the vaginal secretions in the solution. For the visualization of formed elements, a wet mount of the saline suspension is prepared using a microscope slide and coverslip. The wet mount is observed for the presence of trichomonads, clue cells, bacteria, yeast, hyphae, and other fungal cells using both low- and high-power magnification. Clue cells are often readily apparent in these wet preparations. A KOH preparation for yeast, hyphae, and other fungal cells destroys clue cells and trichomonads. When KOH is added and a distinctly foul, fishy odor develops, however, it is indicative of *G. vaginalis* and an anaerobic counterpart (often *Mobiluncus curtisii*).

Fecal Contaminants

Fecal material contaminates urine primarily by two modes: through improper collection technique or through an abnormal connection or fistula between the urinary tract and the bowel. Specimens received from infants and from patients who are extremely ill or physically compromised are most likely to be contaminated with fecal material because of the difficulty in performing the urine collection. With the assistance of a health care worker for ill or physically compromised patients or the use of collection bags for infants, these specimens can be obtained without contamination. In contrast, when a fistula that continually channels fecal material into the urinary tract is present, optimizing the collection technique will not eliminate the contamination. In the latter condition, the patient has a persistent UTI from the constant influx of the normal bacterial flora from the intestine into the urinary tract; food remnants may also be present in the urine sediment.

The fecal contamination of urine specimens is often not grossly apparent. Microscopic examination of the urine sediment will reveal the abnormal presence of partly digested vegetable cells and muscle fibers from ingested foods. One method to confirm a suspected fistular connection is to have the patient ingest charcoal particles. Following ingestion, the patient's urine is collected for 24 hours or more and the entire collection concentrated by centrifugation. The resultant urine sediment is thoroughly screened microscopically for the presence of charcoal particles. If charcoal particles are found, they confirm a diagnosis of a fistula between the bowel and the urinary tract (Fig. 8–89).

Starch

Starch granules originating from body powders or those found in protective gloves worn by health care workers are frequently encountered microscopically in the urine sediment. Starch has unique characteristics that make it easy to identify. Starch granules can vary greatly in size and usually have a centrally located dimple (Fig. 8–90). They are not perfectly round; rather, they have scalloped or faceted edges. Under polarizing microscopy, starch granules exhibit a maltese cross pattern similar to that of cholesterol (Fig. 8–91). Because they are not round like cholesterol droplets, however, the edges of the maltese pattern are less defined. Owing to their visual differences when using bright-field microscopy, starch granules and cholesterol droplets are usually readily differentiated.

Because starch granules are a urine contaminant, they are not reported. Excessive amounts could interfere with the examination, however, and may necessitate specimen recollection.

Fibers

Numerous types of fibers, such as hair, cotton, and other fabric threads, often appear in the urine sediment. They are considered to be urine specimen contaminants and are disregarded during the microscopic examination. It is important to discuss them to ensure their proper identification by the novice microscopist. Fibers can be quite large with distinct edges, and they are often moderately to highly refractile. They may resemble urinary casts; several features aid in their differentiation. Fibers tend to be flat and thicker at

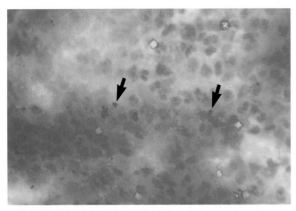

FIGURE 8–89. Charcoal granules *(arrows)* in urine sediment. Note the numerous leukocytes. Cytospin preparation, Wright's stain, brightfield microscopy at a magnification of 400×.

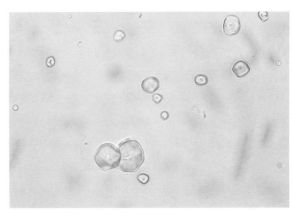

FIGURE 8–90. Starch granules. Brightfield microscopy at a magnification of 400×.

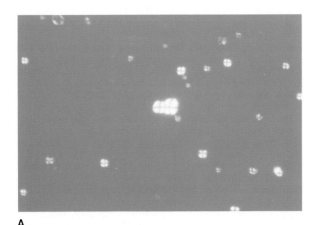

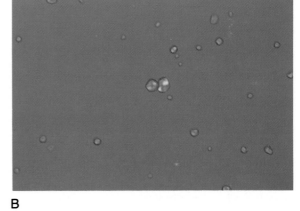

A   B

FIGURE 8–91. Starch granules: *A,* A maltese cross pattern is demonstrated using polarizing microscopy at a magnification of 400×. *B,* Polarizing microscopy with first-order red compensator at a magnification of 400×.

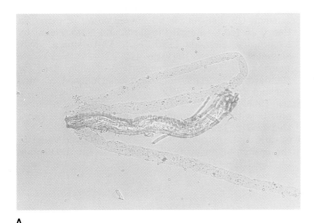

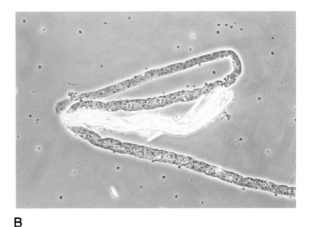

A   B

FIGURE 8–92. Hyaline cast and a fiber. Note the difference in form and refractility. *A,* Phase contrast microscopy at a magnification of 100×. *B,* Brightfield microscopy at a magnification of 100×.

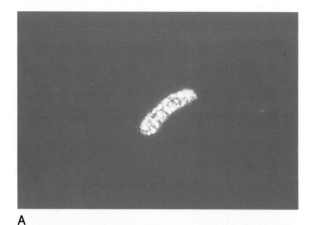

A

B

FIGURE 8–93. *A*, Diaper fiber demonstrating anisotropism with polarizing microscopy at a magnification of 200×. *B*, Polarizing microscopy with first-order red compensator at a magnification of 200×.

their margins, in contrast to casts, which are thicker in the middle (Fig. 8–92). Fibers are anisotropic, and polarizing microscopy will demonstrate their birefringence; casts are not anisotropic (Fig. 8–93).

Parasites

Some parasites and their ova, such as *Entamoeba histolytica* and *Enterobius vermicularis* (pinworm), can be encountered in the urine sediment as a result of fecal contamination. Others, such as *Schistosoma haematobium* ova, can be directly introduced into the urine from the bladder wall mucosa. Regardless of their source, their presence indicates a parasitic infection that requires treatment; therefore, the health care provider is notified of their suspected presence for further investigation. Two frequently observed parasites in the urine sediment are trichomonads and yeast. These parasites are discussed individually in specific sections of this chapter.

References

· ·

Bessis M: Living Blood Cells and Their Ultrastructure, New York, Springer-Verlag, 1973, pp. 50, 145.

Corwin HL, Bray RA, Haber MH: The detection and interpretation of urinary eosinophils. Arch Pathol Lab Med *113:*1256–1258, 1989.

Fairley KF, Birch DF: Hematuria: a simple method for identifying glomerular bleeding. Kidney Int *21:*105, 1982.

Freni SC, Dalderup LM, et al.: Erythrocyturia, smoking and occupation. J Clin Pathol *30:*341, 1977.

Haber MH: Composition of the normal urinary sediment. *In* A Primer of Microscopic Urinalysis (2nd ed.), Garden Grove, California, Hycor Biomedical, Inc., 1991, p. 28.

Mahon CS, Smith LA: Standardization of the urine microscopic examination. Clinical Laboratory Science, Vol. 3, No. 5, 1990.

National Committee for Clinical Laboratory Standards. Routine Urinalysis. Tentative Guideline. NCCLS Document GP16-T (ISBN 1-56238-183-0), *12*(26)2, 1992.

Nolan CR, Anger MS, Kelleher SP: Eosinophiluria: a new method of detection and definition of the clinical spectrum. N Engl J Med *315:*1516–1519, 1986.

Rous P: Urinary siderosis. J Exp Med *28:*645, 1918.

Schumann GB: Cytodiagnostic urinalysis for the nephrology practice. Semin Nephrol *6:*308, 1986.

Schumann GB, Schweitzer SC: Examination of urine. *In* Henry JB (ed.), Clinical Diagnosis and Management by Laboratory Methods (18th ed.), Philadelphia, W.B. Saunders Company, 1991, pp. 412, 421.

Schumann GB, Tebbs RD: Comparison of slides used for standardized routine microscopic urinalysis. J Med Technol *3:*1, 1986.

Sternheimer R, Malbin B: Clinical recognition of pyelonephritis with a new stain for urinary sediments. Am J Med *11:*312, 1951.

Weir MR, Hall-Craggs M, et al.: The prognostic value of the eosinophil in acute allograft rejection. Transplantation *41:*709–712, 1986.

Study Questions

1. **Which of the following are NOT standardized when commercial systems are used for the processing and microscopic examination of urine sediment?**

   A. The microscopic variables, e.g., the number of focal planes
   B. The concentration and volume of the urine sediment prepared
   C. The volume of the urine sediment dispensed for microscopic viewing
   D. The identification and enumeration of the formed elements in the urine sediment

2. **When urine sediment is viewed, stains and various microscopic techniques are used to**

   1. enhance the observation of fine detail.
   2. confirm the identity of suspected components.
   3. differentiate formed elements that look alike.
   4. facilitate the visualization of low-refractile components.

      A. 1, 2, and 3 are correct.
      B. 1 and 3 are correct.
      C. 4 is correct.
      D. All are correct.

3. **The microscopic identification of hemosiderin is enhanced when the urine sediment is stained with**

   A. Gram stain.
   B. Hansel stain.
   C. Prussian blue stain.
   D. Sudan III stain.

4. **When the laboratorian performs the microscopic examination of urine sediment, which of the following are enumerated using low-power magnification?**

   A. Bacteria   C. Red blood cells
   B. Casts   D. Renal tubular cells

5. **A urine sediment could have which of the following formed elements and still be considered "normal"?**

   A. 0 to 2 hyaline casts
   B. 5 to 10 red blood cells
   C. A few bacteria
   D. A few yeast cells

6. **Which of the following statements about red blood cells in urine is true?**

   A. Red blood cells crenate in hypotonic urine.
   B. Red blood cell remnants are called "ghost cells."
   C. Alkaline and hypotonic urine promotes red blood cell disintegration.
   D. Dysmorphic red blood cells are often associated with renal tubular disease.

7. **Hemoglobin is a protein and will**

   A. not react in the protein reagent strip test.
   B. interfere with the protein reagent strip test, producing erroneous results.
   C. always contribute to the protein reagent strip result regardless of the amount of hemoglobin present.
   D. contribute to the protein reagent strip result only when large concentrations of hemoglobin are present.

8. **Which urinary sediment component can resemble red blood cells?**

   A. Yeast
   B. Air bubbles
   C. Oil droplets
   D. Calcium oxalate crystals

      A. 1, 2, and 3 are correct.
      B. 1 and 3 are correct.
      C. 4 is correct.
      D. All are correct.

9. **Which of the following is NOT a characteristic of neutrophils found in the urine sediment?**

   A. They are approximately 10 to 14 μm in diameter.
   B. They form "ghost cells" in hypotonic urine.
   C. They shrink in hypertonic urine, but do not crenate.
   D. As they disintegrate, vacuoles and blebs form and their nuclei fuse.

10. **How do increased numbers of leukocytes usually get into the urine?**

    A. Through a renal bleed
    B. By passive movement through pores in the vascular epithelium
    C. By active ameboid movement through tissues and epithelium
    D. Through damage to the integrity of the normal vascular barrier

11. **Which statement regarding lymphocytes found in urine sediment is correct?**

    A. They are not normally present in the urine.
    B. They produce a positive leukocyte esterase test.
    C. Their number is increased in patients with a drug hypersensitivity.
    D. Their number is increased in patients experiencing kidney transplant rejection.

12. **Which of the following urinary tract structures is NOT lined with transitional epithelium?**

    A. The bladder
    B. The nephrons
    C. The renal pelves
    D. The ureters

13. **Match the number of the epithelial cell type to its characteristic feature. Only one type is correct for each feature.**

Characteristic Feature	Epithelial Cell Type
_____ A. Large and flagstone-shaped; can be anucleated	1. Collecting tubular cell
_____ B. Oblong or cigar-shaped; small eccentric nucleus	2. Distal tubular cell
_____ C. Polygonal; large nucleus	3. Proximal tubular cell
_____ D. Oval to round; small nucleus that is centered or slightly eccentric	4. Squamous epithelial cell
_____ E. Round, pear-shaped, or columnar with a small oval to round nucleus	5. Transitional epithelial cell

14. **Which of the following can be observed in the urine sediment as an intact fragment or sheet of cells?**

    1. The collecting tubular epithelium
    2. The distal tubular epithelium
    3. The transitional epithelium
    4. The proximal tubular epithelium

       A. 1, 2, and 3 are correct.
       B. 1 and 3 are correct.
       C. 4 is correct.
       D. All are correct.

15. **Urinary casts are formed in the**

    A. distal and collecting tubules.
    B. distal tubules and the loops of Henle.
    C. proximal and distal tubules.
    D. proximal tubules and the loops of Henle.

16. **Urinary casts are formed with a core matrix of**

    A. albumin.
    B. Bence Jones protein.
    C. Tamm-Horsfall mucoprotein.
    D. transferrin.

17. **Which of the following does NOT contribute to the size, shape, or length of a urinary cast?**

    A. The concentration of protein in the cast's core matrix
    B. The configuration of the tubule in which the cast is formed
    C. The diameter of the tubular lumen in which the cast is formed
    D. The duration of time the cast is allowed to form in the tubule

18. **All of the following will enhance urinary cast formation EXCEPT**

    A. an alkaline pH.
    B. urinary stasis.
    C. an increase in the ultrafiltrate's solute concentration.
    D. an increase in the amount of plasma proteins in the ultrafiltrate.

19. **When the laboratorian is using brightfield microscopy, a urinary cast that appears homogeneous with well-defined edges, blunt ends, and cracks is most likely a**

    A. fatty cast.   C. hyaline cast.
    B. granular cast.   D. waxy cast.

20. **All of the following can be found incorporated into a cast matrix EXCEPT**

    A. bacteria.
    B. crystals.
    C. transitional epithelial cells.
    D. white blood cells.

21. **Which of the following urinary casts are diagnostic of glomerular or renal tubular damage?**

    A. Bacterial casts
    B. Red blood cell casts
    C. Renal tubular cell casts
    D. White blood cell casts

22. **Which of the following most differentiates waxy casts from fibers that contaminate the urine sediment?**

    A. Waxy casts do not polarize light; fibers do.
    B. Waxy casts are more refractile than fibers.
    C. Waxy casts have rounded ends; fibers do not.
    D. Waxy casts are thicker at their margins; fibers are thicker in the middle.

23. **Which of the following does NOT affect the formation of urinary crystals in the nephrons?**

    A. The pH of the ultrafiltrate
    B. The diameter of the tubular lumen
    C. The flow of the urine through the tubules
    D. The concentration of solutes in the ultrafiltrate

24. **The formation of urinary crystals is associated with a specific urine pH. Match the urine pH that facilitates crystalline formation to the crystal type. More than one number can be used.**

Crystal Type	Urine pH
_____ A. Ammonium biurate	1. Acid
_____ B. Amorphous urates	2. Neutral
_____ C. Amorphous phosphates	3. Alkaline
_____ D. Calcium oxalate	
_____ E. Cholesterol	
_____ F. Cystine	
_____ G. Radiographic contrast media	
_____ H. Sulfonamides	
_____ I. Triple phosphate	
_____ J. Tyrosine	
_____ K. Uric acid	

25. **Match the crystal composition to the microscopic description that best describes it.**

Microscopic Description	Crystal Composition
_____ A. Colorless "coffin lid" form	1. Ammonium biurate
_____ B. Colorless hexagonal plates	2. Amorphous urates
_____ C. Colorless "envelope" form	3. Amorphous phosphates
_____ D. Colorless rectangular plates with notched corners	4. Calcium oxalate
	5. Cholesterol
_____ E. Yellow-brown "thorny apple" form	6. Cystine
_____ F. Colorless to yellow; diamond- or lemon-shaped; flat or rosettes	7. Sulfonamide
	8. Triple phosphate
_____ G. Yellow-brown sheaves of wheat	9. Uric acid

26. **Which of the following crystals, when found in the urine sediment, most likely indicates an abnormal metabolic condition?**

    A. Bilirubin
    B. Sulfonamide
    C. Triple phosphate
    D. Uric acid

27. **During the microscopic examination of a urine sediment, cystine crystals are found. The laboratorian must perform which of the following before reporting the presence of these crystals?**

    1. Perform a confirmatory chemical test
    2. Ensure that the urine specimen has an acid pH
    3. Enumerate the number of crystals per low-power field
    4. Check the current medications that the patient is taking

       A. 1, 2, and 3 are correct.
       B. 1 and 3 are correct.
       C. 4 is correct.
       D. All are correct.

28. **Mucus threads can be difficult to differentiate from**

    A. fibers.
    B. hyaline casts.
    C. pigmented casts.
    D. waxy casts.

29. **Which of the following is NOT a distinguishing characteristic of yeast in the urine sediment?**

    A. Motility
    B. Budding forms
    C. Hyphae formation
    D. Colorless ovoid forms

30. **Fats can be found in the urine sediment in all of the following forms EXCEPT**

    A. within casts.
    B. within cells.
    C. as free-floating globules.
    D. within hemosiderin granules.

31. **Which of the following statements regarding the characteristics of urinary fats is true?**

    A. Cholesterol droplets stain with Sudan III stain.
    B. Triglycerides or neutral fat stain with Oil Red O stain.
    C. Cholesterol droplets do not form a maltese cross pattern under polarized light.
    D. Triglycerides or neutral fat are anisotropic and form a maltese cross pattern under polarized light.

32. **Which of the following statements regarding the microscopic examination of urine sediment is FALSE?**

    A. If large numbers of leukocytes are present microscopically, then bacteria are present.

    B. If urinary fat is present microscopically, then the chemical test for protein should be positive.

    C. If large numbers of casts are present microscopically, then the chemical test for protein should be positive.

    D. If large numbers of red blood cells are present microscopically, then the chemical test for blood should be positive.

33. **The following are initial results obtained during a routine urinalysis. Which results should be investigated further?**

    A. Negative protein; 2 to 5 waxy casts

    B. Cloudy, brown urine; 2 to 5 red blood cells

    C. Urine pH 7.5; ammonium biurate crystals

    D. Clear, colorless urine; specific gravity 1.010

34. **The following are initial results obtained during a routine urinalysis. Which results should be investigated further?**

    A. Negative protein; 0 to 2 hyaline casts

    B. Urine pH 6.0; calcium oxalate crystals

    C. Cloudy, yellow urine; specific gravity 1.050

    D. Amber urine with yellow foam; negative bilirubin by reagent strip; positive Ictotest (Chapter 7)

35. **Which of the following when found in the urine sediment from a female patient is NOT considered a vaginal contaminant?**

    A. Fat

    B. Clue cells

    C. Spermatozoa

    D. Trichomonads

Renal and Metabolic Disease

. . . .

LEARNING OBJECTIVES

After studying this chapter, the student should be able to

1. Discuss the pathogenesis of glomerular damage and describe four morphologic changes that occur in the glomeruli.

2. Describe the clinical features associated with glomerular disease and discuss factors that affect the degree to which they are present.

3. Describe briefly the morphologic appearances of the glomeruli, the mechanisms of glomerular damage, and the clinical presentations of the following glomerular diseases:
   - acute glomerulonephritis
   - chronic glomerulonephritis
   - rapidly progressive glomerulonephritis (RPGN)
   - focal proliferative glomerulonephritis
   - focal segmental glomerulosclerosis (FSG)
   - IgA nephropathy
   - membranoproliferative glomerulonephritis (MPGN)
   - membranous glomerulonephritis (MGN)
   - minimal change disease (MCD)

4. Describe the pathologic mechanisms of glomerular damage in the following systemic diseases:
   - systemic lupus erythematosus (SLE)
   - diabetes mellitus
   - amyloidosis

5. State at least five clinical features that characterize the nephrotic syndrome and identify diseases that are associated with this syndrome.

6. Differentiate between ischemic and toxic acute tubular necrosis (ATN) and discuss the clinical presentation and urinalysis findings associated with this disease.

7. Describe the renal dysfunction and clinical features of the following renal tubular disorders:
   - cystinosis
   - cystinuria
   - Fanconi's syndrome
   - renal glycosuria
   - renal phosphaturia
   - renal tubular acidosis (RTA)

8. Compare and contrast the etiology, clinical features, and typical urinalysis findings in the following tubulointerstitial diseases and urinary tract infections:
   - acute and chronic pyelonephritis
   - acute interstitial nephritis (AIN)
   - lower urinary tract infections
   - yeast infections

9. Describe briefly the effects of vascular disease on renal function.

10. Compare and contrast the etiology and clinical features of acute and chronic renal failure.

11. Summarize the pathogenesis of calculi formation; discuss four factors that influence the formation of urinary tract calculi and briefly review current treatment options.

12. Describe briefly the physiologic mechanism, clinical features, and role of the urinalysis laboratory in the diagnosis of the following amino acid disorders:
    - cystinuria and cystinosis
    - homogentisic acid (alkaptonuria)
    - maple syrup urine disease (MSUD)
    - phenylketonuria (PKU)
    - tyrosinuria and melanuria

13. **Describe briefly the physiologic mechanisms, clinical features, and typical urinalysis findings in the following carbohydrate disorders:**
   - glucosuria
   - diabetes mellitus
   - galactosuria

14. **Describe briefly the physiologic mechanisms, clinical features, and typical urinalysis findings in the following metabolic disorders:**
   - diabetes insipidus
   - porphyrin disorders

- -

KEY TERMS

acute interstitial nephritis (AIN): an acute inflammatory process that develops 3 to 21 days following exposure to an immunogenic drug (e.g., sulfonamides, penicillins) and results in injury to the renal tubules and interstitium. It is characterized by fever, skin rash, leukocyturia (particularly eosinophiliuria), and acute renal failure. Discontinuation of the offending agent can result in full recovery of renal function.

acute poststreptococcal glomerulonephritis: a type of glomerular inflammation occurring 1 to 2 weeks after a group A beta-hemolytic streptococcal infection. Onset is sudden, and the glomerular damage is immune mediated.

acute pyelonephritis: an inflammatory process involving the renal tubules, interstitium, and renal pelvis. It is most often due to a bacterial infection and is characterized by the sudden onset of symptoms, e.g., flank pain, dysuria, frequency of micturition, and urinary urgency.

acute renal failure (ARF): a renal disorder characterized by a sudden decrease in the glomerular filtration rate that results in azotemia and oliguria. It is a consequence of numerous conditions and can be categorized as prerenal (e.g., decrease in renal blood flow), renal (e.g., acute tubular necrosis), or postrenal (e.g., urinary tract obstruction). The disease course varies greatly, and survivors usually regain normal renal function.

acute tubular necrosis (ATN): a group of renal diseases characterized by destruction of the renal tubular epithelium. It is classified into two types: ischemic ATN, due to decreased renal perfusion that results in tissue ischemia,

and toxic ATN, resulting from the ingestion, inhalation, or injection of nephrotoxic substances.

alkaptonuria: a rare recessively inherited disease characterized by excretion of large amounts of homogentisic acid (i.e., alcapton bodies) owing to a deficiency of the enzyme homogentisic acid oxidase.

aminoaciduria: the presence of increased amounts of amino acids in the urine.

amyloidosis: a group of systemic diseases characterized by the deposition of amyloid, a proteinaceous substance, between cells in numerous tissues and organs.

calculi (also called **stones**): solid aggregates or concretions of chemicals, usually mineral salts, that form in secreting glands of the body.

chronic glomerulonephritis: a slowly progressive glomerular disease that develops years after other forms of glomerulonephritis. It usually leads to irreversible renal failure, requiring dialysis or kidney transplantation.

chronic pyelonephritis: a renal inflammatory process involving the tubules, interstitium, renal calyces, and renal pelves, most often due to reflex nephropathies that cause chronic bacterial infections of the upper urinary tract. This chronic inflammation results in fibrosis and scarring of the kidney and eventually loss of renal function.

chronic renal failure (CRF): a renal disorder characterized by the progressive loss of renal function due to an irreversible and intrinsic renal disease. The glomerular filtration rate decreases progressively. CRF concludes with end-stage renal disease, characterized by

isosthenuria, significant proteinuria, variable hematuria, and numerous casts of all types, particularly waxy and broad casts.

cystinosis: an inherited recessive disorder characterized by intracellular deposition of the amino acid cystine throughout the body. Cystine deposition within renal tubular cells results in their dysfunction and the development of extensive renal disease.

cystinuria: an autosomal recessive inherited disorder characterized by the inability to reabsorb the amino acids cystine, arginine, lysine, and ornithine in the renal tubules, as well as in the intestine. This results in the presence of cystine and the other dibasic amino acids in the urine, despite normal cystine metabolism. Because cystine is insoluble in an acid pH, it readily precipitates in the renal tubules, resulting in formation of calculi. The other dibasic amino acids are freely soluble and are easily excreted.

diabetes insipidus: a metabolic disease characterized by polyuria and polydipsia due to either defective antidiuretic hormone production (neurogenic) or lack of renal tubular response to antidiuretic hormone (nephrogenic).

diabetes mellitus: a metabolic disease characterized by the inability to metabolize glucose, resulting in hyperglycemia, glucosuria, and alterations in fat and protein metabolism. The cause is either defective insulin production or the formation of dysfunctional insulin by the pancreas. The disease is classified into types I or II, depending on age of onset, initial presentation, insulin requirements, and other factors.

focal proliferative glomerulonephritis: a type of glomerular inflammation characterized by cellular proliferation in a specific part of the glomeruli (segmental) and limited to a specific number of glomeruli (focal).

focal segmental glomerulosclerosis (FSG): a type of glomerular disease characterized by sclerosis of the glomeruli. Not all glomeruli are affected, hence the term *focal*, and of those that are, only certain portions become diseased, hence the term *segmental*.

galactosuria: the presence of galactose in the urine.

glomerulonephritides (GN): a group of nephritic conditions characterized by damage and inflammation of the glomeruli. Causes are varied and include immunologic, metabolic, and hereditary disorders.

IgA nephropathy: a type of glomerular inflammation characterized by the deposition of IgA in the glomerular mesangium. It often occurs 1 to 2 days following a mucosal infection of the respiratory, gastrointestinal, or urinary tract.

maple syrup urine disease (MSUD): a rare autosomal recessive inherited defect or deficiency in the enzyme responsible for the oxidation of the branched-chain amino acids — leucine, isoleucine, and valine. As a result, these amino acids along with their corresponding α-keto acids accumulate in the blood, cerebrospinal fluid, and urine. The name derives from the subtle maple syrup odor of the urine from these patients.

melanuria: the increased excretion of melanin in the urine.

membranoproliferative glomerulonephritis (MPGN): a type of glomerular inflammation characterized by cellular proliferation of the mesangium, with leukocyte infiltration and thickening of the glomerular basement membrane. Immunologically based, it is slowly progressive.

membranous glomerulonephritis (MGN): a type of glomerular inflammation characterized by the deposition of immunoglobulins and complement along the epithelial side (podocytes) of the basement membrane. It is associated with numerous immune-mediated diseases and is the major cause of nephrotic syndrome in adults.

minimal change disease (MCD): a type of glomerular inflammation characterized by the loss of the podocyte foot processes. Believed to be immune mediated, it is the major cause of nephrotic syndrome in children.

phenylketonuria (PKU): an autosomal recessive inherited enzyme defect or deficiency characterized by the inability to convert phenylalanine to tyrosine. As a result, phenylalanine is converted to phenylketones, which are excreted in the urine.

porphyria: the increased production of porphyrin precursors or porphyrins.

rapidly progressive glomerulonephritis (RPGN) (also called **crescentic glomerulonephritis**): a type of glomerular inflammation characterized

by cellular proliferation into Bowman's space to form "crescents." Numerous disease processes can lead to its development, including systemic lupus erythematosus, vasculitis, and infections.

renal phosphaturia: a rare hereditary disease characterized by the inability of the distal tubules to reabsorb inorganic phosphorus.

renal tubular acidosis (RTA): a renal disorder characterized by the inability of the renal tubules to secrete adequate hydrogen ions. Four types are recognized, and they can be inherited or acquired. Patients are unable to produce an acidic urine, regardless of the acid-base status of the blood plasma.

systemic lupus erythematosus (SLE): an autoimmune disorder that affects numerous organ systems and is characterized by autoantibodies. It is a chronic disease, frequently insidious, often febrile, involving varied neurologic, hematologic, and immunologic abnormalities. Renal involvement, as well as pleuritis and pericarditis, is common. The clinical presentation is extremely varied and is associated with a constellation of symptoms such as joint pain, skin lesions, leukopenia, hypergammaglobulinemia, antinuclear antibodies, and LE cells.

tyrosinuria: the presence of the amino acid tyrosine in the urine.

yeast infection: an inflammatory condition that results from the proliferation of a fungi, most commonly *Candida* species.

. . . .

For centuries, the study of urine has been used to provide information about the health status of the body. From the time of Hippocrates to the present, the diagnoses of renal diseases and many metabolic diseases are aided by the performance of a routine urinalysis. Because the onset of disease can be asymptomatic, a urinalysis may often detect abnormalities before the patient exhibits any clinical manifestations. In addition, urinalysis provides a means of monitoring disease progression and the effectiveness of treatments. This chapter discusses the clinical features of renal and metabolic diseases and the typical urinalysis results associated with them. Because extensive coverage of these diseases is beyond the scope of this text, the reader should see the bibliography section for sources of information.

Renal Diseases

· ·

Diseases of the kidney are often classified into four types based on the morphologic component initially affected: glomerular, tubular, interstitial, or vascular. Initially, renal disease may affect only one morphologic component; however, with disease progression, other components are involved because of their close structural and functional interdependence. Susceptibility to disease varies with each structural component. Glomerular diseases are most often immunologically mediated, whereas tubular and interstitial diseases result from infectious or toxic substances. In contrast, vascular diseases cause a reduction in renal perfusion that subsequently induces both morphologic and functional changes in the kidney.

Glomerular Disease

Diseases that damage glomeruli are varied and include immunologic, metabolic, and hereditary disorders (Table 9–1). The systemic disorders are technically *secondary* glomeru-

T A B L E 9 – 1. GLOMERULAR DISEASES

Primary glomerular diseases
  Acute glomerulonephritis (AGN)
    Poststreptococcal
    Nonpoststreptococcal
  Crescentic glomerulonephritis
  Membranous glomerulonephritis
  Minimal change disease (lipoid nephrosis)
  Focal glomerulosclerosis
  Membranoproliferative glomerulonephritis
  IgA nephropathy
  Focal glomerulonephritis
  Chronic glomerulonephritis
Secondary glomerular diseases
  Systemic diseases
    Diabetes mellitus
    Systemic lupus erythematosus
    Amyloidosis
    Vasculitis; e.g., polyarteritis nodosa
    Bacterial endocarditis
  Hereditary disorders
    Alport's syndrome
    Fabry's disease

lar diseases because they principally involve other organs; the glomeruli are involved only as a consequence of the primary disease's progression. In contrast, *primary* glomerular diseases specifically affect the kidney, which often is the only organ involved. Primary glomerular disorders are termed primary **glomerulonephritides (GN)** and consist of several types, discussed below.

Morphologic Changes in the Glomerulus

Essentially four distinct morphologic changes of the glomeruli are recognized: cellular proliferation, leukocytic infiltration, glomerular basement membrane thickening, and hyalinization with sclerosis. One or more of these changes accompany glomerulonephritis, thus assisting in characterizing the various types of glomerular diseases.

In the glomerular tuft, cellular proliferation is characterized by increased numbers of endothelial cells (capillary endothelium), mesangial cells, and epithelial cells (podocytes). This proliferation may be *segmental*, involving only a part of each glomerulus. At the same time, it can be *focal*, involving only a certain number of glomeruli, or *diffuse*, involving all glomeruli.

Drawn by a local chemotactic response, leukocytes, particularly neutrophils and macrophages, can readily infiltrate glomeruli. Present in some types of acute glomerulonephritis, leukocyte infiltration may also be accompanied by cellular proliferation.

Glomerular basement membrane thickening includes any process that results in the enlargement of the basement membrane. Most commonly, thickening results from the deposition of precipitated proteins (e.g., immune complexes, fibrin) on either side of or within the basement membrane. However, in diabetic glomerulosclerosis, the basement membrane thickens without evidence of deposition of any material.

Hyalinization of glomeruli is characterized by the accumulation of a homogeneous, eosinophilic extracellular material in the glomeruli. As this amorphous substance accumulates, glomeruli lose their structural detail and become sclerotic. Various glomerular diseases lead to these irreversible changes.

Pathogenesis of Glomerular Damage

The primary mode of glomerular injury results from immunologic processes. Both circulating antigen-antibody complexes and complexes that result from antigen-antibody reactions occurring within the glomerulus (i.e., in situ) play a role in glomerular damage.

Circulating immune complexes are created in response to either endogenous (e.g., tumor antigens, thyroglobulin) or exogenous (e.g., viruses, parasites) antigens. These circulating immune complexes become trapped within the glomeruli. The antibodies associated with them have no specificity for the glomeruli; rather, they are found there because of glomerular hemodynamic characteristics and physicochemical factors (e.g., molecular charge, shape, size). The end result is that the immune complexes, now entrapped in the glomeruli, bind complement that subsequently causes glomerular injury.

A second immune mechanism involves antibodies that react directly with glomerular tissue antigens (e.g., in antiglomerular basement membrane disease) or with nonglomerular antigens that currently reside in glomerular tissue. These latter nonglomerular antigens can originate from a variety of sources such as drugs and infectious agents (i.e., viral, bacterial, parasitic). Because immune complexes, immunoglobulins, and complement retain reactive sites even after their deposition, their presence in the glomeruli actually induces further immune complexation.

Glomerular injury results not from the immune complexes, but from the chemical mediators and toxic substances that they produce. Complement, neutrophils, monocytes, platelets, and other factors at the site produce proteases, oxygen-derived free radicals, and arachidonic acid metabolites. These substances, along with others, stimulate a local inflammatory response that further induces the glomerular tissue damage. The coagulation system also plays a role, with fibrin frequently present in these diseased glomeruli. Fibrinogen that has leaked into Bowman's space also induces cellular proliferation.

Clinical Features of Glomerular Diseases

Glomerular damage presents with characteristic clinical features, also termed syndromes (i.e., a group of symptoms or findings that occur together). The syndromes heralding glomerular damage are found in patients suffering from primary glomerular disease, as well as in patients that have glomerular injury secondary to a systemic disorder. It is the clinician's task to differentiate between the diseases.

The features characterizing glomerular damage include hematuria, proteinuria, oliguria, azotemia, edema, and hypertension (Table 9-2). The severity of each feature and the combination present varies depending on the number of glomeruli involved, the mechanism of injury, and the rapidity of disease onset. The acute nephritic syndrome is characterized by all of these features; the classic example of this syndrome is acute poststreptococcal glomerulonephritis. Some cases of glomerulonephritis are asymptomatic and are detected only when routine screening reveals microscopic hematuria or subnephrotic proteinuria (e.g., membranoproliferative glomerulonephritis or focal proliferative glomerulonephritis). The nephrotic syndrome, described later in this chapter, is a frequent manifestation of glomerular diseases. Each of

TABLE 9-2. SYNDROMES INDICATING GLOMERULAR INJURY

SYNDROME	CLINICAL FEATURES
Acute nephritis	Hematuria, proteinuria, oliguria, azotemia, edema, hypertension
Asymptomatic hematuria or proteinuria	Variable hematuria, subnephrotic proteinuria
Nephrotic syndrome	Proteinuria (>3 g/d), lipiduria, hypoproteinemia, hyperlipidemia, edema

these syndromes can eventually develop into chronic renal failure; once this happens, 80 percent to 85 percent of the kidneys' normal functioning ability is gone. Table 9–3 presents a summary of typical urinalysis results found in selected glomerular diseases.

Types of Glomerulonephritis

Glomerulonephritis can be classified on the basis of the characteristic anatomic alterations to the glomeruli. These morphologic and immunologic changes are apparent in renal biopsy specimens either by light microscopy or by the use of special stains (e.g., an immunofluorescent stain) and microscopic techniques (e.g., fluorescent or electron microscopy). The different types of glomerulonephritis are not disease-specific. For example, a patient recovering from an infection can present with glomerulonephritis of the crescentic type, typical acute glomerulonephritis, or minimal change disease. In addition, although initial presentation may be of one type of glomerular disease, the disease can progress into that of another. The classic example is the eventual development of chronic glomerulonephritis in 90 percent of patients with crescentic or rapidly progres-

sive glomerulonephritis. Table 9–4 summarizes the predominant forms of primary glomerulonephritis discussed in this section.

ACUTE GLOMERULONEPHRITIS. Acute poststreptococcal glomerulonephritis is a relatively common glomerular disease that follows 1 to 2 weeks after a streptococcal infection of the throat or skin. Although it occurs most often in children, acute glomerulonephritis can affect individuals at any age. Only certain strains of group A beta-hemolytic streptococci—those with the M protein in their cell walls—induce this nephritis. The delay between the streptococcal infection and the clinical presentation of glomerulonephritis correlates with the time required for antibody formation.

Morphologically, all glomeruli show cellular proliferation of the mesangium and endothelium, as well as leukocytic infiltration. Swelling of the interstitium owing to edema and inflammation obstructs capillaries and tubules. As a result, fibrin forms in the capillary lumina, and red blood cell casts form in the tubules. In addition, deposits of immune complexes, complement, and fibrin can be shown in the mesangium and along the basement membrane using special staining and microscopy techniques.

TABLE 9–3. TYPICAL URINALYSIS FINDINGS WITH SELECTED GLOMERULAR DISEASES

DISEASE	PHYSICAL AND CHEMICAL EXAMINATION	MICROSCOPIC EXAMINATION*
Acute glomerulonephritis	Protein—mild (<1.0 g/d), can reach nephrotic levels (>3–3.5 g/d) Blood—positive (degree variable)	↑ RBCs, often dysmorphic ↑ WBCs ↑ Renal tubular epithelial cells ↑ Casts—RBC, hemoglobin casts (pathognomonic), granular; occasional WBC and renal cell casts
Chronic glomerulonephritis	Protein—heavy (>2.5 g/d) Blood—positive (usually small) Specific gravity—low and fixed	↑ RBCs ↑ WBCs ↑ Casts—all types, particularly granular, waxy, broad ↑ Renal epithelial cells
Nephrotic syndrome	Protein—severe (>3.5 g/d) Blood—positive (usually small)	Lipiduria—oval fat bodies, free fat globules ↑ Casts—all types, particularly fatty, waxy, renal cell casts ↑ Renal epithelial cells ↑ RBCs

* ↑ = increased.

TABLE 9-4.   SUMMARY OF PREDOMINANT FORMS OF PRIMARY GLOMERULONEPHRITIS

DISEASE	TYPICAL CLINICAL PRESENTATION	PATHOGENESIS	GLOMERULAR CHANGES
Acute poststreptococcal glomerulonephritis	Acute nephritis	Antibody-mediated	Cellular proliferation (diffuse); leukocytic infiltration; interstitial swelling
Crescentic glomerulonephritis (RPGN)	Acute nephritis	Antibody-mediated; often anti-GBM*	Cellular proliferation to form characteristic "crescents"; leukocytic infiltration; fibrin deposition; GBM* disruptions
Membranous glomerulonephritis (MGN)	Nephrotic syndrome	Antibody-mediated	Basement membrane thickening owing to Ig and complement deposits; loss of foot processes (diffuse)
Minimal change disease (MCD) or lipoid nephrosis	Nephrotic syndrome	T-cell immunity dysfunction; loss of glomerular polyanions	Loss of foot processes
Focal segmental glomerulosclerosis (FSG)	Proteinuria variable; subnephrotic to nephrotic	Unknown; possibly a circulating systemic factor	Sclerotic glomeruli with hyaline and lipid deposits (focal and segmental); *diffuse* loss of foot processes; focal IgM and C3 deposits
Membranoproliferative glomerulonephritis (MPGN)	Depends on type: nephrotic syndrome or hematuria or proteinuria	Immune complex or complement activation	Cellular proliferation (mesangium); leukocytic infiltration; IgG and complement deposits
IgA nephropathy	Recurrent hematuria and proteinuria	IgA-mediated; complement activation	Deposition of IgA in mesangium; variable cellular proliferation
Chronic glomerulonephritis	Chronic renal failure	Variable	Hyalinized glomeruli

GBM = glomerular basement membrane.

Typically, the onset of acute glomerulonephritis is sudden and includes fever, malaise, nausea, oliguria, hematuria, and proteinuria. Edema may be present, often around the eyes (periorbital), knees, or ankles, and hypertension is usually mild to moderate. Because this disease is immune mediated, any blood or urine cultures for infectious agents are negative. Blood tests reveal an elevated ASO (antistreptolysin O) titer, a decrease in serum complement, and the presence of cryoglobulins. In addition, the creatinine clearance is decreased and the blood urea nitrogen–to-creatinine ratio is increased. Serum albumin levels can be normal; however, if large amounts of protein are being excreted, the levels are decreased.

Over 95 percent of the children suffering from acute poststreptococcal glomerulonephritis recover either spontaneously or with minimal therapy. Only about 60 percent of adults recover rapidly. Many of the rest of the infected adults eventually recover but others develop chronic glomerulonephritis.

Acute glomerulonephritis caused by nonstreptococcal agents, although rare, has been reported. It has been associated with other bacteria (e.g., pneumococci), viruses (e.g., mumps, hepatitis B), and parasitic infections (e.g., malaria). The clinical features of these diseases are the same; only the etiologic agent inducing the immune complex formation differs.

CRESCENTIC GLOMERULONEPHRITIS. This type of glomerulonephritis is characterized by cellular proliferation in Bowman's space to form "crescents," from which its name is derived. These cellular crescents within the glomerular tuft cause pressure changes and can even occlude the entrance to the proximal tubule. Infiltration with leukocytes and fibrin deposition within these crescents are also characteristic of this type of glomerulonephritis. As a result of these degenerative changes of the glomeruli, characteristic wrinkling and disruptions in the glomerular basement membrane are evident by electron microscopy.

Crescentic glomerulonephritis is also termed **rapidly progressive glomerulonephritis (RPGN)**. It develops 1) following an infection; 2) secondary to a systemic disease, such as systemic lupus erythematosus or vasculitis; and 3) idiopathically (usually following a flulike episode). Hematuria is present and the level of proteinuria is variable. Edema or hypertension may or may not be present. Although an antibody to the basement membrane can be demonstrated in the majority of patients with RPGN, others may show few or no immune deposits in the glomeruli. This fact supports the theory of multiple pathways leading to severe glomerular damage. Regardless of therapy, 90 percent of patients exhibiting RPGN eventually develop chronic glomerulonephritis and require long-term dialysis or kidney transplantation.

MEMBRANOUS GLOMERULONEPHRITIS. The deposition of immunoglobulins and complement along the epithelial (podocytes) side of the basement membrane characterizes **membraneous glomerulonephritis (MGN)**. With time, these deposits cause the loss of the foot processes and a thickening of the basement membrane that encloses the immune deposits. Eventually, the basement membrane's thickening severely reduces the capillary lumen and causes glomerular hyalinization and sclerosis. No cellular proliferation or leukocytic infiltration is evident.

This type of glomerulonephritis is the major cause of the nephrotic syndrome in adults. Complement activation (specifically the action of C5b-9, the membrane-attack complex of complement) is responsible for the glomerular damage that results in leakage of large amounts of protein into the renal tubules.

MGN is associated with numerous antibody-antigen mediated diseases. The antigens implicated can be exogenous *(Treponema)* or endogenous (thyroglobulin, deoxyribonucleic acid). Many antigens remain unknown. MGN frequently occurs secondary to other conditions, such as systemic lupus erythematosus, diabetes mellitus, or thyroiditis, or following exposure to metals (e.g., gold, mercury) or drugs (e.g., penicillamine). However, in approximately 85 percent of the patients, MGN is idiopathic.

Sudden onset of the nephrotic syndrome is the usual clinical presentation of MGN. Hematuria and mild hypertension may be present. The clinical course of the disease varies, with no resolution of the proteinuria in up to 90 percent of the patients. Although it may take many years to develop, eventually 50 percent of the MGN patients progress to chronic glomerulonephritis. Only 10 percent to 30 percent of MGN patients show complete or partial recovery.

MINIMAL CHANGE DISEASE. Minimal change disease (MCD) is characterized by glomeruli that look normal by light microscopy; however, the loss of the podocyte foot processes is apparent with electron microscopy. The foot processes are replaced by a simplified structure, and their cytoplasm shows vacuolization. No leukocyte infiltration or cellular proliferation is present.

Despite the absence of any immunoglobulin or complement deposits, MCD is believed to be immunologically based, involving a dysfunction of T-cell immunity. Various factors support this belief; the most notable factor is MCD's onset following infections or immunizations and its rapid response to corticosteroid therapy. The T-cell dysfunction results in loss of the glomerular "shield of negativity" or polyanions (e.g., heparin sulfate proteoglycan). Remember, albumin can readily pass through the glomerular filtration barrier if the negative charge is removed; hence, MCD is characterized by the nephrotic syndrome, i.e., massive proteinuria.

MCD is responsible for the majority of cases of nephrotic syndrome in children. However, no hypertension or hematuria is associated with it. Clinically, its differentiation from MGN is based on its dramatic response to corticosteroid therapy. Although patients may become steroid-dependent to keep the disease in check, the prognosis for recovery is excellent for both children and adults.

FOCAL SEGMENTAL GLOMERULOSCLEROSIS. Focal segmental glomerulosclerosis (FSG) is characterized by the sclerosis of glomeruli. The process is focal, occurring in only a certain number of glomeruli, as well as segmental, affecting only a specific area within each of the affected glomeruli. Morphologically, the sclerotic glomeruli show hyaline and lipid deposition, collapsed basement membranes, and proliferation of the mesangium. FSG is characterized most by diffuse damage to the epithelium (podocytes) that is not readily apparent. Electron microscopy reveals the loss of the foot processes (i.e., diffuse) in both sclerotic and nonsclerotic glomeruli. The glomerular hyalinization and sclerosis results from the mesangial response to the accumulation of plasma proteins and fibrin deposits. In addition, IgM and C3 are evident by immunofluorescence in these sclerotic areas.

FSG may be 1) a primary glomerular disease; 2) associated with another glomerular disease, such as IgA nephropathy; or 3) secondary to other disorders. Heroin abuse, acquired immunodeficiency syndrome (AIDS), reflux nephropathy, and analgesic abuse nephropathy are some conditions that can precede secondary FSG.

FSG presents as the nephrotic syndrome in 10 percent to 15 percent of the patients; the remaining patients exhibit moderate-to-heavy proteinuria. Hematuria, reduced glomerular filtration rate (GFR), and hypertension may also be present. Patients with FSG have little or no response to corticosteroid therapy, which helps to differentiate them from patients with MCD. Many patients develop chronic glomerulonephritis at variable rates. It is interesting to note that FSG can recur following renal transplantation (25 percent to 50 percent), sometimes within days, suggesting a circulating systemic factor as the causative agent.

MEMBRANOPROLIFERATIVE GLOMERULONEPHRITIS (MPGN). Membranoproliferative glomerulonephritis (MPGN) is characterized by cellular proliferation, particularly of the mesangium, along with leukocyte infiltration and thickening of the glomerular basement membrane. As a result of the increased numbers of mesangial cells, the glomeruli take on a "lobular" appearance, which is apparent microscopically. Ultrastructural characteristics subdivide MPGN into two types, types I and II.

An immunologic basis underlies the majority of MPGN cases. The basis can be in the form of immune complex formation in the glomeruli or the deposition in glomeruli of complement and its activation.

MPGN is a slow, progressive disease, with 50 percent of the patients developing chronic renal failure. It accounts for 5 percent to 10 percent of the patients who present with the nephrotic syndrome. It has a varied presentation pattern, however; some patients may show only hematuria or subnephrotic proteinuria (less than 3 to 3.5 g/d). In renal transplant recipients, MPGN has an unusually high incidence of recurrence.

IgA NEPHROPATHY. The deposition of IgA in the glomerular mesangium characterizes IgA nephropathy, one of the most prevalent types of glomerulonephritis. IgA deposits, however, are detectable only using special staining and microscopy techniques (e.g., immunofluorescence). Apparently, circulating IgA complexes or aggregates become trapped and engulfed by mesangial cells. It is known that aggregated IgA is capable of activating the alternative complement pathway, which results in glomerular damage. Morphologically, the glomerular lesions are varied. Some may appear normal, whereas others may show evidence of either focal or diffuse cellular proliferation.

A common finding is recurrent hematuria in a range from gross to microscopic amounts. Proteinuria is usually present, varying in degree from mild to severe. IgA nephropathy often occurs 1 to 2 days following a mucosal infection of the respiratory, gastrointestinal, or urinary tract from infectious agents (e.g., bacteria, viruses) that stimulate mucosal IgA synthesis. As a result, serum IgA levels are frequently elevated, and circulating IgA immune complexes are present in these patients.

IgA nephropathy primarily affects children and young adults. It is slowly progressive and results in chronic renal failure in 50 percent of the patients. The patient develops renal failure more quickly when disease onset occurs in old age or when it is associated with severe proteinuria and hypertension.

FOCAL PROLIFERATIVE GLOMERULONEPHRITIS. Focal proliferative glomerulonephritis is characterized by cellular proliferation in a specific part of the glomeruli (i.e., segmental) and is limited to a specific number or portion of them (i.e., focal). In addition, focal cellular necrosis, as well as fibrin deposition, can occur.

Primary focal proliferative glomerulonephritis often presents with mild or subclinical features such as recurrent hematuria (microscopic or gross) or subnephrotic proteinuria. It also presents secondarily to numerous systemic diseases, such as systemic lupus erythematosus, polyarteritis nodosa, and bacterial endocarditis.

CHRONIC GLOMERULONEPHRITIS. In time, numerous glomerular diseases result in the development of **chronic glomerulonephritis.** Morphologically, the glomeruli have become hyalinized, appearing as acellular eosinophilic masses. In addition, the renal tubules atrophy, fibrosis is evident in the renal interstitium, and infiltration by lymphocytes may occur.

About 80 percent of the patients that develop chronic glomerulonephritis have previously presented with some other form of glomerulonephritis (Table 9–5). The remaining 20 percent of cases represent forms of glomerulonephritis that were unrecognized or subclinical in their presentation. The development of chronic glomerulonephritis is slow and silent, taking many years to progress. Some patients may present with edema, leading to the discovery of the underlying renal disease; other clinical findings include proteinuria, hypertension, and azotemia. Occasionally cerebral or cardiovascular conditions, along with hypertension, manifest first clinically. Death resulting from uremia and from the pathologic changes it causes in other organs (e.g., uremic pericarditis, uremic gastroenteritis) will occur if patients are not maintained on dialysis or do not undergo renal transplantation.

Systemic Diseases and Glomerular Damage

Systemic lupus erythematosus (SLE) presents clinically with a constellation of lesions and clinical manifestations. Almost all SLE patients show some type of renal involvement. The pathogenesis of the glomerular damage is due to immune complex deposition, specifically, deoxyribonucleic acid (DNA) and anti-DNA complexes, and complement activation. There are five recognized morphologic patterns of lupus nephritis; however, none of them is diagnostic or unique to SLE. In other words, any of the clinical syndromes such as recurrent hematuria, acute nephritis, or the nephrotic syndrome may be exhibited by patients with SLE. It is important to note that chronic renal failure is a leading cause of death in these patients.

Diabetes mellitus is another systemic disorder that frequently results in renal disease. It presents most commonly as a glomerular syndrome; however, vascular lesions of the arterioles and frequently associated hypertension, as well as an enhanced susceptibility to pyelonephritis and papillary necrosis, account for other forms of renal disease in the diabetic patient. Consequently, it is not surprising that renal disease is a major cause of death in the diabetic patient. Proteinuria, ranging from subnephrotic to nephrotic levels, eventually develops in up to 55 percent of diabetic patients, whereas thickening

TABLE 9–5. PERCENTAGE OF GLOMERULAR DISEASES RESULTING IN CHRONIC GLOMERULONEPHRITIS

DISEASE	APPROXIMATE PERCENTAGE
Crescentic (rapidly progressive) glomerulonephritis	90%
Focal glomerulosclerosis	50%–80%
Membranous glomerulonephritis	50%
Membranoproliferative glomerulonephritis	50%
IgA nephropathy	30%–50%
Poststreptococcal glomerulonephritis	1%–2%

of the glomerular basement membrane, evident only by electron microscopy, occurs in all diabetics. Within 10 to 20 years of disease onset, pronounced cellular proliferation of the glomerular mesangium eventually results in glomerulosclerosis (Fig. 9–1). Chronic renal failure usually develops within 4 to 5 years following the onset of persistent proteinuria and requires long-term renal dialysis or transplantation.

The development of diabetic glomerulosclerosis occurs more often in type I (insulin-dependent) than in type II (non-insulin-dependent) diabetics. It is believed that the development of diabetic renal disease results directly from either insulin deficiency or hyperglycemia. Therefore, it is speculated that tight control of blood glucose levels may be able to prevent the development and progression of diabetic nephropathy.

Amyloidosis is a group of systemic diseases that involves many organs. It is characterized by the deposition of amyloid, a pathologic proteinaceous substance, between cells in numerous tissues and organs. Amyloid is made up of about 90 percent fibril protein and 10 percent glycoprotein. Microscopically in tissue, amyloid initially appears as an eosinophilic hyaline substance. It is differentiated from hyaline (e.g., collagen, fibrin) by Congo red staining, which imparts amyloid with a characteristic green birefringence with polarizing microscopy.

The deposition of amyloid within the glomeruli eventually destroys them. As a result, patients with amyloidosis present clinically with heavy proteinuria or nephrotic syndrome. With time and the continual destruction of glomeruli, renal failure and uremia develop.

Nephrotic Syndrome

The nephrotic syndrome is a group of clinical features that occur simultaneously. Representing the increased permeability of the glomeruli to the passage of plasma proteins, most notably albumin, it is characterized by heavy proteinuria (3.5 g/d or more). Additional features include hypoproteinemia, hyperlipidemia, lipiduria, and edema. Plasma albumin levels are usually less than 3 g/dL because liver synthesis is unable to compensate for the large amounts of protein being excreted. Albumin is the predominant protein lost because of its high plasma concentration. However, proteins of equal or smaller size, such as immunoglobulins, low-molecular-weight complement components, and anticoagulant cofactors, are also excreted in increased amounts. As a result, patients with the nephrotic syndrome are more susceptible to infections and thrombotic complications.

Hyperlipidemia in the nephrotic syndrome is due to increased plasma levels of triglycerides, cholesterol, phospholipids, and very low density lipoproteins (VLDL). Whereas the exact mechanisms causing the hyperlipidemia are still unknown, it is at least partly caused by an increased synthesis of these lipids by the liver and compounded by a decrease in their catabolism. Because of the increased glomerular permeability, these lipids are able to cross the glomerular filtration barrier and appear in the urine. They may be present as free-floating fat globules,

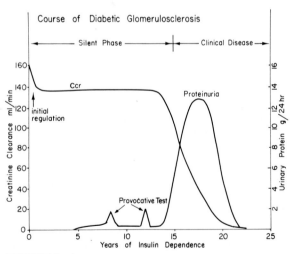

FIGURE 9–1. A composite drawing showing the course of diabetic nephropathy. Exercise and other stress will cause intermittent proteinuria before a sustained protein leak, which may lead to nephrotic syndrome. Initial regulation indicates initiation of insulin therapy. (From Friedman EA, Shieh SD: Clinical management of diabetic nephropathy. *In* Friedman EA, L'Esperance FA [eds]: Diabetic Renal-Retinal Syndrome, New York, Grune-Stratton, 1980. (Used with permission.)

found within renal epithelial cells or macro-phages (i.e., oval fat bodies), or encased in casts.

The generalized edema present with the nephrotic syndrome is characteristically soft and pitting (i.e., when the flesh is depressed, the indentation remains). Its development is due primarily to the decreased excretion of sodium (de Wardener, 1985). Whereas the exact mechanism is not clearly understood, it is due partly to the increased reabsorption of sodium and water by the distal tubules. The loss of protein and protein's associated on-cotic pressure from the blood plasma also re-sults in the movement of fluid into the inter-stitial tissues; however, its role is minor compared to that of sodium in the develop-ment of edema in these patients. Edema is usually apparent around the eyes (perior-bital) and in the legs, but severe cases can also develop pleural effusions and ascites.

Along with the heavy proteinuria and li-piduria in these patients, the urine micro-scopic examination often shows a mild mi-croscopic hematuria. In addition, pathologic casts such as fatty, waxy, and renal tubular casts are often present (see Table 9–3).

Nephrotic syndrome occurs in patients with minimal change disease (lipoid nephro-sis), membranous glomerulonephritis, focal segmental glomerulosclerosis, and membrano-proliferative glomerulonephritis. These glo-merular diseases account for about 90 per-cent of all nephrotic syndrome cases in children and about 75 percent of those in adults. Systemic diseases that can present with the nephrotic syndrome include diabetes mellitus, systemic lupus erythematosus, amy-loidosis, malignant neoplasms, and infections, as well as renal responses to nephrotoxic agents (e.g., drugs, poisons).

Tubular Disease

Acute Tubular Necrosis

Acute tubular necrosis (ATN) is character-ized by the destruction of renal tubular epi-thelial cells. The causes are varied. ATN can be classified into two distinct types: ischemic ATN and toxic ATN. Ischemic ATN follows a hypotensive event (e.g., shock) that results in decreased perfusion of the kidneys and is-chemia. In contrast, renal tubular cell dam-age in toxic ATN results from nephrotoxic agents that have been ingested, injected, or inhaled. The tubular damage that results from either type of ATN can be reversed once normal renal function has been restored. It is interesting to note that approximately 45 percent of all cases of ATN result from surgical procedures.

The three principal causes of ischemic ATN are sepsis, shock, and trauma. However, any obstruction to renal blood flow or occlu-sion of renal arteries or arterioles can result in renal hypoperfusion and tissue ischemia. Examples of sepsis and shock include exten-sive bacterial infections and severe burns; examples of trauma include crushing injuries, and numerous surgical procedures.

Myoglobin and hemoglobin are two pig-mented heme proteins that are known to be toxic to the renal tubules. Myoglobinuria is a result of severe muscle damage (rhabdomyo-lysis) as well as of nontraumatic causes such as alcohol abuse, heat stroke, and drug use. Hemoglobinuria follows a severe hemolytic episode in which haptoglobin—the plasma protein that normally binds hemoglobin to prevent its loss in the urine—has been de-pleted and free hemoglobin readily passes the glomerular filtration barrier into the tubules. Despite the nephrotoxicity of hemoglobin and myoglobin, the development of ATN in their presence is actually caused by the associated dehydration and renal ischemia that accom-panies their excretion (Cotran, 1989).

Toxic ATN is caused by numerous nephrotoxic agents that fall principally into two categories: drugs and toxins. Drugs in-clude antibiotics (aminoglycosides, cephalo-sporins), anesthetics (methoxyflurane), radio-graphic contrast media, and chemotherapeutic drugs (cyclosporine). Toxins include heavy metals (mercury, lead), organic solvents (car-bon tetrachloride, ethylene glycol) and other poisons (mushrooms, pesticides). The tubular necrosis induced by these toxic substances can result in oliguria and acute renal failure.

Morphologically, ischemic ATN affects short segments (i.e., focal) of the tubules in random areas throughout the nephron, from the medullary segments of the proximal tubules and ascending loops of Henle to the collecting tubules. The tubular basement membrane is often disrupted (i.e., tubulorrhexis) as a result of the complete necrosis of the tubular cells; consequently, the renal interstitium is exposed to the tubular lumen. As a result, renal cell fragments are sloughed into the urine. These cell fragments consist of three or more tubular cells shed intact and usually originate in the collecting duct. In contrast, toxic ATN causes tubular necrosis primarily in the proximal tubules and does not usually involve their basement membranes. Convoluted renal tubular epithelial cells are found in the urine sediment; finding these distinctively large proximal tubular epithelial cells is indicative of toxic ATN. In addition to tubular cell death, nephrotoxins in high concentrations often cause renal vasoconstriction. Because of this, patients may also present with characteristics typical of ischemic ATN. Both types of ATN show cast formation within the distal convoluted and collecting tubules. Compared to toxic ATN, however, ischemic ATN shows an increased number and variety of casts in the urine sediment, including granular, renal tubular cell, waxy, and broad casts.

The clinical presentation of ATN is often divided into three phases: onset, renal failure, and recovery. The onset of ATN may be abrupt following a hypotensive episode, or deceptively subtle in a previously healthy individual following the exposure to a toxin or the administration of a nephrotoxic drug. This variable presentation develops into a renal failure phase with azotemia, hyperkalemia, and metabolic acidosis. At this time, approximately 50 percent of patients have a reduction in urine output to below 400 mL/d (oliguria). The recovery phase is indicated by a steady increase in urine output and may reach levels of 3 L/d. This diuretic state is exhibited by both oliguric and nonoliguric patients. It is best explained by the return to normal of the glomerular filtration rate (GFR) before full recovery of the damaged tubular epithelium. This increased diuresis results in the loss of large amounts of water, sodium, and potassium until tubular function completely returns. At the same time, the azotemia resolves. Full renal tubular function and concentrating ability return in about 6 months.

Tubular Dysfunction

Renal tubular dysfunctions may result from a primary renal disease or may be induced secondarily. The dysfunction may involve a single pathway with only one solute type affected, or it may involve multiple pathways, thereby affecting a variety of tubular functions. Tables 9–6 and 9–7 summarize tubular dysfunctions according to the tubular segment involved and the disorders associated with them. Isolated portions of the tubule (e.g., proximal tubule) can be affected while the remaining nephron segments retain essentially normal function. Similarly, these renal tubular disorders do not affect glomerular function; thus, GFR is usually normal. This section discusses some of the more commonly encountered tubular dysfunctions, and typical urinalysis findings are outlined in Table 9–8. For more extensive coverage of renal tubular dysfunctions, the reader should see the bibliography section.

RENAL GLUCOSURIA. Glucosuria may be a result of a lowered *maximal tubular reabsorptive capacity* (T_m) for glucose. Normally, the T_m for glucose is approximately 350 mg/min by the proximal tubules. Renal glucosuria is an inherited condition that results in the excretion of glucose in the urine despite normal blood glucose levels. This glucosuria, caused by a reduction in the glucose T_m in these patients, is a benign condition.

CYSTINURIA. Cystinuria is characterized by the urinary excretion of large amounts of the amino acid cystine, as well as the dibasic amino acids arginine, lysine, and ornithine. In this disease, inherited as an autosomal recessive trait, the proximal tubules are unable to reabsorb these amino acids, despite normal cystine metabolism. At the same time, pa-

TABLE 9–6.   PROXIMAL TUBULAR DYSFUNCTIONS

DYSFUNCTION	DISEASE
Single defect in proximal tubular function	
Impaired ability to reabsorb glucose	Renal glucosuria
Impaired ability to reabsorb specific amino acids	Cystinuria (cystine and dibasic amino acids)
	Hartnup disease (monoamino-monocarboxylic amino acids)
Impaired ability to reabsorb sodium	Bartter syndrome
Impaired ability to reabsorb bicarbonate	Renal tubular acidosis type II
Impaired ability to reabsorb calcium	Idiopathic hypercalciuria
Excessive reabsorption of calcium	Hypocalciuric familial hypercalcemia
Excessive reabsorption of sodium	Gordon syndrome
Excessive reabsorption of phosphate	Pseudohypoparathyroidism
Multiple defects in proximal tubular function	Inherited diseases
	Cystinosis
	Tyrosinemia
	Wilson disease
	Galactosemia
	Hereditary fructose intolerance
	Glycogen storage disease
	Metabolic diseases
	Bone diseases, e.g., osteomalacia, primary hyperparathyroidism, vitamin D–dependent rickets
	Renal diseases
	Amyloidosis
	Nephrotic syndrome
	Transplant rejection
	Renal vascular injury
	Toxin induced
	Heavy metals, e.g., lead, mercury, cadmium
	Drugs, e.g., aminoglycosides, cephalosporins, mercaptopurine, expired tetracycline

TABLE 9–7.   DISTAL TUBULAR DYSFUNCTIONS

DYSFUNCTION	DISEASE
Impaired ability to reabsorb phosphate	Familial hypophosphatemia (vitamin D–resistant rickets)
Impaired ability to reabsorb calcium	Idiopathic hypercalciuria
Impaired ability to acidify urine	Renal tubular acidosis types I and IV
Impaired ability to retain sodium	Renal salt-losing disorders
Impaired ability to concentrate urine	Nephrogenic diabetes insipidus
Excessive reabsorption of sodium	Liddle syndrome

tients with cystinuria have defective intestinal absorption of these amino acids. Because cystine readily precipitates at an acid pH when the tubular filtrate becomes concentrated, the patient frequently presents with renal calculi made of cystine. The other amino acids excreted are soluble and therefore do not form calculi. To prevent cystine stone formation, patients are instructed to stay well-hydrated, particularly during the night when the urine becomes the most concentrated and acidic. This requires that the patient awaken in the middle of the night to drink water and even then is not always successful in preventing stone formation. Treatment may involve oral administration of D-

TABLE 9–8.   TYPICAL URINALYSIS FINDINGS WITH SELECTED TUBULAR DISEASES

DISEASE	PHYSICAL AND CHEMICAL EXAMINATION	MICROSCOPIC EXAMINATION*
Acute tubular necrosis	Protein—mild (<1 g/d) Blood—positive Specific gravity—low	↑ RBCs ↑ WBCs ↑ Renal epithelial cells, including renal cell fragments; proximal tubular cells in toxic ATN; collecting tubular cells in ischemic ATN ↑ Casts: renal cell, granular, waxy, and broad
Cystinuria and cystinosis	Blood—positive (usually small) *Cystinosis:* Protein—mild (<1 g/d)	↑ RBCs Cystine crystals
Renal tubular acidosis†	pH > 5.5	Unremarkable
Fanconi syndrome	Protein—moderate (<2.5 g/d) Glucose—positive; amount variable	Unremarkable

* ↑ = *increased.*
† *RTA patients can develop Fanconi syndrome.*

penicillamine. This drug converts cystine to a highly soluble form—penicillamine-cysteine-disulfide; however, there are disadvantages. D-penicillamine is very expensive and has several undesirable side effects including fever, rash, proteinuria, and nephrotic syndrome.

FANCONI SYNDROME. The term "Fanconi syndrome" is used to characterize any condition that presents with a generalized loss of proximal tubular function. As a result of this dysfunction, amino acids, glucose, water, phosphorus, potassium, and calcium are lost in the urine. A spectrum of disorders can result in the presentation of this syndrome, including inherited diseases (e.g., cystinosis), toxin exposure (e.g., lead), metabolic bone diseases (e.g., rickets), and renal diseases (e.g., amyloidosis).

CYSTINOSIS. Cystinosis is an inherited recessive trait that results in the intracellular deposition of cystine throughout the body. These crystals accumulate within the proximal tubular cells, causing generalized proximal tubular dysfunction and development of Fanconi syndrome. Late in the disease, when the distal tubules become involved, patients with cystinosis are unable to concentrate or to acidify their urine.

This hereditary disease is evident during the first year of life. These patients show growth retardation, rickets, and acidosis, as well as polydipsia and polyuria. Without renal dialysis or a kidney transplant, these patients die by the time they are 10 years old as a result of the extensive renal damage.

RENAL PHOSPHATURIA. Renal phosphaturia is an uncommon hereditary disorder characterized by an inability of the distal tubules to reabsorb inorganic phosphorus. The tubular defect appears to be two-fold: a hypersensitivity of the distal tubules to the parathyroid hormone that causes increased phosphate excretion, and a decreased proximal tubular response to lowered plasma phosphate levels. Because of the low plasma phosphate levels, bone growth and mineralization decrease. Renal phosphaturia patients may be asymptomatic or can exhibit signs of severe deficiency such as osteomalacia or rickets and growth retardation. Inherited as a dominant sex-linked characteristic, this disorder is often termed familial hypophosphatemia or vitamin D–resistant rickets.

RENAL TUBULAR ACIDOSIS. Renal tubular acidosis (RTA) is characterized by the inability of the tubules to secrete adequate hydrogen ions despite a normal glomerular filtration rate. As a result, these patients are unable to produce acidified urine below a pH of 5.3, even when in an acidotic state. RTA can be inherited as an autosomal dominant trait, with partial or complete expression, or can occur secondary to a variety of diseases.

Several forms of RTA (types I, II, III, and IV) are identified based on their renal tubular defect(s). In type I RTA, the tubular dysfunction appears to be two-fold: an inability to maintain the normal hydrogen ion gradient, and an inability to increase tubular ammonia secretion to compensate. The defect in maintaining the hydrogen ion gradient results either from a tubular secretory defect or from increased back-diffusion of hydrogen ions in the distal tubules. Regardless, RTA patients become acidotic and their bodies compensate by removing calcium carbonate ($CaCO_3$) from bone to buffer the retained acids. Consequently, the patients develop osteomalacia and hypercalcemia. The resultant hypercalciuria causes nephrocalcinosis, the precipitation of calcium salts in the tubules and renal parenchyma.

Type II RTA is characterized by decreased proximal tubular reabsorption of bicarbonate. As a result, an increased amount of bicarbonate is presented to the distal tubules for reabsorption. To compensate, most of the hydrogen ions that the distal tubule secretes are used to retain this bicarbonate rather than being eliminated in the urine. Consequently, hydrogen ion excretion decreases and the urinary pH increases. This type of RTA is rarely seen without additional abnormalities of the proximal tubule (e.g., Fanconi syndrome).

Type III RTA patients express characteristics of both type I and type II RTA. Type IV RTA is characterized by an impaired ability to exchange sodium for potassium and hydrogen in the distal tubule.

Numerous conditions can give rise to acquired RTA. Approximately 30 percent of acquired RTA type I patients have an autoimmune disorder that has an associated hypergammaglobulinemia, such as biliary cirrhosis or thyroid disease. Drugs, nephrotoxins, and kidney transplant rejection can also result in the development of RTA, as can inborn errors of metabolism such as Wilson's disease or cystinosis.

Individualized treatment for RTA consists of reducing the acidemia by oral administration of alkaline salts (e.g., sodium bicarbonate) and potassium. This serves to raise the plasma pH toward normal and replace lost potassium (primarily in RTA types I and II). Other clinical problems such as the development of renal calculi (stones) and upper urinary tract infections may require additional treatment regimens.

Tubulointerstitial Disease and Urinary Tract Infections

Because of their close structural and functional relationship, a disease process affecting the renal interstitium inevitably involves the tubules, leading to tubulointerstitial disease. Numerous conditions or factors are capable of causing a tubulointerstitial disease process, and the pathogenic mechanism for each can differ (Table 9–9). Tubulointerstitial disease and lower urinary tract infections can be intimately involved because the latter represents the principal mechanism leading to the development of acute pyelonephritis. Typical routine urinalysis findings in selected urinary tract infections and tubulointerstitial diseases are outlined in Table 9–10.

TABLE 9–9. CAUSES OF TUBULOINTERSTITIAL DISEASES

Infection
  Acute pyelonephritis
  Chronic pyelonephritis
Toxins
  Drugs
    Acute interstitial nephritis (AIN)
    Analgesic nephritis
  Heavy metal poisonings, e.g., lead
Metabolic disease
  Urate nephropathy
  Nephrocalcinosis
Vascular diseases
Irradiation
  Radiation nephritis
Neoplasms
  Multiple myeloma
Transplant rejection

TABLE 9–10.   TYPICAL URINALYSIS FINDINGS IN SELECTED URINARY TRACT INFECTIONS AND TUBULOINTERSTITIAL DISEASES

DISEASE	PHYSICAL AND CHEMICAL EXAMINATION*	MICROSCOPIC EXAMINATION†
Lower urinary tract infection Cystitis	Protein—small (<0.5 g/d) Blood—positive (usually small) Leukocyte esterase—±; usually + Nitrite—±; usually +	↑ WBCs ↑ Bacteria: variable, small to large numbers ↑ RBCs ↑ Transitional epithelial cells
Tubulointerstitial disease (Upper urinary tract infection) Acute pyelonephritis	Protein—mild (<1 g/d) Blood—positive (usually small) Leukocyte esterase—±; usually + Nitrite—±; usually + Specific gravity—normal to low	↑ WBCs, often in clumps; macrophages ↑ Bacteria: variable, small to large numbers ↑ Casts: WBC (pathognomonic), granular, renal cell, waxy ↑ RBCs ↑ Renal epithelial cells
Chronic pyelonephritis	Protein—moderate (<2.5 g/d) Leukocyte esterase—± Specific gravity—low	↑ WBCs, macrophages ↑ Casts: granular, waxy, broad; few WBC and renal cells
Acute interstitial nephritis	Protein—mild (<1 g/d) Blood—positive (degree variable) Leukocyte esterase—±; usually +	↑ WBCs, macrophages; differential reveals increased eosinophils ↑ RBCs ↑ Casts: leukocyte (eosinophil) cast, granular, hyaline, renal cell ↑ Renal epithelial cells (Crystals—drug crystals possible, if drug is inducing the disease)

* ± = *either positive or negative;* + = *positive;* − = *negative.*
† ↑ = *increased.*

Urinary Tract Infections

Urinary tract infections (UTIs) involve either the upper or lower urinary tract. A lower UTI can involve the urethra (urethritis), the bladder (cystitis), or both, whereas an upper UTI can involve the renal pelvis alone (pyelitis) or with the interstitium (pyelonephritis). UTIs are very common and affect females approximately 10 times more than males. This predisposition is due to several factors: the shorter urethra in females; hormonal influences enhancing bacterial adherence to mucosa; the "milking" of bacteria up the urethra during sexual intercourse; and the lack of the antibacterial action present in prostatic fluid.

Normally, urine and the urinary tract are sterile, except for the normal bacterial flora at the extreme distal portion of the urethra. The continual flushing of the urethra during the voiding of urine normally prevents the movement of bacteria into the sterile portions of the urinary tract. In spite of this, UTIs develop most often from bacteria present in the patient's normal fecal flora and are considered endogenous infections (i.e., the infecting agent originated from within the organism). In other words, owing to various factors, these intestinal organisms, the fecal flora, are introduced into the urinary tract, where they proliferate and cause an infection. Approximately 85 percent of all UTIs are due to the gram-negative rods present in normal feces. The most common pathogen is *Escherichia coli;* however, *Proteus, Klebsiella, Enterobacter,* and *Pseudomonas* are other gram-negative rods often encountered. *Streptococcus faecalis* (enterococci) and *Staphylococcus aureus* are gram-positive organisms that have also been implicated in UTIs. It is worth noting, however, that essentially any bacterial or fungal agent can cause a UTI.

Lower UTIs are characterized by pain or burning on urination (dysuria) and occasionally lower abdominal pain. A routine urinalysis will reveal leukocyturia and bacteriuria. Of particular note is the absence of casts, differentiating a lower UTI from one of the upper urinary tract, where casts are present. A quantitative urine culture is used to establish the diagnosis, with a finding of 10^5 colonies per mL indicating infection. Minimal hematuria and proteinuria may be present. Increased numbers of transitional epithelial cells may also be sloughed and noted microscopically.

The clinical presentation and findings of an upper urinary tract infection are discussed in the next section on acute pyelonephritis, the most common upper UTI encountered.

Acute Pyelonephritis

Acute pyelonephritis is a bacterial infection involving the renal tubules, interstitium, and renal pelvis. Two different mechanisms can lead to this renal infection: bacteria moving from the lower urinary tract to the kidneys, or bacteria in the blood localizing in the kidneys (hematogenous infection). The most common cause is the ascending urinary tract infection resulting from gram-negative organisms that are normal intestinal tract flora. Usually, when bacteria reach the bladder, they are kept from ascending the ureters because of the continual flushing of urine during voiding as well as other antibacterial mechanisms. However, when voiding is incomplete (e.g., obstruction, dysfunction), allowing bacterial proliferation in the bladder, or when anatomic abnormalities in the urinary tract facilitate bacterial movement up the ureters (e.g., vesicoureteral reflux), infections of the kidney can occur.

Acute pyelonephritis is usually associated with predisposing conditions that en-hance the proliferation and movement of bacteria to the kidneys. These conditions include catheterization, urinary obstruction, pregnancy, vesicoureteral reflux, diabetes mellitus, and immunosuppressive conditions, as well as the patient's age and sex. Once in the kidney, bacteria multiply predominantly in the interstitium, causing an acute inflammation that eventually involves the tubules. The tubules become necrotic, and bacterial toxins along with leukocytic enzymes cause abscesses to form in the tubules. Large numbers of neutrophils accumulate in these tubules in an attempt to prevent further spread of the infection. The glomeruli are rarely involved in this infection.

Clinically, acute pyelonephritis has a sudden onset characterized by flank pain (the costovertebral angle), dysuria, and a frequency of micturition that includes nocturia and urgency. The patient may also present with fever, nausea, headache, and generalized malaise. A urinalysis reveals bacteria and large numbers of leukocytes (leukocyturia) and other inflammatory cells (e.g., macrophages) that derive from the inflammatory infiltrate in the kidney. The presence of leukocyte casts, as well as other casts (e.g., granular, renal tubular cell, broad), is pathognomonic of renal involvement (i.e., an upper UTI). Minimal-to-mild proteinuria and hematuria are present, and the urine specific gravity is usually low.

Acute pyelonephritis lasts 1 to 2 weeks and is most often benign. With appropriate antibiotic therapy, symptoms disappear within a few days. If predisposing conditions are not resolved, repeat infections can lead to eventual permanent renal damage.

Chronic Pyelonephritis

Chronic tubulointerstitial inflammation results in the permanent scarring of renal tissue and can eventually involve the renal calyces and pelvis, which is then termed **chronic pyelonephritis.** Many diseases can cause chronic tubulointerstitial disease; however, most do not involve the renal calyces and pelvis. Both chronic obstruction and reflux nephropathies can cause chronic pyelonephritis; in children, reflux nephropathy is the most frequent cause. The reflux nephropathies involved are either a vesicoureteral or an intrarenal reflux. Vesicoureteral reflux is due to a congenital, inherited anatomic variation at the junction of the ureter and bladder that allows the backward flow of urine up the ureters. Intrarenal reflex occurs within the renal pelvis and is due to anatomic variations of renal papillae. It results in the movement of urine back up the collecting ducts into the renal cortex. In either condition, any bacteria present readily spread into the renal interstitium, causing an upper UTI. This chronic inflammation results in fibrosis and the scarring of the parenchyma. In addition, the renal calyces become dilated and deformed, characteristic of chronic pyelonephritis.

The most common cause of chronic pyelonephritis is reflux nephropathy. The onset of reflux nephropathy is usually insidious and is often detected by a routine urinalysis or following the development of renal insufficiency and hypertension. The urinalysis reveals increased leukocytes and proteinuria; bacteria may or may not be present. Whereas casts are present in early stages, they are usually absent in the later chronic stages. Polyuria and nocturia develop as tubular function is lost; hence, the urine specific gravity is low. With disease progression and the development of hypertension, renal blood flow and the glomerular filtration rate are affected. Approximately 10 percent to 15 percent of patients with chronic pyelonephritis develop chronic renal failure (end-stage renal disease) and require dialysis.

Acute Interstitial Nephritis

Acute interstitial nephritis (AIN) occurs in response to various drugs and toxins. Three modes of renal injury are associated with these agents: 1) an immediate allergic response in the renal interstitium (e.g., sulfonamides, penicillins); 2) direct and acute damage to tubules (e.g., heavy metals, aminoglycosides); or 3) over time, the slow destruction of tubular function (e.g., analgesic abuse). The first mechanism of renal injury, an allergic response, results in the development of AIN.

Most notably the sulfonamide and penicillin families of antibiotics are associated with AIN; however, many other drugs such as furosemide, rifampin, phenylbutazone, and cimetidine have also been implicated. As these various drugs are removed by tubular secretion, they become immunogenic and induce an immune response involving the renal tubular epithelium. As a result, antibodies and cell-mediated immune reactions cause injury. The renal interstitium becomes edemic and infiltrated with leukocytes, particularly lymphocytes, macrophages, eosinophils, and neutrophils. Varying degrees of tubular necrosis can result, whereas the glomeruli and renal vasculature are usually not involved and retain their normal functioning ability. A routine urinalysis reveals hematuria, mild proteinuria, and leukocyturia without bacteria (i.e., sterile leukocyturia). A differential analysis of the leukocytes present reveals increased numbers of eosinophils (eosinophiluria). Leukocyte or eosinophil casts may also be demonstrated.

The development of AIN usually begins 3 to 21 days following the initiation of drug therapy. It is characterized by a fever and, in some patients (25 percent), a skin rash. Discontinuation of the offending drug can result in full recovery of renal function; however, irreversible damage can occur, especially in elderly individuals.

Yeast Infections

The urinary tract of both men and women is susceptible to **yeast infection,** although such infection occurs more commonly in the vagina. *Candida* species (e.g., *Candida albicans*) are normal flora in the gastrointestinal tract and vagina, and their proliferation is kept in check by the other normal flora in these areas. When this bacterial flora is disrupted by antibiotics or pH changes, however, yeasts will proliferate. Urinary and blood catheters provide a mode of inoculating these organisms into the urinary tract or bloodstream. *Candida* has a predilection for renal tissue and can cause either an upper or lower UTI. These yeast infections are particularly severe in immunocompromised patients.

Vascular Disease

Because the kidneys' functioning is directly related to receiving 25 percent of the cardiac output, any disruption in this blood supply will affect renal function. Likewise, any changes in the vasculature of the kidney directly affect the close interrelationship and interdependence of these blood vessels and the renal interstitium and tubules. As a result, disorders that affect the supply of blood to the kidney or the blood vessels themselves cause renal disease. Atherosclerosis of intrarenal arteries causes a reduction in renal blood flow, whereas hypertension, polyarteritis nodosa, eclampsia, diabetes, and amyloidosis often cause significant changes in the arterioles and glomerular capillaries such that severe and fatal renal ischemia can result.

The kidneys play an active role in the control of blood pressure by influencing vascular resistance and blood volume; hence, hypertension is a frequent finding in various renal disorders. Some diseases that affect the glomerular vasculature such as glomerulosclerosis and systemic lupus erythematosus, have already been discussed. Many others exist. Discussion of the kidneys' role in blood pressure regulation and the mechanisms of renal hypertension are beyond the scope of this text; hence, the reader is directed to the bibliography section for additional information.

Acute and Chronic Renal Failure

Acute Renal Failure

Acute renal failure (ARF) is characterized clinically by a sudden decrease in the glomerular filtration rate (GFR), azotemia, and oliguria (i.e., urine output less than 400 mL). Usually there is no histologic abnormality of the nephrons; rather, they are functionally abnormal. Often the initial oliguria leads to anuria and, despite the fact that ARF is usually reversible, it has a high mortality rate.

The three principal mechanisms that cause ARF are classified as prerenal, renal, and postrenal. Approximately 25 percent of ARF cases are prerenal, resulting from a decrease in renal blood flow (RBF). Any event that reduces the mean arterial blood pressure in the afferent arterioles below 80 mm Hg will cause a reduction in the GFR. The most common initiator is a decreased cardiac output causing a decrease in renal perfusion. If this condition lasts long enough, tissue ischemia results. In fact, ischemic ATN is the most common cause of ARF. Other conditions that cause a sudden reduction in blood volume and are associated with this type of ARF include hemorrhages, burns, and surgical procedures, as well as acute diarrhea and vomiting. In response to a decreased blood pressure, the kidneys increase sodium and water reabsorption in an attempt to restore normal blood volume and perfusion. If this process is unsuccessful, ischemic renal injury can result, and the development of a renal type ARF will be superimposed on the initiating prerenal cause.

The urine sediment in prerenal ARF is not distinctive. It is the urine electrolytes that provide more information to aid in identifying this disease process. The urine sodium is low because an increased amount of sodium is being reabsorbed. Despite this, the urine osmolality is usually greater than the serum osmolality. In addition, the BUN-to-creatinine ratio is significantly increased.

Renal causes of ARF account for approximately 65 percent of cases. Characterized by renal damage, ARF can result from any glomerular, tubular, or vascular disease process. The majority of patients (99 percent) present clinically with ATN. As ATN progresses, the renal tubular destruction results in a loss of water and electrolytes (e.g., sodium, potassium). This increased urinary excretion of sodium from renal ARF contrasts with the decreased urine sodium from prerenal causes of ARF and aids in the differentiation of the causes.

Postrenal causes of ARF are due to obstructions in urine flow and account for approximately 10 percent of ARF patients. Mechanical obstruction within the kidney can result from various sources such as crystalline deposition (e.g., drugs, amino acids, solutes) and neoplasms. Regardless, the obstruction causes an increase in the hydrostatic pressure within the tubules and Bowman's space. As a result, the normal filtration pressures across the glomerular filtration barrier are disrupted and the GFR decreases. Eventually, the tubules become damaged and renal function is lost.

Regardless of the cause of ARF, the urinalysis findings are not characteristically diagnostic. However, careful examination is important to aid in the diagnosis of the underlying cause (e.g., ATN, obstruction, myoglobinuria, nephrotoxin). The clinical course of ARF varies greatly; patients who survive usually regain normal renal function. The monitoring of the patient's fluids and electrolytes is crucial during the course of ARF, with dialysis often needed to control the azotemia. If a patient becomes overhydrated, edema and heart failure may result. The high mortality of ARF is due principally to concomitant infections or potassium intoxication.

Chronic Renal Failure

The progressive loss of renal function owing to an irreversible and intrinsic renal disease characterizes **chronic renal failure (CRF)**. With CRF, the GFR slowly but continuously decreases, the decrease becoming clinically recognizable only after 80 percent to 85 percent of normal renal function (i.e., a GFR of approximately 15 to 20 mL/min) has been lost. Hence, the course of CRF is often described as "slow and silent." Early in the course of CRF, the remaining healthy nephrons hypertrophy to compensate for those destroyed and in doing so are able to maintain apparently normal renal function.

Numerous diseases result in CRF, with the glomerulonephropathies accounting for 50 percent to 60 percent of cases. Diabetic nephropathy, chronic pyelonephritis, hypertension, collagen vascular diseases (e.g., systemic lupus erythematosus), and congenital abnormalities are some other causes.

Clinically, CRF presents with azotemia, acid-base imbalance, water and electrolyte imbalance, and abnormal calcium and phosphorus metabolism. Periodic determinations of the GFR assist the clinician in monitoring CRF. Other clinical features include anemia, bleeding tendencies, hypertension, weight loss, nausea, and vomiting. Eventually, CRF progresses to an advanced renal disease often termed end-stage renal disease or end-stage kidneys. When patients reach this stage, they require dialysis or renal transplantation in order to survive.

Urinalysis findings associated with end-stage renal disease include a fixed specific gravity (isothenuria, at 1.010), significant proteinuria, minimal-to-moderate hematuria, and the presence of all types of casts, particularly waxy and broad casts.

Calculi

Pathogenesis

Calculi are solid aggregates of chemicals, usually mineral salts, that form within the body. They may be found in any secreting gland, including the pancreas, gallbladder, salivary gland, lacrimal gland, and urinary tract. This discussion will focus primarily on calculi, or "stones," of the urinary tract. They are found primarily in the renal calyces, pelvis, ureter, or bladder.

Only about 0.1 percent of the population develop renal calculi, and approximately 75 percent of these calculi contain calcium (Table 9–11). Calculi are rarely composed of a single chemical component; rather, they are most often a mixture that includes calcium, oxalate, or both. Magnesium ammonium phosphate ("triple phosphate"), phosphate, uric acid, and cystine are also frequently involved. All calculi have an organic mucoprotein matrix. Whether changes in urinary mucoproteins that form this matrix cause or enhance stone formation is unknown.

Underlying metabolic or endocrine disorders, as well as infections and isohydria (fixed urinary pH), cause or enhance calculi formation. When the urine becomes supersat-

TABLE 9–11. RENAL CALCULI COMPOSITION

CHEMICAL COMPONENT	APPROXIMATE FREQUENCY
Calcium	75%
with oxalate	35%
with phosphate	15%
with others	25%
Magnesium ammonium phosphate	15%
Uric acid	6%
Cystine	2%
All others	<1%

urated with chemical components (i.e., the components' solubility is exceeded) and the pH is optimal, renal calculi form. Stone formation may or may not be associated with a concomitant increase of these solutes in the blood. For example, about 25 percent of individuals who develop calcium stones do not have hypercalcemia or hypercalciuria; similarly, more than 50 percent of patients with uric acid stones do not have hyperuricemia or hyperuricosuria. Patients with hypercalciuria, hyperoxaluria, and hyperuricemia are at a risk of developing renal calculi, however. Renal tubular reabsorption mechanisms may be dysfunctional, allowing increased urinary excretion of the chemical constituent; alternatively, increased intestinal absorption resulting from dietary increases or from hereditary conditions can account for the increased urinary amounts present. It is postulated that calculi formation may also be affected by the absence of natural inhibitors. These inhibitors may include pyrophosphate, diphosphonate, citrate, and nephrocalcin; however, conclusive evidence of their role in calculi formation has yet to be confirmed. It is believed that these substances, when deficient or absent, may induce calculi formation.

Factors Influencing Formation

Essentially four factors influence renal calculi formation: 1) an increase in concentration of the chemical salts; 2) changes in urinary pH; 3) urinary stasis; and 4) the presence of a foreign body seed.

Increases in concentration of urinary solutes can be due to external causes, endocrine disorders, or metabolic conditions. External causes include dehydration, in which the urinary solutes are excreted in as small amount of water as possible to conserve body water. Dietary excess as seen in vegetarians whose diets are high in oxalates or in individuals ingesting megadoses of ascorbic acid, as well as increased intestinal absorption present in patients with inflammatory bowel disease, can lead to increased urinary concentrations of particular solutes. Medications, particularly cytotoxic drugs, can also result in increases of urinary solutes. For example, drug regimens used to combat leukemias use medications that destroy blast cells, causing an increase in nucleic acid breakdown. As a result, the uric acid concentration in the blood and urine is increased. If the urine formed is sufficiently acidified by the distal tubules, uric acid crystals will readily precipitate out of solution. Endocrine disorders, such as hyperparathyroidism, cause reabsorption of calcium from bone and subsequently hypercalcemia and hypercalciuria. Metabolic conditions such as gout (hyperuricemia), inborn errors of metabolism (e.g., cystinuria), or primary oxaluria can also produce urines supersaturated with some chemical constituents.

Changes in urinary pH play an important role in calculi formation. Without the proper pH, even high concentrations of chemicals can remain soluble. Calculi formation is enhanced when a patient experiences isohydruria (i.e., a constant and unchanging urinary pH), losing the body's normal "acid-alkaline tide." The inorganic salts—calcium, magnesium, ammonium, phosphate, and oxalate—are less soluble in neutral or alkaline urine. In contrast, organic salts such as uric acid, cystine, and bilirubin are less soluble in an acidic urine. RTA, which is associated with many renal disorders and was discussed earlier in this chapter, is also linked to calculi formation. With RTA, the patient's tubules are unable to acidify the urine (i.e., excrete hydrogen ions), and to compensate, increased amounts of urinary calcium are excreted. As a result, patients with RTA have an increased chance of forming renal calculi. Patients with UTIs owing to urea-splitting organisms such as *Proteus* have alkaline urine because of the bacterial conversion of urinary urea to ammonia. As a result, these individuals form magnesium ammonium phosphate stones. These "staghorn" stones are some of the largest renal stones ever formed and derive their name from their branching shape that matches the renal pelvis in which they were formed. Almost without exception, staghorn stones are associated with an upper urinary tract infection.

Urinary stasis (e.g., malformations) enhances renal calculi formation by increasing the chances of supersaturation and precipitation. The presence of a foreign body seed provides a nucleus that stimulates crystalline deposition. This seed may be a clump of bacteria, a fibrin clot, an epithelial cell, or a bit of debris.

The formation of renal stones is most often discovered when the urinary tract becomes obstructed or the stones produce ulceration and bleeding. Small stones can pass from the renal pelvis into the ureters where they can cause obstruction and produce intense pain, often referred to as renal colic. This pain is intense, beginning in the kidney region and radiating forward and downward to include the abdomen, genitalia, and legs. The patient often experiences nausea, vomiting, sweating, and a frequent urge to urinate. Large stones unable to pass into the ureter (or urethra) remain in the renal pelvis (or bladder) and are discovered only from the trauma they produce, which is usually manifested by hematuria.

Prevention and Treatment

Increasing fluid intake to produce a dilute urine and modifying the diet to eliminate excesses in certain solutes are two easy ways to prevent future calculi formation. Urinary pH can be controlled by the ingestion of acids (e.g., ammonium chloride) or alkalis (e.g., sodium bicarbonate) to ensure solubility of the offending solute. Sometimes drugs are used to convert a solute to a more soluble form. For example, D-penicillamine converts cys-

tine to a soluble compound, whereas allopurinol administered to patients who form uric acid stones inhibits an enzyme necessary for its formation and forces the production of soluble hypoxanthine instead. Eliminating the causative agent can also prevent stone formation. This includes administering an appropriate antibiotic to eliminate urea-splitting bacteria or discontinuing drug administration when it is the cause (e.g., sulfonamides).

Once a stone has formed, several techniques are available for its destruction or removal. Currently, lithotripsy—the use of sound waves to break up the stone in vivo—is used and is rapidly replacing once-common surgical procedures. If the stone is located in the lower third of the ureter or in the bladder, cystoscopy can be used to crush and remove the stone. However, if the patient is in danger of progressive deterioration or if an obstruction is present, surgical removal is performed.

Metabolic Diseases

A routine urinalysis can also provide important information regarding metabolic diseases. These diseases vary and may be characterized by an increased excretion of a normal urinary constituent or by the appearance in the urine of a substance that is not normally present. Because some metabolic diseases are linked to long-lasting detrimental effects, such as mental retardation or nervous system degeneration, early detection is paramount. Although the urinalysis laboratory may detect or suspect the presence of a particular substance in a patient's urine, more accurate quantitative procedures are available in clinical chemistry laboratories to specifically identify them. For example, a pediatric urine specimen contains a reducing sugar other than glucose. This information must be conveyed rapidly and clearly to the physician so that additional testing, such as the identification of reducing sugars by thin-layer chromatography, can be performed. Early intervention in galactosuria prevents its associated severe liver damage and mental retardation. Hence, the role of the urinalysis laboratory is to screen for abnormal substances or increased amounts of normal solutes and to alert the physician to their presence.

Amino Acid Disorders

The liver and kidneys are actively involved in the metabolism of amino acids. They interconvert amino acids by transamination and degrade them by deamination. The latter results in ammonium ions, which are used to form urea. The urea is subsequently eliminated from the body by the kidneys. Normally, amino acids readily pass the glomerular filtration barrier and are reabsorbed by the proximal tubule. This reabsorption, an active transport mechanism, is threshold-limited and facilitated by membrane-bound carriers.

The three types of **aminoaciduria,** differentiated by their causes, include overflow, no-threshold, and renal aminoacidurias. Overflow aminoaciduria is due to an increase in the plasma levels of the amino acid(s) such that the amino acids' renal threshold for reabsorption is exceeded and the additional amino acids are excreted in the urine. The second type, no-threshold aminoaciduria, also has an overflow mechanism. The difference is that the amino acids in this type are not normally reabsorbed by the tubules; any increase in the blood produces an increased amount in the urine. The third type, renal aminoaciduria, occurs when the plasma levels of amino acids are normal, but because of a tubular defect (congenital or acquired), they are not reabsorbed and appear in the urine in increased amounts.

Aminoacidurias can occur as either a primary or a secondary disease. The primary diseases are also known as inborn errors of metabolism and result from an inherited defect. Two types of defects are possible; either 1) an enzyme is defective (or deficient) in the specific metabolic pathway of the amino acid, or 2) there is tubular reabsorption dysfunction. Secondary aminoacidurias are in-

duced most notably by severe liver disease or through generalized renal tubular dysfunction (e.g., Fanconi's syndrome).

Cystinuria and Cystinosis

These diseases are discussed in the renal disease section of this chapter because they cause renal tubular dysfunction. Cystinuria is an inherited autosomal recessive disorder that is characterized by the defective tubular reabsorption of cystine and the amino acids arginine, lysine, and ornithine, which are specifically affected by this disorder. Cystinosis is a metabolic disease that involves the intracellular deposition of cystine in the lysosomes of all cells of the body, particularly the kidney, eye, bone marrow, and spleen. Its effect on the proximal renal tubules is secondary. Cystinosis is inherited as a recessive trait, and when cystine crystals accumulate within the proximal tubular cells, the patient develops Fanconi's syndrome with a generalized aminoaciduria and glucosuria. When the distal tubules become involved, cystinosis patients are unable to concentrate or to acidify their urine. This hereditary disease is evident during the first year of life. Patients with cystinosis show growth retardation, rickets, and acidosis, as well as polydipsia and polyuria. Without renal dialysis or a transplant, these patients die by age 10 years as a result of the extensive renal damage.

Maple Syrup Urine Disease

Maple syrup urine disease (MSUD) is a rare autosomal recessive inherited disease. It is characterized by the accumulation of the branched-chain amino acids—leucine, isoleucine, and valine—and their corresponding α-keto acids in the blood, cerebrospinal fluid, and urine. These acids accumulate as a result of an inherited defect or deficiency in the enzyme responsible for their normal oxidative decarboxylation to acyl-CoA derivatives (fatty acids). Both neonatal screening using a Guthrie microbial inhibition test and prenatal screening using cultured amniotic cells can detect this inherited disorder.

Although they appear normal at birth, infants with MSUD demonstrate symptoms of the disease within the first few weeks of life. An acute ketoacidosis develops along with vomiting, seizures, and lethargy. If not diagnosed and treated appropriately, mental retardation or death can result. The increased amounts of urinary keto acids account for the distinctive maple syrup or carmelized sugar odor associated with this disease. Although assessment of urine odor is not routinely performed in a routine urinalysis, the laboratorian should make the physician aware of such an unusual feature. Diagnosis of MSUD is usually made following amino acid analysis using high-performance liquid chromatography. Treatment consists of dietary restriction of the branched-chain amino acids, along with daily monitoring of urinary keto acids using the dinitrophenylhydrazine (DNPH) screening test.

Phenylketonuria

Inherited as an autosomal recessive disease, **phenylketonuria (PKU)** is characterized by an increased urinary excretion of phenylpyruvate (a ketone) and its metabolites. Normally, phenylalanine is converted to tyrosine by the major metabolic pathway depicted in Figure 9–2. However, in "classic" PKU, the enzyme phenylalanine hydroxylase is deficient or defective and the minor metabolic pathway is stimulated, producing phenylketones. Other forms of PKU result from a defect or decrease in the enzyme's cofactor, tetrahydrobiopterin.

Without detection and treatment, PKU results in severe mental retardation. As with other aminoacidurias, affected children appear normal at birth. Nonspecific initial symptoms include delayed development and feeding difficulties such as severe vomiting.

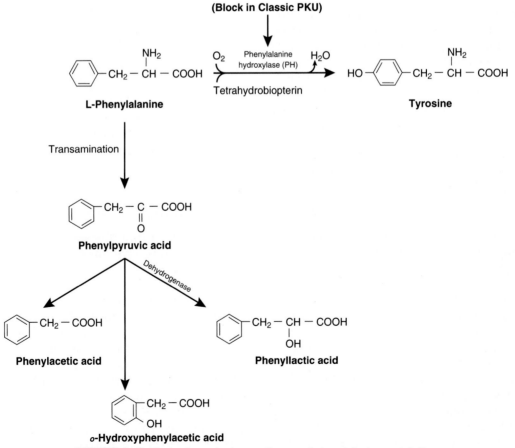

FIGURE 9–2. The major and minor pathways of phenylalanine metabolism.

Within the infant's first 2 to 3 weeks of life, high plasma levels of phenylalanine cause brain injury, with the maximal effect achieved by the time the patient is 9 months old. The mousy or musty odor associated with the urine and sweat from PKU patients is due to the phenylpyruvate present in these fluids. An additional feature of PKU patients is decreased skin pigmentation, resulting from the competitive inhibition of the enzyme tyrosinase by phenylalanine. This inhibition decreases the production of tyrosine and its pigmentation metabolite, melanin.

Neonatal screening tests for PKU use blood for the detection of increased levels of phenylalanine for two related reasons: permanent mental retardation occurs within the first few weeks of life, and the urinary excretion of phenylpyruvic acid does not occur until there has been substantial plasma accumulation of phenylalanine, i.e., after 2 or more weeks. Hence, if urinary detection methods were used, the detrimental and irreversible effects of the disorder would have already taken place. A Guthrie microbial inhibition test is widely used, and screening for PKU is mandated by all states on all newborns.

Treatment consists of dietary modification to eliminate phenylalanine from the diet. Mental retardation can be avoided completely with early diagnosis and treatment; however, even late detection (when the patient is 4 to 6 months old) can often avoid further mental deterioration. Routine monitoring is usually performed on the patient's blood plasma; however, the ferric chloride test provides a rapid qualitative means of screening urine for phenylpyruvate levels greater than 10 mg/dL. It is important to note that the ferric chloride test is a nonspecific test that can produce positive results owing to a variety of amino acids and medications.

Alkaptonuria

Alkaptonuria is a rare, recessive disease characterized by the excretion of large amounts of homogentisic acid (dihydroxyphenylacetic acid), a substance not normally present in urine. This disease was called alkaptonuria because of the unusual darkening of the urine when alkali is added. Homogentisic acid is normally oxidized to maleylacetoacetic acid by the enzyme homogentisic acid oxidase (Fig. 9–3). When this liver enzyme is deficient or absent, homogentisic acid is unable to proceed down the remaining steps of its normal metabolic pathway. As a result, homogentisic acid accumulates in the cells and body fluids and is excreted in the urine. By binding to collagen in cartilage and

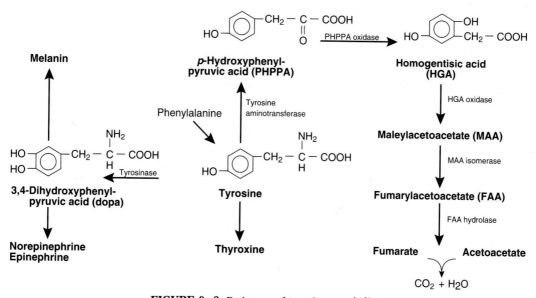

FIGURE 9–3. Pathways of tyrosine metabolism.

other connective tissues, homogentisic acid causes an abnormal dark blue or black tissue pigmentation and the development of degenerative arthritis.

Alkaptonuria is not usually diagnosed until middle age, when arthritis and pigmentation in the ears (ochronosis) becomes apparent. However, it can be detected in neonates if the dark color that develops on their diapers is noted and investigated. Urine with homogentisic acid will darken with standing, with exposure to air or sunlight, or with the addition of alkali. This urine darkening or coloration requires further investigation and differentiation from other substances such as melanin, indican (indoxyl sulfate), and gentisic acid (a salicylate metabolite). Several rapid screening tests based on the reducing ability of homogentisic acid include an ammoniacal silver nitrate test and Benedict's test. In the ferric chloride test, homogentisic acid produces a transient dark blue color. Regardless of the test used, confirmatory identification of homogentisic acid requires either thin-layer or high-performance liquid chromatography.

Treatment for alkaptonuria is limited to dietary restrictions of tyrosine and phenylalanine; however, the benefit of this regimen has yet to be established.

Tyrosinuria and Melanuria

Tyrosinuria, the presence of urinary tyrosine, is due to the overflow of this amino acid from the blood plasma. Several forms of tyrosinemia are possible; the form most frequently seen is a transient form in neonates. Others include severe liver diseases that can produce a generalized amino acid disorder with tyrosine excretion and the rare inherited disorder, hereditary tyrosinemia.

Because tyrosine is the metabolic precursor of several compounds—melanin, thyroxine, and the catecholamines—various defects may affect one product and not another (see Fig. 9–3). The principal metabolic pathway involves the formation of homogentisic acid and ends in the formation of CO_2 and water from fumarate and acetoacetate. Transient neonatal tyrosinemia results from an immature liver in infants and is characterized by the infant's inability to synthesize adequate enzymes. As the liver matures, normal enzyme levels are established and the tyrosinemia resolves within 4 to 8 weeks. Severe liver disease with dramatically decreased enzyme synthesis can also produce a tyrosinemia similar to the transient neonatal form.

Lastly, the rare, inherited tyrosinemias can be divided into two types, type I and type II. Type I, also termed tyrosinosis, is due to a defect in the enzyme fumarylacetoacetate hydrolase (FAA). Type II tyrosinemia is due to a defect with the enzyme tyrosine aminotransferase. Both types result in liver damage and renal disease characterized by a generalized aminoaciduria. Both types have high levels of tyrosine in the blood and urine and are usually fatal within the patient's first decade of life.

In these cases of tyrosinuria, the microscopic examination may reveal the presence of tyrosine and leucine crystals in acid urines. The nonspecific nitrosonaphthol test can be used to screen for abnormally high levels of tyrosine in urine; however, diagnosis is made following quantitative procedures (e.g., chromatographic methods) of serum.

Melanin is produced from tyrosine by melanocytes and is the pigment responsible for the color of hair, skin, and eyes. When inherited defects result in defective melanin production, hypomelanosis or albinism results. Conversely, increased production of melanin and its colorless precursors (e.g., 5,6-dihydroxyindole) results in increased urinary excretion of melanin, or **melanuria.** A malignant neoplasm of melanocytes (also called a melanoma) in the skin, mucous membranes, or retina will produce melanuria. When melanin and its precursors are present in the urine, the urine color will darken with exposure to air or sunlight. The extent of darkening varies with melanin concentration and exposure time; in extreme cases, the urine can turn black. Because homogentisic acid can also cause similar coloration, further investigation is required to confirm the identity of the darkening substance.

Carbohydrate Disorders

Glucose and Diabetes Mellitus

Diabetes mellitus is not a single disorder but actually several disorders, each affecting the metabolism of carbohydrate, fat, and protein. It is characterized by chronic hyperglycemia and glucosuria, both of which are evidence of an impaired ability to utilize glucose. The actual defect varies between being either a deficiency in the production of pancreatic insulin or the production of dysfunctional insulin.

Diabetes mellitus is classified as type I, insulin-dependent diabetes mellitus (IDDM), or as type II, noninsulin-dependent diabetes mellitus (NIDDM). This classification was developed in 1979 by the National Diabetes Data Group of the National Institutes of Health to standardize the identification and naming of various diabetic conditions. Type I diabetes mellitus can occur at any age; however, most individuals present before 40 years of age (hence, IDDM was formerly referred to as juvenile-onset diabetes). Classic symptoms of this form of diabetes include polyuria, polydipsia, ketonuria, and rapid weight loss. Accounting for about 10 percent to 20 percent of patients with diabetes, type I diabetes mellitus often presents suddenly as an acute illness with ketoacidosis. These individuals require insulin to maintain and utilize normal blood glucose levels. In contrast, type II diabetes mellitus usually presents after 40 years of age (hence, NIDDM was formerly termed adult-onset diabetes). The disorder progresses slowly and often is initially detected during a routine wellness screening or during testing for other clinical concerns. While obesity is very common and often associated with type II diabetes mellitus, it is not found in all type II patients. Type II diabetes mellitus accounts for 80 percent to 90 percent of patients with diabetes. Usually dietary regimens are used to control blood glucose levels, and most of these diabetic patients do not require exogenous insulin.

Another difference between patients with type I and type II diabetes mellitus is the tendency to develop serious complications. Over time, type I diabetics tend to develop numerous complications of the eyes (retinopathy), nerves (neuropathy), blood vessels (angiopathy), and kidneys (nephropathy). For example, the incidence of cataracts is up to six times greater in a type I diabetic than in a nondiabetic individual, and 40 percent to 50 percent of type I diabetics will eventually develop renal failure. Varying degrees of neuropathy are found in all type I diabetics, and in 10 percent of these individuals it is a serious concern. In contrast, most of these complications do not develop in type II diabetes mellitus patients, with one exception: the development of angiopathy of the macrovasculature causes both type I and II diabetes mellitus patients to be at a higher risk for strokes and heart attacks. Table 9–12 summarizes some differentiating characteristics

TABLE 9–12. CHARACTERISTICS OF TYPE I AND TYPE II DIABETES MELLITUS

TYPE	CLINICAL FEATURES
Type I, insulin-dependent diabetes mellitus (IDDM)	Presents before 40 years of age Onset usually sudden, acute Inadequate production of insulin Patient requires insulin injections Patient tends to develop ketoacidosis Patient tends to develop complications 　Retinopathy 　Neuropathy 　Nephropathy 　Angiopathy (both the micro- and macrovasculature)
Type II, noninsulin-dependent diabetes mellitus (NIDDM)	Presents after 40 years of age Onset slow and insidious Insulin levels variable Dietary regimens aid in control of hyperglycemia; insulin injections not necessary Obesity very common Angiopathy of macrovasculature common

of type I and type II diabetes mellitus patients.

Regardless of the type of diabetes mellitus, when inadequate or dysfunctional insulin is present, these individuals experience polydipsia and polyuria. Their urine appears dilute, but the specific gravity is significantly increased owing to the large amounts of urinary glucose present. This glucosuria indicates that the renal tubular resorptive ability (i.e., the renal threshold for glucose Tm_g) has been exceeded. With insufficient utilization of glucose, these patients metabolize fat; hence, keto acids or ketones will also be detected in their urine.

Galactosuria

Two autosomal recessive inherited diseases result in the development of galactosemia and **galactosuria.** They result from different enzymatic defects in the galactose metabolic pathway. As a result, galactose, which is derived from lactose in the diet, cannot be converted to glucose. Instead, galactose accumulates, and a minor metabolic pathway results in the formation of galactitol and galactonate. These toxic intermediate products of galactose metabolism are responsible for the clinical manifestations of this disease. In early infancy, patients with galactosuria present clinically with diarrhea, vomiting, and a failure to thrive. Evidence of liver dysfunction, such as hepatomegaly and jaundice, may be present; in addition, cataracts are often present shortly after birth. If galactosuria is allowed to go untreated, mental retardation will be evident by 3 to 4 months old. Early intervention with dietary restrictions can prevent the development of cataracts and mental retardation and permit normal growth.

Prenatal detection of galactosuria can be done using cultured amniotic cells. Some states perform mass screening tests to detect infants with this disease. In a routine urinalysis laboratory, urine specimens from children who are less than 2 years old should be screened for the presence of reducing substances. If a reducing substance is present and glucose and ascorbic acid are not, galac-

tose, lactose, fructose, or pentose should be suspected. Thin-layer chromatography should be employed to positively identify the reducing sugar present.

Diabetes Insipidus

Diabetes insipidus derives its name "diabetes" from the copious amounts of urine (polyuria) that this disorder produces. Insipidus refers to the urine's bland taste (in contrast to diabetes mellitus, in which the urine tastes sweet). Diabetes insipidus is a disorder characterized by either 1) the decreased production of antidiuretic hormone (ADH) by the posterior pituitary (neurogenic diabetes insipidus) or 2) the lack of renal tubular response to ADH (nephrogenic diabetes insipidus). In either case, water is not adequately reabsorbed by the renal tubules, resulting in polyuria, which in turn induces polydipsia. Compulsive water drinking and certain drugs (e.g., lithium, demeclocycline) can also induce diabetes insipidus. In contrast to the urine from diabetes mellitus patients, the dilute-appearing urine of diabetes insipidus patients has a low specific gravity. As long as these patients are able to replace the large amounts of water being excreted, they remain healthy with normal plasma tonicity. Despite supervised fluid restrictions, these patients are unable to produce a concentrated urine. Dehydration in these patients can be life-threatening; it causes them to rapidly become hypertonic and go into shock.

Porphyrin Disorders

Porphyrins (uroporphyrin, coproporphyrin, protoporphyrin) are intermediate compounds that form during the production of heme (see Fig. 7–6). They are derived from porphin by the addition of organic groups in the eight peripheral positions on its four pyrrole rings (Fig. 9–4). Normally, heme synthesis is so closely regulated that only trace amounts of porphyrins are formed. The porphyrins result from the spontaneous and irreversible oxidation of their respective porphyrinogens. Once this process has taken place, the por-

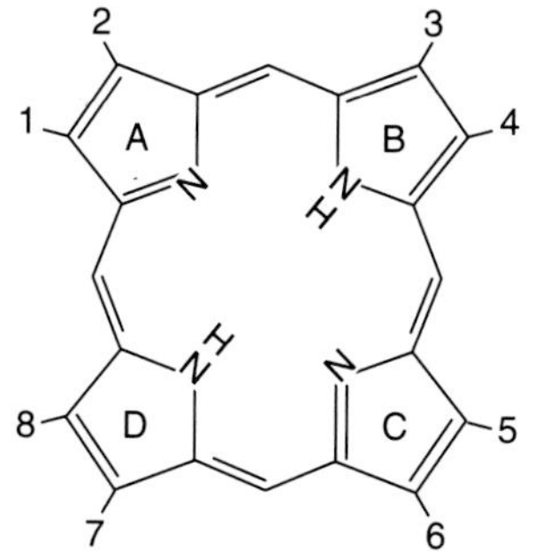

Porphyrin

FIGURE 9-4. The basic structure of porphyrins.

phyrins cannot re-enter the heme synthetic pathway, have no biological function, and must be excreted.

Each porphyrin differs with respect to its polarity and therefore its solubility. Uroporphyrin (UP) is excreted almost exclusively in the urine; coproporphyrin (CP), being of intermediate solubility, is excreted in both the urine and the feces; and protoporphyrin (PP), the least water soluble, is excreted only in the feces. The porphyrin precursors—porphobilinogen (PBG) and δ-aminolevulinic acid (ALA)—appear principally in the urine, because they are rapidly removed from the blood by glomerular filtration and have a low renal threshold.

The porphyrin precursors (PBG and ALA) and the porphyrinogens (uroporphyrinogen, coproporphyrinogen, protoporphyrinogen) are colorless and nonfluorescent compounds. In contrast, their oxidative forms (UP, CP, PP) are dark red or purple and intensely fluores-

cent. Increased amounts of these substances can be detected or suspected when a routine urinalysis is performed. Porphobilin, the oxidative form of PBG, is dark red. As a result, urine containing porphobilin and porphobilinogen may appear dark red, often described as "port wine." When a urine of this color tests negative for the presence of blood and when medications have been ruled out, porphyria should be considered and screening performed. Other urine specimens may initially have a normal color but after standing change color (i.e., become deep red) because of the photo-oxidation of PBG.

The porphyrins and heme are produced by all mammalian cells; however, the major sites of synthesis are the bone marrow and liver. As discussed in Chapter 7 with porphobilinogen, various inherited or induced disorders can result in **porphyria,** the increased urinary excretion of porphyrin precursors or porphyrins (Table 9-13). These disorders reflect a deficiency or inhibition of an enzyme required in heme biosynthesis. As intermediate compounds accumulate behind the pathway defect, they are found in increased amounts in the blood, feces, or urine. Porphyrias can be classified as hepatic or erythropoietic based on the site of the metabolic abnormality; however, classification based on clinical presentation is often more practical and readily applicable (Table 9-14). All porphyrias are rare, with porphyria cutanea tarda being the most common type found in North America. All show autosomal dominant inheritance with the exception of

TABLE 9-13. CLASSIFICATION OF PORPHYRIAS

	ENZYME DEFECT	TRANSMISSION
Inherited disorders		
Acute intermittent porphyria	Uroporphyrinogen I synthase deficiency	Autosomal dominant
Congenital erythropoietic porphyria	Uroporphyrinogen cosynthase deficiency	Autosomal recessive
Porphyria cutanea tarda	Uroporphyrinogen decarboxylase deficiency	Autosomal dominant
Protoporphyria	Ferrochelatase deficiency	Autosomal dominant
Coproporphyria	Coproporphyrinogen oxidase deficiency	Autosomal dominant
Porphyria variegata	Protoporphyrinogen oxidase deficiency	Autosomal dominant
Induced disorders		
Coproporphyrinuria, due to lead poisoning, tyrosinemia, alcoholism, drugs (e.g., sedatives, hypnotics)		
Protoporphyrinemia, due to lead poisoning, iron deficiency anemias		

T A B L E 9–14.   SUMMARY OF PORPHYRIA CHARACTERISTICS

CLINICAL PRESENTATION	DISORDER	ONSET	PORPHYRINS INCREASED*
Neurologic symptoms	Acute intermittent porphyria	Acute	ALA, PBG, UP
Cutaneous symptoms (photosensitive)	Congenital erythropoietic porphyria	Chronic	UP, CP, Bl-P, F-P
	Porphyria cutanea tarda	Chronic	UP, 7-COOH P
	Protoporphyria	Chronic	Bl-PP, F-PP
Neurologic and cutaneous symptoms	Coproporphyria	Acute	ALA, PBG, CP, F-CP
	Porphyria variegata	Acute	ALA, PBG, CP, F-CP, F-PP

* ALA = Urinary δ-aminolevulinic acid; PBG = urinary porphobilinogen; UP = urinary uroporphyrin; CP = urinary coproporphyrin; Bl-P = blood porphyrins; F-P = fecal porphyrins; 7-COOH P = urinary 7-COOH porphyrin; Bl-PP = blood protoporphyrin; F-PP = fecal protoporphyrin; F-CP = fecal coproporphyrin.

congenital erythropoietic porphyria, the rarest form of porphyria. Induced disorders are generally classified into one of two types: those that result in the accumulation and excretion of coproporphyrin in the urine, and those that result in the accumulation of protoporphyrin in the blood and its excretion in feces. Chronic lead poisoning can cause the development of both features, whereas other disorders, such as iron deficiency anemia or tyrosinemia, are associated with only one of these features. Induced porphyria-like disorders also produce excesses of other porphyrins or porphyrin precursors to varying degrees.

Clinically, the porphyrias manifest themselves quite differently. Disorders that result in the accumulation of the precursors (ALA and PBG) present with primarily neurologic symptoms, because these substances are neurotoxins. In contrast, when porphyrins are the major accumulation product, photosensitivity is the distinguishing clinical feature. In these cases, the porphyrins absorb light, causing the formation of toxic free radicals that cause cutaneous lesions (e.g., extensive blistering or bullous lesions) or a burning sensation and inflammatory skin reaction.

Diagnosis is based on the amount and type of porphyrin precursors and porphyrins present in the blood and those excreted in the urine and feces. In Chapter 7, various tests used in the urinalysis laboratory for porphyria screening, particularly for the detection of increased excretion of PBG, are discussed. Measurement of the specific defective enzyme may be required because the levels of porphyrin precursors and porphyrins can be normal during an acute attack. Clinically, porphyrias that present with primarily neurologic symptoms can be difficult to diagnose. For example, acute intermittent porphyria can present with symptoms similar to those in patients with gastrointestinal or mental health problems. In an acute presentation, porphyria patients may complain of abdominal pain, nausea, constipation, depression, muscle weakness, hypertension, and tachycardia. In addition, they may present with neuropsychiatric problems such as hysteria, psychosis, or seizures.

Acute porphyria attacks can be initiated by the ingestion of drugs, particularly barbiturates and oral contraceptives. Other precipitating agents include ingestion of alcohol, stress, hormonal changes, starvation, and infections. Some of these same factors, most notably a history of excessive alcohol ingestion, can induce chronic porphyrias.

In all cases of porphyria, treatment consists of identifying and removing any precipitating factors. In acute porphyrias, supportive measures include the maintenance of fluid and electrolyte balance and the use of analgesics to relieve pain. Acute intermittent porphyria patients benefit from an intravenous infusion of hematin, which inhibits the activity of ALA synthetase: the rate-limiting step in heme synthesis. (See the porphobilinogen section in Chapter 7 for more discussion of this enzyme's role in the heme biosynthetic pathway.) Patients with the porphyrias characterized by photosensitivity should avoid direct sunlight and use barrier skin lotions that provide protection from the sun's ultraviolet rays.

References
. . . .

Cotran RS, Kumar V, Robbins SL: Robbins Pathologic Basis of Disease (4th ed.), Philadelphia, W. B. Saunders Company, 1989, pp. 1048–1049.

de Wardener HE: The Kidney (5th ed.), New York, Churchill Livingstone, 1985, p. 163.

Bibliography
. . . .

Cotran RS, Leaf A: Renal Pathophysiology (3rd ed.), New York, Oxford University Press, 1985.

Henry, JB (ed.), Clinical Diagnosis and Management by Laboratory Methods (18th ed.), Philadelphia, W. B. Saunders Company, 1991.

Marshall WJ: Illustrated Textbook of Clinical Chemistry, Philadelphia: J. B. Lippincott Company, 1988.

Tietz, NW (ed.), Fundamentals of Clinical Chemistry (3rd ed.), Philadelphia, W. B. Saunders Company, 1987.

Walmsley RN, White GH: A Guide to Diagnostic Clinical Chemistry (2nd ed.), Melbourne, Blackwell Scientific Publications, 1988.

Study Questions

1. **Which of the following statements about renal diseases is true?**

   A. Glomerular renal diseases are usually immune mediated.
   B. Vascular disorders induce renal disease by increasing renal perfusion.
   C. All structural components of the kidney are equally susceptible to disease.
   D. Tubulointerstitial renal diseases usually result from antibody-antigen and complement interactions.

2. **In glomerular diseases, morphologic changes in the glomeruli include all of the following EXCEPT**

   A. cellular proliferation.
   B. erythrocyte congestion.
   C. leukocyte infiltration.
   D. glomerular basement membrane thickening.

3. **When "all" renal glomeruli are affected by a morphologic change, this change is described as**

   A. diffuse.
   B. focal.
   C. differentiated.
   D. segmental.

4. **In glomerular renal disease, the glomerular damage results from**

   A. deposition of infectious agents.
   B. a decrease in glomerular perfusion.
   C. changes in glomerular hemodynamics.
   D. toxic substances produced by immune complex formation.

5. **Clinical features that are characteristic of glomerular damage include all of the following EXCEPT**

   A. edema.   C. proteinuria.
   B. hematuria.   D. polyuria.

6. **Which of the following frequently occurs following a bacterial infection of the skin or throat?**

   A. Acute glomerulonephritis
   B. Chronic glomerulonephritis
   C. Membranous glomerulonephritis
   D. Rapidly progressive glomerulonephritis

7. **Which of the following is characterized by cellular proliferation into Bowman's space to form cellular "crescents"?**

   A. Chronic glomerulonephritis
   B. Membranous glomerulonephritis
   C. Focal proliferative glomerulonephritis
   D. Rapidly progressive glomerulonephritis

8. **Which of the following is the major cause of nephrotic syndrome in adults?**

   A. Focal proliferative glomerulonephritis
   B. Membranoproliferative glomerulonephritis
   C. Membranous glomerulonephritis
   D. Rapidly progressive glomerulonephritis

9. **Which of the following glomerular diseases is the major cause of nephrotic syndrome in children?**

   A. IgA nephropathy
   B. Minimal change disease
   C. Membranous glomerulonephritis
   D. Rapidly progressive glomerulonephritis

10. **Which of the following statements regarding IgA nephropathy is true?**

    A. It often follows a mucosal infection.
    B. It is associated with nephrotic syndrome.
    C. It is characterized by leukocyte infiltration of the glomeruli.
    D. It often occurs secondary to systemic lupus erythematosus.

11. **Eighty percent of patients who develop chronic glomerulonephritis previously had some type of glomerular disease. Which of the following is most frequently implicated in the development of chronic glomerulonephritis?**

    A. IgA nephropathy
    B. Membranous glomerulonephritis
    C. Poststreptococcal glomerulonephritis
    D. Rapidly progressive glomerulonephritis

12. **Chronic renal failure often develops in each of the following diseases EX-
     CEPT**

     A. amyloidosis.
     B. diabetes mellitus.
     C. diabetes insipidus.
     D. systemic lupus erythematosus.

13. **Which of the following characterizes nephrotic syndrome?**

     1. Proteinuria
     2. Edema
     3. Hypoalbuminemia
     4. Hyperlipidemia
         A. 1, 2, and 3 are correct.
         B. 1 and 3 are correct.
         C. 4 is correct.
         D. All are correct.

14. **In a patient with nephrotic syndrome, the microscopic examination of the
     urine sediment often reveals**

     A. granular casts.
     B. leukocyte casts.
     C. red blood cell casts.
     D. waxy casts.

15. **Which of the following has NOT been associated with acute tubular necrosis?**

     A. Antibiotics
     B. Galactosuria
     C. Hemoglobinuria
     D. Surgical procedures

16. **Which formed element in urine sediment is characteristic of toxic acute tubu-
     lar necrosis and aids in its differentiation from ischemic acute tubular necro-
     sis?**

     A. Collecting tubular cells
     B. Granular casts
     C. Proximal tubular cells
     D. Waxy casts

17. **Which of the following disorders is characterized by the urinary excretion of
     large amounts of arginine, cystine, lysine, and ornithine?**

     A. Cystinosis
     B. Cystinuria
     C. Lysinuria
     D. Tyrosinuria

18. **A generalized loss of proximal tubular function is a characteristic of**

   A. Fanconi's syndrome.
   B. nephrotic syndrome.
   C. renal glucosuria.
   D. renal tubular acidosis.

19. **Which of the following is NOT associated with renal tubular acidosis?**

   A. Decreased glomerular filtration rate.
   B. Decreased renal tubular secretion of hydrogen ions.
   C. Decreased proximal tubular reabsorption of bicarbonate.
   D. Increased back-diffusion of hydrogen ions in the distal tubules.

20. **Which of the following is considered a "lower" urinary tract infection?**

   A. Cystitis
   B. Glomerulonephritis
   C. Pyelitis
   D. Pyelonephritis

21. **Most urinary tract infections are due to**

   A. yeast, e.g., *Candida* sp.
   B. gram-negative rods.
   C. gram-positive rods.
   D. gram-positive cocci.

22. **Which of the following formed elements found in urine sediment is most indicative of an "upper" urinary tract infection?**

   A. Bacteria
   B. Casts
   C. Erythrocytes
   D. Leukocytes

23. **The most common cause of chronic pyelonephritis is**

   A. cystitis.
   B. bacterial sepsis.
   C. drug-induced nephropathies.
   D. reflux nephropathies.

24. **Eosinophiluria, fever, and skin rash are characteristic clinical features of**

   A. acute pyelonephritis.
   B. acute interstitial nephritis.
   C. acute glomerulonephritis.
   D. chronic glomerulonephritis.

25. **Cessation of the administration of a drug is the fastest and most effective treatment for**

    A. acute pyelonephritis.
    B. acute interstitial nephritis.
    C. acute glomerulonephritis.
    D. chronic glomerulonephritis.

26. **Yeast is considered part of the normal flora in each of the following locations EXCEPT in the**

    A. gastrointestinal tract.
    B. oral cavity.
    C. urinary tract.
    D. vagina.

27. **Acute renal failure can be caused by all of the following EXCEPT**

    A. hemorrhage.
    B. acute tubular necrosis.
    C. acute pyelonephritis.
    D. urinary tract obstruction.

28. **Which of the following is a feature of chronic renal failure?**

    A. It can be reversed by appropriate treatment regimens.
    B. It eventually progresses to end-stage renal disease.
    C. It is monitored by periodic determinations of renal blood flow.
    D. Its onset involves a sudden decrease in the glomerular filtration rate.

29. **Isosthenuria, significant proteinuria, and numerous casts of all types describes the urinalysis findings from a patient with**

    A. acute renal failure.
    B. acute tubular necrosis.
    C. chronic renal failure.
    D. renal tubular acidosis.

30. **Approximately 75% of the renal calculi that form in patients contain**

    A. calcium.
    B. cystine.
    C. oxalate.
    D. uric acid.

31. **The formation of renal calculi is enhanced by**

    A. an increase in urine flow.
    B. the body's natural "acid-alkaline" tide.
    C. increases in protein in the urine ultrafiltrate.
    D. increases in chemical salts in the urine ultrafiltrate.

32. An "overflow" mechanism is responsible for the aminoaciduria present in

   A. cystinosis.
   B. cystinuria.
   C. tyrosinuria.
   D. phenylketonuria.

33. Which of the following hereditary diseases results in the accumulation and excretion of large amounts of homogentisic acid?

   A. Alkaptonuria
   B. Melanuria
   C. Phenylketonuria
   D. Tyrosinuria

34. Which of the following substances oxidizes with exposure to air, causing the urine to turn brown or black?

   A. Melanin
   B. Porphyrin
   C. Tyrosine
   D. Urobilinogen

35. Which of the following diseases is related to tyrosine production or metabolism?

   1. Tyrosinuria
   2. Melanuria
   3. Phenylketonuria
   4. Alkaptonuria
      A. 1, 2, and 3 are correct.
      B. 1 and 3 are correct.
      C. 4 is correct.
      D. All are correct.

36. Which of the following diseases can result in severe mental retardation if not detected and treated in the infant?

   1. Phenylketonuria
   2. Maple syrup urine disease
   3. Galactosuria
   4. Alkaptonuria
      A. 1, 2, and 3 are correct.
      B. 1 and 3 are correct.
      C. 4 is correct.
      D. All are correct.

37. **Which of the following is a characteristic feature of type II diabetes mellitus?**

    A. Daily insulin injections are necessary.
    B. Onset of the disease is usually sudden.
    C. The patient has a strong tendency to develop ketoacidosis.
    D. The disease usually presents after 40 years of age.

38. **Which of the following is NOT a clinical feature of an infant with galacto-suria?**

    A. Cataract formation
    B. Liver dysfunction
    C. Mental retardation
    D. Polyuria

39. **Galactose is produced in the normal metabolism of**

    A. fructose.
    B. glucose.
    C. lactose.
    D. sucrose.

40. **Which of the following is NOT a characteristic of diabetes insipidus?**

    A. Polyuria
    B. Polydipsia
    C. Increased production of ADH
    D. Urine with a low specific gravity

41. **Porphyria is characterized by**

    A. increased heme degradation.
    B. increased heme formation.
    C. decreased globin synthesis.
    D. decreased iron catabolism.

42. **Which of the following statements regarding porphyrin and porphyrin precursors is true?**

    1. Porphyria can be inherited or induced.
    2. Porphyrin precursors are neurotoxins.
    3. Porphyrins can be dark red or purple.
    4. Porphyrin precursor accumulation causes skin photosensitivity.
        A. 1, 2, and 3 are correct.
        B. 1 and 3 are correct.
        C. 4 is correct.
        D. All are correct.

Fecal Analysis

LEARNING OBJECTIVES

After studying this chapter, the student should be able to

1. Describe the composition and formation of normal fecal material.

2. Describe the effect of abnormal intestinal water reabsorption on the consistency of the feces formed.

3. Classify the condition of diarrhea according to the physiologic mechanisms involved.

4. Differentiate between secretory and osmotic diarrhea using the fecal osmolality.

5. Identify at least three causes of secretory and osmotic diarrhea.

6. Compare and contrast the mechanisms of maldigestion and malabsorption and the relationship of each to diarrhea.

7. Differentiate steatorrhea from diarrhea and discuss the physiologic conditions that result in steatorrhea.

8. Describe the following types of fecal collections and give an example of a test requiring each type:
   - a random stool collection, with and without dietary restrictions
   - a 3-day fecal collection, with and without dietary restrictions

9. Describe the normal macroscopic characteristics of normal feces.

10. List the major causes of abnormal fecal color, consistency, and odor.

11. State the primary purpose of the microscopic examination for fecal leukocytes.

12. Discuss the microscopic examination for fecal fat.

13. Compare the qualitative and quantitative fecal fat results obtained from tests on a patient with normal feces and with those on a patient with steatorrhea.

14. List at least five causes of blood in the feces and state the importance of fecal occult blood detection.

15. Discuss the advantages and disadvantages of the different indicators used on commercial slide tests for fecal occult blood.

16. Compare and contrast the following methods for the detection of fecal blood:
    - slide tests
    - quantitative chemical tests
    - immunologic assays
    - radiometric assays

17. Describe the chemical principle employed when feces or vomitus is screened for fetal hemoglobin.

18. Discuss the effect disaccharidase deficiency has on fecal characteristics and formation.

19. State two methods for the qualitative detection of abnormal amounts of fecal carbohydrates.

20. State the purpose of and describe the principle behind the xylose absorption test.

KEY TERMS

acholic stools: pale, gray, or clay-colored stools. They result when production of the normal fecal pigments —stercobilin, mesobilin, and urobilin— is partially or completely inhibited.

constipation: infrequent and difficult bowel movements, compared to an individual's normal bowel movement pattern. The fecal material produced is made up of hard, small, frequently spherical masses.

diarrhea: an increase in the volume, liquidity, and frequency of bowel movements compared to an individual's normal bowel movement pattern.

disaccharidase deficiency: a lack of sufficient enzymes (disaccharidases) for the metabolism of disaccharides in the small intestine. This deficiency can be hereditary or acquired (e.g., resulting from diseases, drug therapy).

malabsorption: the inadequate intestinal absorption of processed foodstuffs despite normal digestive ability.

maldigestion: the inability to convert foodstuffs in the gastrointestinal tract into readily absorbable substances.

melena: the excretion of dark or black, pitchy-looking stools owing to the presence of large amounts (50 to 100

mL/d) of blood in the feces. The coloration is due to hemoglobin oxidation by intestinal and bacterial enzymes in the gastrointestinal tract.

occult blood: small amounts of blood, not visually apparent, in the feces.

steatorrhea: the excretion of greater than 6 g/d of fat in the feces.

urobilins: orange-brown pigments that impart to feces its characteristic color. Specifically, they are stercobilin, mesobilin, and urobilin, which result from spontaneous intestinal oxidation of the colorless tetrapyrroles stereobilinogen, mesobilinogen, and urobilinogen.

The examination of feces provides important information that aids in the differential diagnosis of various gastrointestinal (GI) tract disorders. GI disorders range from maldigestion and malabsorption to bleeding or infestation by bacteria, viruses, or parasites. Hepatic and biliary conditions that result in decreased bile secretion, as well as pancreatic diseases that cause insufficient digestive enzymes, can also be identified by fecal analysis. By far the most common test currently performed on feces is the chemical test for "occult," or hidden, blood. Occult blood is recognized as the earliest and most frequent initial symptom of colorectal cancer. It is recommended that fecal blood testing be performed routinely on all individuals that are 40 years old and older. Bleeding anywhere in the GI tract, from the mouth to the anus, can result in a positive fecal blood test; additional follow-up testing is required, however,

to identify the specific cause of the bleeding. Fecal analysis is also valuable in determining the presence of increased fecal lipids (steatorrhea) and in the differential diagnosis of diarrhea. This chapter discusses the macroscopic, microscopic, and chemical examinations of feces routinely performed in the laboratory.

Fecal Formation

Normally, about 100 to 200 g of fecal material is passed each day. The feces consist of undigested foodstuffs (e.g., cellulose), sloughed intestinal epithelium, intestinal bacteria, GI secretions (e.g., digestive enzymes), bile pigments, electrolytes, and water. Because of the slow movement of the fecal material in the large intestine, it normally takes 18 to 24 hours for the contents presented to it by the small intestine to be excreted as feces.

The small intestine's function is the digestion and absorption of foodstuffs, whereas the large intestine's principal function is the absorption of water, sodium, and chloride. Approximately 9000 mL of fluid enters the GI tract from food, water, saliva, gastric secretions, bile, pancreatic secretions, and small intestinal secretions. Only 500 to 1500 mL actually enters the large intestine each day, however, with a final excretion of only about 150 mL of fluid in normal feces. Because the large intestine has a limited ability to absorb liquid (up to about 2700 mL), a volume of fluid presented to it that exceeds this capacity will cause watery stools (diarrhea). Similarly, if water absorption is inhibited or if inadequate time is allowed for the absorption process, diarrhea will result. In contrast, stationary bowel contents (or decreased intestinal motility) permits increased water absorption and results in **constipation.** Fecal specimens from constipated individuals are typically small, hard, frequently spherical masses (scybala) that are often difficult and painful to excrete.

Fermentation by intestinal bacteria in the large intestine results in the production of intestinal gas or flatus. It is normally produced at a rate of about 400 to 700 mL/day. Certain types of carbohydrates that are not completely digested by intestinal enzymes (e.g., brown beans) are readily metabolized by intestinal bacteria to produce large amounts of gas. Increased gas production and its incorporation into the feces can result in foamy and floating stools. Although these stools can be normal, they are often present in patients with the conditions of lactose intolerance and steatorrhea.

Diarrhea

Diarrhea is defined as an increase in the volume, liquidity, and frequency of bowel movements compared to an individual's normal bowel movement pattern. It can be classified into three types: secretory diarrhea, osmotic diarrhea, or diarrhea owing to intestinal hypermotility (Table 10–1). With both secretory and osmotic diarrhea, the presence of an unabsorbed solute draws and retains water in the intestinal lumen. The origin of this osmotically active solute differs. Secretory diarrhea results from increased intestinal secretion of a solute; osmotic diarrhea results from ingestion of an osmotically active solute (e.g., lactose).

Fecal osmolality determinations to differentiate these two conditions require the determination of the fecal osmolality, fecal sodium, and fecal potassium levels. The observed fecal osmolality is compared to the "calculated" fecal osmolality using the fecal sodium and potassium results and Equation 10–1.

(10–1)
$$\text{Calculated fecal osmolality} = 2 \times (Na^+_{fecal} + K^+_{fecal})$$

If the difference between the measured and calculated fecal osmolality exceeds 20 mOsm/kg, the patient is experiencing osmotic diarrhea. If the measured and calculated fecal osmolalities agree within 10 to 20 mOsm/kg, the patient is experiencing secretory diarrhea.

Secretory diarrhea is characteristic of infestation with numerous enterotoxin-producing organisms. These microbes release substances that stimulate intestinal secretions, which are rich in electrolytes. Similarly, intestinal mucosal damage, either drug-induced or disease-related, can also result in secretory diarrhea.

Conditions characterized by maldigestion or malabsorption present with osmotic diarrhea. **Maldigestion,** the inability to convert foodstuffs into readily absorbable substances, most often results from various pancreatic and hepatic diseases. With these disorders, the pancreatic digestive enzymes or bile salts needed for fat emulsification and lipase activation are deficient or lacking. The absence of other digestive enzymes, such as dissacharidases (e.g., lactase) in the small intestine, can also result in maldigestion. In contrast, intestinal **malabsorption** is characterized by normal digestive ability, but inadequate intestinal absorption of the already

T A B L E 10–1. CLASSIFICATION OF DIARRHEA

TYPE	MECHANISM	COMMON CAUSES
Secretory diarrhea	Increased solute secretions by the intestine cause increased fluid to be presented to the large intestine; the large intestine's absorptive capacity is exceeded	Enterotoxin-producing organisms (e.g., *Vibrio cholera, Salmonella, Shigella, Escherichia coli, Clostridium, Staphylococcus, Protozoa*) Mucosal involvement (e.g., viral gastroenteritis, ulcerative colitis, drugs) Neoplasms Drugs or hormones (e.g., caffeine, prostaglandin, vasoactive intestinal peptide)
Osmotic diarrhea	Increased amounts of osmotically active solutes remain in the lumen, causing the secretion of water and electrolytes into the intestine; the large intestine's absorptive capacity is exceeded	Maldigestion (e.g., lactase deficiency, lipase deficiency) Malabsorption of nonelectrolytes (e.g., mucosal diseases) Laxative action of some drugs (e.g., antacids, sorbitol, tetracycline, lincomycin) Parasitic infestations (e.g., giardiasis, strongyloidiasis) Surgical procedures (e.g., small bowel resection)
Intestinal hypermotility	An increase in intestinal motility decreases the time allowed for the intestinal absorptive processes	Secretory and osmotic diarrhea Parasympathetic nerve activity Laxatives (e.g., castor oil) Emotions (e.g., stress) Cardiovascular drugs (e.g., digitalis, quinidine)

processed foodstuffs. Some parasitic infestations, mucosal diseases (e.g., celiac sprue, tropical sprue, ulcerative colitis), hereditary diseases (e.g., disaccharidase deficiencies), surgical procedures, or drugs can cause malabsorption and osmotic diarrhea. In summary, both maldigestion and malabsorption present an abnormally increased amount of foodstuffs to the large intestine. These osmotically active substances (i.e., the foodstuffs) cause the retention of large amounts of water and electrolytes in the intestinal lumen and the excretion of a watery stool or diarrhea.

Intestinal hypermotility results in diarrhea when the transit time for the intestinal contents is too short to allow normal intestinal absorption to take place. Normally, intestinal motility is stimulated by intestinal distention. Foodstuffs that are bulky, such as dietary fiber, produce a natural laxative effect because of the intestinal distention they cause. Intestinal motility can also be altered by chemicals, nerves, hormones, and emotions. Laxatives (e.g., castor oil) and para-

sympathetic nerve activity increase intestinal motility, whereas sympathetic nerve activity decreases intestinal motility. During secretory and osmotic diarrhea, the increased lumen fluid causes intestinal distention, thereby increasing intestinal motility and compounding the diarrheal condition.

When severe, diarrhea decreases the blood volume (hypovolemia) and disrupts the body's acid-base balance. The large fluid loss and the accompanying electrolyte depletion (particularly sodium, bicarbonate, and potassium) can result in metabolic acidosis.

Steatorrhea
. . . .
Normally, the fecal excretion of fat is less than 6 g each day (usually measured as fatty acids). This fat originates from several sources: the diet, GI secretions, bacterial byproducts of metabolism, and sloughed intestinal epithelium. The amount of dietary fat ingested has a minor effect on the total amount of fecal lipids excreted; in addition,

T A B L E 10–2.   A COMPARISON OF DIARRHEA AND STEATORRHEA

CONDITION	FECAL CHARACTERISTICS	FECAL VOLUME	FECAL FREQUENCY	CAUSE	CLINICAL FEATURES
Diarrhea	Watery; odor normal or unremarkable	Increased	Increased	Disruption in water and electrolyte absorption	Water and electrolyte imbalance; acidosis; hypovolemia
Steatorrhea	Greasy; foul odor; spongy consistency	Increased	Normal or increased	Maldigestion or malabsorption of dietary fat	Malnutrition; weight loss

the types of lipid (fatty acid salts, neutral fat) excreted can vary significantly from the dietary fat ingested (Kao, 1991).

Fecal fat excretion exceeding 6 g per day, termed **steatorrhea,** is a common feature of patients with malabsorption syndromes. Steatorrheal fecal specimens are characteristically pale, greasy, bulky, spongy or pasty in consistency, and extremely foul smelling. They vary in fluidity and may float or be foamy owing to the presence of large amounts of gas within them. This latter feature is not particularly significant because normal stools may also contain gas.

It is very important clinically that steatorrhea be differentiated from diarrhea (Table 10–2). Although macroscopic examination of the feces can be highly suggestive of steatorrhea, some diarrheal conditions can make differentiation difficult. Therefore, to diagnose steatorrhea, a fecal fat determination must be performed (see the section on the chemical examination of feces). Any condition that alters fat digestion or fat absorption will present with steatorrhea (Table 10–3).

Conditions producing steatorrhea can occur simultaneously with diarrhea. In order for appropriate patient management to begin, the cause of the diarrhea, steatorrhea, or both must be identified. Usually, this is achieved by following an algorithm similar to that in Figure 10–1. Because a definitive diagnosis may not be readily apparent, a good patient history is invaluable. It can provide information that directly relates to the cause of the patient's condition (e.g., diet, environment, recent exposure or contacts). For example, following the algorithm in Figure 10–1 to a negative stool culture rules out

specific bacteria but does not exclude parasites, viruses, or other inflammatory conditions. A good patient history might reveal that the patient was in a foreign country and exposed to contaminated water sources, or that the patient recently ingested fresh oysters while in New Orleans.

Specimen Collection

Patient Education

Unlike with urination, individuals have limited control in the timing of fecal excretion. In addition, collecting fecal specimens is

T A B L E 10–3.   CAUSES OF STEATORRHEA

TYPE	CAUSE
Maldigestion	Decreased pancreatic enzymes
	Pancreatitis
	Cystic fibrosis
	Pancreatic cancer
	Zollinger-Ellison syndrome
	Ileal resection
	Decreased bile acid micelle formation
	Hepatocellular disease (severe)
	Bile duct obstruction; biliary cirrhosis
	Bile acid deconjugation owing to stasis (e.g., strictures, blind-loop syndrome, diabetic visceral neuropathy)
Malabsorption	Damaged intestinal mucosa
	Celiac disease
	Tropical sprue
	Biochemical defect
	a-β-lipoproteinemia
	Lymphatic obstruction
	Lymphoma
	Whipple's disease

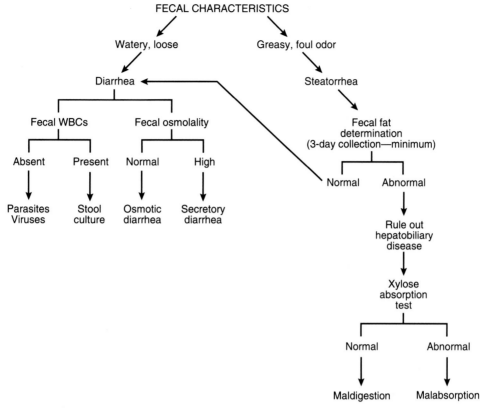

FIGURE 10–1. An algorithm to aid in the evaluation of diarrhea and steatorrhea.

probably highly undesirable for the patient. In light of these considerations, it is of utmost importance that the patient be educated regarding the importance of a properly collected fecal specimen. Both verbal and written instructions should be provided to the patient along with an appropriate specimen container.

Specimen Containers

Fecal specimen containers vary depending on the amount of specimen to be collected. Essentially any clean, nonbreakable container that is sealable and leakproof is acceptable. For specimen collections over multiple days, large containers such as paint cans are frequently used. Single, random collections can be placed in routine urine cups or other suitable containers. Often the entire stool is not required for analysis, which again necessitates properly instructing the patient about what portion of the stool to test or to trans-

port to the laboratory. Some commercial fecal collection kits are available for the recovery of feces after they are passed into the toilet onto a sheet of floating tissue paper. These kits have greatly facilitated fecal collection by patients. After a portion of the feces is sampled, the patient can flush the remainder.

Type and Amount Collected

The type and amount of specimen collected will vary with the test to be performed. Fecal analysis for occult blood, white blood cells, or qualitative fecal fat requires only a small amount of a randomly collected specimen. In contrast, quantitative tests for the daily fecal excretion of any substance requires a minimum of a 3-day fecal collection. This 3-day collection is necessary because the daily excretion of feces does not correlate well with the amount of food ingested by the patient in the same 24-hour period. In addition, to ensure an optimum specimen, some fecal collections require dietary restrictions prior to the collection (e.g., tests for occult blood, quantitative fecal fat).

Contaminants to Avoid

Contamination of the fecal specimen with urine, toilet tissue, or toilet water must be avoided. The detection of protozoa can be adversely affected by contaminating urine, and the strong cleaning agents used in toilets can interfere with chemical testing. Patients must also be instructed to avoid contaminating the exterior of collection containers or applying too much sample to occult blood slides.

Gas Formation

Fecal specimens produce gas owing to bacterial fermentation, both in vivo and in vitro. Therefore, closed containers of fecal specimens should be covered with a disposable tissue or toweling and opened slowly. This covering will retard spattering of fecal matter should gas build-up cause the sudden release of the fecal contents when the container is opened.

Macroscopic Examination

Color

The macroscopic examination of feces involves the visual assessment of color, consistency, and form. Other notable substances within the feces include mucus and undigested matter. The normal brown color of feces results from bile pigments. When conjugated bilirubin is secreted as bile into the small intestine, it is hydrolyzed back to its unconjugated form. Intestinal anaerobic bacteria subsequently reduce it to the three colorless tetrapyrroles collectively called the urobilinogens—stercobilinogen, mesobilinogen, and urobilinogen. These urobilinogens spontaneously oxidize in the intestine to produce the **urobilins**—stercobilin, mesobilin, and urobilin—which are orange-brown and impart color to the feces. With conditions in

which bile secretion into the small intestine is partially or completely inhibited, the color of the feces changes. Pale or clay-colored stools, also termed **acholic stools,** are characteristic of these posthepatic obstructions. Be aware that similarly colored fecal specimens resulting from barium sulfate contamination can be obtained following a diagnostic procedure to evaluate GI function (i.e., a barium enema). Unusual fecal colors are also encountered owing to the ingestion of certain foodstuffs or medications or to the presence of blood. Table 10–4 summarizes various macroscopic characteristics observed in feces.

Consistency and Form

The consistency of feces ranges from loose and watery stools (diarrhea) to small, hard masses **(constipation).** Normal feces are usually formed masses; soft stools indicate an increase in fecal water content. The latter can be normal, can be related to the intake of laxatives, or can accompany GI disorders; a good patient history helps the healthcare provider to determine if the patient has noticed a change in the consistency of his or her stools. Feces may be bulky because of undigested matter or increased gas throughout the stool. Undigested substances such as seed casings, vegetable skins, or proglottids from intestinal parasites may also be observed. Normal stools are formed cylindrical masses; in contrast, the excretion of long, ribbon-like stools can indicate intestinal obstruction or lumen narrowing as a result of strictures.

Mucus

Mucus, a translucent gelatinous substance, is not present in normal feces. When present, it can vary dramatically from a small amount to massive quantities found in patients with villous adenoma. Mucus has been associated with benign conditions, such as straining during bowel movements or constipation, and with several GI diseases such as colitis, intestinal tuberculosis, ulcerative diverticulitis,

TABLE 10–4. FECAL MACROSCOPIC CHARACTERISTICS

	CHARACTERISTIC	CAUSE
Color	Clay-colored or gray, pale yellow, or white	Posthepatic obstruction
		Barium (ingestion or enema)
	Red	Blood (from lower GI tract)
		Beets
		Food dyes
		Drugs (e.g., BSP* dye, rifampin)
	Brown	Normal
	Black	Blood (from upper GI tract)
		Charcoal
		Iron therapy
		Bismuth (e.g., medications, suppositories)
	Green	Green vegetables (e.g., spinach)
		Biliverdin (during antibiotic therapy)
Consistency	Formed	Normal
	Hard	Constipation (i.e., scybalum)
	Soft	Increased fecal water content
	Watery	Diarrhea, steatorrhea
Form	Cylindrical	Normal
	Narrow, ribbon-like	Bowel obstruction
		Intestinal narrowing (e.g., strictures)
	Small, round	Constipation
	Bulky	Steatorrhea
Other	Foamy, floating	Increased gas incorporated into the stool
	Greasy, spongy	Steatorrhea
	Mucus	Constipation, straining
		Disease (e.g., colitis, villous adenoma)

* BSP = bromsulphalein.

bacillary dysentery, villous adenoma, neoplasms, and rectal inflammation.

Odor

The normal odor of feces is a result of the metabolic by-products of the intestinal bacterial flora. If the normal flora is disrupted or the foodstuffs presented to it change dramatically, however, a change in the fecal odor may be noticed. For example, steatorrhea results in distinctively foul-smelling feces owing to the bacterial breakdown of the undigested lipids.

Microscopic Examination

The microscopic examination of the feces is performed on an aliquot of a stool suspension and can aid in differentiating the cause of diarrhea or in screening for steatorrhea. Microscopically, white blood cells (WBCs) and undigested foodstuffs such as fats, meat fibers, and vegetable fibers can be identified. Although this examination is only qualitative, it is easy to perform and can provide diagnostically useful information.

Fecal Leukocytes

The presence of fecal leukocytes (WBCs) or pus (an exudate containing WBCs) aids in the differential diagnosis of diarrhea. Generally, when the intestinal wall is infected or inflamed, fecal leukocytes are present in an inflammatory exudate. In contrast, if the mucosal wall is not compromised, fecal leukocytes are usually not present. Table 10–5 lists disorders in which a microscopic examination for fecal leukocytes aids in the differential diagnosis of diarrhea. Normally, leukocytes are not present in feces; hence, the presence of even a small number (1 to 3 per

TABLE 10–5. DISEASE DIFFERENTIATION BASED ON THE PRESENCE OF FECAL LEUKOCYTES (WBCs)

WBCs PRESENT	WBCs ABSENT
Ulcerative colitis	Amebic colitis
Bacillary dysentery	Viral gastroenteritis
Ulcerative diverticulitis	
Intestinal tuberculosis	
Abscesses or fistulas	

high-power field) is indicative of an invasive and inflammatory condition. To enhance the identification of leukocytes in feces, wet preparations can be stained using either Wright's or methylene blue stains.

Fecal Fat

The presence of increased amounts of fat can be indicated macroscopically and confirmed both microscopically and chemically. Steatorrhea (fecal fat excretion that exceeds 6 g/d) is a common feature of maldigestion or malabsorption. Whereas good correlation has been observed between the qualitative assessment and the quantitative chemical determination of fecal fat, the latter should be performed to confirm steatorrhea.

Using Sudan III, Sudan IV, or Oil Red O stains, neutral fat (triglycerides) can be readily identified in a fecal suspension by its characteristic orange-to-red staining. The laboratorian can perform a simple two-slide qualitative procedure to identify fecal fats. To detect neutral fats, a suspension of the feces is placed on a microscope slide with several drops of ethanol (95 percent). The stain is added to the slide, and the wet preparation is coverslipped and observed for the characteristically staining fat globules (Fig. 10–2). Normal feces contains less than 60 globules of neutral fat per high-power field.

On a second slide, another aliquot of the fecal suspension is acidified with acetic acid and heated. This slide provides an estimation of total fecal fat content—neutral fats plus fatty acids and fatty acid salts (soaps). Acidification hydrolyzes soaps to their respective fatty acids, and heating causes the fatty acids to absorb the stain. Because fatty acids and their salts (soaps) are present in normal feces, an increased number of orange-red–staining fat globules are observed on the second slide when compared to the first. Both the number of fat globules and their size (diameter) are important. Normally, less than 100 globules per high-power field should be observed, and they should not exceed 4 μm in diameter (about half the size of a red blood

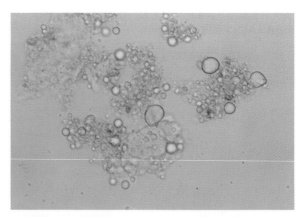

FIGURE 10–2. Numerous globules of neutral fat stained with Sudan III. Note characteristic orange-red coloration. Present in fecal suspension during qualitative fecal fat microscopic examination. Brightfield microscopy, 200×.

cell) (Drummey, 1961). Increased numbers of globules, as well as extremely large globules (i.e., 40 to 80 μm), are common with steatorrhea (Fig. 10–3). Maldigestion can often be differentiated from malabsorption by evaluating the results obtained from the two slides. A normal amount of fecal neutral fat (on the first slide) compared with an increased amount of total fat (on the second slide) is indicative of intestinal malabsorption. In other words, the increased fat present is made up of fatty acids and soaps that were not absorbed by the small intes-

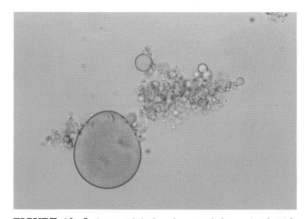

FIGURE 10–3. Large globule of neutral fat stained with Sudan III. Note characteristic orange-red coloration. Brightfield microscopy, 200×.

tine. In contrast, if the amount of neutral fat is increased (the first slide), maldigestion is indicated.

Prior to a fecal fat determination, it is important that the patient maintain a normal dietary intake of fat. In addition, the contamination of the fecal specimen with mineral oils or creams that can produce false positive results must be avoided.

Meat Fibers

Undigested foodstuffs, such as meat and vegetable fibers, can be identified in feces microscopically. Meat fibers are rectangular and have characteristic cross striations (Fig. 10–4). Often their identification and the qualitative assessment of their numbers is included with a qualitative fecal fat examination; while screening the first fecal fat slide for neutral fat globules, the laboratorian also estimates the presence of meat fibers. An alternative approach is to apply a few drops of a fecal suspension to a slide and stain it with a solution of eosin in 10 percent alcohol. Increased numbers of fecal meat fibers (creatorrhea) correlates with impaired digestion and rapid intestinal transit.

Chemical Examination
. . . .

Fecal Blood

Bleeding anywhere in the GI tract from the mouth (bleeding gums) to the anus (hemorrhoids) can result in detectable blood in the feces. Because fecal blood is a frequent and early symptom of colorectal cancer, annual screening is recommended by the American Cancer Society on all individuals over 40 years old. Of all GI tract cancers, more than 50 percent are colorectal, with early detection and treatment directly related to a good prognosis. In addition to cancer, bleeding gums, esophageal varices, ulcers, hemorrhoids, inflammatory conditions, and various drugs that irritate the intestinal mucosa (e.g.,

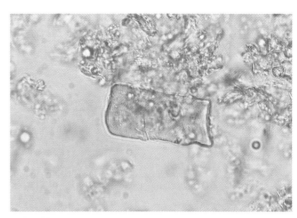

FIGURE 10–4. Meat fiber (note striations on fiber) present in fecal suspension during qualitative fecal fat microscopic examination. Brightfield microscopy, 400×.

aspirin, iron supplements) can result in a positive fecal blood test.

When present in large amounts, fecal blood may be readily identified macroscopically. With bleeding in the lower GI tract, bright-red blood can coat the surface of the stools; in contrast, bleeding in the upper GI tract may cause the stool to appear dark or mahogany. The excretion of dark or black, pitchy stools resulting from the presence of large amounts of fecal blood (50 to 100 mL/d) is termed **melena.** This dark fecal coloration is due to the degradation of hemoglobin (heme oxidation) by intestinal and bacterial enzymes.

Small amounts of fecal blood are often not visually apparent and are termed **occult blood.** Normally, less than 2.5 mL of blood is lost each day in the feces (or approximately 2 mg of hemoglobin per gram of stool). Any increase in fecal blood is significant and requires further investigation to discover its source. Therefore, chemical tests using commercially prepared slides are routinely employed to detect fecal blood. Because GI bleeding is often intermittent and blood is frequently hidden within the stool, patients must be instructed to sample several portions of the same stool in order to maximize its detection. To facilitate this, occult blood slides usually have two windows for the placement of feces from two different areas of the same specimen. These slide tests take advantage of the pseudoperoxidase activity of hemoglobin (Equation 10–2).

(10–2)

$$H_2O_2 + \underset{\text{(colorless)}}{\text{Indicator*}} \xrightarrow[\text{or peroxidase}]{\text{pseudo-peroxidase\dagger}} \underset{\text{(colored)}}{\text{Oxidized indicator}} + H_2O$$

*Indicators used: benzidine, orthotoluidine, and guaiac
† Possible pseudoperoxidases and peroxidases: hemoglobin, myoglobin, bacterial peroxidases, fruit and vegetable peroxidases

Any substance with peroxidase or pseudoperoxidase activity can participate in this reaction to give positive results. Hence, the sensitivity of these slide tests has been adjusted to account for both the normal amount of fecal blood that can be present and the peroxidase activity of various foodstuffs.

The indicators used in qualitative chemical fecal blood tests differ in their sensitivity and include benzidine, orthotoluidine, and guaiac. Although benzidine is the most sensitive, it is also carcinogenic and is no longer routinely employed. Orthotoluidine is second in sensitivity, with guaiac the least sensitive of the three. Because myoglobin and hemoglobin in meats and fish and peroxidases from intestinal bacteria or from ingested fruits and vegetables can produce false positive results, guaiac has become the indicator of choice. Its use reduces the number of false positive results obtained owing to these dietary factors (Table 10–6). An alternative approach is to reduce the sensitivity of the other indicators by decreasing their concentration or purity.

Numerous commercial occult blood slide tests use guaiac as the indicator: Hemoccult II (SmithKline Diagnostics), Quik-Cult and Tri-Slide (Laboratory Diagnostics), Colo-Screen (Helena Laboratories) and Seracult (Propper Manufacturing Co.). These slide tests consist of guaiac-impregnated paper enclosed in a rigid cardboard holder. The patient opens the holder or slide, applies a fecal sample to the exposed paper using an applicator stick, closes the holder or slide, and returns the slide to the laboratory for pro-

TABLE 10–6. INGESTED SUBSTANCES ASSOCIATED WITH ERRONEOUS FECAL OCCULT BLOOD DETERMINATIONS

FALSE POSITIVE RESULTS	FALSE NEGATIVE RESULTS
Red or rare cooked meats and fish	Ascorbic acid
Vegetables,* e.g., turnips, broccoli, cauliflower, horseradish	
Fruits,* e.g., cantaloupe, bananas, pears, plums	
Drugs, e.g., aspirin and other GI irritants	

* Adequate cooking can destroy the peroxidase activity of vegetables and fruits.

cessing. In the laboratory, the back of the slide is opened to reveal the guaiac-impregnated paper behind the fecal specimen, and developer (hydrogen peroxide) is applied. If hemoglobin or any other pseudoperoxidase or peroxidase is present in adequate amounts, the indicator is oxidized, resulting in a color change. The intensity of the color is proportional to the amount of enzymatic activity present.

Numerous factors can interfere with fecal occult blood testing. Improper specimen collection includes the application of too much feces or not enough, or the use of a fecal specimen that has been contaminated with chemicals from the toilet. Specimen contamination with menstrual blood or hemorrhoidal blood is another source of interference. Medications can interfere, causing either false positive or false negative results. Drugs that irritate the intestinal mucosa, such as salicylates and iron supplements, cause increased GI tract bleeding and false positive results, whereas antacids and ascorbic acid (vitamin C) interfere with the chemical reaction to produce false negative results. Defective guaiac or peroxide developer and the storage of fecal specimens or prepared slides beyond 6 days have also produced false negative results.

Once hemoglobin has been degraded, its pseudoperoxidase activity is lost and it is no longer detectable by these chemical slide tests. This heme degradation can take place within the intestinal tract or during storage of the fecal specimen, whether by itself or already applied to the test slide. Studies have shown that false positive results are obtained if the fecal specimen on the slide is hydrated with water prior to testing (Ahlquist, 1984). As a result, the American Cancer Society recommends that slides are tested within 6 days of collection and are *not* rehydrated prior to testing.

Another chemical method for the detection of fecal blood is the HemoQuant test (SmithKline Diagnostics). This quantitative test is based on the chemical conversion of nonfluorescing heme to intensely fluorescent porphyrins. It enables the detection and quantitation of total fecal hemoglobin, including both the portion converted to porphyrin in the intestine and the portion remaining as hemoglobin. The routinely used occult blood slide tests are unable to detect the intestinally converted portion; this portion is often the major fraction of fecal hemoglobin present or can increase with specimen storage. HemoQuant measures only heme and heme-derived porphyrins and is not affected by those substances that interfere with the qualitative occult blood slide tests, e.g., diet, ascorbic acid, and specimen storage or dehydration. Besides providing reproducible quantitative results, HemoQuant has an additional advantage in that it can be automated.

Immunologic methods (e.g., immunodiffusion, enzyme-linked immunoassay) for fecal blood detection using antibodies to human hemoglobin are available. These techniques eliminate many of the interferences associated with the blood detection slide tests; however, because these techniques are very sensitive, many false positive results are obtained with normal amounts of fecal blood. Therefore, these techniques are not yet suitable for routine screening for fecal occult blood.

Radiometric assays using radioactive chromium (^{51}Cr) are available to detect and localize a GI bleed. With this method, an aliquot of the patient's red blood cells is bound with radioactive chromium (^{51}Cr) and injected back into the patient. Subsequently, comparisons are made between the amount of radioactivity recovered in the feces (resulting from intestinal bleeding) and the radioactivity remaining in the blood. To localize the bleed, GI fluid is removed from various portions of the intestinal lumen and assessed for blood staining and radioactivity. Any advantages this procedure may have are outweighed by its disadvantages: it is expensive, time-consuming, and invasive.

Fetal Hemoglobin in Feces (Apt Test)

Newborn infants may excrete stools or vomitus containing blood. This blood can originate from maternal blood ingested during delivery or can derive from the GI tract of the neonate. Differentiation between these two sources is crucial. By using the alkaline resistance of fetal hemoglobin, a qualitative assessment of the blood in neonatal feces or vomitus can be made. A fresh, bloody fecal specimen from the neonate or a soiled, bloody diaper can be used. Black, tarry stools are not acceptable because they indicate that hemoglobin degradation to hematin has taken place. With the Apt test, a suspension of the feces (or vomitus) with water is made and centrifuged. Five milliliters of the resultant pink supernatant is aliquoted into two tubes. To one tube, the laboratorian adds 1 mL of sodium hydroxide (0.25 mol/L). If the original pink color changes to yellow or brown within 2 minutes, the hemoglobin present in the fecal material is maternal hemoglobin (Hb A). If the pink color remains, it indicates that fetal hemoglobin (Hb F) is present. The second tube is used as a color reference to evaluate changes in the treated tube. Control specimens must be run each time a specimen is tested. Positive controls can be made using infant peripheral or cord blood, and negative controls can be made using any adult blood sample. This test is frequently called the Apt test after its developer, L. Apt (Apt, 1955).

Quantitative Fecal Fat

The quantitative determination of fecal fat is the definitive test for steatorrhea. Although this chemical test confirms that abnormal amounts of dietary lipids are being excreted, it does not identify the cause of the excretion. For 2 days prior to the specimen collection, as well as throughout the test period, patients are provided with special dietary instructions to ensure adequate fat and caloric intake. In addition, they are requested not to skip any meals or take any medications. During the test, the patient collects all feces excreted for 3 (minimum) to 6 days in large, preweighed collection containers (e.g., paint cans). The fecal collection is brought to the laboratory, where it is weighed and homogenized using a mechanical shaker (e.g., a paint can shaker). An aliquot of the fecal specimen is removed for chemical analysis of the lipid content by either a titrimetric or a gravimetric method. Both methods employ a solvent extraction to remove the lipids from the fecal specimen. With the titrimetric method (Van de Kamer, 1949), neutral fats and soaps are converted to fatty acids prior to extraction. The resultant solution of fatty acids is extracted and titrated with sodium hydroxide. Because this titrimetric technique is unable to completely recover medium chain fatty acids, it measures approximately 80 percent of the total fecal lipid content. In contrast, the gravimetric method extracts and quantifies all of the fecal lipids present.

Fecal fat content is reported as grams of fat excreted per day, with a normal adult excreting 1 to 6 g/d. If the fecal fat excretion is borderline or if a standard 100-g fat diet is not used (e.g., with small children), the determination of the coefficient or percentage of fat retention is helpful. This requires careful recording of dietary intake; its determination is expressed in Equation 10–3.

(10–3)

$$\frac{\%\ \text{Fat}}{\text{retention}} = \frac{\text{Dietary fat} - \text{fecal fat}}{\text{Dietary fat}} \times 100$$

Normally, both children (3 years old and older) and adults retain at least 95 percent of the dietary fat ingested. Values below 95 percent are indicative of steatorrhea in these individuals.

Fecal Carbohydrates

When there are insufficient enzymes for disaccharide metabolism in the small intestine, these sugars are presented to the large intestine and excreted. Because these unhydrolyzed disaccharides are osmotically active, they cause large amounts of water to be retained in the intestinal lumen and produce an osmotic diarrhea.

Hereditary **disaccharidase deficiency** is uncommon but should be considered and ruled out in infants that present with diarrhea and a failure to gain weight. Secondary disaccharidase deficiency owing to disease (e.g., celiac disease, tropical sprue) or drug effects (e.g., oral neomycin or kanamycin) is an acquired condition; it usually affects more than one disaccharide and is only temporary. Lactose intolerance in adults is relatively common, particularly in African and Asian populations. These individuals were able to adequately digest lactose as children but develop a progressive inability to do so as adults. Consequently, for these individuals, the ingestion of lactose results in bloating, flatulence, and explosive diarrhea. These clinical manifestations of dissacharidase deficiency result from intestinal bacteria actively fermenting the carbohydrates present in the intestinal lumen. This fermentation results in the production of large amounts of intestinal gas and diarrheal stools with a characteristically decreased pH (of approximately 5.0 to 6.0). Normally, feces are alkaline (pH greater than 7.0) because of pancreatic and other intestinal secretions. A rapid qualitative determination of the fecal pH can be obtained using pH paper and the diarrheal stool supernatant.

Diarrheal stools can be screened for the presence of carbohydrates using the Clinitest tablet test for reducing substances (Ames Company) discussed in Chapter 7. Although the Clinitest is not advocated for use on fecal specimens by the manufacturer (i.e., FDA approval has not been requested), its use to detect fecal reducing substances is widely employed and documented in the literature (Kerry, 1964). To perform the Clinitest on feces, a 1:3 dilution of the supernatant from a diarrheal stool is used. Fecal excretion of reducing substances greater than 250 mg/dL is considered to be abnormal. A positive Clinitest indicates the presence of a reducing substance but does not specifically identify the substance being excreted. Note that sucrose is undetectable by this method because it is not a reducing sugar. In order to quantitate or specifically identify the sugar(s) present in fecal material, chromatographic or specific chemical methods must be employed.

The most diagnostic test for determining an intestinal enzyme deficiency (e.g., lactase deficiency) involves specific histochemical examination of the intestinal epithelium. A more convenient approach is to perform an oral tolerance test using specific sugars (e.g., lactose, sucrose). An oral tolerance test involves the ingestion of a measured dose of a specific disaccharide (e.g., lactose, sucrose) by the patient. If the patient has adequate amounts of the appropriate intestinal disaccharidase (e.g., lactase), the disaccharide (e.g., lactose) is hydrolyzed to its corresponding monosaccharides (e.g., glucose and galactose) and is absorbed into the patient's blood. An increase in blood glucose greater than 30 mg/dL above the patient's fasting glucose level indicates adequate enzyme activity (e.g., lactase); an increase less than 20 mg/dL above the patient's fasting glucose level indicates deficiency of the enzyme.

The presence of carbohydrates in the feces can also be a result of inadequate intestinal absorption. To differentiate carbohydrate malabsorption from carbohydrate maldigestion, a xylose absorption test is performed. Xylose is a pentose that does not depend on liver or pancreatic function for digestion and is readily reabsorbed in the small intestine. Normally, xylose is not present in significant levels in the blood, nor is it metabolized by the body. In addition, xylose readily passes through the glomerular filtration barrier for excretion in the urine. This xylose absorption test involves the patient's ingestion of a dose of xylose, followed by the collection of a 2-hour blood sample and a 5-hour urine specimen. The concentration of xylose is quantitatively determined in both the blood and the urine. Depending on the size of the initial oral dose, at least 16 percent to 24 percent of the ingested dose of xylose is normally excreted by adults.

References

Ahlquist DA, McGill DB, et al.: HemoQuant—a new quantitative assay for fecal hemoglobin. Ann Intern Med *101*:297–302, 1984.

Apt L, Downey WS: Melena neonatorium: swallowed blood syndrome. A simple test for the differentiation of adult and fetal hemoglobin in bloody stools. J Pediatr *47*:5, 1955.

Bradley GM: Fecal analysis: much more than an unpleasant necessity. Diagn Med *3*(2):64, 1980.

Drummey GD, Benson JA, Jones GM: Microscopical examination of the stool for steatorrhea. N Engl J Med *264*:85, 1961.

Kao YS, Liu FJ: Laboratory diagnosis of gastrointestinal tract and exocrine pancreatic disorders. *In* Henry JB (ed.): Clinical Diagnosis and Management by Laboratory Methods (18th ed.), Philadelphia, W. B. Saunders Company, 1991, pp. 519–549.

Kerry KR, Anderson CM: A ward test for sugar in feces. Lancet *1*:981, 1964

Van de Kamer JH, Ten Bokel Huinink H, Weyers HW: Rapid method for the determination of fat in feces. J Biol Chem *177*:347, 1949.

Study Questions

1. Which of the following substances is NOT a component of "normal" feces?

   A. Bacteria
   B. Blood
   C. Electrolytes
   D. Water

2. All of the following will result in watery or diarrheal stools EXCEPT

   A. decreased intestinal motility.
   B. the inhibition of water reabsorption.
   C. inadequate time allowed for water reabsorption.
   D. an excessive volume of fluid presented for reabsorption.

3. Lactose intolerance owing to the lack of sufficient lactase will primarily present with

   A. steatorrhea.
   B. osmotic diarrhea.
   C. secretory diarrhea.
   D. intestinal hypermotility.

4. Which of the following tests assists most in the differentiation of secretory from osmotic diarrhea?

   A. Fecal fat
   B. Fecal carbohydrates
   C. Fecal occult blood
   D. Fecal osmolality

5. The inability to convert dietary foodstuffs into readily absorbable substances is called intestinal

   A. inadequacy.
   B. hypermotility.
   C. malabsorption
   D. maldigestion.

6. **Intestinal motility is stimulated by each of the following EXCEPT**

   A. castor oil.
   B. dietary fiber.
   C. intestinal distention.
   D. sympathetic nerve activity.

7. **Which of the following conditions is characterized by the excretion of greasy, pale, foul-smelling feces?**

   A. Steatorrhea
   B. Osmotic diarrhea
   C. Secretory diarrhea
   D. Intestinal hypermotility

8. **The daily amount of fat excreted in the feces is normally less than**

   A. 0.6 g.
   B. 6 g.
   C. 60 g.
   D. 600 g.

9. **Which of the following tests is required in order to diagnose steatorrhea?**

   A. Fecal fat
   B. Fecal carbohydrates
   C. Fecal occult blood
   D. Fecal osmolality

10. **Which of the following statements regarding feces is true?**

    A. The normal color of feces is primarily due to urobilinogens.
    B. The amount of feces produced in 24 hours correlates poorly with food intake.
    C. The normal odor of the feces is usually due to metabolic by-products of intestinal protozoa.
    D. The consistency of the feces is primarily determined by the amount of fluid intake.

11. **Fecal specimens are often tested for all of the following EXCEPT**

    A. fat.
    B. blood.
    C. bilirubin.
    D. carbohydrates.

12. **Which of the following is responsible for the characteristic color of normal feces?**

    A. Bilirubin
    B. Hemoglobin
    C. Urobilins
    D. Urobilinogens

13. **Which of the following statements regarding fecal tests is true?**

    A. A fecal fat determination identifies the cause of steatorrhea.
    B. A fecal leukocyte determination aids in differentiating the cause of diarrhea.
    C. A fecal Clinitest identifies the enzyme deficiency that prevents sugar digestion.
    D. A fecal blood screen aids in differentiating bacterial from parasitic infestations.

14. **Which of the following types of fat readily stain with Sudan III or Oil Red O stains?**

    1. Fatty acids
    2. Cholesterol
    3. Soaps (fatty acid salts)
    4. Neutral fats (triglycerides)

        A. 1, 2, and 3 are correct.
        B. 1 and 3 are correct.
        C. 4 is correct.
        D. All are correct.

15. **Which of the following types of fat require acidification and heat before they are stained with Sudan III or Oil Red O stains?**

    1. Fatty acids
    2. Cholesterol
    3. Soaps (fatty acid salts)
    4. Neutral fats (triglycerides)

        A. 1, 2, and 3 are correct.
        B. 1 and 3 are correct.
        C. 4 is correct.
        D. All are correct.

16. **With the two-slide qualitative fecal fat determination, the first slide produces a normal amount of staining fat present, whereas the second slide, following acid addition and heat, produces an abnormally increased amount of fat present. These results are indicative of**

    A. malabsorption.
    B. maldigestion.
    C. parasitic infestation.
    D. disaccharidase deficiency.

17. **Mass screening in adults for occult blood in the feces is primarily performed to detect**

    A. ulcers.
    B. hemorrhoids.
    C. colorectal cancer.
    D. esophageal varices.

18. **Which of the following dietary substances can cause a false negative fecal occult blood slide test?**

    A. Fish
    B. Red meat
    C. Ascorbic acid
    D. Fruits and vegetables

19. **Which of the following can cause a false positive fecal occult blood slide test?**

    A. The rehydration of the specimen on the slide before testing
    B. The degradation of hemoglobin to porphyrin
    C. The storage of fecal specimens before testing
    D. The storage of slides with the specimen already applied

20. **Which of the following is the indicator of choice in fecal occult blood slide tests?**

    A. Guaiac
    B. Benzidine
    C. Orthotoluidine
    D. Tetramethylbenzidine

21. **Which of the following conditions can result in the excretion of small amounts of occult blood in the feces?**

    1. Hemorrhoids
    2. Bleeding gums
    3. Peptic ulcers
    4. Intake of iron supplements

        A. 1, 2, and 3 are correct.
        B. 1 and 3 are correct.
        C. 4 is correct.
        D. All are correct.

22. **Which of the following statements regarding the test for fetal hemoglobin in the feces (the Apt test) is true?**

    A. Any adult hemoglobin present should be resistant to alkali treatment.

    B. The Apt test is used to differentiate various hemoglobinopathies in the newborn.

    C. Hemoglobin degraded to hematin usually produces a positive test result.

    D. A pink color following alkali treatment indicates the presence of fetal hemoglobin.

23. **Which of the following are clinical manifestations of disaccharidase deficiency?**

    1. A positive fecal Clinitest

    2. Constipation and gas

    3. A fecal pH of 5.0

    4. A positive fecal occult blood test

        A. 1, 2, and 3 are correct.

        B. 1 and 3 are correct.

        C. 4 is correct.

        D. All are correct.

24. **Which of the following tests can differentiate inadequate carbohydrate metabolism from inadequate carbohydrate absorption?**

    A. The fecal Clinitest

    B. The xylose absorption test

    C. Oral carbohydrate tolerance tests

    D. Carbohydrate thin-layer chromatography

Seminal Fluid Analysis

LEARNING OBJECTIVES

After studying this chapter, the student should be able to

1. Discuss the composition of seminal fluid and briefly describe the function of each of the following structures in seminal fluid formation:
   - the epididymis
   - the interstitial cells of Leydig
   - the prostate gland
   - the seminal vesicles
   - the seminiferous tubules

2. Outline the maturation of spermatozoa and identify the morphologic structures in which each maturation phase occurs.

3. Summarize the collection of seminal fluid for analysis, including the importance of timing and the recovery of a complete specimen.

4. Describe the performance of the physical examination (appearance, volume, and viscosity) of seminal fluid and the results expected from a normal specimen.

5. Describe the procedures employed to evaluate the following characteristics of spermatozoa in seminal fluid; state the normal range for each parameter; and relate each function to male fertility:
   - agglutination
   - concentration
   - morphology
   - motility
   - viability

6. Identify and describe the morphologic appearance of normal and abnormal forms of spermatozoa.

7. Discuss the origin and clinical significance of cells other than spermatozoa in the seminal fluid.

8. Discuss briefly the role of quantifying the following biochemical substances in seminal fluid and identify the structure whose function each evaluates:
   - acid phosphatase
   - citric acid
   - fructose
   - pH
   - zinc

KEY TERMS

epididymis: a long coiled tubular structure attached to the upper surface of each testis and continuous with the vas deferens. It is the site of final spermatozoa maturation and the development of motility. Spermatozoa are concentrated and stored here until ejaculation.

interstitial cells of Leydig: the cells located in the interstitial space between the seminiferous tubules of the testes. These cells produce and secrete the hormone testosterone.

liquefaction: the physical conversion of seminal fluid from a coagulum to a liquid following ejaculation.

prostate gland: a lobular gland surrounding the male urethra immediately after it exits the bladder. It is an

332

accessory gland of the male reproductive system. The prostate is testosterone dependent and produces a mildly acidic secretion rich in citric acid, enzymes, proteins, and zinc.

seminal fluid also called **semen:** a complex body fluid that transports spermatozoa. It is composed of secretions from the testes, the epididymis, the seminal vesicles, and the prostate gland.

seminal vesicles: paired glands that secrete a slightly alkaline fluid, rich in fructose, into the ejaculatory duct. Most of the fluid in the ejaculate originates in the seminal vesicles.

seminiferous tubules: numerous coiled tubules located in the testes; the seminiferous tubules are collectively the site of spermatogenesis. Immature and immotile spermatozoa are released into the seminiferous tubular lumen and are carried by its secretions to the epididymis for maturation.

viscosity: a measure of fluid flow or its resistance to flow. Low-viscosity fluids (e.g., water) flow freely and will form discrete droplets when expelled drop by drop from a pipette. In contrast, high-viscosity fluids (e.g., corn syrup) flow less freely and will not form discrete droplets; rather, they momentarily form threads or strings as they are expelled from a pipette.

. . . .

Seminal fluid or semen is a complex body fluid used to transport spermatozoa. It is routinely analyzed to evaluate infertility and to follow up a vasectomy to ensure its effectiveness. Other reasons for its analysis include the evaluation of semen quality for donation and forensic applications (e.g., the presence of sperm in vaginal secretions, DNA fingerprinting). Familiarity with the male reproductive tract and the functions of each of its components facilitates understanding of the physical, microscopic, and biochemical abnormalities that can occur in semen.

Physiology

Semen is composed primarily of secretions from the testes, the epididymis, the seminal vesicles, and the prostate gland, with a very small amount derived from the bulbourethral glands. The biochemical composition of semen is complex. Although the specific functions of some components (e.g., fructose) are known, others (e.g., prostaglandins) remain uncertain. The testes are paired glands suspended in the scrotum and located outside the body (Fig. 11–1). Their external location allows for the lower organ temperature that is necessary for spermatozoa formation. Each testis is composed of numerous coiled **seminiferous tubules.** The epithelium of these tubules consists of Sertoli and germ cells. The undifferentiated germ cells (spermatogonia) continuously undergo mitotic division to produce more germ cells. At the same time, some of them move slowly toward the tubular lumen, changing in size and undergoing meiotic (reduction) division until they form spermatids. Figure 11–2 depicts spermatogenesis in the seminiferous tubular epithelium. Note that all stages of spermatogenesis are depicted in Figure 11–2, from spermatogonia (germ cell) to spermatocyte, to early and late spermatids. With nuclear modification and cellular restructuring, spermatids ultimately differentiate into immotile spermatozoa and are released into the tubular lumen.

Sertoli cells of the seminiferous tubular epithelium have several functions. Owing to their tight interconnections, they essentially form a barrier separating the epithelium into two distinct compartments: the basal compartment (i.e., the germ cell layer) and the adluminal compartment (the epithelium nearest the tubular lumen). As a result, these cells effectively limit the movement of chemical substances from the blood into the tubular lumen and serve as "gate keepers," controlling the movement of spermatocytes from the basal compartment into the adluminal compartment. Sertoli cells also play a role in supplying the nutrients, hormones, and other substances necessary for normal spermatogenesis, as well as in continuously producing

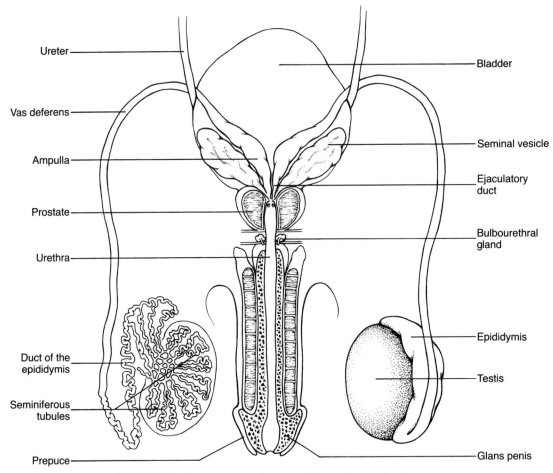

FIGURE 11–1. A schematic diagram of the male reproductive tract.

the lumen fluid that carries the immotile sperm into the epididymis.

Located in the interstitium of the testes, between the seminiferous tubules, are the **interstitial cells of Leydig.** These interstitial cells perform a primary endocrine function: the production and secretion of the male sex hormone testosterone. Hence, the testes perform both an exocrine (the secretion of spermatozoa) and an endocrine (the secretion of testosterone) function, and the cells responsible for these functions are distinctly different. These two functions of the testes are closely interdependent and are regulated by two pituitary hormones, follicle stimulating hormone and luteinizing hormone.

When Sertoli cells release spermatozoa into the lumen of the seminiferous tubules, the spermatozoa are nonmotile and still im-

mature. Luminal fluid from Sertoli cells carries the spermatozoa into the tubular network of the **epididymis,** where they undergo final maturation and become motile. The epididymis also adds carnitine and acetylcarnitine to the lumen fluid. Although the exact function of these chemicals remains to be elucidated, abnormal levels of the chemicals have been associated with infertility. Other functions of the epididymis include concentration of the semen by the absorption of lumen fluid and storage until ejaculation. Following a vasectomy, the epididymis is the site of leukocyte infiltration and phagocytization of accumulated spermatozoa.

The epididymis ultimately forms a single duct that joins the vas deferens. The vas deferens is a thick-walled muscular tube that transports sperm from the epididymis to the

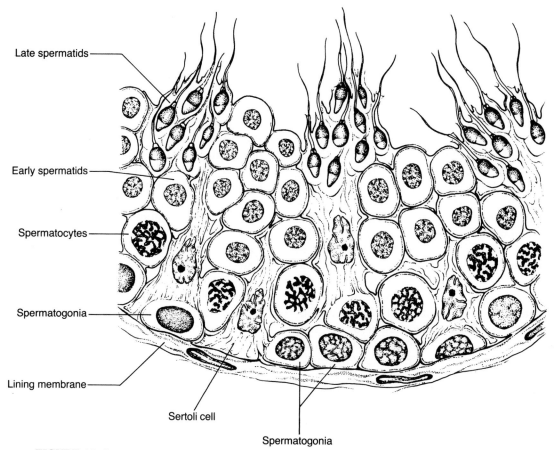

Late spermatids

Early spermatids

Spermatocytes

Spermatogonia

Lining membrane

Sertoli cell

Spermatogonia

FIGURE 11–2. A schematic diagram of spermatogenesis from germ cells in the seminiferous tubules.

ejaculatory duct—the dilated end of the vas deferens located inferior to the bladder. Secretions from the seminal vesicles are added at the ejaculatory duct. Both ejaculatory ducts then pass through the prostate gland and empty into the prostatic urethra along with secretions from the prostate. All structures preceding the prostate gland are paired (e.g., two ejaculatory ducts, two seminal vesicles).

The **seminal vesicles** and the **prostate gland** are considered accessory glands of the male reproductive system and are testosterone dependent. They produce and store fluids that provide the principal transport medium of the sperm. Seminal vesicle fluid accounts for the bulk of the ejaculate and is high in flavin. Flavin imparts the characteristic gray or opalescent appearance to semen and is responsible for semen's green-white fluores-

cence under ultraviolet light (Kjeldsberg, 1986). Another characteristic of seminal vesicle fluid is its high concentration of fructose, believed to serve as a nutrient for the spermatozoa. Various proteins secreted by the seminal vesicles play a role in the coagulation of the ejaculate; the function of the prostaglandins in the semen remains under investigation. (Prostaglandins were originally thought to be a prostatic gland secretion; hence, their misnaming.)

Prostatic fluid secretions account for approximately 25 percent of the ejaculate volume. The principal components of this milky, slightly acidic fluid are citric acid; enzymes, particularly acid phosphatase and proteolytic enzymes; proteins; and zinc. Semen is unique in its extremely high concentration of the enzyme acid phosphatase. Hence, acid phosphatase activity can be used to positively identify the presence of this body fluid. Proteins and some enzymes in prostatic fluid secretions play a role in the coagulation of the ejaculate, whereas the proteolytic enzymes present are responsible for its liquefaction. Zinc is primarily added to the semen by the prostate gland; however, the testes and spermatozoa also contribute zinc. A decreased amount of zinc in seminal fluid has been associated with disorders of the prostate gland; hence, semen zinc levels can be used to evaluate prostate function.

In summary, semen is a highly complex transport medium for spermatozoa. The paired seminal vesicles and the single prostate gland are the major fluid contributors to the semen. Spermatozoa, produced by the testes and matured and concentrated in the epididymis, make up only a small percentage of an ejaculate. The dilution of the spermatozoa by the relatively large volume of seminal fluid enhances sperm motility. Without adequate dilution, sperm motility is significantly reduced. The entire process of spermatogenesis and maturation (i.e., from primary spermatocyte to mature motile spermatozoon) takes approximately 90 days.

Specimen Collection

Because the sperm concentration in normal seminal fluid can vary significantly, two or more samples of seminal fluid should be analyzed for evaluating male fertility. Specimen collections should take place within a 3-month period and at least 7 days apart. Sexual abstinence for at least 2 days (48 hours), but not exceeding 7 days, should precede the collection. The specimen is collected by the patient through masturbation, and the entire ejaculate is collected in a clean, wide-mouth sterile plastic or glass container. Although some plastic containers are toxic to spermatozoa, others are not. Sterile urine specimen or similar containers are often satisfactory but must be evaluated by the laboratory before their use (Amelar, 1977). The collection container should be at room temperature or warmed before the collection to avoid the

possibility of cold-shock to the spermatozoa. The container can easily be warmed by holding it next to the patient's body or under the arm for several minutes before the collection. This technique can also be used to control the temperature of specimens being transported in cold climates. Specimen containers and request forms must be labeled with the patient's name, the period of sexual abstinence and the date and time of specimen collection. The time of actual specimen collection is crucial in evaluating liquefaction and sperm motility.

Lubricants should not be used during specimen collection, and ordinary condoms are not acceptable, because both lubricants and condoms have spermicidal properties. For patients unable to collect a specimen through masturbation, special nonspermicidal (e.g., Silastic) condoms can be provided for specimen collection.

The collection of seminal fluid requires sensitivity and professionalism. Written and verbal instructions should be provided to the patient, as well as a comfortable and private room near the laboratory. If the specimen is to be collected elsewhere and delivered to the laboratory, clearly written instructions regarding specimen transportation conditions must also be provided to the patient. Specimens must be received in the laboratory within 1 hour following the collection, and the specimen must be protected from extreme temperatures, i.e., maintained between 20° and 40°C (WHO, 1992). If these criteria are not met, the specimen will not be satisfactory for sperm function tests, and an abnormally low sperm motility can result. Because the ejaculate differs in its composition, with the first portion often the most concentrated with spermatozoa, only complete collections are acceptable for analysis. Patient instructions must state this clearly; patients should be asked whether any portion of the specimen was lost.

As with all body fluids, seminal fluid represents a potential biohazard and must be handled accordingly. Because seminal fluid may contain infectious agents such as hepatitis virus, human immunodeficiency virus (HIV), herpesvirus, and others, Universal

Precautions must be adhered to by all personnel when handling these specimens.

Physical Examination

Appearance

Normal semen is gray-white and opalescent. A brown or red hue may indicate the presence of blood, whereas a yellow coloration has been associated with certain drugs. If large numbers of leukocytes are present, the seminal fluid may appear more turbid with less translucence. In contrast, the specimen may appear almost clear when the concentration of spermatozoa is very low. Mucus clumps or strands may be present. Semen has a distinctive odor, which is sometimes described as musty. Although infections in the male reproductive tract can modify this odor, this change is rarely noted or reported. Table 11–1 summarizes the expected physical, microscopic, and chemical parameters of a normal seminal fluid specimen.

TABLE 11–1.   NORMAL VALUES FOR SEMEN ANALYSIS

PHYSICAL EXAMINATION

Appearance	Gray-white, opalescent, opaque
Volume	2 to 5 mL
Viscosity/liquefaction	Discrete droplets (watery) within 60 minutes

MICROSCOPIC EXAMINATION

Motility	50% or more with moderate to rapid linear (forward) progression
Concentration	20 to 250 $\times$ 10^6 spermatozoa/mL of ejaculate
Morphology	50% or more have normal morphology
Viability	50% or more are alive
Leukocytes	Less than 1 $\times$ 10^6/mL of ejaculate

CHEMICAL EXAMINATION

pH	7.2 to 7.8
Acid phosphatase (total)	$\geq$200 U per ejaculate at 37°C (p-nitrophenylphosphate)
Citric acid (total)	$\geq$52 μmol per ejaculate
Fructose (total)	$\geq$13 μmol per ejaculate
Zinc (total)	$\geq$2.4 μmol per ejaculate

Semen is a homogeneous viscous fluid that immediately coagulates after ejaculation. Within 30 minutes, it again liquefies (becomes watery). It is necessary to know the time of actual specimen collection to evaluate this **liquefaction.** Although liquefaction may take longer, any delay beyond 60 minutes is considered abnormal and must be noted. Because complete liquefaction is necessary to perform the rest of the analysis, semen specimens that do not completely liquefy must be treated. The laboratorian must physically break up any mucus and clumps or add chemicals (e.g., amylase, bromelin). Following normal liquefaction, undissolved particles or gel-like granules may be noted in the specimen. A small amount of this particulate matter is considered to be normal.

Volume

The physical and microscopic analyses of seminal fluid should take place immediately following liquefaction or within 1 hour after collection (for specimens collected away from the laboratory). If a semen culture for bacteria is to be performed, sterile technique and materials must be employed. Specimen volume is measured to one decimal place (0.1 mL) using a graduated cylinder or a serologic pipette. Normally, a complete ejaculate collection recovers 2 to 5 mL of seminal fluid. Volumes less than and greater than this range have been associated with infertility.

Viscosity

After complete liquefaction, the **viscosity** of the semen is evaluated by using a Pasteur pipette and observing the droplets that form when the fluid is expelled. A normal specimen will be watery and form into discrete droplets. Abnormal viscosity or fluid thickness is indicated by the formation of a string or thread (greater than 2 cm in length) as a drop of fluid is expelled from the pipette (WHO, 1992). Alternative techniques employing a syringe or a glass rod may also be used. Grading viscosity varies among laboratories, with most applying numerical values from 0, indicating a normal watery (i.e., forming discrete drops) specimen, to 4, indicating a gel-like specimen (Overstreet, 1987).

Microscopic Examination

As in other laboratory areas, the standardization of procedures and techniques is necessary to enhance the precision and reproducibility of semen analysis. Once achieved, this standardization enables both intralaboratory and interlaboratory comparisons of data. Appropriate quality control measures must also be in place whenever applicable. The World Health Organization (WHO) publication entitled "The WHO Laboratory Manual for the Examination of Human Semen and Semen-Cervical Mucus Interaction" is an excellent reference for any laboratory performing semen analysis. The microscopic examination includes the determination of sperm motility, concentration, morphology, and viability; the concentration of other cells present; and the presence of agglutination. Some laboratories use a single stain for the evaluation of several parameters (e.g., eosin-nigrosin for sperm viability and morphology and the identification of other cells), whereas others use different stains that specifically enhance each parameter to aid in the identification and evaluation of spermatozoa and other cells.

Motility

Motility is one of the most important characteristics of sperm because immotile sperm, even in high concentrations, will be unable to reach an ovum. Traditionally, the evaluation of sperm motility has been assessed subjectively by experienced technologists. In the last decade, numerous computerized videomicrography and time-elapsed photomicrography applications have been developed for semen evaluation. This advanced technology enables the objective evaluation of sperm motility and morphology; however, the

equipment's high cost precludes routine laboratories from acquiring it.

Routinely, sperm motility is subjectively and semiquantitatively evaluated using phase contrast microscopy (brightfield microscopy can also be used with appropriate condenser adjustments). After complete liquefaction, the semen sample is mixed well to ensure its homogeneity. A consistent volume of the specimen is evaluated, either using a standardized system (e.g., a Makler counting chamber) or pipetting a fixed volume of the specimen onto a microscope slide. With the latter technique, the specimen volume (10 to 20 μL) is dispensed with a calibrated micropipette and covered with a predetermined sized coverslip (e.g., 18 $\times$ 18 mm). These wet mounts should be prepared in duplicate and allowed to settle for about 1 minute before evaluation. Because sperm motility is adversely affected by temperature, some laboratories control the temperature of the microscope slide at 37°C using an air curtain incubator (Overstreet, 1987). Others perform the analysis at room temperature, i.e., 22 $\pm$ 2°C.

Initially, each wet preparation should be screened to ensure uniformity in spermatozoa movement throughout the preparation. Next, sperm motility is subjectively graded from 0 to 4 using 200$\times$ (or 400$\times$) magnification. Table 11–2 shows typical grading criteria used to evaluate sperm motility. Some laboratories use a cell counter and evaluate the motility characteristics in 100 sperm, whereas others grade the sperm encountered in 6 to 10 high-power fields (400$\times$). Both the sperm's speed and forward progression are evaluated. In normal semen, evaluated within 60 minutes of collection, 50 percent or more of the sperm will show moderate to strong

TABLE 11–2.   SPERM MOTILITY GRADING CRITERIA

0	Immotile
1	Motile, without forward progression
2	Motile, with slow nonlinear or meandering progression
3	Motile, with moderate linear (forward) progression
4	Motile, with strong linear (forward) progression

linear or forward progression. The practice of reassessing sperm motility at additional intervals serves no purpose and has no clinical significance, because following ejaculation, the spermatozoa leave the seminal fluid within minutes and enter the cervical mucus.

Concentration

The actual number of spermatozoa is not as important for fertility purposes as are their other characteristics. This assumption is supported by studies of fertile men with extremely low sperm counts (less than 1 million/mL) (Barfield, 1979). The concentration of sperm in an ejaculate is considered normal if 20 to 250 million/mL of spermatozoa are present, values below or above this range are considered abnormal and are associated with infertility. The variation in the sperm concentration within a single individual can be significant. It is partially dependent on the period of sexual abstinence but can also be affected by viral infections and stress. For these reasons, multiple specimens should be evaluated to reliably assess spermatozoa quantity and quality.

The concentration of spermatozoa is routinely determined using a hemacytometer and a manual dilution of the semen specimen. A 1:20 dilution is routinely prepared. If during initial microscopic examination the laboratorian notes that the sperm concentration is exceptionally high or low, however, the dilution can be adjusted accordingly. The appropriate dilution is made using a calibrated micropipette to deliver the sample quantitatively to a premeasured amount of diluent (e.g., Isoton Plus). Note that a hematology white blood cell pipette is not accurate for use with seminal fluid and should not be used (WHO, 1992). The resultant dilution is mixed well and placed in a hemacytometer. After filling, the hemacytometer is placed in a humidifying chamber and allowed to settle for approximately 3 to 5 minutes before counting. The type of hemacytometer, the specimen dilution used, and the areas counted determine the conversion factor necessary to obtain the concentration of spermatozoa in millions per milliliter (see Appendix C for procedural details). An alternative method is to use a Makler counting chamber designed specifically for semen analysis (Makler, 1980). This technique does not require dilution of the specimen; hence, the sperm concentration, motility, and morphology can be determined using the same wet preparation.

Morphology

Sperm morphology, like motility, is routinely assessed subjectively. Hence, this qualitative determination is subject to both intralaboratory and interlaboratory variations. To minimize these variations, standardized procedures and grading criteria must be established by each laboratory and adhered to by all laboratorians. Because the technical ability to identify and classify various morphologic forms requires experience, new staff members must be appropriately trained and their initial work evaluated to ensure accuracy and consistency in reporting. Subtle abnormalities in spermatozoa are easily missed by an inexperienced observer. The computerized techniques currently available to evaluate sperm motility can also be used to evaluate sperm morphology. Sperm morphometry—the measurement of the sperm head length, width, circumference, and area—enables the generation of objective data; however, "normal" ranges for these parameters have yet to be established. Nevertheless, studies have shown statistically significant differences in the ratio of sperm head length to head width in the ejaculates of fertile and infertile men (Katz, 1986).

The current subjective method for the evaluation of sperm morphology is complicated by the wide variation of abnormal forms that can be encountered. Human sperm have three distinct areas: the head, the midpiece, and the tail. Viewed from the top, normal human sperm have oval heads that are 2 to 3 μm in width and 3 to 5 μm in length. When viewed from the side, they appear to be arrowhead-shaped (Fig. 11–3). The mid-

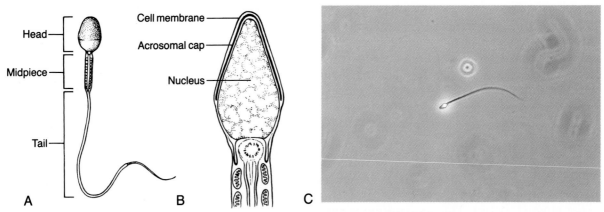

FIGURE 11–3. Spermatozoon or sperm. *A,* A schematic of a top view. *B,* A schematic of a side view. *C,* A photomicrograph using phase contrast microscopy at magnification of 400×.

piece, located between the head and tail, is about 7 to 8 μm long, whereas the tail is slender, uncoiled, and at least 45 μm long. Spermatozoa are often classified into six categories: normal, large head, pin head, tapering head, double or duplicate heads, and amorphous forms. The latter term encompasses any mature sperm types that do not fall into the other categories. Figure 11–4 shows several forms of morphologically abnormal spermatozoa that are frequently seen.

To evaluate sperm morphology, smears of fresh semen are made and stained. The smears are made similarly to traditional blood smears, using a drop (10 to 15 μL) of semen placed near one side of a clean microscope slide. Using the edge of another slide, the drop is allowed to spread along the second slide's edge; then, the edge of the second slide is moved forward, dragging the semen sample across the surface of the first slide and producing a smear. Staining enhances

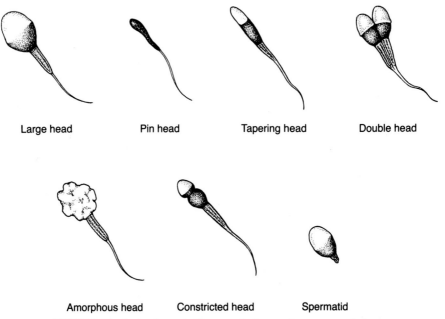

FIGURE 11–4. A schematic diagram of abnormal sperm morphology.

the visualization of sperm morphology and enables the identification and differentiation of white blood cells, epithelial cells of the urethra, and immature spermatogenic cells (i.e., spermatids, spermatocytes, and spermatogonia). Giemsa, Wright, and Papanicolaou stains are frequently employed. These stains differ with respect to complexity and turnaround time; hence, laboratories select the stain that best suits their needs and resources.

Using oil immersion (1000×), 100 to 200 sperm are classified morphologically. Morphologically abnormal spermatozoa are found in all semen specimens. Abnormalities may involve all or only one region of the spermatozoon and can affect its size, shape, or both. In addition, numerous variations are found within a single ejaculate. Although some morphologic abnormalities have been associated with particular disorders (e.g., tapered heads with varicocele), most abnormalities are nonspecific. Regardless, semen specimens with 50 percent or more sperm of normal morphology are considered normal.

Viability

Supravital staining of a fresh semen smear enables rapid differentiation of live and dead spermatozoa. Because dead sperm have damaged plasma membranes, these cells take up the stain; viable sperm do not (Fig. 11–5).

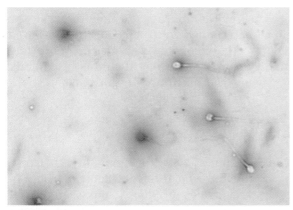

FIGURE 11–5. Sperm viability using Blom's stain. White sperm are viable; pink-stained sperm are dead. Brightfield microscopy at a magnification of 400×.

When a large percentage of immotile sperm are observed, this evaluation determines if the sperm are immotile because they are dead or because of a structural abnormality (e.g., a defective flagellum).

Eosin alone or an eosin-nigrosin (a modification of Blom's technique) combination is frequently used to determine sperm viability. Using either brightfield or phase contrast microscopy and 1000× (or 400×), 100 spermatozoa on a stained smear are evaluated. The percentage of dead sperm cells should not exceed the percentage of immotile sperm. In other words, if 65 percent of the sperm in a semen specimen are dead, the motility cannot exceed 35 percent. Hence, the viability evaluation provides a convenient cross-check of the motility evaluation. In fresh normal semen, 50 percent or more of the sperm are alive.

Cells Other Than Spermatozoa

An ejaculate is a complex mixture biochemically and cellularly. It normally contains cells other than spermatozoa, such as urethral epithelial cells, leukocytes, and immature spermatogenic cells (i.e., spermatids, spermatocytes, and spermatogonia), as well as particulate matter and cellular debris. Because of size and nuclear pattern similarities, these cells can be difficult to differentiate. A peroxidase stain can aid in this evaluation, because neutrophils are peroxidase-positive cells, whereas lymphocytes and spermatogenic cells are peroxidase-negative cells. (Wright stain may be preferred, however, because many peroxidase stains require special handling owing to the carcinogenicity of their chemicals).

The presence of greater than 1 million leukocytes per milliliter of ejaculate is indicative of an inflammatory process, most often involving the male accessory glands (e.g., the seminal vesicle, the prostate). However, a normal leukocyte count does not rule out an infection. The concentration of leukocytes and spermatogenic cells can be determined by using a hemacytometer after performing the sperm count (see Appendix C). If the concentration of these cells exceeds 1 million/mL, a stained smear (e.g., Wright or peroxidase stain) of the fresh ejaculate is evaluated. Using this smear, the number of leukocytes and immature spermatogenic cells is counted in the same fields used to count 100 mature spermatozoa. Knowing the sperm count (S) and using the following equation, the concentration (C) of these cell types (N) can be determined (WHO, 1992) (Equation 11–1).

(11–1)

$$C = \frac{N \times S}{100}$$

Immature spermatogenic cells are present in the semen when they are prematurely exfoliated from the germinal epithelium of the seminiferous tubules. Distinguishing between an increase in leukocytes and an increase in immature spermatogenic cells is necessary in the evaluation of infection and infertility.

The presence of red blood cells and bacteria in semen should be reported. These entities, normally not present in seminal fluid, are apparent during various aspects of the microscopic evaluation.

Agglutination

Agglutination, the sticking together of motile sperm, is evident by microscopic examination of a wet preparation. Although some clumping of the sperm may occur in normal semen specimens, the observation of distinct head to head, head to tail, or tail to tail orientation of spermatozoa is associated with the presence of sperm agglutinating antibodies. Clumping of spermatozoa with other entities, such as mucus and other cell types, is not identified as agglutination. The extent of true agglutination is often graded as "few," "moderate," or "many." Even a small amount of true agglutination is significant and indicates the need for further evaluation.

Both IgG and IgA antibodies binding to sperm have been identified and correlated with reduced fertility: immunologic infertility. Either the man or the woman can produce these antibodies. If the man is producing them, the antibodies are present on the surface of the sperm before intercourse; if the woman is producing them, the spermato-

zoa are coated with antibodies after ejaculation and their deposition in the cervical mucus. Macroscopic (mixed antiglobulin or the MAR-test) and microscopic techniques (the Immunobead test) are available for the detection and immunoglobulin-class determination of sperm antibodies (WHO, 1992). In both tests, normal semen will show less than 10 percent of the spermatozoa associated with the immunoparticles or immunobeads.

Chemical Examination

pH

The pH of fresh normal semen ranges from 7.2 to 7.8. Fresh specimens with a pH less than 7.2 can be obtained from individuals with abnormalities of the epididymis, the vas deferens, or the seminal vesicles. In contrast, fresh specimens exceeding pH 7.8 suggest an infection in the male reproductive tract. Specimens not tested within 1 hour of collection can show changes in the pH for several reasons. An increase in pH can occur because of a loss of carbon dioxide; conversely, a decrease in pH can occur because of the accumulation of lactic acid, particularly in specimens with a high sperm count (Amelar, 1977).

Despite the limited usefulness of a seminal fluid pH, it is easy to determine and may be included in a seminal fluid analysis. Using commercial reagent strip tests (or pH paper), a drop of semen is placed on the reagent test area. After the appropriate time interval, the pH is determined by comparing the test area color to the color key provided. Appropriate quality control solutions should be used daily to ensure the accuracy of the reagent strips used.

Fructose

The determination of seminal fluid fructose is a commonly performed chemical test. Because fructose is produced and secreted by the seminal vesicles, its presence in semen reflects the secretory function of this gland, as well as the functional integrity of the ejaculatory ducts and vas deferens. The fructose level is most often determined when the sperm count reveals azoospermia (i.e., the absence of sperm in semen). Obstruction of the ejaculatory ducts or abnormalities of the seminal vesicles and the vas deferens will produce both low fructose levels and azoospermia.

Normally, semen fructose levels are equal to or greater than 13 μmol per ejaculate. Several quantitative, spectrophotometric procedures are available for fructose determinations. A rapid and easy qualitative tube test based on the development of an orange-red color in the presence of fructose can also be performed (Amelar, 1977). In this assessment, failure of the specimen to develop an orange-red color indicates the absence of fructose. This technique is qualitative, relies on the visual assessment of color, and lacks sensitivity to decreased fructose levels, but its ease of performance and rapid turnaround time make it a useful tool.

Other Biochemical Indicators

The quantitative determinations of zinc and citric acid levels in the seminal fluid can be used to evaluate the secretory function of the prostate gland. The usefulness of zinc and citric acid measurements as markers of biochemical function is ongoing; clinicians are attempting to establish correlations with disease processes (e.g., low zinc levels with prostatitis). Quantitation of zinc in seminal fluid can be performed by either spectrophotometric or atomic absorption spectroscopy techniques. In normal semen, the total zinc concentration is equal to or greater than 2.4 μmol per ejaculate.

Citric acid, the major anion in semen, can be quantitated using spectrophotometric methods (Kjeldsberg, 1986). Decreased levels indicate dysfunction of the prostate gland. The total citric acid concentration in normal semen is equal to or greater than 52 μmol per ejaculate.

Acid phosphatase activity is a useful marker to assess the secretory function of the prostate gland. Normally, seminal fluid contains 200 units of activity or more per ejaculate, whereas other body fluids contain insignificant amounts of activity. Because of this uniquely high concentration, prostatic acid phosphatase measurements are often used to determine if semen is present in vaginal fluid specimens obtained from women following an alleged rape or sexual assault. Even washings of the skin and stained clothing can reveal significant levels of prostatic acid phosphatase, which positively identify the presence of seminal fluid.

Other biochemical substances are being investigated in an attempt to identify and establish specific markers for male reproductive tract abnormalities. For example, L-carnitine and α-glucosidase are being evaluated as indicators of epididymal function, whereas specific lactate dehydrogenase isoenzymes of spermatozoa are being examined for their clinical utility in the evaluation of male fertility.

References

Amelar RD, Dubin L: Semen Analysis. *In* Amelar RD, Dubin L, Walsh PC (eds.): Male Infertility, Philadelphia, W.B. Saunders Company, 1977, pp. 105–140.

Barfield A, Melo J, et al: Pregnancies associated with sperm concentrations below 10 million/mL in clinical studies of a potential male contraceptive method, monthly depot medroxyprogesterone acetate and testosterone esters. Contraception *20*:121–127, 1979.

Katz DF, Overstreet JW, et al.: Morphometric analysis of spermatozoa in the assessment of human male fertility. J Androl *7*(4):203–210, 1986.

Kjeldsberg CR, Knight JA: Body Fluids (2nd ed.), Chicago, American Society of Clinical Pathologists Press, 1986, p. 118.

Makler A: The improved ten-micrometer chamber for rapid sperm count and motility evaluation. Fertil Steril *33*:337–338, 1980.

Overstreet JW, Katz DF, et al.: A simple inexpensive method for the objective assessment of human sperm movement characteristics. Fertil Steril *31*:162–172, 1979.

World Health Organization (WHO) Laboratory Manual for the Examination of Human Semen and Semen-cervical Mucus Interaction (3rd ed) New York, Cambridge University Press, 1992 pp. 5–6.

Bibliography

Amelar RD: The semen analysis. *In:* Infertility in Men: Diagnosis and Treatment, Philadelphia, F.A. Davis Company, 1966, pp. 30–53.

Freund M: Standards for the rating of human sperm morphology. Int J Fertil *11*:97–180, 1966.

Overstreet JW, Katz DF: Semen analysis. Urol Clin North Am *14*(3):441–449, 1987.

Study Questions

1. **Seminal fluid analysis is routinely performed to evaluate which of the following?**

    A. Prostate cancer
    B. Postvasectomy status
    C. Penile implant status
    D. Premature ejaculation

2. **Which of the following structures contribute(s) secretions to seminal fluid?**

    1. The epididymis
    2. The prostate gland
    3. The seminal vesicles
    4. The seminiferous tubules

    A. 1, 2, and 3 are correct.
    B. 1 and 3 are correct.
    C. 4 is correct.
    D. All are correct.

3.. **Which of the following structures performs both an endocrine and an exocrine function?**

    A. The testes
    B. The epididymis
    C. The prostate gland
    D. The seminal vesicles

4. **The primary function of seminal fluid is to**

    A. nourish the spermatozoa.
    B. coagulate the ejaculate.
    C. transport the spermatozoa.
    D. stimulate spermatozoa maturation.

5. **Match the number of the structure to the feature that best describes it. Only one structure is correct for each feature.**

Descriptive Feature		Structure	
_____	A. Produces and secretes testosterone	1.	Bulbourethral gland
_____	B. The site of spermatogenesis	2.	Ejaculatory duct
_____	C. Concentrates and stores sperm	3.	Epididymis
_____	D. Secretes fluid rich in zinc	4.	Interstitial cells of Leydig
_____	E. Secretes fluid high in fructose	5.	Prostate gland
_____	F. Transports sperm to the ejaculatory duct	6.	Seminal vesicles
		7.	Seminiferous tubules
		8.	Vas deferens

6. **Which of the following is a requirement when collecting seminal fluid specimens?**

   A. The patient should abstain from sexual intercourse for at least 2 days following the collection.

   B. Only complete collections of the entire ejaculate are acceptable for analysis.

   C. A single seminal fluid specimen is sufficient for the evaluation of male fertility.

   D. Seminal fluid specimens must be evaluated within 3 hours following collection.

7. **Which of the following will adversely affect the quality of a seminal fluid specimen?**

   A. The use of Silastic condoms

   B. The time of day the collection is obtained

   C. The collection of the specimen in a glass container

   D. The storage of the specimen at refrigerator temperatures

8. **Which of the following statements regarding seminal fluid is true?**

   A. Seminal fluid usually coagulates within 30 minutes after ejaculation.

   B. It is abnormal for seminal fluid to liquefy before 60 minutes.

   C. Following liquefaction, the viscosity of normal seminal fluid is similar to that of water.

   D. Following liquefaction, the presence of particulate matter is highly indicative of a bacterial infection.

9. **Which of the following statements regarding the evaluation of spermatozoa motility is NOT true?**

   A. Spermatozoa motility is most often subjectively graded.

   B. Spermatozoa motility is adversely affected by temperature.

   C. Spermatozoa motility appraises both speed and forward progression.

   D. Spermatozoa motility should be evaluated initially and at 2 hours after collection.

10. **Which of the following statements regarding sperm motility is true?**

    A. Sperm concentration within a single individual is usually constant.
    B. Sperm concentration is dependent solely on the period of abstinence.
    C. Sperm concentration in a normal ejaculate ranges from 20 to 250 million/mL.
    D. Sperm concentration is more important than sperm motility for fertility.

11. **Which of the following statements regarding sperm morphology is true?**

    A. Sperm morphology is usually assessed using computerized techniques.
    B. Stained smears of fresh semen are used to evaluate sperm morphology.
    C. Sperm morphology is evaluated using 400X (high-power) magnification.
    D. Normal seminal fluid contains at least 80 percent sperm with normal morphology.

12. **Which of the following parameters directly relates to and provides a check of the spermatozoa motility evaluation?**

    A. The agglutination evaluation
    B. The concentration determination
    C. The morphology assessment
    D. The viability assessment

13. **Microscopically, immature spermatogenic cells are often difficult to distinguish from**

    A. bacteria.
    B. erythrocytes.
    C. leukocytes.
    D. epithelial cells.

14. **A seminal fluid pH greater than 7.8 is associated with**

    A. premature ejaculation.
    B. obstruction of the vas deferens.
    C. abnormal seminal vesicle function.
    D. infection of the male reproductive tract.

15. **Fructose in seminal fluid assists in the evaluation of which of the following?**

    1. The secretory function of the seminal vesicles
    2. The functional integrity of the epididymis
    3. The functional integrity of the vas deferens
    4. The secretory function of the prostate gland

       A. 1, 2, and 3 are correct.
       B. 1 and 3 are correct.
       C. 4 is correct.
       D. All are correct.

16. **Which of the following can be used to evaluate the secretory function of the prostate gland?**

    A. Carnitine
    B. Fructose
    C. pH
    D. Zinc

17. **The concentration of which of the following substances can be used to positively identify a fluid as seminal fluid?**

    A. Acid phosphatase
    B. Citric acid
    C. Fructose
    D. Zinc

Amniotic Fluid Analysis

LEARNING OBJECTIVES

After studying this chapter, the student should be able to

1. Discuss amniotic fluid formation and the interactive role the fetus has in the amniotic fluid's composition.

2. State at least four indications for performing an amniocentesis and the stage in pregnancy best suited for each analysis.

3. Identify at least four sources of error in amniotic-fluid testing caused by inappropriate specimen handling or chemical contamination.

4. Differentiate amniotic fluid from urine.

5. Compare and contrast the following tests for fetal pulmonary maturity:
   - the lecithin/sphingomyelin ratio
   - phosphatidylglycerol
   - foam stability index
   - microviscosity by fluorescence polarization

6. Describe the analysis of bilirubin in the amniotic fluid (ΔA_{450}) and this value's relationship to fetal distress.

KEY TERMS

erythroblastosis fetalis: a hemolytic disease of the newborn that results from a blood group incompatibility between the mother and the infant.

fluorescence polarization: an analytical technique based on the change in polarization observed in fluorescent light emitted compared to the incident polarized fluorescent light. The observed changes in the polarization of light directly result from the molecular size of the fluorophore-tagged complex. Large molecules cannot randomly orient as rapidly as small molecules. Hence, fluorophores tagged to large molecular complexes will emit more fluorescence in the same polarized plane as the initial incident light than will fluorophores tagged to small molecular complexes.

hydramnios (also called **polyhydramnios**): an abnormally increased amount of amniotic fluid in the amniotic sac. It is often associated with central nervous system or gastrointestinal tract malformations of the fetus.

meconium: a dark green, gelatinous or mucus-like material representing swallowed amniotic fluid and intestinal secretions that is excreted by the near-term or full-term infant. The infant normally passes meconium as the first bowel movement shortly after birth.

oligohydramnios: a decreased amount of amniotic fluid in the amniotic sac.

With the use of ultrasound, amniocentesis is now a common and safe obstetric procedure. Advancements in technology have provided new technical methods and clinical applications for amniotic fluid analysis. The study of amniotic fluid is primarily performed for three reasons: to allow antenatal diagnosis of genetic and congenital disorders early in fetal gestation (at 15 to 18 weeks), and, later in the pregnancy (at 20 to 42 weeks), to assess fetal pulmonary maturity or to estimate the degree of fetal distress owing to isoimmunization or infection. By far the most frequently performed tests in the routine clinical laboratory evaluate the amniotic fluid for fetal pulmonary maturity and fetal distress, and these are discussed in this chapter. The detection of numerous inherited metabolic disorders and chromosomal abnormalities requires specialized laboratory techniques and is beyond the intent and scope of this text.

Physiology and Composition

Function

Amniotic fluid is the liquid medium that bathes the fetus throughout its gestation (Fig. 12–1). The amnion, a membrane composed of a single layer of cuboidal epithelial cells, surrounds the fetus and is filled with this fluid. Amniotic fluid serves several functions. It protects the fetus and enables fetal movement, and it plays a role in various biochemical processes. Fetal cellular constituents and numerous biochemical compounds, such as electrolytes, nitrogenous compounds, proteins, enzymes, lipids, and hormones, are present in the amniotic fluid. Although studies have investigated many substances as potential biochemical markers of disease, relatively few substances have demonstrated reliable clinical utility (e.g., phospholipids).

Formation

The dynamics of amniotic fluid formation and its composition change throughout fetal gestation. Initially, amniotic fluid is produced by the amnion and the placenta, and its composition is similar to a dialysate of plasma. As gestation progresses, however, the fetus plays more of an active role in the fluid's composition. Water and solutes exchange between the fetus and its surrounding medium through several mechanisms: 1) intestinal ab-

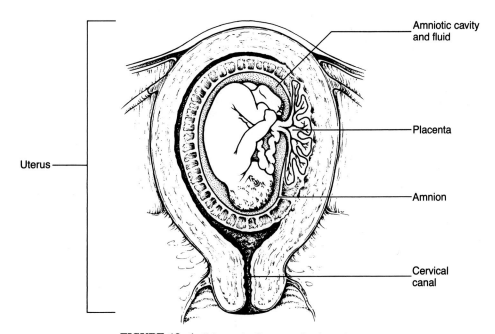

Amniotic cavity and fluid

Placenta

Amnion

Cervical canal

Uterus

FIGURE 12–1. Schematic diagram of a fetus in utero.

sorption following fetal swallowing of amniotic fluid; 2) capillary exchange in the pulmonary system, as the alveoli of the fetus' lungs are bathed with amniotic fluid; and 3) fetal urination. Early in gestation (before the keratinization of the skin), a transudate passes through the skin of the fetus and makes a small contribution to the amniotic fluid volume. Because of fetal respiration of amniotic fluid in utero, fetal pulmonary surfactants produced by the alveolar epithelial cells of the fetus' lungs mix with and can be evaluated from the amniotic fluid. In the later stages of pregnancy, fetal swallowing and urination play a major role in the volume and composition of the amniotic fluid. Water and electrolytes removed by the fetus from the amniotic fluid are replaced with metabolic by-products such as urea, creatinine, and uric acid. In addition to the exchange between the amniotic fluid and the fetus, a comparable exchange between the amniotic fluid and the maternal plasma results in a complete exchange of the amniotic fluid volume every 2 to 3 hours (Greene, 1987).

Volume

The volume of amniotic fluid increases steadily throughout pregnancy, from approximately 25 to 50 mL at 12 weeks' gestation to a maximum volume of 1100 to 1500 mL at 36 weeks' gestation. Abnormally increased amounts of amniotic fluid, termed **hydramnios,** is associated with decreased fetal swallowing and often indicates congenital fetal malformations. Abnormally decreased amounts of amniotic fluid, termed **oligohydramnios,** can occur with congenital malformations and other conditions, such as the premature rupture of the membranes.

Specimen Collection

The Timing of and Indications for Amniocentesis

Amniotic fluid is collected either transabdominally or vaginally with simultaneous ultrasonic examination. Using real-time ultra-

sound allows the clinician to identify a maternal tapping site that will yield amniotic fluid and at the same time avoid injury to the fetus or the placenta. Transabdominal amniocentesis is preferred because vaginal amniocentesis is associated with an increased risk of infection and can also result in the contamination of the fluid with vaginal cells and bacteria. Normally, amniocentesis can be performed anytime after 14 weeks' gestation; however, the purpose of performing the procedure usually dictates when it is to be done (Table 12-1). For example, an amniocentesis for the purpose of genetic studies is usually performed between 15 and 18 weeks' gestation. This allows enough time for culture of the fetal cells recovered from the amniotic fluid, performance of chromosomal and biochemical studies, and consideration of pregnancy termination if the fetus is determined to be abnormal. An amniocentesis later in pregnancy is used to assess the health status of the fetus, because several maternal conditions can adversely affect fetal health such as rhesus factor (Rh) isoimmunization, toxemia, and diabetes mellitus. Often these conditions necessitate early termination of a pregnancy and the delivery of a premature infant. If results indicate an immature fetal pulmonary system, elective delivery can be

TABLE 12-1. INDICATIONS FOR AMNIOCENTESIS

When to Perform Amniocentesis	Indications
14 to 18 weeks	Mother's age is 35 years or more
	Parent with known chromosomal abnormality
	Previous child with chromosomal abnormality
	Previous child with a neural tube defect
	Parent is a carrier of a metabolic disorder
	Elevated maternal alpha-fetoprotein
20 to 42 weeks	Assessment of fetal distress owing to
	• Rh or other isiommunization
	• Infection
	Assessment of fetal pulmonary maturity

postponed or premature labor suppressed. Amniocentesis provides a means of determining the maturity of the fetal pulmonary system by analyzing the surfactants present in the amniotic fluid.

Collection and Specimen Containers

Using aseptic technique, the physician pierces the abdominal and uterine walls with a long sterile needle and aspirates approximately 10 to 20 mL of amniotic fluid into several sterile syringes. A series of numbered syringes (usually two or three) are used to prevent contamination of the entire collection with blood that can be encountered initially. The blood can originate from piercing of a blood vessel in the maternal abdominal wall or the myometrium of the uterus, or from piercing of the placenta, umbilical cord, or fetus. Ideally, the amniotic fluid will show no evidence of blood.

Immediately following its collection, the amniotic fluid should be carefully transferred into sterile plastic containers for transport to the laboratory. Glass containers should be avoided because cells tend to adhere to glass. Amber-colored containers or aluminum foil should be used to protect the specimen from light, thereby preventing the photo-oxidation of bilirubin if present. The amniotic fluid must be processed aseptically if cytogenetic or microbial studies are to be performed.

Specimen Transport, Storage, and Centrifugation

Transporting of the specimen to the laboratory should take place as soon as possible to ensure the preservation of both cellular and biochemical constituents. Specimens for cell culture and chromosomal studies must be maintained at body or room temperature, whereas those for phospholipid analysis should be transported on ice. Maintaining amniotic fluid at room temperature without centrifugation can result in a significant loss of phospholipids (e.g., lecithin and sphingomyelin) because of cellular metabolic processes. If the fluid is centrifuged at $500 \times g$ and the supernatant removed, the phospholipids are not significantly metabolized. Therefore, all amniotic fluid specimens for chemical analysis that must be stored for any length of time should be centrifuged. If storage for more than 24 hours is necessary, the specimen should be frozen.

The speed and duration of centrifugation can significantly alter the composition of the amniotic fluid supernatant and pellet. Low centrifuge speeds (approximately $140 \times g$) are used for recovering fetal cells from amniotic fluid for cell culture. A centrifugation speed of $500 \times g$ is used to prepare the supernatant for the analysis of amniotic fluid phospholipids. Higher centrifugation speeds are associated with a loss of phospholipids into the pellet and erroneous lecithin/sphingomyelin results. For spectrophotometric assays, centrifugation speeds of 1500 to $2000 \times g$ for 5 to 15 minutes are used to maximally clear the supernatant of turbidity. If desired, the laboratorian can also filter the specimen to remove residual turbidity, but this can result in a significant loss of sample volume.

Differentiation from Urine

At times it may be necessary to determine if the fluid collected is actually amniotic fluid or if it is urine aspirated from the bladder. Physical examination alone will not distinguish them because urine can have the same appearance as amniotic fluid. Urine contains characteristically high concentrations of creatinine and urea, and essentially no protein or glucose. In contrast, amniotic fluid contains protein (approximately 2 to 8 g/L) and glucose. Hence, these substances serve as a means of positively identifying the fluid collected. Amniotic fluid has creatinine values similar to those of normal plasma. Late in pregnancy (approximately 37 or more weeks' gestation), however, as fetal renal function gradually begins, the amniotic fluid creatinine value can be two to three times that of normal plasma. Nevertheless, if creatinine values are greater than 4 mg/dL, the fluid collected is either urine or amniotic fluid contaminated with urine. Similarly, if a reagent strip test for glucose and protein is used, a positive test result identifies the fluid collected as amniotic fluid. These latter results should be confirmed with a creatinine or urea determination because diabetes and renal disease can cause protein and glucose to be present in the urine.

Physical Examination

Color

The physical examination of amniotic fluid should take place immediately after its receipt in the laboratory. The examination consists of a visual assessment of the fluid's color and turbidity. Normally, amniotic fluid is colorless or very pale yellow. Distinctive yellow or amber coloration is associated with the presence of bilirubin, whereas a green color indicates the presence of meconium. **Meconium** is a gelatinous or mucus-like material resulting from swallowed amniotic fluid and intestinal secretions by the fetal intestine. Biliverdin is responsible for meconium's dark green color. Meconium is normally excreted as the first bowel movement of term infants.

Blood contamination can cause amniotic fluid to appear anywhere from pinkish to red. If blood is present in the amniotic fluid sample, the specimen should be centrifuged immediately to remove any intact red blood cells before hemolysis occurs. Hemolysis results in the formation of oxyhemoglobin, which can interfere with several biochemical tests.

Turbidity

All amniotic fluid is turbid to some degree depending on the stage of pregnancy. Early in pregnancy, little particulate matter is present; hence, the fluid is not very turbid. As pregnancy progresses, however, increased amounts of fetal cells, hair, and vernix are sloughed and remain suspended in the amniotic fluid. Either centrifugation or filtration can be used to remove the particulate matter causing the fluid's turbidity.

Chemical Examination

Fetal Lung Maturity Tests

When premature delivery is anticipated or desired because of fetal distress or various complications of pregnancy, it is important to ensure that the fetus will be viable outside of the mother's uterus. The measurement of various analytes, the microscopic examination of the amniotic fluid epithelial cells, and an ultrasound examination have all been used to evaluate fetal maturity. To date, no single test or procedure is able to unequivocally ascertain that a fetus is mature. Because the pulmonary system is one of the last systems to mature, however, tests that evaluate the lungs' functional status are primarily used to assess fetal maturity and viability.

Respiratory distress syndrome (RDS) is the most common cause of death in the newborn and the primary concern when a preterm delivery is imminent. RDS results from an insufficient production of surfactant at the alveolar surfaces in the newborn's lungs. Normally, alveolar epithelial cells of the lungs produce and secrete lipid and protein compounds that act as surfactants, thus preventing the collapse of the alveoli at expiration and reducing the amount of pressure required to open the alveoli at inspiration. Gluck and Kulovich discovered the correlation between fetal lung maturity and the concentrations of specific phospholipids in amniotic fluid (Gluck, 1971). Despite the many phospholipids present in amniotic fluid, currently only three phospholipids are routinely used to evaluate fetal lung maturity — lecithin (phosphatidylcholine), sphingomyelin, and phosphatidylglycerol.

Lecithin/Sphingomyelin (L/S) Ratio and Phosphatidylglycerol

Lecithin is the major pulmonary surfactant; in contrast, the role of sphingomyelin, found in numerous cell membranes, has yet to be established. Until approximately 33 weeks' gestation, lecithin and sphingomyelin are produced by the fetal pulmonary system in relatively equal concentrations. At 34 to 36 weeks' gestation, the concentration of sphingomyelin decreases in the amniotic fluid, whereas that of lecithin significantly increases (Fig. 12–2). These observations led to the calculation of the lecithin/sphingomyelin (L/S) ratio and its subsequent use in evaluating fetal pulmonary status.

An L/S ratio less than 2.0 is associated with immaturity of the fetal pulmonary system, whereas one equal to or greater than 2.0 indicates fetal pulmonary system maturity. These values depend on the thin-layer chromatography (TLC) procedure used in determining the relative concentrations of the phospholipids. Numerous variations of the original TLC procedure exist; hence, the assessment of fetal lung maturity requires a comparison of the L/S ratio obtained to the criteria established at each institution performing the procedure. Because lecithin and sphingomyelin are also present in blood and meconium, amniotic fluid specimens contaminated with these substances are of limited value and must be interpreted with caution.

The L/S ratio is a better predictor of fetal lung maturity than of immaturity. In other words, a few infants (2 percent to 5 percent) with an L/S ratio greater than 2.0 still develop RDS, despite a "mature" L/S ratio. In contrast, 30 percent to 40 percent of infants with an L/S ratio between 1.5 and 2.0 will not develop RDS and are falsely identi-

fied as having an "immature" pulmonary system.

Phosphatidylglycerol (PG), another lipid component of the pulmonary surfactants, is normally not detectable in amniotic fluid until 35 weeks' gestation. It can be measured using the same TLC procedures as lecithin and sphingomyelin, or by agglutination slide tests. Even though the rapid and simple semi-quantitative slide tests are specific for PG, they produce a high number of false negative results. Therefore, positive slide test results can indicate pulmonary maturity, but the value of a negative slide test result is questionable. Measurement of PG, however, is more sensitive and reliable using TLC methods. A distinct advantage of PG detection tests, regardless of the method used, is that results are not affected by the presence of blood or meconium in the amniotic fluid.

Along with the L/S ratio, PG detection assists the physician in evaluating complicated pregnancies, particularly in patients with diabetes mellitus. Studies have shown that in pregnant women with diabetes mellitus, when the L/S ratio is greater than 2.0 and PG is absent, a significant number of infants still develop RDS. In contrast, if PG is present, there is essentially no risk for the infants' development of RDS. Another advantage to PG detection is that its detection is not affected by the presence of blood or meconium in the amniotic fluid, in contrast to the L/S ratio, which must be interpreted with care if these substances are present. In summary, the simultaneous determination of both the L/S ratio and the presence of PG is currently the best means of assessing fetal maturity based on pulmonary surfactants.

Foam Stability Index (FSI)

Although the L/S ratio and PG detection are based on measurements of the chemical surfactants in the amniotic fluid, the FSI or "shake test" is based on the physical or functional characteristics that the surfactants impart to amniotic fluid. In other words, if adequate surfactants are present in the amniotic fluid, a foam can be produced by shaking vigorously with ethanol, and the bubbles will remain stable at the air-liquid

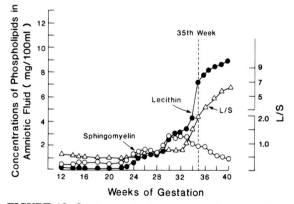

FIGURE 12–2. Changes in the concentrations of lecithin and sphingomyelin and changes in the lecithin/sphingomyelin ratio during normal pregnancy. (Adapted from Gluck L, Kulovich MV: Am J Obstet Gynecol 115:539–546, 1973.)

interface in the tube. Because this indirect assessment of surfactant concentration is rapid and easy to perform, it is frequently used when chromatographic methods are not available.

Determining the FSI involves mixing equal volumes of amniotic fluid with differing volumes of ethanol, followed by vigorous shaking. The concentration of ethanol in each tube represents the possible index values, ranging from 0.43 to 0.55. The highest concentration of ethanol with a "stable foam" present is the FSI for that specimen. A stable foam is one in which the bubbles remain around the entire meniscus of the tube 15 minutes after shaking. An FSI of 0.48 or greater correlates with fetal pulmonary maturity and is analogous to an L/S ratio of 2.0.

A significant disadvantage of the FSI is the inaccurate results obtained when blood or meconium contaminates the amniotic fluid. These substances cause a falsely high or "mature" index value, when in fact the amount of functional pulmonary surfactant present is inadequate. Therefore, a "mature" FSI (i.e., 0.48 or greater) obtained on a contaminated specimen is of no clinical value; in contrast, an "immature" index on a contaminated specimen is clinically useful, indicating inadequate pulmonary surfactant.

Microviscosity Tests

The microviscosity of amniotic fluid is related to the amount of pulmonary surfactants present. **Fluorescence polarization,** which measures microviscosity indirectly, can be used to evaluate the amniotic fluid content of pulmonary surfactant relative to albumin. In this assay technique, a fluorophore (i.e., fluorescent dye) is mixed with the amniotic fluid and becomes associated with albumin and with the liposomes of the surfactants (i.e., aggregates of phospholipids) present. Fluorophores associated with albumin are not able to rotate as freely as fluorophores associated with the surfactant liposomes; consequently, the measured fluorescence polarization is high in amniotic fluid containing low levels of surfactants. The ability of the fluorophore to rotate also depends on the surfac-

tant content of the liposomes that it associates with. Fluorophores with liposomes of high sphingomyelin content yield higher fluorescence polarization values than do fluorophores with liposomes of high lecithin content. Consequently, as the concentration of lecithin in amniotic fluid increases compared to the concentration of sphingomyelin (i.e., the L/S ratio is increasing) and as the concentration of surfactants relative to the albumin concentration increases, the microviscosity of the amniotic fluid decreases, as does the fluorescence polarization of an added fluorophore. Therefore, in this method, the amount of polarized fluorescent light emitted relates directly to the composition of the surfactants present in the amniotic fluid if the concentration of albumin remains unchanged. Because the amount of albumin normally present in amniotic fluid during the third trimester of pregnancy is constant, albumin serves as an internal standard against which the surfactant content is compared. By measuring microviscosity using fluorescence polarization and comparing it to a standard curve obtained using calibrators of known surfactant/albumin content, the concentration of surfactant/albumin in amniotic fluid can be determined.

Blood- and meconium-contaminated specimens cannot be accurately assessed by this method. In addition, amniotic fluid specimens should not be centrifuged prior to analysis because phospholipids can be removed during centrifugation, resulting in a falsely decreased surfactant/albumin ratio. If particulate matter needs to be separated from the amniotic fluid, filtration techniques should be used.

Amniotic Fluid Bilirubin (or ΔA_{450} Determination)

Normally throughout fetal gestation, the bilirubin concentration in the amniotic fluid is low and essentially undetectable (approximately 10 to 30 μg/dL). During normal erythrocyte destruction in the fetus, unconjugated bilirubin is produced and rapidly removed into the maternal circulation by the placenta.

Because the fetus has an immature liver, when a hemolytic disease process causes increased and persistent hemolysis of fetal erythrocytes, the production of unconjugated bilirubin is significantly increased. As a result, an increased amount of unconjugated bilirubin enters the amniotic fluid through a mechanism that remains unclear, and its presence is detectable spectrophotometrically. Hemolytic disease of the newborn, or **erythroblastosis fetalis,** is caused when maternal antibodies cross the placenta into the fetal circulation and destroy large numbers of fetal red blood cells. These isoimmune diseases can involve any erythrocyte antigen and indicate that, at some point during the current pregnancy or in a previous one, the maternal circulation was exposed to fetal blood cells and developed an antibody against them. By far the most commonly encountered hemolytic disease results from the sensitization of an Rh-negative mother to the Rh_o (D) antigen. Its prevalence has decreased significantly because of methods (e.g., Rh_o [D] immune globulin) currently available that prevent the Rh-negative mother from becoming sensitized to the Rh antigen.

The amount of bilirubin present in the amniotic fluid relates directly to the severity of hemolysis. When normal amniotic fluid is scanned spectrophotometrically from 350 to 580 nm, the spectral curve obtained is essentially a straight line between 365 and 550 nm that gradually decreases in absorbance (Fig. 12–3*A*). Bilirubin shows maximum absorbance at 450 nm. Therefore, as the concentration of bilirubin in the amniotic fluid increases, the absorbance of the spectral curve at 450 nm also increases proportionally (Fig. 12–3*B*). The ΔA_{450}, or the change in absorbance at 450 nm, is obtained by hand-drawing a straight baseline for the spectral curve between 365 and 550 nm and calculating the difference in absorbance (between the hand-drawn baseline and the spectral curve) at 450 nm (Fig. 12–3*C*).

From numerous studies performed in the 1950s and 1960s, a relationship between the amniotic fluid's ΔA_{450} and the severity of hemolytic disease was established (Liley, 1961). Using a semilogarithmic plot of the ΔA_{450} values against the fetal gestational age, three zones were determined to represent the severity of the hemolytic disease that the fetus is experiencing in utero (Fig. 12–4). Note that the ΔA_{450} values indicated by each zone decrease with increasing fetal gestational age. Therefore, before the ΔA_{450} can be evaluated, the gestational age must be known.

ΔA_{450} values that fall into zone I are considered normal, representing a minimally affected fetus. Zone II, the middle zone, represents moderate hemolysis. If repeated amniocentesis shows values increasing in zone II, however, then marked hemolysis is taking place. Values in the uppermost region, zone III, indicate that the fetus is experiencing severe hemolysis and will die without intervention. Currently, when an immunologic incompatibility between the fetus and the mother is suspected, amniocentesis is initially performed around 22 weeks' gestation and is repeated at periodic intervals thereafter. A decreasing ΔA_{450} in subsequent determinations is a good prognostic sign, whereas equivalent or increasing values indicate a worsening of the fetal health status.

Amniotic fluid specimens contaminated with blood are generally not acceptable because of interference caused by oxyhemoglobin absorbance peaks at 412 and 540 nm. If bloody specimens are processed immediately and the blood is removed before significant hemolysis has taken place, however, the spectral curve obtained may not be significantly affected. The magnitude of the oxyhemoglobin contamination can be determined by calculating the difference in the absorbance at 412 nm. If there is a significant overlap of the oxyhemoglobin and bilirubin absorbance curves, the ΔA_{450} results are not valid. Similarly, meconium-contaminated amniotic fluid specimens are not acceptable for ΔA_{450} measurements because meconium absorbs maximally between 350 and 400 nm. Both blood and meconium interfere with the drawing of the spectral baseline, and the ΔA_{450} results produced will indicate falsely low amounts of bilirubin in these contaminated specimens. Another source of error in bilirubin detection is not protecting the spec-

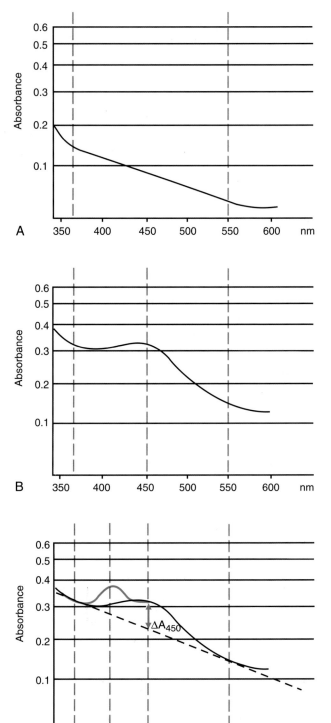

FIGURE 12-3. The determination of Δ A$_{450}$ in amniotic fluid. *A*, Normal amniotic fluid. *B*, Amniotic fluid with a bilirubin peak at 450 nm. *C*, Amniotic fluid with a bilirubin peak at 450 nm and contaminated with oxyhemoglobin, which peaks at 412 nm. The dashed line indicates the baseline drawn between the linear portions of the curve (i.e., between 365 and 550 nm). The red line indicates oxyhemoglobin absorbance.

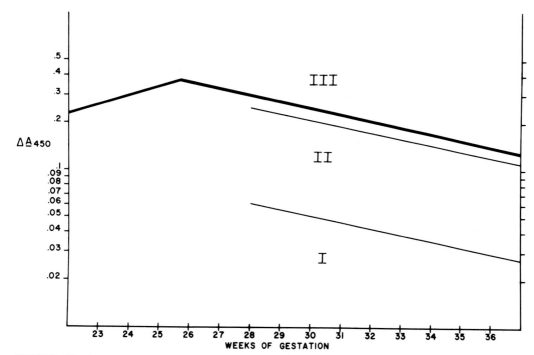

FIGURE 12–4. Liley's three-zone chart (with modification) for the interpretation of amniotic fluid ΔA_{450} values. The dark line extending from 22 to 38 weeks' gestation represents the upward revision of the "danger line" by Dr. Irving Umansky. (Redrawn from Reid DE, Ryan KJ, Benirschke K: Principles and Management of Human Reproduction, Philadelphia, W. B. Saunders Company, 1972.)

imen from light immediately following its collection and throughout its transport and processing. The loss of bilirubin owing to light exposure will also result in falsely low ΔA_{450} values.

References

Gluck L, Kulovich MV, et al.: Diagnosis of the respiratory distress syndrome by amniocentesis. Am J Obstet Gynecol 109:440–445, 1971.

Greene MF, Fencl MdeM, Tulchinsky D: Biochemical aspects of pregnancy. *In* Tietz NW (ed.): Fundamentals of Clinical Chemistry (3rd ed.), Philadelphia, W.B. Saunders Company, 1987, p. 917.

Liley AW: Liquor amnii analysis in the management of pregnancy complicated by rhesus sensitization. Am J Obstet Gynecol 82:1359–1370, 1961.

Bibliography

Amenta JS, Silverman JA: Amniotic fluid lecithin, phosphatidylglycerol, L/S ratio, and foam stability test in predicting respiratory distress in the newborn. Am J Clin Pathol 79:52–64, 1983.

Clements JA, Platzker ACG, et al.: Assessment of the risk of the respiratory-distress syndrome by a rapid test for surfactant in amniotic fluid. N Engl J Med 286:1077–1081, 1972.

Cox KH, Ross JBA, et al.: Fetal lung maturity assessed by fluorescence polarization: evaluation of predictive value correction for endogenous fluorescence, and comparison with L/S ratio. Clin Chem 29:346–349, 1983.

Freer DE, Statland BE: Measurement of amniotic fluid surfactant. Clin Chem 27:1629–1641, 1981.

Garite TJ, Yabusaki KK, et al.: A new rapid-slide agglutination test for amniotic fluid phosphatidylglycerol: laboratory and clinical correlation. Am J Obstet Gynecol 147:681–686, 1983.

Gluck L, Kulovich MV: Lecithin/sphingomyelin ratios in amniotic fluid in normal and abnormal pregnancies. Am J Obstet Gynecol 115:539–546, 1973.

Kjeldsberg CR, Knight JA: Body Fluids (2nd ed.), Chicago, American Society of Clinical Pathologists Press, 1986, pp. 1–30.

Liley AW. Errors in the assessment of hemolytic disease from amniotic fluid. Am J Obstet Gynecol 86:485–494, 1963.

Russell JC: A calibrated fluorescence polarization assay for assessment of fetal lung maturity. Clin Chem 33:1177–1184, 1987.

Russell PT: Pregnancy and fetal function. *In* Kaplan LA, Pesce AJ (eds.): Clinical Chemistry Theory, Analysis, and Correlation (2nd ed.), St. Louis, C. V. Mosby Company, 1989, pp. 569–586.

van Voorst tot Voorst EJGM. Effects of centrifugation, storage, and contamination of amniotic fluid on its total phospholipid content. Clin Chem 26:232–234, 1980.

Study Questions

1. **Which of the following is NOT a function of the amniotic fluid that surrounds a developing fetus?**

   A. It provides protection of the fetus.
   B. It enables the movement of the fetus.
   C. It is a medium for exchange of oxygen.
   D. It is a source of water and solute exchange.

2. **Amniocentesis is usually performed at 15 to 18 weeks' gestation to determine which of the following?**

   A. Fetal distress
   B. Fetal maturity
   C. Genetic disorders
   D. Infections in the amniotic fluid

3. **Through which of the following mechanism(s) does solute and water exchange occur between the fetus and the amniotic fluid?**

   1. Fetal swallowing of the amniotic fluid
   2. Transudation across the fetal skin
   3. Fetal urination into the amniotic fluid
   4. Respiration of amniotic fluid into the fetal pulmonary system

      A. 1, 2, and 3 are correct.
      B. 1 and 3 are correct.
      C. 4 is correct.
      D. All are correct.

4. **Select the term used to describe a decreased volume of amniotic fluid present in the amniotic sac.**

   A. Ahydramnios
   B. Hydramnios
   C. Oligohydramnios
   D. Polyhydramnios

5. **Amniotic fluid is immediately protected from light to preserve which of the following substances?**

   A. Bilirubin
   B. Fetal cells
   C. Meconium
   D. Phospholipids

6. **Which of the following substances, when present in amniotic fluid, is adversely affected by refrigeration?**

   A. Bilirubin
   B. Fetal cells
   C. Protein
   D. Phospholipids

7. **High centrifugation speeds in processing amniotic fluid must be avoided to prevent the loss of**

   A. bilirubin.
   B. fetal cells.
   C. meconium.
   D. phospholipids.

8. **Analysis for which of the following substances can aid in the differentiation of amniotic fluid from urine?**

   1. Urea
   2. Glucose
   3. Creatinine
   4. Protein

      A. 1, 2, and 3 are correct.
      B. 1 and 3 are correct.
      C. 4 is correct.
      D. All are correct.

9. **Which of the following statements about amniotic fluid is true?**

   A. Amniotic fluid is normally clear and colorless.
   B. Amniotic fluid normally contains fetal hair, cells, and vernix.
   C. Amniotic fluid and urine can be distinguished by a physical examination of the fluid.
   D. Amniotic fluid contaminated with meconium takes on a yellow or amber coloration.

10. **Which of the following is NOT a test to evaluate the surfactants present in the fetal pulmonary system?**

    A. ΔA_{450}
    B. Lecithin/sphingomyelin ratio
    C. Phosphatidylglycerol detection
    D. Foam stability index

11. **Which of the following test results would indicate fetal lung immaturity?**

    1. An L/S ratio of less than 2.0
    2. An L/S ratio of more than 2.0
    3. An L/S ratio of more than 2.0, with PG absent
    4. An L/S ratio of less than 2.0, with PG present

        A. 1, 2, and 3 are correct.
        B. 1 and 3 are correct.
        C. 4 is correct.
        D. All are correct.

12. **Which of the following causes erythroblastosis fetalis?**

    A. Immaturity of the fetal liver
    B. Decreased amounts of amniotic fluid
    C. Inadequate fetal pulmonary surfactants
    D. Maternal immunization by fetal antigens

13. **A ΔA_{450} value that falls into zone III indicates that the fetus is experiencing**

    A. no hemolysis.
    B. mild hemolysis.
    C. moderate hemolysis.
    D. severe hemolysis.

Cerebrospinal Fluid Analysis

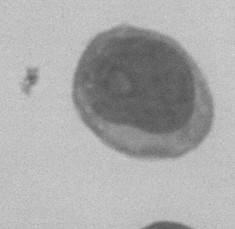
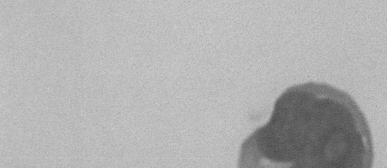

LEARNING OBJECTIVES

After studying this chapter, the student should be able to

1. Describe the formation of cerebrospinal fluid (CSF) and state at least three functions that the CSF performs.

2. Describe the procedure for lumbar puncture and the proper collection technique for CSF.

3. Discuss the importance of timely processing and testing of CSF and state at least three adverse effects of time delay on CSF specimens.

4. State the physical characteristics of normal CSF and discuss how each characteristic can be modified in disease states.

5. Discuss the clinical importance of the microscopic examination of CSF.

6. Compare and contrast the concentration of the following constituents of CSF in health and in disease states:
   - albumin
   - glucose
   - IgG
   - lactate
   - total protein

7. Describe briefly protein electrophoretic patterns of CSF and the abnormal presence of oligoclonal banding.

8. Calculate the CSF/serum albumin index and the CSF IgG index and state the clinical importance of each index.

9. Discuss the proper microbiologic examination of CSF and its importance in the diagnosis of infectious diseases of the central nervous system.

10. Explain briefly the role of CSF immunologic tests in the diagnosis of meningitis.

blood-brain barrier: the physiologic interface between the vascular system and the cerebrospinal fluid. Changes in the normal regulating conditions of the blood-brain barrier result in changes in the normal chemical and cellular composition of the cerebrospinal fluid.

cerebrospinal fluid (CSF): the normally clear, colorless fluid found between the arachnoid and pia mater in the brain and spinal cord. It is formed primarily from plasma by selective secretions of the choroid plexus and, to a lesser extent, by intrathecal synthesis by ependymal cells of the ventricles.

choroid plexus: the highly vascular folds of capillaries, nerves, and ependymal cells in the pia mater. Located in the four ventricles of the brain, the choroid plexus actively synthesizes cerebrospinal fluid.

meninges: the three membranes that surround the brain and spinal cord. The innermost membrane is the pia mater, the outermost membrane is the dura mater, and the centrally located membrane is the arachnoid mater.

meningitis: inflammation of the meninges.

oligoclonal bands: multiple discrete bands in the gamma region noted during electrophoresis of plasma or other body fluids (e.g., CSF).

pleocytosis: the presence of a greater than normal number of cells in the cerebrospinal fluid.

STAT: an abbreviation for the Latin word *statim*, which means "immediately."

subarachnoid space: the space between the arachnoid and the pia mater.

ventricles: the four fluid-filled cavities in the brain lined with ependymal cells. The choroid plexus is located here.

xanthochromia: the pink, orange, or yellowish discoloration of supernatant cerebrospinal fluid following centrifugation.

Physiology and Composition

Cerebrospinal fluid (CSF) bathes the brain and spinal cord. The CSF is produced primarily (70 percent) from secretions into the four **ventricles** of the brain by the highly vascular **choroid plexus** (vascular fringe-like folds in the pia mater). The ependymal cells that line the brain and spinal cord also play a minor role in the production of CSF. The formation of CSF can be described as a selective secretion from plasma, not as an ultrafiltrate. This is evidenced by higher CSF concentrations of some solutes (e.g., sodium, chloride, magnesium) and lower CSF concentrations of other solutes (e.g., potassium, total calcium) compared with plasma. If simple ultrafiltration were responsible for CSF production, these solute concentration differences would not exist.

The brain and spinal cord are surrounded by three membranes, collectively termed the **meninges.** The tough outermost membrane, the dura mater, is next to the bone. The arachnoid mater, or middle layer, derives its name from its visual resemblance to a spider web. The innermost membrane, the pia mater, adheres to the surface of the neural tissues (Fig. 13–1). CSF flows in the space between the arachnoid and the pia mater, called the **subarachnoid space,** where it bathes and protects the delicate tissues of the central nervous system. From its initial formation in the ventricles, the CSF circulates to the brain stem and spinal cord, principally through pressure changes caused by postural, respiratory, and circulatory pressures (Fig. 13–2). It eventually flows in the subarachnoid space to the top outer surface of the brain and is reabsorbed into the blood via small one-way valves in the arachnoid villi. CSF formation, circulation, and reabsorption into the blood make up a dynamic process that constantly turns over about 20 mL each hour (McComb, 1983). If the flow path between CSF's production and its reabsorption into the blood is obstructed for any reason, CSF will accumulate, producing hydrocephalus; the intracranial pressure can in-

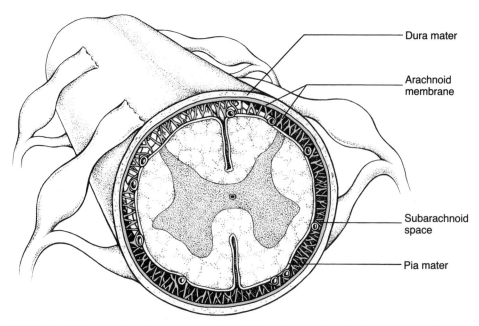

FIGURE 13-1. A schematic representation of the spinal cord and the meninges that surround it.

Dura mater

Arachnoid membrane

Subarachnoid space

Pia mater

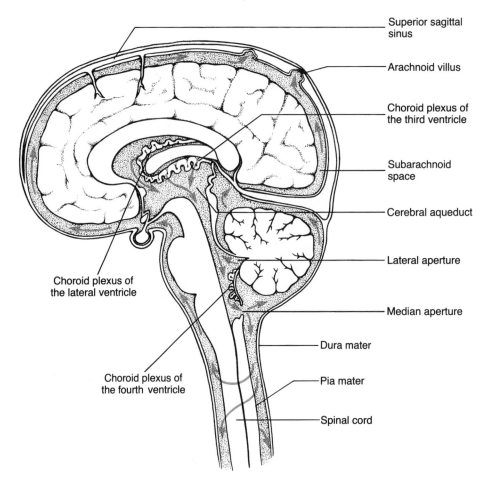

Superior sagittal sinus

Arachnoid villus

Choroid plexus of the third ventricle

Subarachnoid space

Cerebral aqueduct

Lateral aperture

Median aperture

Dura mater

Pia mater

Spinal cord

Choroid plexus of the lateral ventricle

Choroid plexus of the fourth ventricle

FIGURE 13-2. A schematic representation of the brain and spinal cord, including the circulation of the cerebrospinal fluid.

crease, causing brain damage, mental retardation, or death if left untreated. Normally, the total volume of CSF in an adult ranges from 85 to 150 mL. The volume in neonates is significantly smaller, ranging from 10 to 60 mL.

The CSF protects and supports the brain and spinal cord, and provides a medium for the transport and exchange of nutrients and metabolic wastes. The capillary endothelium in contact with the CSF enables the transfer of substances from the blood into the CSF and vice versa. This capillary endothelium differs from the endothelium in other tissues by the presence of tight junctions between adjacent endothelial cells. These tight junctions significantly reduce the extracellular passage of substances from the blood plasma into the CSF. In other words, all substances that enter or leave the CSF must pass through the membranes and cytoplasm of the capillary endothelial cells. This modulating interface between the blood and the CSF is called the **blood-brain barrier** and accounts for the observed concentration differences of electrolytes, proteins, and other solutes. An example of the selectivity and effectiveness of this blood-brain barrier is the failure of some antibiotics (e.g., penicillins), given intravenously, to enter the CSF, although these antibiotics freely penetrate all other tissues of the body.

In healthy individuals, the chemical composition of CSF is closely regulated and includes low-molecular-weight proteins. Changes in this chemical composition or in the cellular components present can aid in the diagnosis of disease. Protein, glucose, and lactate are routinely measured in CSF. Although numerous other parameters (e.g., sodium, potassium, chloride, magnesium, pH, PCO_2, enzymes) have been evaluated for diagnostic use, they have yet to prove their diagnostic value. In addition to chemical analysis, CSF is routinely cultured for microbial organisms, examined microscopically to evaluate the cellular components present, and tested for the presence of specific antigens. These cytologic, microbiologic, and immunologic studies can provide valuable diagnostic information.

Specimen Collection

CSF specimens are collected specifically for the diagnosis or treatment of disease (Table 13–1). Although the lumbar puncture principally used to obtain CSF specimens is fairly routine, it involves significant patient discomfort, and it may cause complications. Therefore, once a CSF specimen has been collected, it is imperative that it is properly labeled and handled both at the bedside and in the laboratory.

Usually the physician performs the lumbar puncture in the third or fourth lumbar interspace (or lower) in adults or the fourth or fifth interspace in children (Fig. 13–3). The puncture site selection can vary if an infection is present at the preferred site. A locally infected site must be avoided to prevent introduction of the infection into the central nervous system. The lumbar puncture

TABLE 13–1. INDICATIONS AND CONTRAINDICATIONS FOR LUMBAR PUNCTURE AND CSF EXAMINATION

INDICATIONS
Infections
   Meningitis
   Encephalitis
   Brain abscess
Hemorrhage
   Subarachnoid
   Intracerebral
Neurologic disease
   Multiple sclerosis
   Guillain-Barré syndrome
Malignancy
   Leukemia
   Lymphoma
   Metastatic carcinoma
Tumor
   Brain
   Spinal cord
Treatments
   Chemotherapy
   Anesthetics
   Radiographic contrast media
   Antibiotic therapy

CONTRAINDICATIONS
Septicemia
Systemic infections
Localized lumbar infection

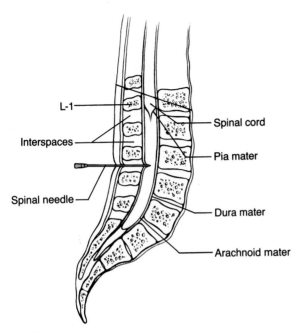

FIGURE 13-3. A schematic representation of a lumbar puncture procedure.

procedure is performed aseptically after thorough cleansing of the patient's skin and the application of a local anesthetic. The spinal needle is advanced into the lumbar interspace, and often a "pop" is heard as the dura mater is penetrated. Immediately after the dura mater has been entered and before any CSF has been removed, the physician takes the initial or "opening" pressure of the CSF using a manometer that attaches to the spinal needle. Normal CSF pressures for an adult in a lateral recumbent position range from 50 to 180 mm Hg, with slightly higher pressures obtained from individuals in a sitting position. If the pressure is in the normal range, up to 20 mL of CSF (approximately 15 percent of the estimated total CSF volume) can be removed safely. If the CSF pressure is less than or greater than normal, only 1 to 2 mL should be removed. Because the total volume of CSF is significantly smaller in infants and children, proportionally smaller volumes are collected from them. After the CSF has been removed and before the spinal needle has been withdrawn, the physician takes the "closing" CSF pressure. Both CSF pressure values and the amount of CSF removed are recorded in the patient's chart.

As CSF is collected, it is dispensed into three (or more) sequentially labeled sterile collection tubes. The first tube is used for chemical and immunologic testing, because any minimal blood contamination resulting from vessel injury during the initial tap normally does not affect these results. The second tube is used for microbial testing, and the third tube is reserved for the microscopic examination of cellular components (i.e., red and white blood cell counts and cytology studies). If only a small amount of CSF is obtained and a single collection tube must be used, the ordering physician prioritizes the tests desired. With these low-volume specimens, the microbiology laboratory receives the specimen first, to ensure the culturing of a sterile specimen. Cell counts, followed by chemical and immunologic testing, should immediately follow the microbiological examination.

The examination and testing of CSF should take place as soon as possible after its collection. Therefore, in most institutions, tests ordered on CSF specimens are considered **STAT.** Delay in testing can cause inaccurate results, such as falsely low cell counts owing to the lysis of white blood cells or falsely high lactate levels owing to glycolysis. In addition, the recovery of viable microbial organisms is jeopardized. When delay is unavoidable, each CSF collection tube must be stored at the temperature that will best ensure the recovery of the constituents of interest (Table 13-2). Any CSF remaining after the initial tests have been performed should be frozen and saved for possible future chemical or immunologic studies.

Physical Examination

Normal CSF is clear and colorless, with a viscosity similar to that of water. Increased viscosity, although rare, can occur as a result of metastatic, mucin-secreting adenocarcinomas. Abnormally increased amounts of fibrinogen in CSF owing to a compromised blood-brain barrier can result in clot formation. Fine delicate clots can form a thin film or pellicle on the surface of CSF after it has been stored

TABLE 13-2. CSF SPECIMEN PROCESSING TEMPERATURE

Chemical and immunologic testing (Tube #1)	Frozen (−15 to −30°C)
Microbiologic studies (Tube #2)	Room temperature (19 to 26°C)
Cell counts and cytology (Tube #3)	Refrigerated (2 to 8°C)

at refrigerator temperatures for 12 or more hours. Most often, clot formation is associated with a traumatic puncture procedure, in which blood and plasma proteins contaminated the CSF. Rarely, no blood is present in the CSF, and clots form as a result of elevated CSF protein with conditions such as Froin syndrome or suppurative or tuberculous meningitis, or as a result of subarachnoid obstruction. Despite the various possibilities for clot formation, clots are rarely encountered even in patients with pathologic conditions. If present, however, clot formation must be noted and reported.

The clarity or turbidity of CSF will depend on its cellularity. **Pleocytosis,** an increase in the number of cells in the CSF, will cause it to appear cloudy to varying degrees. A cloudy CSF specimen is associated with a white blood cell count greater than 200/μL or a red blood cell count exceeding 400/μL. Similarly, microorganisms or an increased protein content can produce cloudy CSF specimens. CSF clarity can be graded semiquantitatively from 0 (clear) to 4+ (newsprint cannot be read through the fluid) using standardized criteria, e.g., the same volume of CSF, the same-diameter clear glass tube. Occasionally, the CSF will appear oily owing to the presence of radiographic contrast media.

Although normal CSF is colorless, in disease states it often appears xanthochromic. Although **xanthochromia** literally means a yellow discoloration, this term is applied to a spectrum of CSF discolorations, including pink, orange, and yellow. A pink supernatant after centrifugation results from oxyhemoglobin, a yellow supernatant results from bilirubin, an orange supernatant results from a combination of these, and a brownish supernatant results from methemoglobin formation. High concentrations of other substances, such as carotene, and protein in concentrations greater than 150 mg/dL, can also cause xanthochromic CSF specimens, as can conditions such as meningeal melanoma or the collection of the CSF 2 to 5 days after a traumatic tap (Table 13-3).

Gross blood in the CSF is visually apparent, and determining its source requires differentiation between a traumatic puncture procedure and a subarachnoid or intracerebral hemorrhage. A couple of observations can be used to make this differentiation. A traumatic tap results in the greatest amount of blood collected in the first specimen tube. Hence, a visual assessment or a comparison of the red blood cell counts obtained in each collection tube will be significantly different. In contrast, a hemorrhage results in a homogeneous distribution of red blood cells throughout all collection tubes. Secondly, following centrifugation of the CSF, a colorless supernatant indicates a traumatic tap, whereas a xanthochromic supernatant reveals a hemorrhage, because about 1 to 2 hours are needed for red blood cells to lyse in CSF (Marton, 1986). The lysis of red blood cells observed in CSF is not osmotically induced because plasma and CSF are osmotically equivalent; rather, it is speculated that the lack of sufficient CSF proteins and lipids needed to stabilize red blood cell membranes causes the lysis. Because lysis can occur in vivo or in vitro, timely processing and testing

TABLE 13-3. CAUSES OF XANTHOCHROMIA IN CSF

Hemorrhage, subarachnoid or intracerebral
Hyperbilirubinemia
Hypercarotenemia
Meningeal melanoma
Normal neonate*
Protein concentration exceeding 150 mg/dL
Previous traumatic tap

* Xanthochromia in neonates results from a combination of increased bilirubin and increased protein owing to immaturity in the blood-brain barrier.

of CSF specimens is necessary. Once red cell lysis has occurred in CSF, xanthochromia, owing initially to oxyhemoglobin and later to bilirubin, will be evident for as long as 4 weeks. Lastly, when the microscopic examination of the CSF reveals macrophages with phagocytosed red blood cells, a hemorrhage has taken place. These erythrophagocytic cells may persist for 4 to 8 weeks following a hemorrhage, will stain positive for hemosiderin, and may include hematoidin crystals.

Because a CSF specimen is collected into three or more specimen tubes and all tubes may not be sent to the same laboratory, each tube must be physically examined and individually assessed for color, clarity, and volume by the testing laboratory.

Microscopic Examination

The CSF of adults normally contains a small number of lymphocytes and monocytes, 0 to 5 cells/μL. Similar low numbers of leukocytes (0 to 10 cells/μL) are expected in children, whereas normal neonates can have up to 30 monocytes and other types of leukocytes/μL, with monocytes predominating. In contrast, red blood cells are not normally present in the CSF. When present, they most often represent CSF contamination with peripheral blood during the lumbar puncture procedure. Rarely, they are present because of a recent (within 1 or 2 hours) subarachnoid or cerebral hemorrhage.

Cell counts on CSF must be performed as soon as possible to ensure the validity of the results. At room temperature, 40 percent of the leukocytes present in CSF will lyse in 2 hours (Chow, 1984). If the specimen is refrigerated, the lysis of leukocytes can be significantly reduced to approximately 15 percent, but not completely prevented. Similarly, erythrocytes do not demonstrate significant lysis at 4°C; therefore, the CSF collection tube for cell counts should be refrigerated if the count must be delayed for any reason.

Depending on the testing institution, different approaches to CSF cell counts are possible. Some laboratories do not perform a total cell count; instead, they perform individual erythrocyte and leukocyte counts. The sum of these two counts is equivalent to a total cell count. In other laboratories, a total cell count and a leukocyte count are performed; the difference between them is the erythrocyte count.

Total Cell Count

Because the number of cells in CSF is normally very low and electronic cell counters are inaccurate in this range (the instrument's background count is higher than the cell count), total cell counts on CSF are performed manually using a hemacytometer. Appendix C describes a procedure for performing cell counts using a hemacytometer. A method for preparing simulated CSF specimens for quality control and teaching purposes was developed by Lofsness and Jensen (Lofsness, 1983).

Total cell counts on CSF are usually made using well-mixed, undiluted CSF. Because of the low viscosity and protein content of CSF, cells settle within 1 minute after filling the hemacytometer chambers. When cells are crowded or overlapping, a dilution of the CSF with saline must be made and used for total cell counting. Dilutions vary according to the concentration of cells present, ranging from a 1:10 dilution for a slightly cloudy specimen to a 1:10,000 dilution for bloody specimens.

Erythrocyte (Red Blood Cell) Count

Erythrocyte counts provide very little diagnostically useful information. They may be performed to aid in the differentiation of a recent hemorrhage from a traumatic puncture procedure, as previously discussed. Another application of the red blood cell count is to correct the white blood cell count and total protein determinations obtained from a CSF specimen known to be contaminated with peripheral blood. These calculated "corrections" have limited accuracy, usually overcorrect the counts, assume that all of the red blood cells present result from contamination, and have little clinical utility. Therefore, this chapter does not describe these corrections in detail; readers are referred to the bibliography for additional information.

As with the total cell count, well-mixed, undiluted CSF is used for the red blood cell count unless the number of cells present requires a dilution owing to cell overlapping and crowding. Because the differentiation between small lymphocytes and crenated erythrocytes can be difficult in unstained wet preparations, some laboratories eliminate this count, replacing it with the difference obtained between the total cell count and the leukocyte count.

Leukocyte (White Blood Cell) Count

Increased CSF leukocyte counts are found in patients with diseases of the central nervous system as well as with a variety of other conditions (Table 13–4). The leukocyte count can vary significantly depending on the etiologic agent. Often the highest CSF leukocyte counts (greater than $50,000/\mu L$) are seen in patients with bacterial meningitis, whereas other patients with the same condition may show no pleocytosis (Fishbein, 1981).

To enhance the visualization of white blood cell nuclei and to eliminate any erythrocytes present, the CSF is exposed to glacial acetic acid before the hemacytometer chambers are filled, and approximately 3 to 5 minutes is allowed for the lysis of erythrocytes. With their nuclei more readily apparent, as the white blood cells are counted they can also be classified as mononuclear or polymorphonuclear cells. This classification of leukocytes during the count, or "chamber differential," has poor precision and is unsatisfactory for reporting; however, it provides a preliminary indication of the cell types present. When the cell numbers are such that a dilution is required for white blood cell counting, an acetic acid and stain (e.g., crystal violet) mixture can be used as the diluent, which enhances the visualization of and facilitates the classification of white blood cells.

Differential Cell Count

Techniques

Useful diagnostic information is provided by a differential cell count. Normally, lymphocytes and monocytes predominate in the CSF, with the percentages of each differing for adults and neonates (Table 13–5). A normal range for children 2 months old to 18 years old has yet to be established because of limited data. Before cytocentrifuge techniques were employed, any neutrophils present were considered abnormal. Currently, with the increased cell recovery obtained using cytospin preparations, neutrophil counts below 10 percent are considered normal (Novak, 1984).

To perform a differential count of the cells present in CSF requires the laboratorian to 1) concentrate the cells; 2) prepare a smear of the concentrate on a microscope slide; and 3) stain the preparation with Wright's stain. Essentially four techniques are available to concentrate the CSF, each having unique advantages and disadvantages. The simplest and most inexpensive technique is centrifugation of the specimen, but cell recovery is variable and cells become damaged and distorted by the high-speed centrifugation. Although sedimentation methods preserve cellular morphology, cell recovery is not very good. In contrast, filtration techniques using commercial filters (e.g., from manufacturers Millipore Corp., Nucleopore, Gelman Instrument Co.) have excellent cellular recovery (approximately 90 percent); however, these techniques are time-consuming, and preparation of a suitable smear requires significant technical skill. On the other hand, the cytocentrifuge technique has good cellular recovery and preservation. It is a rapid and technically simple procedure to perform. Despite the disadvantage of several known cellular distortions that can occur when cytospin specimens are prepared, this technique is currently the most widely used.

Pleocytosis

NEUTROPHILS. With bacterial **meningitis,** as many as 90 percent of the leukocytes present can be neutrophils. This neutrophilic

TABLE 13–4.   CELL TYPES AND CAUSES OF CSF PLEOCYTOSIS

PREDOMINANT CELL TYPE	INFECTIOUS CAUSES	NONINFECTIOUS CAUSES

Neutrophils	Meningitis
	  Bacterial
	  Early viral, tuberculous, fungal
	  Amebic encephalomyelitis
	Cerebral abscess
		Hemorrhage
		  Subarachnoid
		  Intracerebral
		CNS infarct
		Tumor
		Repeated lumbar puncture
		Intrathecal treatments (e.g., drugs, myelography)

Lymphocytes	Meningitis
	  Viral
	  Tuberculous
	  Fungal
	  Syphilitic
	Partially treated bacterial meningitis
	Parasitic infestations
		Multiple sclerosis
		Guillain-Barré syndrome
		Drug abuse

Plasma cells	Same disorders associated with increased lymphocytes, particularly tuberculous and syphilitic meningitis	Multiple sclerosis Guillain-Barré syndrome

Eosinophils	Parasitic infestations
	Fungal infections
	Idiopathic eosinophilic meningitis
		Allergic reaction to
		  Intracranial shunts
		  Radiographic contrast media
		  Intrathecal medications

Macrophages	Tuberculous meningitis
	Fungal meningitis
		Response to erythrocytes and lipid in CSF owing to
		  Hemorrhage
		  Brain abscess, contusion, infarction
		  Blood contamination following lumbar puncture
		Treatments
		  Intrathecal medications
		  Radiographic contrast media
		  Brain irradiation

Malignant cells Blasts		Leukemia Lymphoma
Tumor cells		CNS tumors (medulloblastoma) Metastatic carcinoma (e.g., lung, breast, gastrointestinal tract, melanoma)

TABLE 13–5.   NORMAL CSF DIFFERENTIAL COUNT*

AGE	LYMPHOCYTES	MONOCYTES	NEUTROPHILS
Neonates (0 to 2 mo.)	5% to 35%	50% to 90%	0% to 8%
Adults (>18 y.)	40% to 80%	15% to 45%	0% to 6%
Children (2 mo. to 18 y.)	Not yet established	Not yet established	Not yet established

* *Data apply to CSF differential counts using a cytospin preparation technique.*

pleocytosis also occurs with other infectious and noninfectious conditions (see Table 13–4). Although pronounced neutrophilic pleocytosis frequently occurs in bacterial meningitis, in the early disease stages with some infectious agents only a small percentage of neutrophils (approximately 10 percent) may be present. Noninfectious conditions such as subarachnoid or intracerebral hemorrhage, repeated lumbar punctures, and intrathecal administration of drugs or radiographic contrast media have also been associated with increased neutrophils in the CSF.

LYMPHOCYTES. Increased lymphocytes in the CSF are associated with viral, tubercular, fungal, and syphilitic meningitis. Although initially these conditions may show a mixture of cells (i.e., neutrophils, lymphocytes, monocytes, and plasma cells), in later stages of the disease lymphocytes predominate. Lymphocytes in CSF can become activated in the same way as those in peripheral blood. As a result, a variety of lymphoid cells can be present in the CSF. They can range in size from small typical cells to large cells with basophilic cytoplasm (a transformed lymphocyte or immunoblast). Along with atypical and plasmacytoid lymphocytes, lymphocytes are often found in patients with viral meningitis. Other conditions demonstrating CSF-lymphocytic pleocytosis are listed in Table 13–4.

PLASMA CELLS. Plasma cells are normally not present in CSF. They may be seen in acute viral and chronic inflammatory conditions: many of the same conditions that result in lymphocytic pleocytosis. In some cases of multiple sclerosis, the presence of plasma cells may be the only CSF abnormality.

MONOCYTES. The number of monocytes in CSF may be increased, but monocytes rarely predominate. Usually increased monocytes occur in a mixed pleocytosis pattern with other cell types (i.e., lymphocytes, neutrophils, plasma cells). This mixed pattern may be seen in patients with tuberculous or fungal meningitis, chronic bacterial meningitis, or rupture of a cerebral abscess.

EOSINOPHILS. Few eosinophils are seen in normal CSF, and small increases are not considered clinically significant. Eosinophil pleocytosis (10 percent or greater) is associated with various parasitic and fungal infections. It is also commonly seen, however, as an allergic reaction to malfunctioning intracranial shunts or to the intrathecal injection of foreign substances such as radiographic contrast media or medications. A form of meningitis that results in eosinophil pleocytosis has also been described: when evidence of an etiologic agent or pathogen is not identified, it is termed idiopathic eosinophilic meningitis (Kuberski, 1979).

MACROPHAGES. Macrophages in the CSF originate from monocytes and possibly from stem cells located in the reticuloendothelial tissue of the arachnoid and pia mater. Although they are not present in normal CSF, macrophages are frequently found following hemorrhage and various other conditions because of their active phagocytic ability. Central nervous system procedures such as myelography and pneumoencephalography can stimulate an increase in monocytes and macrophages in the CSF that can persist for 2 to 3 weeks following the procedure. Macrophages are capable of phagocytosing other cells, such as red blood cells and white blood cells, as well as other substances such as lipids, pigments, and microorganisms. Following a subarachnoid or cerebral hemorrhage, recently phagocytosed red blood cells, are readily apparent in macrophages. The engulfed red blood cells rapidly lose their pigmentation, forming vacuoles in the cytoplasm of these large cells. The presence of hemosiderin (i.e., brown pigmented granules from red blood cell hemoglobin), is best observed when iron staining a cytospin preparation. In addition to hemosiderin formation, which takes 2 to 4 days, hematoidin crystals can eventually develop. These yellow or red, often parallelogram-shaped crystals, similar in chemical composition to bilirubin, may also be observed in the cytoplasm of these macrophages. The presence of a small number of erythrophagocytic macrophages does not always indicate a hemorrhage. If a second lumbar puncture is performed within 8 to 12 hours of a previous puncture, peripheral blood that entered the CSF during the initial procedure is responsible for stimulating the observed activity. However, if iron staining reveals hemosiderin- or hematoidin-containing macrophages (siderophages), a hemorrhage in the central nervous system most likely occurred. These macrophages and siderophages can persist for 2 to 8 weeks. Macrophages also actively phagocytose lipids that may be present in the CSF as a result of injury, abscess, or infarction in the central nervous system. These lipid-laden macrophages are often termed lipophages and display a foamy cytoplasm with the nucleus often pushed to one side.

MALIGNANT CELLS. Malignant cells can be present in the CSF as a result of a primary central nervous system tumor (e.g., medulloblastoma) or as a result of metastasis. Most commonly seen are metastatic tumor cells from melanoma, or lung, breast, or gastrointestinal tract cancers. Leukemia, particularly acute lymphoblastic leukemia and acute myeloblastic leukemia, as well as lymphoma, can also result in the presence of malignant cells in the CSF. In patients with lymphoma and acute lymphoblastic leukemia with meningeal infiltration, increased numbers of lymphoblasts are present in the CSF; in patients with acute myeloblastic leukemia, readily identifiable and uniform myeloblasts are seen. The leukemic and lymphoma lymphoblasts are characteristically of uniform size, shape, and appearance, in contrast to transformed reactive lymphocytes in lymphoid-stimulating conditions, which show a significant variation in the types of cells present. The actual number of lymphoblasts present is not of diagnostic importance; even small numbers are clinically significant. Because drugs used in chemotherapy do not pass the blood-brain barrier, malignant cells that enter the central nervous system can proliferate unchecked in the CSF. As a result, most patients with acute lymphoblastic leukemia (approximately 80 percent) and acute myeloblastic leukemia (approximately 60 percent) develop central nervous system involvement at some stage during their disease (Kjeldsberg, 1986).

Malignant tumor cells may appear singly or as cell clumps in the CSF. When cell clumps are present, it is important to positively identify and differentiate malignant cells from clumps of normal cells of the choroid plexus and from the ependymal cells that line the ventricles. These normal cells of the central nervous system closely resemble malignant cells in size, shape, and appearance, but they have no clinical significance. In contrast, malignant cells are always of diagnostic importance.

Chemical Examination

Although numerous chemical constituents of CSF have been evaluated and studied, relatively few have established clinical utility. With advances in technology, methods that were previously inaccurate or unavailable enable accurate analysis and review of the usefulness of these CSF constituents, such as lactate, various enzymes, electrolytes, and proteins. Although historically numerous electrolytes and acid-base indicators, such as chloride, calcium, magnesium, pH, and PCO_2, were analyzed, these analytes now have little clinical value. Instead, assays of glucose, lactate, and various proteins in CSF predominate, providing substantive diagnostic information. This chapter does not discuss those chemical tests with limited clinical utility, such as glutamine quantitation, which reflects CSF ammonia levels and aids in the diagnosis of hepatic encephalopathy resulting from Reye's syndrome, viral hepatitis, or cirrhosis; and it does not discuss lactate dehydrogenase activity with isoenzyme analysis, which aids in the differential diagnosis of various central nervous system disorders.

Protein

The bulk of CSF protein (more than 80 percent) is derived from the transport of plasma proteins (via pinocytosis) through the capillary endothelium in the choroid plexus and meninges; the remainder of the protein results from intrathecal synthesis (Grant, 1987). Because of this transport process of proteins, normally only low-molecular-weight proteins are present in the CSF. Electrophoresis, after concentrating CSF (80 to 100 times), normally reveals only the presence of prealbumin, albumin, and transferrin. Trace amounts of IgG, a relatively high-molecular-weight protein (MW 160,000), can also be demonstrated electrophoretically in some normal CSF specimens.

Total Protein

The total amount of protein in the CSF varies with the age of the individual and the site from which it is obtained. The protein content of CSF obtained from the lumbar region is greater than that obtained from the cisterna or ventricles. In general, CSF total protein concentrations ranging from 15 to 45 mg/dL (150 to 450 mg/L) are considered normal, although infants and adults older than 40 years often have higher protein concentrations.

The CSF total protein is most commonly determined to assess the integrity of the blood-brain barrier and to indicate central nervous system pathology. Increased CSF total protein can result from four different mechanisms: 1) CSF contamination with peripheral blood during the puncture procedure; 2) altered capillary endothelial exchange (change in the blood-brain barrier); 3) decreased reabsorption into the venous blood; or 4) increased synthesis in the central nervous system. Because of the high concentration of proteins in the blood plasma compared with CSF (approximately 1000 : 1), a traumatic tap can result in significant false elevation of the CSF total protein. Formulas to correct for the contribution of plasma protein to CSF after a traumatic tap use the erythrocyte count obtained from the same collection tube. As mentioned earlier, however, these erythrocyte count formulas overestimate the correction, are rough estimates at best, and are not clinically useful.

Changes in the permeability of the blood-brain barrier and decreased reabsorption at the arachnoid villi occur with numerous disorders, such as bacterial, viral, and other forms of meningitis, cerebral infarction, hemorrhage, endocrine disorders, and trauma. Obstruction to the flow of CSF caused by tumors, disc herniations, or abscess prevents the normal circulation of fluid, which enhances water reabsorption in the spinal cord and results in increased CSF protein. Lastly, the infiltration of the CNS with immunocompetent cells that synthesize immunoglobulins can also result in an increased total protein determination (e.g., in multiple sclerosis, neurosyphilis).

Decreased CSF total protein can result from 1) increased reabsorption through the arachnoid villi owing to increased intracranial pressure, or 2) loss of fluid owing to trauma (e.g., a dural tear) or invasive procedures (e.g., pneumoencephalography).

Several methods are available for the determination of CSF total protein. Test selection is dictated by the limited sample volume and the need for sensitivity because CSF protein concentrations are normally low (15 to 45 mg/dL). Most often used are turbidometric procedures based on the precipitation of protein. For a comprehensive discussion of the methodologies available, including the advantages and disadvantages of each, the reader should consult a textbook in clinical chemistry.

Albumin and IgG

Because albumin is not synthesized in the central nervous system, all albumin present in CSF results from passage across the blood-brain barrier, assuming that there is no contamination during the puncture procedure. Therefore, albumin can be used as a reference protein to monitor the permeability of the blood-brain barrier. The permeability is evaluated by determining the CSF/serum albumin index, the ratio of the albumin concentration in the CSF to the concentration of albumin in the plasma (Equation 13–1). Note that the concentration units differ: CSF concentration is reported in mg/dL, whereas serum concentration is reported in g/dL. A CSF/serum albumin index less than 9 is considered normal. Index values between 9.0 and 14.0 represent minimal impairment of the blood-brain barrier, index values between 15 and 100 represent moderate to severe impairment of the barrier; and index values exceeding 100 indicate a complete breakdown of the barrier (Grant, 1987).

(13–1)

$$\text{CSF/Serum albumin index} = \frac{\text{Alb}_{\text{CSF}}, \text{mg/dL}}{\text{Alb}_{\text{Serum}}, \text{g/dL}}$$

In contrast to albumin, IgG is a large-molecular-weight protein that is normally present in very small amounts (approximately 1 mg/dL) in the CSF. In patients with pathologic conditions, increased CSF IgG can result from increased production within the CNS or from increased transport from the blood plasma. To specifically identify those conditions resulting in increased intrathecal synthesis, albumin is used as a reference protein; the following formula is employed to determine the CSF IgG index:

(13–2)

CSF IgG index =

$$\frac{\text{IgG}_{\text{CSF}}, \text{mg/dL}}{\text{IgG}_{\text{Serum}}, \text{g/dL}} \times \frac{\text{Albumin}_{\text{Serum}}, \text{g/dL}}{\text{Albumin}_{\text{CSF}}, \text{mg/dL}}$$

Note that the units of each component differ and that both the serum and the CSF must be analyzed for albumin and IgG. Because this calculation depends on the determinations of both the albumin and IgG, any analytic error is magnified. Therefore, it is imperative that precise quantitative immunochemical methods (e.g., nephelometry) be employed in determining the albumin and IgG concentrations. An IgG index less than 0.77 is considered normal (this can vary with the technical methods employed and the patient population). A value greater than 0.77 is associated with increased intrathecal production of IgG, whereas low values indicate a compromised blood-brain barrier. Because about 90 percent of patients with multiple sclerosis have an IgG index greater than 0.77, this index is diagnostically sensitive for this disease. However, other inflammatory CNS disorders can also cause increased IgG synthesis, which limits the specificity of the index for multiple sclerosis. Regardless, the CSF IgG index is a diagnostically useful tool and is frequently employed.

Protein Electrophoresis

The composition and distribution of proteins in CSF can be revealed by protein electrophoresis. An abnormal distribution of proteins can be present in CSF, despite a normal total protein content. Because of its low protein content, CSF must be concentrated 80- to 100-fold before electrophoresis. This is most commonly achieved using commercial concentrator systems (e.g., Minicon, Amicon Corp.) A normal CSF pattern predominantly demonstrates a prealbumin, an albumin, and two transferrin bands (Table 13–6). In addition, faint bands of α_1-antitrypsin and IgG may also be present. The prealbumin band and the second, slower transferrin band are unique to CSF; therefore, when a CSF pattern is compared to a serum pattern from the same individual, these bands will not be present. The second transferrin band located in the β_2 region is a carbohydrate-deficient form of transferrin synthesized only in the CNS. Its presence positively identifies a fluid as CSF and can be used to diagnose CSF rhinorrhea or otorrhea (i.e., the discharge of CSF through the nose or ears, respectively).

The electrophoresis of CSF is primarily performed to detect **oligoclonal bands** in the gamma region. Oligoclonal banding can vary significantly from a few faint discrete bands to many intense bands. Their presence in CSF and concomitant absence in serum is highly indicative of multiple sclerosis. Because IgG can pass the blood-brain barrier, it is necessary that simultaneous electrophoretic analysis of both serum and CSF take place. Some lymphoproliferative disorders will produce oligoclonal banding in both serum and CSF. In these cases, if only CSF is analyzed, an inaccurate conclusion could be made. In patients with multiple sclerosis, 90 percent demonstrate CSF oligoclonal bands at some time in the course of their disease. Although these bands aid in the diagnosis of multiple sclerosis, their presence or intensity does not correlate with a particular stage of disease, nor can they be used to predict disease progression. In addition, other CNS disorders can also demonstrate CSF oligoclonal banding, such as subacute sclerosing panencephalitis, neurosyphilis, bacterial and viral men-

T A B L E 13–6. CEREBROSPINAL FLUID REFERENCE RANGES*

	CONVENTIONAL UNITS	SI UNITS
Chemical Examination		
Electrolytes		
Calcium	2.0 to 2.8 mEq/L	1.00 to 1.40 mmol/L
Chloride	115 to 130 mEq/L	115 to 130 mmol/L
Lactate	10 to 22 mg/dL	1.1 to 2.4 mmol/L
Magnesium	2.4 to 3.0 mEq/L	1.2 to 1.5 mmol/L
Potassium	2.6 to 3.0 mEq/L	2.6 to 3.0 mmol/L
Sodium	135 to 150 mEq/L	135 to 150 mmol/L
Glucose	50 to 80 mg/dL	2.75 to 4.40 mmol/L
Total protein	15 to 45 mg/dL	150 to 450 mg/L
Albumin	10 to 30 mg/dL	100 to 300 mg/L
IgG	1 to 4 mg/dL	10 to 40 mg/L
Protein electrophoresis		
(percent of total protein)		
Prealbumin	2% to 7%	
Albumin	56% to 76%	
α_1-Globulin	2% to 7%	
α_2-Globulin	4% to 12%	
β-Globulin	8% to 18%	
γ-Globulin	3% to 12%	
Microscopic Examination		
Leukocyte count		
Neonates (<1 year)	0 to 30 cells/μL	0 to 30 $\times$ 10^6/L
1 to 4 years	0 to 20 cells/μL	0 to 20 $\times$ 10^6/L
5 to 18 years	0 to 10 cells/μL	0 to 10 $\times$ 10^6/L
Adults	0 to 5 cells/μL	0 to 5 $\times$ 10^6/L
Differential cell count		
Neonates		
Lymphocytes	5% to 35%	
Monocytes	50% to 90%	
Neutrophils	0% to 8%	
Adults		
Lymphocytes	40% to 80%	
Monocytes	15% to 45%	
Neutrophils	0% to 6%	

* For cerebrospinal fluid specimens obtained by lumbar puncture.

ingitis, and acute necrotizing encephalitis. As a result, CSF oligoclonal banding alone cannot be considered pathognomonic for multiple sclerosis. Instead, a protocol consisting of laboratory tests and a clinical assessment of neurologic dysfunction is used to diagnose multiple sclerosis.

Myelin-Basic Protein

Myelin, a primarily lipid substance (70 percent), surrounds the axons of nerves and is necessary for proper nerve conduction. The remaining 30 percent of myelin is made up of proteins, one of which is myelin-basic protein. With multiple sclerosis and other demyelinating diseases, the myelin sheaths undergo degradation and release myelin-basic protein into the CSF, where it can be detected using sensitive radioimmunoassays. Detection of myelin-basic protein is not specific for multiple sclerosis, and it is present only during acute exacerbation of the disease. Myelin-basic protein determinations, therefore, are primarily used to follow the course of disease or to identify those individuals with multiple sclerosis who do not show oligoclonal banding (approximately 10 percent).

Glucose

The CSF glucose concentration is in a dynamic equilibrium with glucose in the blood plasma. Two mechanisms account for glucose in the CSF: 1) active transport by endothelial cells and 2) simple diffusion along a concentration gradient that exists between the blood plasma and the CSF. Because of the time involved for these processes to occur, a CSF glucose value reflects the plasma glucose concentration 30 to 90 minutes preceding collection of the fluid. Accurately interpreting CSF glucose values requires a plasma glucose drawn 30 to 60 minutes preceding the lumbar puncture, preferably a fasting level. Normally, CSF glucose ranges from 50 to 80 mg/dL (2.75 to 4.40 mmol/L), which is approximately 60 percent to 70 percent of the plasma concentration. If a CSF/plasma glucose ratio is calculated, normal values average 0.6.

Increased CSF glucose levels are found following hyperglycemia and traumatic puncture procedures (owing to peripheral blood contamination), but have no diagnostic significance. In contrast, low CSF glucose values (less than 40 mg/dL) are associated with numerous conditions such as hypoglycemic states, meningitis, and infiltration of the meninges with metastatic or primary tumors. More than 50 percent of meningitis cases have a low CSF glucose level. The mechanism for the low CSF glucose level observed is two-fold: decreased or defective transport across the blood-brain barrier, coupled with increased glycolysis within the CNS.

Lactate

Lactate is normally present in CSF at concentrations ranging from 10 to 22 mg/dL (1.1 to 2.4 mmol/L), and its CSF concentration is essentially unrelated to that of the blood plasma. Increased CSF lactate levels result from anaerobic metabolism within the CNS

owing to tissue hypoxia, decreased oxygenation of the brain. Any condition that impairs the blood supply or the transport of oxygen to the CNS will result in increased CSF lactate levels. Numerous conditions that produce high CSF lactate levels include low arterial PO_2, cerebral infarction, cerebral arteriosclerosis, intracranial hemorrhage, hydrocephalus, traumatic brain injury, cerebral edema, and meningitis.

The determination of CSF lactate can assist in differentiating meningitis owing to bacterial, fungal, or tuberculous agents from viral meningitis. In viral meningitis, the lactate level rarely exceeds 25 to 30 mg/dL; in contrast, other forms of meningitis usually present with CSF lactate levels greater than 35 mg/dL. It is interesting to note that increased CSF lactate levels are also closely associated with low CSF glucose levels; the combined result from both parameters may be a better diagnostic indicator of bacterial meningitis than either parameter alone.

Microbiologic Examination

The microbiology laboratory plays a key role in the diagnosis of and selection of treatment for meningitis. If a limited volume of CSF is obtained, most often microbiologic studies take precedence over all other studies. With the identification of the causative agent responsible for meningitis, appropriate antibiotic therapy can begin. Gram staining and other microscopic techniques may reveal the etiologic agent; a CSF culture can assist in diagnosis, but more often confirms it; and detection of microbial antigens in the CSF using immunologic tests greatly aids in the diagnosis of meningitis.

Usually the second CSF collection tube obtained from a puncture procedure is sent to the microbiology laboratory. This tube or any later tube is preferred because it is less likely than the first tube to contain microbial organisms from the puncture site. The CSF for microbial studies must be maintained at room temperature and should be processed immediately to ensure the recovery of viable organisms. Centrifugation of CSF at 1500 ×

g for 15 minutes should be used to prepare a sediment from which both smears and cultures are prepared (Murray, 1980).

Stains

Because the microscopic examination of concentrated CSF sediment can provide a rapid presumptive diagnosis of meningitis in 60 percent to 80 percent of cases, it is imperative the examination be performed properly by a skilled microbiologist. Routine or cytocentrifuged smears can be prepared, with the latter technique concentrating any organisms present into a well-defined area on the slide, facilitating the microscopic examination. Gram-stained smears can be difficult to interpret. False negatives can occur owing to the presence of only a small number of organisms. On the other hand, precipitated dye and debris, as well as contaminating organisms from reagents and supplies, can result in false positive Gram stain results. Although other stains, such as acridine orange, a fluorescent stain, are being evaluated for their sensitivity, the Gram stain remains the most commonly employed stain to identify microorganisms in CSF.

If tuberculous meningitis is suspected, an acid-fast stain is used to prepare the specimen for the examination. CSF specimens from suspected cases of fungal meningitis are often evaluated using both the Gram stain and an India ink preparation. Because both of these techniques can be insensitive, requiring the presence of numerous organisms, immunologic tests are frequently employed to assist in the diagnosis of various types of meningitis.

Culture

The most common causes of meningitis are *Hemophilus influenzae, Neisseria meningitidis,* and *Streptococcus pneumoniae;* however, numerous other bacteria, fungi, parasites, and viruses can be the etiologic agent. Aerobic culturing of CSF enables the isolation of the common types of bacteria in 80 percent to 90 percent of cases. If antibiotic therapy

preceded the CSF collection, however, the recovery of bacterial isolates from the specimen can be significantly reduced. In suspected cases of tuberculous meningitis, the chance of positive culture increases with repeat CSF cultures. In cases of suspected meningitis, blood cultures should also be performed. These cultures are positive in 40 percent to 60 percent of patients with suspected meningitis and often provide the only clue as to the causative agent (Kjeldsberg, 1986).

Immunologic Examination

Several immunologic assays are currently available to detect the presence of microbial antigens in CSF (and in serum). The various techniques employed include coagglutination, latex agglutination, radioimmunoassay, and counterimmunoelectrophoresis. In these assays, the reagent containing polyclonal antibodies is combined with CSF; if the microbial antigen is present, a positive test result is obtained. As monoclonal antibodies are developed, both the sensitivity and specificity of these assays will improve.

Currently, immunologic tests can be used for the detection of several bacterial and fungal organisms that cause meningitis. The latex slide agglutination test for *Cryptococcus* antigen is widely used because of its high sensitivity (60 percent to 99 percent) and specificity (80 percent to 99 percent). In addition, this test serves as a good prognostic indicator, with increasing titers suggesting spread of the disease and decreasing titers associated with response to treatment. Similarly, immunologic assays for *Coccidioides immitis, Mycobacteria tuberculosis, Hemophilus influenzae, Neisseria meningitidis, Streptococcus pneumoniae,* and group B streptococci are available. Although these assays are generally rapid and easy to perform, each does not have equivalent diagnostic value. Sensitivity and specificity vary with each assay, and false positive nonspecific reactions, as well as false negative reactions, can occur. Hence, despite the clinical utility of microbial antigen detection, CSF Gram stain and culture remains the standard for the diagnosis of bacterial and fungal meningitis.

References

Chow G, Schmidley JW: Lysis of erythrocytes and leukocytes in traumatic lumbar punctures. Arch Neurol *41*:1084–1085, 1984.

Fishbein D, Palmer DL, Porter KM: Bacterial meningitis in the absence of pleocytosis. Arch Intern Med *141*:1369–1372, 1981.

Grant GH, Silverman LM, Christenson RH: Amino acids and proteins. *In* Tietz NW (ed.): Fundamentals of Clinical Chemistry, Philadelphia, W. B. Saunders Company, 1987, pp. 339–342.

Kjeldsberg CR, Knight JA: Body Fluids (2nd ed.), Chicago, American Society of Clinical Pathologists Press, 1986, pp. 1–30.

Kuberski T: Eosinophils in the cerebrospinal fluid. Ann Intern Med *91*:70–75, 1979.

Lofsness KG, Jensen TL: The preparation of simulated spinal fluid for teaching purposes. Am J Med Technol *49*(7):493–497, 1983.

Marton KI, Gean AD: The spinal tap: a new look at an old test. Ann Intern Med 104:840, 1986.

McComb JG: Recent research into the nature of cerebrospinal fluid formation and absorption. J Neurosurg *59*:369–383, 1983.

Murray PR, Hampton CM: Recovery of pathogenic bacteria from cerebrospinal fluid. J Clin Microbiol *12*:554–557, 1980.

Novak RW: Lack of validity of standard corrections for white cell counts of blood contaminated cerebrospinal fluid in infants. Am J Clin Pathol *82*:95–97, 1984.

Bibliography

Fishman RA: Cerebrospinal Fluid in Disease of the Nervous System, Philadelphia, W. B. Saunders Company, 1980.

Glasser L: Tapping the wealth of information in CSF. Diagnostic Medicine *4*(1):23–33, 1981.

Krieg AF, Kjeldsberg CR: Cerebrospinal fluid and other body fluids. *In* Henry JB (ed.): Clinical Diagnosis and Management of Laboratory Methods, Philadelphia, W. B. Saunders Company, 1991, pp. 445–457.

Fishman RA: Cerebrospinal Fluid in Disease of the Nervous System, Philadelphia, W. B. Saunders Company, 1980.

Moriarty G: Central nervous system. *In* Kaplan LA, Pesce AJ (eds.): Clinical Chemistry, Theory, Analysis, and Correlation, St. Louis, C. V. Mosby Company, 1989, pp. 594–606.

Oehmichen M: Cerebrospinal Fluid Cytology, an Introduction and Atlas, Philadelphia, W. B. Saunders Company, 1976.

Study Questions

1. **Cerebrospinal fluid is produced primarily from**

   A. secretions by the choroid plexus.
   B. diffusion from plasma into the central nervous system.
   C. ultrafiltration of plasma in the ventricles of the brain.
   D. excretions from ependymal cells lining the brain and spinal cord.

2. **CSF is found between the**

   A. arachnoid and dura mater.
   B. arachnoid and pia mater.
   C. pia mater and dura mater.
   D. pia mater and choroid plexus.

3. **Which of the following statements regarding CSF is true?**

   A. CSF is constantly being produced.
   B. CSF is reabsorbed into the blood at the choroid plexus.
   C. CSF is essentially composed of diluted plasma.
   D. CSF circulates through the brain and spinal cord because of active and passive diffusion processes.

4. **Which of the following normally does NOT pass through the blood-brain barrier?**

   A. PO_2
   B. Albumin
   C. Glucose
   D. Fibrinogen

5. **During a lumbar puncture procedure, the first collection tube of CSF removed should be used for**

   A. chemistry tests.
   B. cytology studies.
   C. hematology tests.
   D. microbiology studies.

6. **Which of the following is NOT an analytical concern when processing and testing of the CSF is delayed?**

   A. The viability of microorganisms
   B. The lability of the immunoglobulins
   C. The lysis of leukocytes and erythrocytes
   D. Alterations in the chemical composition

7. **Pleocytosis is a term used to describe**

   A. an increased number of cells in the CSF.
   B. a pink, orange, or yellow CSF specimen.
   C. an increased protein content in the CSF owing to cellular lysis.
   D. inflammation and sloughing of the cells from the choroid plexus.

8. **All of the following can cause xanthochromia in CSF EXCEPT**

   A. high concentrations of protein.
   B. high concentrations of bilirubin.
   C. increased numbers of leukocytes.
   D. erythrocytes from a traumatic tap.

9. **In CSF, which of the following indicates a traumatic puncture?**

   A. The presence of erythrophagocytic cells in the CSF
   B. Hemosiderin granules within macrophages in the CSF sediment
   C. An uneven distribution of blood in the CSF collection tubes
   D. A xanthochromic supernatant following CSF centrifugation

10. **How many leukocytes are normally present in the CSF obtained from an adult?**

    A. 0 to 5 cells/μL
    B. 0 to 10 cells/μL
    C. 0 to 20 cells/μL
    D. 0 to 30 cells/μL

11. **Which of the following cells may be present in small numbers in normal CSF?**

    A. Erythrocytes
    B. Lymphocytes
    C. Macrophages
    D. Plasma cells

12. **Which of the following cell types predominate in CSF during a classic case of bacterial meningitis?**

    A. Lymphocytes
    B. Macrophages
    C. Monocytes
    D. Neutrophils

13. **Which of the following cell types predominate in CSF during a classic case of viral meningitis?**

    A. Lymphocytes
    B. Macrophages
    C. Monocytes
    D. Neutrophils

14. **When choroid plexus cells and ependymal cells are present in CSF, they**

    A. are clinically significant.
    B. represent the demyelination of nerve tissue.
    C. closely resemble clusters of malignant cells.
    D. indicate breakdown of the blood-brain barrier.

15. **All of the following proteins are normally present in the CSF EXCEPT**

    A. albumin.
    B. fibrinogen.
    C. prealbumin.
    D. transferrin.

16. **Which of the following will NOT result in an increased CSF total protein?**

    A. A traumatic puncture procedure
    B. Alterations in the blood-brain barrier
    C. Trauma to the central nervous system, resulting in fluid loss
    D. Decreased reabsorption of CSF into the peripheral blood

17. **Which of the following proteins in the CSF is used to monitor the integrity of the blood-brain barrier?**

    A. Albumin
    B. Prealbumin
    C. Transferrin
    D. IgG

18. **An IgG index greater than 0.77 is indicative of**

    A. intrathecal synthesis of IgG.
    B. a compromised blood-brain barrier.
    C. active demyelination of neural proteins.
    D. increased transport of IgG from plasma into the CSF.

19. **An unknown fluid can be positively identified as being CSF by**

    A. determining the lactate concentration.
    B. determining the albumin concentration.
    C. determining the presence of oligoclonal banding on electrophoresis.
    D. determining the presence of carbohydrate-deficient transferrin on electrophoresis.

20. Which of the following statements about oligoclonal bands is false?

A. In the CSF, these bands indicate increased intrathecal concentrations of IgG.

B. The bands usually correlate with the stage of disease and can be used to predict disease progression.

C. The bands are often present in the CSF and serum of individuals with a lymphoproliferative disease.

D. The bands are often present in the CSF but not in the serum of individuals with multiple sclerosis.

21. Which of the following statements about CSF glucose is false?

A. Increased CSF glucose values are diagnostically significant.

B. Glucose enters the CSF by active transport and simple diffusion.

C. Decreased CSF glucose values reflect a defective blood-brain barrier and increased glycolysis.

D. CSF glucose values reflect the plasma glucose concentration 30 to 90 minutes preceding collection.

22. Normal CSF lactate levels (below 25 mg/dL) are commonly found in patients with

A. bacterial meningitis.

B. fungal meningitis.

C. tuberculous meningitis.

D. viral meningitis.

23. Which of the following procedures frequently provides a rapid presumptive diagnosis of bacterial meningitis?

A. A blood culture

B. A CSF culture

C. A CSF Gram stain

D. Immunologic tests for microbial antigens

24. India ink preparations and microbial antigen tests on CSF can aid in the diagnosis of

A. bacterial meningitis.

B. fungal meningitis.

C. tuberculous meningitis.

D. viral meningitis.

Synovial Fluid Analysis

LEARNING OBJECTIVES

After studying this chapter, the student should be able to

1. Describe the formation and function of synovial fluid.

2. Summarize the four principal classifications of joint disease.

3. Classify synovial fluid as normal, noninflammatory, inflammatory, septic, or hemorrhagic using various laboratory results.

4. Discuss appropriate tubes for the collection and distribution of synovial fluid specimens; discuss the importance of timely specimen processing and testing.

5. State the physical characteristics of normal synovial fluid and discuss how each characteristic can be modified in disease states.

6. Correlate the cells and crystals observed during the microscopic examination of synovial fluid with various joint diseases.

7. Compare and contrast the concentrations of selected chemical constituents of synovial fluid from healthy joints to those with joint disease.

8. Discuss the microbiologic examination of synovial fluid and its importance in the diagnosis of infectious joint disease.

KEY TERMS

arthritis: the inflammation of a joint.

arthrocentesis: a percutaneous puncture procedure used to remove synovial fluid from joint cavities.

hyaluronate: a high-molecular-weight polymer of repeating disaccharide units secreted by synoviocytes into the synovial fluid. It imparts the high viscosity to synovial fluid and serves as a lubricant for a joint. It is a salt or ester of hyaluronic acid.

synovial fluid: the fluid that fills joint cavities. It is formed by the ultrafiltration of plasma across the synovial membrane and by secretions from synoviocytes.

synoviocytes: cells of the synovial membrane. There are two types of synoviocytes: one type is actively phagocytic and synthesizes degradative enzymes, and the other type synthesizes and secretes hyaluronate.

Physiology and Composition

In areas of the skeleton where friction could develop, such as the joints, bursae, and tendon sheaths, viscous **synovial fluid** is found. Within articulated diarthroidal joints (e.g., the knee), the ends of apposing bones are covered with articular cartilage, the joint space is lined by a synovial membrane (except in the weight-bearing areas), and synovial fluid bathes and lubricates the joint (Fig. 14–1). The surface of the synovial membrane surrounding the joint consists of numerous microvilli with a layer, one to three cells deep, of synovial cells called **synoviocytes.** Two types of synoviocytes are present in the synovial membrane; the most prevalent type is actively phagocytic and synthesizes degradative enzymes (e.g., collagenases). The second type of synoviocyte synthesizes hyaluronate, a mucopolysaccharide linked with approximately 2 percent protein. The synoviocytes are loosely organized in the synovial membrane and differ from cells in other lining membranes because they have no basement membrane and because adjacent synovial cells are not joined with desmosomes. Beneath the synoviocytes is a thin layer of loose connective tissue containing a vast network of blood vessels, lymphatics, and nerves. Variable numbers of mononuclear cells are also found in this connective tissue layer.

Synovial fluid is formed by the ultrafiltration of plasma across the synovial membrane and from secretions by synoviocytes. The resultant viscous fluid serves as a lubricant for the joint and is the sole nutrient source for the metabolically active articular cartilage, which lacks blood vessels, lymphatics, and nerves. The composition of synovial fluid is unique. Its glucose and uric acid concentrations are equivalent to blood plasma levels, whereas its total protein and immunoglobulin concentrations can vary from one-fourth to one-half those of plasma. Table 14–1 lists reference values for various characteristics and constituents of normal synovial fluid obtained from the knee.

Classification of Joint Disorders

Arthritis and other joint diseases are common, and laboratory analysis of synovial fluid assists in the diagnosis and classification of these conditions. When synovial fluid is removed from a joint space, the laboratory examination enables the classification of the disease process into one of four principal categories: noninflammatory, inflammatory, septic, or hemorrhagic. These general classifications aid in the differential diagnosis of joint disease and are summarized in Table 14–2. It is important to note 1) that these categories overlap somewhat, 2) that several conditions can occur in the joint at the same time, and 3) that variations in test results can occur depending on the stage of the disease process. Consequently, these classifications are used only as a guide for the clinician in the evaluation and diagnosis of joint disease. In contrast to the tentative diagnoses possible based on laboratory findings, a definitive diagnosis can be made when microor-

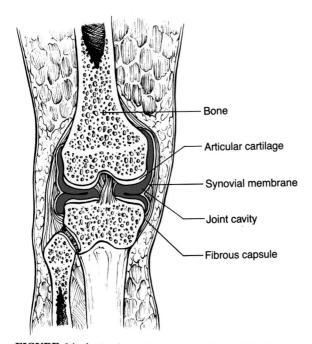

- Bone
- Articular cartilage
- Synovial membrane
- Joint cavity
- Fibrous capsule

FIGURE 14–1. A schematic representation of the knee, a diarthrodial joint.

TABLE 14–1. CHARACTERISTICS OF NORMAL SYNOVIAL FLUID*

PHYSICAL EXAMINATION	
Total volume	0.1 to 3.5 mL
Color	Pale yellow
Clarity	Clear
Viscosity	High; forms "strings" 3 to 6 cm long
Spontaneous clot formation	No
MICROSCOPIC EXAMINATION	
Erythrocyte count	<2000 cells/μL
Leukocyte count	<200 cells/μL
Differential cell count	
Monocytes and macrophages	approximately 60%
Lymphocyes	approximately 30%
Neutrophils	approximately 10%
Crystals	None present
CHEMICAL EXAMINATION	
Glucose	Equivalent to plasma values†
Uric acid	Equivalent to plasma values†
Total protein	1 to 3 g/dL
Lactate	9 to 33 mg/dL**
Hyaluronate	0.3 to 0.4 g/dL

* Values given are for fluid obtained from the knee.

† Synovial fluid values are equivalent to blood plasma values if obtained from a fasting patient.

** Normal lactate values are assumed to be similar to those in blood and cerebrospinal fluid; actual reference intervals have yet to be established.

ganisms (with septic arthritis) or crystals (with crystal synovitis) are identified in the synovial fluid.

Specimen Collection

Synovial fluid is taken from the patient by a process of percutaneous aspiration using aseptic technique, called **arthrocentesis.** Typically, a disposable sterile needle and syringe is used in the procedure to eliminate birefringent contaminants associated with the cleaning and resterilization of reusable supplies. Table 14–3 summarizes synovial fluid volume requirements for analysis. Most often, 3 to 10 mL of the synovial fluid is placed in a sterile collection tube for microbiologic studies, 2 to 5 mL is heparinized for microscopic examination, and the remainder of the specimen is collected into a plain tube (without an anticoagulant) for chemical and immunologic evaluation. Larger volumes of synovial fluid may be used for cultures to enhance the recovery of microbial organisms; similarly, greater volumes of fluid may be used to increase the number of cells recovered for cytology evaluation. The best anticoagulant for synovial fluid is sodium heparin at approximately 25 units/mL of synovial fluid. This will prevent clotting if fibrinogen is present in the fluid. Other anticoagulants (e.g., lithium heparin, oxalate, dry ethylenediaminetetra-acetic acid — EDTA) must be avoided, because they can produce artifacts that interfere with the microscopic examination for crystals. Because synovial fluid specimens are often distributed to different laboratories for testing, the total volume of fluid removed should be recorded on the patient's chart and on the specimen test request forms at the time of fluid collection.

If possible, the patient should have fasted for 4 to 6 hours (or overnight) to allow for the equilibration of some chemical

TABLE 14–2.   CLASSIFICATIONS OF SYNOVIAL FLUID BASED ON LABORATORY EXAMINATION

TEST	NORMAL	GROUP I (NONINFLAMMATORY)	GROUP II (INFLAMMATORY)	GROUP III (SEPTIC)	GROUP IV (HEMORRHAGIC)
Volume (mL)	<3.5	<3.5	>3.5	>3.5	>3.5
Color	Pale yellow	Yellow	Yellow-white	Yellow-green	Red-brown
Viscosity	High	High	Low	Low	Decreased
Leukocyte count (cells/μL)	<200	<3000	3000 to 50,000	>50,000	<10,000
Neutrophils	<25%	<25%	>50%	>75%	>25%
Glucose conc.	Approximately equal to that of plasma	Approximately equal to that of plasma	<that of plasma	<that of plasma	Approximately equal to that of plasma
Glucose: P = SF* difference	<10 mg/dL	<25 mg/dL	>25 mg/dL	>40 mg/dL	<25 mg/dL
Culture	Negative	Negative	Negative	Positive	Negative
Associated diseases	—	Osteoarthritis Osteochondritis Osteochondromatosis Traumatic arthritis Neuroarthropathy	Crystal synovitis† (gout, pseudogout) Rheumatoid arthritis** Reiter's disease Systemic lupus erythematosus††	Bacterial infection Fungal infection Mycobacterial infection	Trauma Blood diseases (e.g., hemophilia, sickle cell disease) Tumor Joint prosthesis

The plasma–synovial fluid difference in glucose concentration in specimens obtained simultaneously.
† With chronic or subsiding conditions, crystal synovitis may present as Group I.
*** Early stages of rheumatoid arthritis may present as Group I.*
†† Systemic lupus erythematosus may also present as Group I.

T A B L E 14–3.   SYNOVIAL FLUID VOLUME REQUIREMENTS FOR ANALYSIS

PHYSICAL EXAMINATION	
Color, clarity, viscosity	approximately 1 mL
MICROSCOPIC EXAMINATION	
Total cell count, differential cell count, crystal identification	2 to 5 mL in sodium heparin
Cytology (e.g., malignant cells)	5 to 50 mL* in sodium heparin
CHEMICAL EXAMINATION	
Glucose	1 to 3 mL (NaFl optional)
Total protein	1 to 3 mL
MICROBIOLOGICAL STUDIES	
Culture	3 to 10 mL†

* No upper limit to the amount of fluid that can be submitted; large volumes of fluid increase the recovery of cellular elements.

† Large fluid volumes may increase the recovery of viable microbial organisms.

constituents between the plasma and synovial fluid; a blood sample should be collected at approximately the same time as the performance of the arthrocentesis procedure.

The volume of synovial fluid in a joint varies with the size of the joint cavity and is normally small, about 0.1 to 3.5 mL (Ropes, 1940). Hence, arthrocentesis of a joint when an effusion (or fluid buildup) is not present can result in a "dry tap," a small yield of synovial fluid. In this case, synovial fluid may be present only in the aspiration needle, requiring that the needle's contents be expressed at the bedside into an appropriate small-volume container or, if desired, directly into culture media. Alternatively, some clinicians insert the needle into a sterile cork and transport the entire syringe to the laboratory for processing. This practice represents a significant potential biohazard, which should be avoided.

As with other body fluids, synovial fluid should be processed and tested as soon as possible after its collection. If processing is delayed, cells in the synovial fluid can alter its chemical composition; the detection of microbial organisms can be jeopardized; and blood cells (i.e., leukocytes and erythrocytes) can undergo lysis.

Following arthrocentesis, if the physician suspects the fluid obtained is not synovial fluid, either a mucin clot test or metachromatic staining with toluidine blue can be used to positively identify synovial fluid. Normal synovial fluid contains no fibrinogen and therefore does not normally clot. If synovial fluid is added to dilute acetic acid (2 percent), however, in a ratio of one part fluid to four parts acid, the hyaluronate present will produce turbidity or cause clot formation. Alternatively, placing a few drops of the fluid onto filter paper followed by 0.2 percent toluidine blue stain will result in metachromatic staining if synovial fluid is present (Goldenberg, 1973). One drawback to this approach is that heparin will also result in strong metachromatic staining; therefore, fluids anticoagulated with heparin cannot be evaluated with toluidine blue stain.

Physical Examination

Color

The hematology laboratory often performs both the physical and microscopic examinations of synovial fluid. The physical examination includes visual assessment for color, clarity, and viscosity. Normally, synovial fluid appears pale yellow or colorless and is clear. Color variations of red and brown are associated with trauma during the arthrocentesis procedure, and with disorders (e.g., joint fracture, tumors, traumatic arthritis) that disrupt the synovial membrane, allowing blood to enter the joint cavity. A traumatic procedure is indicated if the amount of blood in the fluid decreases as the collection continues or if a streak of blood is noticed in the fluid. With some joint disorders, particularly infections, synovial fluid can appear greenish or purulent; with others (e.g., tuberculous arthritis, systemic lupus erythematosus), it may appear milky.

Clarity

The clarity of synovial fluid can be modified by numerous substances. Leukocytes, erythrocytes, synoviocytes, crystals, fat droplets, fibrin, and cellular debris all contribute to the turbidity of a sample. The specific entity or entities within the synovial fluid are usually identified through the microscopic examination.

Viscosity

Synovial fluid has a high viscosity compared with water owing to the relatively high concentration of the mucoprotein **hyaluronate.** This high-molecular-weight polymer of repeating disaccharide units is secreted by synoviocytes and serves as a lubricant for the joint. During inflammatory conditions, hyaluronate in the synovial fluid can be depolymerized by the action of the enzyme hyaluronidase, contained in neutrophils. In addition, disease processes can inhibit the production and secretion of hyaluronate by the synoviocytes. Synovial fluid viscosity can be assessed by observing the synovial fluid as it is expelled from the collection syringe. A drop of normal synovial fluid will "string" out 3 to 6 cm before breaking; the fluid's viscosity is abnormally low when the drop breaks earlier or forms discrete droplets like water. Because more accurate viscosity measurements have little diagnostic or clinical value, they are not performed. The mucin clot test described earlier is also an indirect measure of viscosity because it indicates the degree of hyaluronate polymerization. This

test is now considered obsolete because similar information can be obtained by alternative, more precise, procedures.

Clot Formation

Spontaneous clot formation in synovial fluid indicates the abnormal presence of fibrinogen. Because of its high molecular weight (MW 340,000), fibrinogen is unable to pass through a healthy synovial membrane. Pathologic processes, damage to the synovial membrane, or blood contamination during a traumatic procedure can result in fibrinogen in the synovial fluid, and, as a result, clot formation. To eliminate potential fibrin clots that interfere with the microscopic examination, a portion of the synovial fluid should always be anticoagulated, preferably with sodium heparin.

Microscopic Examination

Using a hemacytometer, the microscopist usually performs the microscopic examination of synovial fluid on well-mixed undiluted fluid (see Appendix C for procedural details). If the fluid is significantly turbid, any dilutions made must use normal saline (0.85 percent), not acetic acid. Because of the fluid's high concentration of hyaluronate, adding acetic acid will cause the formation of a mucin clot and the clumping of cells, which will interfere with the microscopic examination. Because of the fluid's high viscosity, an extended period of time may be needed for the cells to settle in the hemacytometer chamber before the cell count. Highly viscous specimens can be diluted with a hyaluronidase buffer solution, which will reduce the fluid's viscosity and enhance the even distribution of cells in the cell-counting chamber (Kjeldsberg, 1986).

Total Cell Count

Normally, the number of erythrocytes in synovial fluid is less than 2000/μL. Some erythrocytes originate from the procedure itself;

those resulting from hemorrhagic effusions are usually obvious from their large numbers and the fluid's initial physical appearance. If the number of erythrocytes present requires that they be eliminated so that the leukocyte and differential counts can be performed, the fluid can be diluted using hypotonic saline (0.3 percent), which will cause the erythrocytes to lyse.

Leukocytes are normally present in synovial fluid, with cell counts below 200 per microliter considered normal. Although leukocyte counts greater than $2000/\mu L$ are typically associated with bacterial arthritis, leukocytosis also occurs in other conditions such as acute gouty arthritis and rheumatoid arthritis. Hence, total leukocyte counts have limited value in identifying the specific disease process.

Differential Cell Count

Synovial fluid can be concentrated by several techniques; however, cytocentrifugation preserves cellular morphology better than routine centrifugation procedures (Villanueva, 1987). Normally, about 60 percent of the synovial fluid leukocytes are monocytes or macrophages, approximately 30 percent are lymphocytes, and approximately 10 percent are neutrophils (Cohen, 1985). Differential counts have limited clinical value because they can differ not only with the disease process but also with the stage of the disease. A leukocyte differential with more than 80 percent neutrophils is associated with bacterial arthritis and urate gout, regardless of the total cell count. An increase in the lymphocyte percentage is often seen in the early stages of rheumatoid arthritis, whereas neutrophils predominate in later stages. An increased eosinophil count (greater than 2 percent) has been associated with a variety of disorders, including rheumatic fever, parasitic infestations, and metastatic carcinoma, and it often follows treatments such as arthrography and radiation therapy.

Other cells that may be present in synovial fluid include lupus erythematosus cells in patients with the disease; cells with hemosiderin inclusions owing to a hemorrhagic process; multinucleated cartilaginous cells in patients with osteoarthritis; malignant cells in patients with metastatic tumor; and normal synoviocytes from the synovial membrane.

Crystal Identification

One of the most important laboratory tests routinely performed on synovial fluid is the microscopic examination for crystals. Identification of some crystals is pathognomonic of a specific joint disease, thereby enabling a rapid definitive diagnosis (Table 14–4). Because both crystal formation and solubility are affected by temperature and pH changes, synovial fluid specimens should be examined as soon as possible after their collection. Time delays before the microscopic examination can result in inaccurate results if crystals form during storage and the leukocytes actively phagocytose the crystals.

Wet Preparation

The microscopist makes a wet preparation by dispensing a drop of the synovial fluid onto an alcohol-cleaned microscope slide and coverslipping it. The specimen should just fill the area beneath the coverslip; too much specimen will cause the coverslip to float. The coverslip edges can be sealed with fingernail polish or melted paraffin to eliminate evaporation, thereby allowing time for a thorough microscopic examination. Thorough examination of synovial fluid preparations by a skilled microscopist is imperative to ensure visualization and proper identification of synovial fluid crystals. This is necessary because 1) the number of crystals present can vary significantly with disease (i.e., only a few small crystals may be present); 2) the differentiation of crystals is difficult, because different types of crystals closely resemble each other; 3) free crystals can get enmeshed in fibrin or debris and be easily overlooked; and 4) numerous artifacts are

T A B L E 14–4. SYNOVIAL FLUID CRYSTAL IDENTIFICATION, MICROSCOPIC CHARACTERISTICS, AND ASSOCIATED CLINICAL CONDITIONS

CRYSTAL	MICROSCOPIC CHARACTERISTICS*	CLINICAL CONDITION
Monosodium urate monohydrate (MSU)	Fine, needle-like, with pointed ends; strong negative birefringence	Urate arthritis (gouty arthritis)
Calcium pyrophosphate dihydrate (CPPD)	Rod-like or rhombic; weak positive birefringence	Pseudogout (i.e., chondrocalcinosis)
Cholesterol	Flat, plate-like, with notched corners; negative birefringence; intensity varies with crystal thickness	Chronic arthritic conditions (e.g., rheumatoid arthritis)
Hydroxyapatite (HA)	Requires electron microscopy for visualization; not birefringent	Apatite-associated arthropathies
Corticosteroid	Varies with corticosteroid preparation used	Indicates previous intra-articular injection

These are characteristics of typical crystalline forms; however, other crystalline forms may also be present in synovial fluid.

birefringent and must be identified as such. In addition, synovial fluid findings in infectious arthritis and crystal synovitis can be similar, making the microscopic examination for crystals an important tool in their differentiation.

The wet preparation is viewed microscopically using both direct and compensated polarizing microscopy (see Chapter 1 for discussion of polarizing microscopy). Under polarizing microscopy, birefringent substances appear as bright objects against a black background, and the intensity of their birefringence varies with the substance. For example, monosodium urate and cholesterol crystals are bright and easy to visualize compared with calcium pyrophosphate dihydrate crystals. Compensated polarizing microscopy (using a red compensator plate) enables the identification and differentiation of positively and negatively birefringent substances based on the different colors produced when the crystals are oriented parallel and perpendicular to the axis of the compensator.

MSU Crystals

Monosodium urate (MSU) crystals in synovial fluid are indicative of gouty arthritis. Present intracellularly in leukocytes during acute stages of the disease, these needle-like

crystals (see Fig. 8–55) with pointed ends can distend the leukocytes' cytoplasm to accommodate themselves. Free-floating crystals enmeshed in fibrin may also be present. Under polarizing microscopy, MSU crystals are strongly birefringent, appearing bright against a black background. When a red compensator or full-wave plate is used, these negatively birefringent crystals will appear yellow when their longitudinal axes are parallel to the axis of the red compensator plate and blue when their longitudinal axes are perpendicular to it (Fig. 14–2). This characteristic facilitates the differentiation of MSU crystals from other similarly appearing crystals (e.g., EDTA crystals, betamethasone acetate).

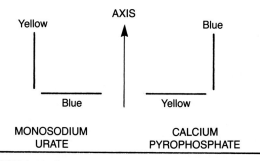

FIGURE 14–2. A two-dimensional schematic representation of monosodium urate and calcium pyrophosphate crystals when viewed under polarized light with a red compensator. The axis indicated is that of the compensator.

CPPD Crystals

A group of diseases is associated with calcium pyrophosphate dihydrate (CPPD) crystals (see Fig. 8–70) in synovial fluid. These conditions, often referred to as pseudogout or chondrocalcinosis, are associated with the calcification of articular cartilages and include degenerative arthritis and arthritides accompanying metabolic diseases (e.g., hypothyroidism, hyperparathyroidism, diabetes mellitus). Several characteristics enable the differentiation of CPPD crystals from MSU crystals. CPPD crystals are smaller and blunter, rod-like, or rhomboid. With compensated polarizing microscopy, they display weak positive birefringence: the CPPD crystals appear blue when their longitudinal axes are parallel to the red compensator plate and yellow when their longitudinal axes are perpendicular to it (see Fig. 14–2).

Cholesterol Crystals

Cholesterol crystals usually appear as flat, rectangular plates with notched corners (see Fig. 8–61*B*). However, rhomboid or needle-like forms that resemble MSU and CPPD crystals have also been observed in synovial fluid. Under polarizing microscopy, cholesterol crystals exhibit strong birefringence that varies with the thickness of the crystal. Associated with chronic inflammatory conditions (e.g., rheumatoid arthritis), cholesterol crystals are considered nonspecific and frequently occur in chronic effusions found in other body cavities.

HA Crystals

Hydroxyapatite (HA) crystals, present intracellularly in leukocytes, require electron microscopy to be visualized. They are extremely small, needle-like crystals and are not birefringent. HA crystals are associated with conditions characterized by calcific deposition and are collectively termed "apatite-associated arthropathies." Apatite is the principal component of bone and is also present in cartilage. In crystalline form, HA crystals can induce an acute inflammatory reaction similar to that caused by MSU and CPPD crystals (Glasser, 1980).

Corticosteroid Crystals

Because corticosteroid crystals may be found in synovial fluid for months following intra-articular injection, the laboratory must be informed of any injections when requested to do a synovial fluid microscopic examination. Depending on the corticosteroid preparation used, these crystals can closely resemble MSU or CPPD crystals. In fact, laboratories can use betamethasone acetate as a microscopic control because the crystals resemble MSU morphologically and exhibit similar negative birefringence. Corticosteroid crystals have no clinical significance other than indicating previous instillation of the drug in the joint.

Artifacts

Numerous artifacts in synovial fluid show birefringence under polarizing microscopy, and the artifacts' differentiation from crystals is necessary. Birefringent artifacts include anticoagulant crystals, starch granules from examination gloves, cartilage and prosthesis fragments, collagen fibers, fibrin, and dust particles. The experienced microscopist is able to differentiate artifacts based on their irregular or indistinct morphologic appearance compared to crystals. Anticoagulant crystals (e.g., calcium oxalate, lithium heparin) can be phagocytosed by leukocytes; therefore, only sodium heparin, which does not form crystals, should be used as an anticoagulant for synovial fluid specimens.

Chemical Examination

Although numerous chemical constituents can be analyzed in synovial fluid, relatively few analytes provide diagnostically useful information to the clinician. Some analytes, such as uric acid, maintain the same concentration in the synovial fluid as in the blood plasma, regardless of joint disease. These analytes are often assessed and monitored through blood plasma measurements. In contrast, joint diseases can cause other analytes (e.g., glucose) to differ in their concentrations in blood plasma and synovial fluid; therefore, determination of the plasma–synovial fluid difference can aid in the identification and differentiation of joint disease.

Glucose

To evaluate synovial fluid glucose concentrations, a blood sample must be drawn at the same time that the arthrocentesis is performed. In a normal, fasting patient, the glucose concentrations in the blood and synovial fluid are equivalent. Hence, the glucose concentrations obtained from the blood plasma and synovial fluid specimens (i.e., the plasma–synovial fluid glucose difference) will be within 10 mg/dL of each other. Because of the time required for this dynamic equilibrium to occur, the plasma–synovial fluid glucose differences in the nonfasting patient can exceed 10 mg/dL. With various joint diseases, the concentration of glucose in the synovial fluid is decreased; hence, the plasma–synovial fluid glucose difference is increased. Generally, plasma–synovial fluid glucose differences that exceed 25 mg/dL are associated with inflammatory conditions, and glucose differences that exceed 40 mg/dL indicate sepsis. In a nonfasting patient, the synovial fluid glucose is considered significantly low if the fluid's glucose concentration is less than half the plasma's glucose value.

Synovial fluid specimens for glucose quantitation should be assayed immediately or, if the quantitation is delayed, sodium fluoride should be used as a preservative. These precautions will eliminate falsely low glucose values resulting from the glycolytic activity of leukocytes that may also be present in the fluid.

Total Protein

Normally, the total protein concentration of synovial fluid is approximately one-third the protein concentration of the blood plasma.

An increased amount of protein in the synovial fluid results from changes in the permeability of the synovial membrane or from increased synthesis within the joint. A variety of joint diseases (e.g., rheumatoid arthritis, crystal synovitis, septic arthritis) routinely have increased protein levels. However, determination of the synovial fluid protein content does not assist in the differential diagnosis of joint disease or in its treatment. Rather, increased total protein in synovial fluid indicates only the presence of an inflammatory process in the joint. Consequently, synovial fluid protein determinations are not routinely performed.

Uric Acid

The uric acid concentration in synovial fluid is equivalent to that in blood plasma. Hence, determining the plasma's uric acid level usually enables the clinician to establish a diagnosis of gout, in which both synovial fluid and plasma uric acid concentrations are increased. Gout is frequently diagnosed by microscopically examining synovial fluid for crystals. Plasma or synovial fluid uric acid levels can be particularly valuable in cases in which MSU crystals are not observed microscopically, however.

Lactate

Increased synovial fluid lactate concentrations are believed to result from anaerobic glycolysis in the synovium. With severe inflammatory conditions, there is an increased demand for energy, and tissue hypoxia can occur. Although the lactate level in the synovial fluid can be determined relatively easily, its clinical utility remains uncertain. Some conditions of the joint, particularly septic arthritis, have been associated with significantly increased synovial fluid lactate levels. In contrast, gonococcal arthritis presents with normal or low lactate levels. Despite numerous studies, the clinical value of routine lactate quantitation in synovial fluid has yet to be established.

Microbiologic Examination

. . . .

Gram Stain

To aid in the differential diagnosis of joint disease, the routine examination of synovial fluid includes a Gram stain and a culture. Gram stains, when positive, provide immediately useful clinical and diagnostic information. Most infectious agents in synovial fluid are bacterial and originate from the blood; other agents in the fluid include fungi, viruses, and mycobacteria. The sensitivity of the Gram stain depends on the organism involved; approximately 75 percent of patients with staphylococcal infections, 50 percent of patients with gram-negative organisms, and 40 percent of patients with gonococcal infections are identified as positive by Gram stain. Other bacteria commonly involved in infectious arthritis include *Streptococcus pyogenes*, *Streptococcus pneumoniae*, and *Hemophilus influenzae*.

Culture

Whether or not the Gram stain is positive, all synovial fluid specimens should be cultured. In most cases of bacterial arthritis, the synovial fluid culture is positive. Recovery of microbial organisms requires careful and rapid processing of a fresh synovial fluid specimen. Special culture media considerations are required if fungal, mycobacterial, and anaerobic organisms are suspected; hence, consultation between the clinician and the microbiology laboratory is very important.

the microbiology laboratory is very important.

References

. . . .

Cohen AS, Goldenberg D: Synovial fluid. *In* Laboratory Diagnostic Procedures in the Rheumatic Diseases (3rd ed.), New York, Grune and Stratton, 1985, p. 6.

Glasser L: Reading the signs in synovia. Diagn Med *3*(4):35–50, 1980.

Goldenberg DL, Brandt KD, Cohen AD: Rapid, simple detection of trace amounts of synovial fluid. Arthritis Rheum *16:*487–490, 1973.

Kjeldsberg CR, Knight JA: Synovial fluid. *In* Body Fluids (2nd ed.), Chicago, American Society of Clinical Pathologists Press, 1986, pp. 129–152.

Ropes MW, Rossmeisl EC, Bauer W: The origin and nature of normal human synovial fluid. J Clin Invest *19:*795, 1940.

Villanueva TG, Schumacher HR, Jr: Cytologic examination of synovial fluid. Diagn Cytopathol *3:*141, 1987.

Bibliography

. . . .

Eisenberg JM, Schumacher HR, et al.: Usefulness of synovial fluid analysis in the evaluation of joint effusions. Arch Intern Med *144:*715, 1984.

Gatter RA: A Practical Handbook of Joint Fluid Analysis, Philadelphia, Lea & Febiger, 1991, pp. 24–38.

Glasser L: Extravascular biological fluids. *In* Kaplan LA, Pesce AJ (eds.), Clinical Chemistry, Theory, Analysis, and Correlation, St. Louis, C. V. Mosby Company, 1989, pp. 591–593.

Kalish RI, Cheskin HS, Blumenfeld TA: Body fluid specimens. *In* Slockbower JM, Blumenfeld TA (eds.), Collection and Handling of Laboratory Specimens, Philadelphia, J. B. Lippincott Company, 1983, pp. 125–135.

Krieg AF, Kjeldsberg CR: Cerebrospinal fluid and other body fluids. *In* Henry JB (ed.), Clinical Diagnosis and Management of Laboratory Methods, Philadelphia, W. B. Saunders Company, 1991, pp. 457–462.

Phelps P, Steele AD, McCarty DJ: Compensated polarized light microscopy. JAMA *203:*166–179, 1968.

Study Questions

1. **Which of the following is a function of synovial fluid?**
   1. Providing lubrication for a joint
   2. Assisting in the structural support of a joint
   3. Transporting nutrients to articular cartilage
   4. Synthesizing hyaluronate and degradative enzymes

   A. 1, 2, and 3 are correct.
   B. 1 and 3 are correct.
   C. 4 is correct.
   D. All are correct.

2. **Which of the following is a characteristic of normal synovial fluid?**

   A. It is viscous.
   B. It is slightly turbid.
   C. It is dark yellow.
   D. It forms small clots upon standing.

3. **Which of the following is NOT normally present in synovial fluid?**

   A. Fibrinogen
   B. Neutrophils
   C. Protein
   D. Uric acid

4. **Which of the following substances will NOT increase the turbidity of synovial fluid?**

   A. Fat
   B. Crystals
   C. Hyaluronate
   D. Leukocytes

5. **Abnormally decreased viscosity in synovial fluid results from**

   A.   mucin degradation by leukocytic lysosomes.
   B.   overproduction of synovial fluid by synoviocytes.
   C.   autoimmune response of synoviocytes in joint disease.
   D.   depolymerization of hyaluronate by neutrophilic enzymes.

6. **A synovial specimen is received in the laboratory 2 hours following its collection. Which of the following changes to the fluid will most likely have taken place?**

   A.   The specimen will have clotted.
   B.   The uric acid concentration will have decreased.
   C.   Crystals may have precipitated or dissolved.
   D.   The lactate concentration will have decreased owing to anaerobic glycolysis.

7. **Which of the following anticoagulants should be used with a synovial fluid specimen when needed?**

   A.   Sodium citrate
   B.   Sodium heparin
   C.   Lithium heparin
   D.   Liquid EDTA

8. **A synovial fluid specimen has a high cell count and requires dilution to be counted. Which of the following diluents should be used?**

   A.   Normal saline
   B.   Dilute acetic acid, e.g., a 2 percent solution
   C.   Dilute methanol, e.g., a 1 percent solution
   D.   Phosphate buffer solution, e.g., 0.050 mol/L

9. **Which of the following results from synovial fluid analysis indicates a joint disease process?**

   A.   A few synoviocytes present in the fluid
   B.   A leukocyte count of less than 200 cells/μL
   C.   An erythrocyte count of less than 2000 cells/μL
   D.   A differential count showing greater than 25 percent neutrophils

10. **Differentiation of synovial fluid crystals, based on their birefringence, is achieved using**

   A.   transmission electron microscopy.
   B.   phase contrast microscopy.
   C.   direct polarizing microscopy.
   D.   compensated polarizing microscopy.

11. **The microscopic examination of synovial fluid for crystals can be difficult because**

   1. numerous artifacts are also birefringent.
   2. few crystals may be present.
   3. free-floating crystals can get enmeshed or hidden in fibrin.
   4. different crystals can closely resemble each other morphologically.

       A. 1, 2, and 3 are correct.
       B. 1 and 3 are correct.
       C. 4 is correct.
       D. All are correct.

12. **Which of the following crystals is characteristically seen in patients with gout?**

       A. Cholesterol crystals
       B. Hydroxyapatite crystals
       C. Monosodium urate monohydrate crystals
       D. Calcium pyrophosphate dihydrate crystals

13. **In synovial fluid, which of the following crystals is NOT birefringent?**

       A. Cholesterol crystals
       B. Hydroxyapatite crystals
       C. Monosodium urate monohydrate crystals
       D. Calcium pyrophosphate dihydrate crystals

14. **Assuming the patient is fasting, which of the following analytes is normally present in the synovial fluid in essentially the same concentration as in the blood plasma?**

   1. Glucose
   2. Lactate
   3. Uric acid
   4. Protein

       A. 1, 2, and 3 are correct.
       B. 1 and 3 are correct.
       C. 4 is correct.
       D. All are correct.

15. **Which of the following provides a definitive diagnosis of a specific joint condition?**

       A. Staphylococcal bacteria identified by Gram stain
       B. Corticosteroid crystals identified during the microscopic examination
       C. A plasma–synovial fluid glucose difference exceeding 20 mg/dL
       D. Greater than 25 leukocytes/μL observed during the microscopic examination

16. **An analysis of a synovial fluid specimen reveals the following:**

- **a cloudy, yellow-green fluid of low viscosity**
- **a total leukocyte count of 98,000 cells/μL**
- **a plasma–synovial fluid difference of 47 mg/dL**

This specimen would most likely be classified as

A. noninflammatory.
B. inflammatory.
C. septic.
D. hemorrhagic.

17. **An analysis of a synovial fluid specimen reveals the following:**

- **a yellow fluid of high viscosity**
- **a total leukocyte count of 300 cells/μL**
- **a plasma–synovial fluid difference of 17 mg/dL**

This specimen would most likely be classified as

A. noninflammatory.
B. inflammatory.
C. septic.
D. hemorrhagic.

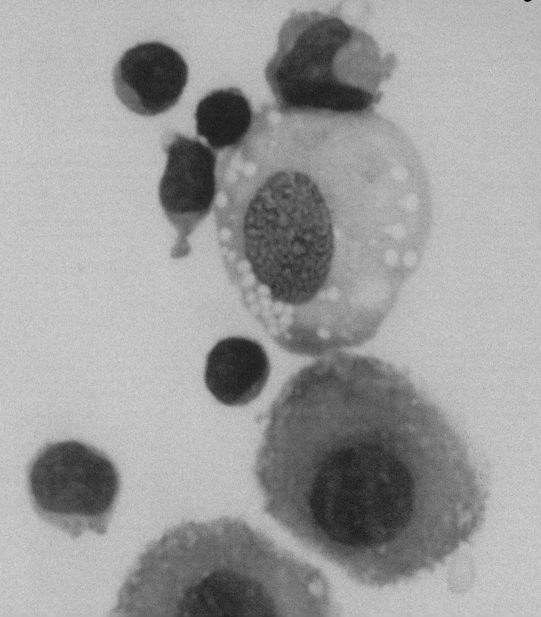

Pleural, Pericardial, and Peritoneal Fluid Analysis

LEARNING OBJECTIVES

After studying this chapter, the student should be able to

1. Describe the function of serous membranes as it relates to the formation and absorption of serous fluid.

2. Describe four pathologic changes that lead to the formation of an effusion.

3. Discuss appropriate collection requirements for serous fluid specimens.

4. Classify a serous fluid effusion as a transudate or an exudate based on the examination of its physical, microscopic, and chemical characteristics.

5. Compare and contrast chylous and pseudochylous effusions.

6. Correlate the microscopic examination and the differential cell count of serous fluid analyses with diseases that affect the serous membranes.

7. Correlate the concentration of selected chemical constituents of serous fluids with various disease states.

8. Discuss the microbiologic examination of serous fluids and its importance in the diagnosis of infectious diseases.

KEY TERMS

ascites: the excessive accumulation of serous fluid in the peritoneal cavity.

chyle: a milky-appearing emulsion of lymph and chylomicrons (triglyceride) that originates from intestinal lymphatic absorption during digestion.

effusion: an accumulation of fluid in a body cavity as a result of a pathologic process.

exudate: an effusion in a body cavity caused by increased capillary permeability or decreased lymphatic absorption.

It is identified by a fluid-to-serum total protein ratio greater than 0.5, a fluid-to-serum lactate dehydrogenase ratio greater than 0.6, or both.

mesothelial cells: flat cells that form a single layer of epithelium, which covers the surface of serous membranes (i.e., the pleura, pericardium, and peritoneum).

paracentesis: a percutaneous puncture procedure used to remove fluid from a body cavity, e.g., the pleural, pericardial, or peritoneal cavity.

pseudochylous effusion: an effusion that appears milky but does not contain chylomicrons and has a low (less than 50 mg/dL) triglyceride content.

serous fluid: a fluid that has a composition similar to that of serum.

transudate: an effusion in a body cavity caused by increased hydrostatic pressure (i.e., blood pressure) or decreased plasma oncotic pressure. It is identified by a fluid-to-serum total protein ratio of less than 0.5 *and* a fluid-to-serum lactate dehydrogenase ratio of less than 0.6.

Physiology and Composition

The lungs, the heart, and the abdominal organs are surrounded by a thin, continuous, serous membrane; the internal surfaces of the body cavity wall also are lined with this serous membrane. These lining membranes form a space or cavity, filled with fluid, between the portion of the membrane that covers the organ (visceral membrane) and the portion of the membrane that lines the body wall (parietal membrane) (Fig. 15–1). Each cavity is separate and named for the organ or organs it encloses. Each lung is surrounded by a pleural cavity; the heart is surrounded by the pericardial cavity; and the abdominal organs are enveloped by the peritoneal cavity. The serous membranes that line these cavities consist of a thin layer of connective tissue covered by a single layer of flat **mesothelial cells.** Within the membrane is an intricate network of capillary and lymphatic vessels. Each membrane is firmly attached to the body wall and the organ it surrounds; however, the membranes' opposing surfaces—despite close contact—are not attached to each other. Instead, the space between the opposing surfaces (i.e., between the visceral and parietal membranes) is filled with a small amount of fluid that serves as a lubricant between the membranes, permitting free movement of the enclosed organ. This fluid is created and maintained through plasma ultrafiltration in the parietal membrane and absorption by the visceral membrane. The name **serous fluid** is a general term frequently used to describe these fluids, the composition of which is similar to that of serum.

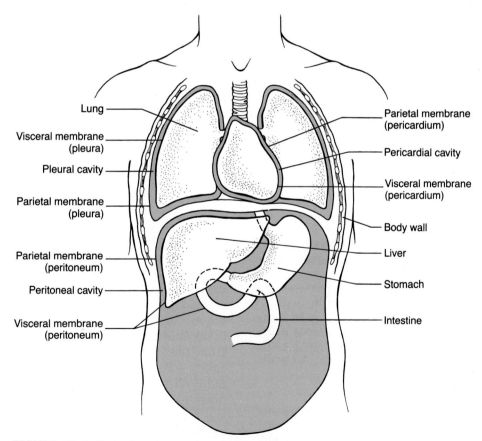

FIGURE 15–1. Parietal and visceral membranes of the pleural, pericardial, and peritoneal cavities. Parietal membranes line the body wall, whereas visceral membranes enclose organs. The two membranes are actually one continuous membrane. The space between opposing surfaces is identified as the body cavity (i.e., pleural cavity, pericardial cavity, peritoneal cavity).

The process of fluid formation and absorption in the pleural, pericardial, and peritoneal cavities is dynamic. Fluid formation is simultaneously controlled by four factors: 1) the permeability of the capillaries in the parietal membrane; 2) the hydrostatic pressure in these capillaries; 3) the oncotic pressure (or colloid osmotic pressure) produced by the presence of plasma proteins within the capillaries; and 4) the absorption of fluid by the lymphatic system (Table 15–1). Hydrostatic pressure (i.e., blood pressure) forces a plasma ultrafiltrate to form in the cavity; at the same time, plasma proteins in the capillaries produce a force (oncotic pressure) opposing this filtration. The permeability of the capillary endothelium regulates the rate of ultrafiltrate formation and its protein composition. For example, increased permeability of the endothelium causes an increased movement of protein from the blood into the cavity fluid. This now protein-rich extravascular fluid further enhances fluid accumulation outside of the vascular system and in the cavity. An accumulation of fluid in a body cavity is termed an **effusion** and indicates a pathologic process. The fourth component involved in cavity fluid formation, the lymphatic system, is primarily involved in the absorption of fluid out of the cavity. If the lymphatic vessels become obstructed or impaired, fluid is not adequately removed from the cavity and it builds up, resulting in an effusion. Other mechanisms that cause effusions, including a decrease in the hydrostatic pressure (e.g., congestive heart failure) and a decrease in the oncotic pressure (i.e., hypoproteinemia), result from various primary and secondary disease processes.

A diagnosis of a pleural, pericardial, or peritoneal effusion is usually made by a physician following a physical examination of the patient or the performance of radiographic imaging, ultrasound, or echocardiography studies. Collection and clinical testing of pleural, pericardial, and peritoneal fluids are very important, however, in identifying the type of effusion present and determining its cause.

Specimen Collection

The term **paracentesis** refers to the percutaneous puncture of a body cavity for the aspiration of fluid. Other anatomically descriptive terms denote fluid collection from specific body cavities. Thoracentesis, for example, refers to the surgical puncture of the chest wall into the pleural cavity to collect pleural fluid, whereas pericardiocentesis and peritoneocentesis (or abdominal paracentesis) identify the puncture procedures into the pericardial and peritoneal cavities, respectively, to collect pericardial and peritoneal fluids. The term **ascites** refers to an effusion in the peritoneal cavity, and ascitic fluid is another term for peritoneal fluid.

The collection of effusions from a body cavity is an invasive surgical procedure performed by a physician using sterile technique. Unlike cerebrospinal fluid and synovial fluid collections, serous fluid collections from the pleural, pericardial, and peritoneal cavity effusions often yield large volumes of fluid. This provides adequate fluid for the diagnostic tests required and often eliminates the need for additional puncture procedures, except when the repeated removal of the effusion is desired for therapeutic purposes (i.e., when the effusion is compressing or inhibiting the movement of vital organs).

T A B L E   15–1.   FORCES INVOLVED IN NORMAL PLEURAL FLUID FORMATION AND ABSORPTION

FORCES FAVORING FLUID FORMATION

Hydrostatic pressure (systemic capillary)	+30 mmHg
Oncotic pressure (systemic capillary)	−26 mmHg
Intrapleural pressure	+ 5 mmHg
Net pressure favoring fluid formation in the pleural cavity	+ 9 mmHg

FORCES FAVORING FLUID ABSORPTION

Hydrostatic pressure (pulmonary capillary)	−11 mmHg
Oncotic pressure (pulmonary capillary)	+26 mmHg
Intrapleural pressure	− 5 mmHg
Net pressure favoring fluid absorption from the pleural cavity	+10 mmHg

TABLE 15–2.   SEROUS FLUID VOLUME REQUIREMENTS

PHYSICAL EXAMINATION
Color and clarity	Recorded at bedside by physician and noted on test request form.

MICROSCOPIC EXAMINATION
Cell count, differential	5 to 8 mL EDTA or sodium heparin
Cytology (e.g., malignant cells)	25 to 50 mL* in sodium heparin (periodic acid–Schiff stain and cell block)
	10 to 20 mL EDTA

CHEMICAL EXAMINATION
Glucose	3 to 5 mL plain tube (NaFl optional)
Protein, lactate dehydrogenase, amylase, triglyceride, others	5 to 10 mL plain tube
pH (pleural)	1 to 3 mL heparinized syringe

MICROBIOLOGIC STUDIES
Gram and acid-fast stains, culture	10 to 20 mL† in sodium heparin, sterile

* No upper limit to the amount of fluid that can be submitted; large volumes of fluid increase the recovery of cellular elements.
† Large fluid volumes may increase the recovery of viable microbial organisms.

Serous fluids collected from body cavities should be transported to the laboratory as soon as possible after their collection to eliminate potential chemical and cellular changes. Prior to the collection procedure, the laboratory should be consulted to ensure that appropriate collection containers are used and suitable volumes obtained (Table 15–2). In microbiologic studies, the percentage of positive cultures obtained increases when a larger volume of specimen (10 to 20 mL) is used or when a concentrated sediment from a centrifuged specimen (50 mL or more) is used to inoculate cultures. Normally, serous fluids do not contain blood or fibrinogen, but a traumatic puncture procedure, a hemorrhagic effusion, or an active bleed (e.g., from a ruptured blood vessel) can result in serous fluid that appears bloody and will clot spontaneously. Therefore, to prevent clot formation that entraps cells and microorganisms, sterile tubes coated with an anticoagulant such as sodium heparin or ethylenediaminetetra-acetic acid (EDTA) are used to collect fluid specimens for the microscopic examination and microbiologic studies. In contrast, serous fluid for the chemical examination is placed into plain collection tubes and allowed to clot. When the paracentesis is performed, a serum sample should be collected for chemical comparison studies.

Transudates and Exudates

An effusion, particularly in the pleural or peritoneal cavity, is classified as either a **transudate** or an **exudate.** This classification can be based on several criteria, including appearance, leukocyte count, total protein concentration, albumin concentration, and cholesterol concentration; however, owing to the overlap between the categories, no single parameter differentiates a transudate from an exudate in all patients (Krieg, 1991). Classifying an effusion as a transudate or exudate is important because this information assists the physician in identifying its cause (Table 15–3). Transudates primarily result from a systemic disease that causes either an increase in hydrostatic pressure or a decrease in the plasma oncotic pressure in the parietal membrane capillaries. These changes are noninflammatory and are frequently associated with congestive heart failure, hepatic cirrhosis, and nephrotic syndrome (i.e., hypoproteinemia). Once an effusion has been

TABLE 15-3.   DIFFERENTIATION OF TRANSUDATES AND EXUDATES

PARAMETER	TRANSUDATES	EXUDATES
Cause	Increased hydrostatic pressure Decreased oncotic pressure	Increased capillary permeability Decreased lymphatic absorption
Physical examination		
Clarity	Clear	Cloudy
Color	Pale yellow	Variable; e.g., yellow, greenish, pink, red
Clots spontaneously	No	Variable; often yes
Microscopic examination		
Leukocyte count	<1000 cells/μL (pleural) <300 cells/μL (peritoneal)	Variable; usually >1000 cells/μL (pleural) >500 cells/μL (peritoneal)
Differential count	Mononuclear cells predominate	Early, neutrophils predominate; late, mononuclear cells predominate
Chemical examination		
Glucose	Equal to serum level	Less than or equal to serum level
Total protein	<50% of serum	>50% of serum
Total protein ratio (fluid-to-serum)	<0.5	>0.5
Lactate dehydrogenase (LD) activity	<60% of serum	>60% of serum
Lactate dehydrogenase (LD) ratio (fluid-to-serum)	<0.6	>0.6

identified as a transudate, further laboratory testing is usually not necessary.

In contrast, exudates result from inflammatory processes that increase the permeability of the capillary endothelium in the parietal membrane or decrease the absorption of fluid by the lymphatic system. Numerous disease processes such as infections, neoplasms, systemic disorders, trauma, or inflammatory conditions can cause exudates. Exudates require more laboratory testing than do transudates, such as microbiologic studies to identify pathologic organisms or cytologic studies to evaluate a suspected malignant neoplasm.

Table 15-4 summarizes various causes of pleural, pericardial, and peritoneal effusions. Unlike pleural and peritoneal effusions, pericardial effusions are not usually classified as a transudate or an exudate. Most often, pericardial effusions result from pathologic changes of the parietal membrane (e.g., owing to infection, damage) that cause an increase in capillary permeability. Hence, the majority of pericardial effusions could be considered exudates.

Physical Examination

Reference values for the characteristics of normal serous fluid in the pleural, pericardial, and peritoneal cavities are not available because, in healthy individuals, the fluid volume in these cavities is small and fluid is not normally collected. Only effusions are routinely collected and are then categorized as a transudate or exudate (see Table 15-3). Transudates are usually clear fluids, pale yellow to yellow, that have a viscosity similar to that of serum. Because transudates do not contain fibrinogen, they do not clot spontaneously. In contrast, exudates are usually cloudy, vary from yellow, green, pink, to red, and may have a shimmer or sheen to them. Because exudates often contain fibrinogen, they can form clots, thus requiring an anticoagulant (e.g., sodium heparin) when they are collected. The effusion's physical appearance is usually recorded on the patient's chart by the physician after paracentesis and should be transcribed onto all test request forms. If this information has not been provided, the laboratory performing the microscopic examination should note and record the physical characteristics of the fluid.

Cloudy paracentesis fluid most often indicates the presence of large numbers of leukocytes or other cells, chyle, lipids, or a combination of these substances. A characteristic milky appearance in pleural or peritoneal fluid usually indicates the presence of **chyle** (i.e., an emulsion of lymph and chylomicrons) in the effusion produced by obstruction of or damage to the lymphatic system. Chronic effusions (as seen with rheumatoid arthritis, tuberculosis, and myxedema) may have a similar appearance owing to the breakdown of cellular components and a characteristically high cholesterol content. Chronic effusions are also termed **pseudochylous effusions** and can be differentiated from true chylous effusions based on their lipid composition (i.e., triglyceride, chylomicron content). Lipoprotein electrophoresis will show an elevated triglyceride level (i.e., greater than 110 mg/dL) and chylomicrons present in a chylous effusion, whereas a pseudochylous effu-

sion has a low triglyceride level (less than 50 mg/dL) and no chylomicrons present.

Blood may be present in both transudates and exudates owing to a traumatic paracentesis procedure. As with other body fluids (e.g., cerebrospinal fluid, synovial fluid), the origin of the blood is determined by the blood's distribution during paracentesis. If the amount of blood decreases during the collection and small clots form, a traumatic tap is suspected as its cause. If the blood is homogeneously distributed in the fluid and the fluid does not clot (indicating that the fluid has been defibrinogenated in the body cavity, a process that takes several hours), the patient has a hemorrhagic effusion.

Microscopic Examination

The microscopic examination of pleural, pericardial, and peritoneal fluids may include a total erythrocyte and leukocyte count, a differential leukocyte count, and cytologic stud-

TABLE 15–4. CAUSES OF PLEURAL, PERICARDIAL, AND PERITONEAL EFFUSIONS

PLEURAL EFFUSIONS	PERICARDIAL EFFUSIONS	PERITONEAL EFFUSIONS

Transudates
Decreased hydrostatic pressure
  Congestive heart failure
Decreased oncotic pressure
  Hepatic cirrhosis
  Nephrotic syndrome
	Infections, e.g., bacterial, viral, fungal, tuberculous
	Cardiovascular disease, e.g., myocardial infarction, aneurysm
	Neoplasms, e.g., metastatic cancer
	Hemorrhage, e.g., trauma, anticoagulant therapy
	Systemic diease, e.g., systemic lupus erythematosus, rheumatoid arthritis
		Transudates
		Decreased hydrostatic pressure
		  Congestive heart failure
		Decreased oncotic pressure
		  Hepatic cirrhosis
		  Nephrotic syndrome

Exudates
Increased capillary permeability
  Infections, e.g., bacterial, tuberculous, fungal, viral
  Neoplasms, e.g., lung, metastatic cancers
  Systemic disease, e.g., rheumatoid arthritis, systemic lupus erythematosus
  Gastrointestinal disease, e.g., pancreatitis
Decreased lymphatic absorption
  Neoplasms, e.g., lymphoma
  Trauma
  Surgery
		Exudates
		Increased capillary permeability
		  Infections, e.g., bacterial, tuberculous
		  Neoplasms, e.g., hepatic and metastatic cancers
		  Pancreatitis
		  Metabolic disease, e.g., uremia
		
		Decreased lymphatic absorption
		  Neoplasms, e.g., lymphoma, metastasis
		  Trauma
		  Tuberculosis

ies. Cell counts are performed manually using a hemacytometer (see Appendix C for procedural details). As with other body fluids, normal saline must be used as the diluent when cloudy effusions require a dilution for cell counting. Acetic acid diluents will cause cells to clump, preventing accurate counting.

Total Cell Counts

Total erythrocyte and leukocyte counts have little differential diagnostic value in the analysis of pleural, pericardial, and peritoneal fluids. No single value for a leukocyte count can be used reliably to differentiate transudates from exudates; hence, these counts have limited clinical utility. However, leukocyte counts in transudates usually are less than 1000 cells/μL, whereas those in exudates generally exceed 1000 cells/μL.

With pericardial fluid, a leukocyte count of greater than 1000 cells/μL suggests pericarditis; erythrocyte counts or hematocrits assist in identifying hemorrhagic effusions (i.e., cases in which the count or hematocrit is less than that of the peripheral blood). With pleural fluid, erythrocyte counts can also be used to identify hemorrhagic effusions; however, high erythrocyte counts (greater than 10,000 cells/μL) are alsofrequently associated with neoplasms and trauma of the pleura. With peritoneal fluid, a leukocyte count exceeding 500 cells/μL with a predominance of neutrophils (greater than 50 percent) is suggestive of bacterial peritonitis. However, the volume of peritoneal fluid (or ascites) can change significantly because of extracellular fluid shifts. These fluid shifts can significantly affect the cell count obtained. Hence, a wide range of leukocyte counts may be encountered in an effusion throughout the course of the disease.

Differential Cell Count

The clinical value of a differential leukocyte count varies with the origin of the paracentesis fluid. At most, the differential count provides limited diagnostic information. In pleural fluid, neutrophils predominate in about 90 percent of effusions caused by acute inflammation (i.e., exudates). Lymphocytes predominate in 90 percent of effusions caused by tuberculosis, neoplasms, and systemic diseases. Similarly, in peritoneal fluid, neutrophils predominate (greater than 25 percent) in most exudates, suggesting bacterial infection. In peritoneal transudates and in exudates caused by decreased lymphatic absorption (e.g., tuberculosis, neoplasms, lymphatic obstruction), lymphocytes predominate. Pericardial fluid differential counts are often not performed because a variety of conditions (e.g., bacterial and viral pericarditis, postmyocardial infarction) can produce the same cell differential; hence, a pericardial fluid differential count provides little diagnostic information.

Various cell types are found in pleural, pericardial, and peritoneal fluids and include neutrophils, eosinophils, lymphocytes, monocytes, macrophages, plasma cells, mesothelial cells (the lining cells of the serous membrane), and malignant cells. The majority of these cells are easily identified in effusions. Increased numbers of eosinophils (greater than 10 percent) have been observed in pleural, pericardial, and peritoneal fluids as a result of a variety of conditions. Rarely, lupus erythematosus (LE) cells are present in the fluids.

Mesothelial cells lining the serous membrane are routinely sloughed off and often appear in effusions. They are large cells (12 to 30 μm in diameter) with often eccentric nuclei and smooth, regular nuclear membranes; their nuclear chromatin pattern is loose and homogeneous; and one to three nucleoli may be present. Often mesothelial cells have abundant cytoplasm, and they sometimes resemble plasma cells. Because they can vary in appearance, such as appearing singly or in clumps, can be multinucleated, and can show reactive or degenerative changes, mesothelial cells can be difficult to differentiate from malignant cells and macrophages.

Malignant cells in effusions are common in patients with neoplastic disease, although the number of malignant cells found can vary significantly. Several characteristics aid in the identification of malignant cells; in particular, 1) they tend to form cell clumps; 2) their nuclear membrane is irregular or jagged; 3) their nuclear chromatin is unevenly distributed; they contain 4) prominent, frequently multiple nucleoli with irregular membranes; and 5) their nuclear-to-cytoplasmic ratio is higher than normal. The proper identification of malignant cells in effusions is crucial and is performed during a cytologic examination by a skilled professional.

Cytologic Examination

When malignant disease is suspected, large volumes (10 to 200 mL) of the pleural, pericardial, or peritoneal effusion should be submitted for cytologic examination. The fluid should be concentrated to increase the yield of cells, and a cell block and cytospin smears can be prepared. The cytologic examination is an important, sensitive, and specific procedure in the diagnosis of primary and metastatic neoplasms.

Chemical Examination

. . . .

The chemistry tests selected to evaluate pleural, pericardial, and peritoneal fluids assist the physician in establishing or confirming a diagnosis for the cause of an effusion. Once a diagnosis has been established, appropriate treatment can be initiated and further testing is usually not required. A specific diagnosis based on laboratory findings from serous fluids is limited to 1) malignancy, when malignant cells are recovered and identified; 2) systemic lupus erythematosus, when characteristic LE cells are found during the microscopic examination; and 3) infectious disease, when microorganisms (e.g., bacteria, fungi) are identified by Gram stain or culture. Several disease processes may occur simultaneously, each contributing to the development of an effusion. Therefore, chemistry tests initially classify the effusion as a transudate or an exudate. Transudates usually require no further chemical analysis,

whereas exudates are tested further to identify their etiologic agents or cause. A systematic approach in serous fluid testing greatly facilitates this diagnostic process.

Total Protein and Lactate Dehydrogenase Ratios

No single test can specifically identify the disease process causing effusions in the pleural, pericardial, and peritoneal cavities. Historically, transudates and exudates were classified by the total protein content or specific gravity of the fluid alone. Because of the significant overlap found with these criteria (i.e., exudates with protein content or specific gravity values that were equivalent to transudates', and vice versa), a better discriminator was needed. Currently, the most useful tests for classifying a serous fluid as a transudate or an exudate are simultaneous determinations of the serum and serous fluid total protein (TP) concentration and lactate dehydrogenase (LD) activity. From these values, the fluid-to-serum TP ratio and the fluid-to-serum LD ratio can be determined as follows:

(15–1)

$$\text{TP ratio} = \frac{\text{TP}_{\text{fluid}}}{\text{TP}_{\text{serum}}}$$

(15–2)

$$\text{LD ratio} = \frac{\text{LD}_{\text{fluid}}}{\text{LD}_{\text{serum}}}$$

These ratios together provide the most reliable means of distinguishing a transudate from an exudate. If the TP ratio is less than 0.5 *and* the LD ratio is less than 0.6, the fluid is classified as a transudate. In contrast, exudates are those fluids with a TP ratio greater than 0.5, an LD ratio greater than 0.6, *or* both.

Glucose

Following appropriate classification, several chemical tests can be used to further evaluate exudates. The tests selected and their usefulness vary with the origin of the fluid.

The simultaneous measurement of serum and serous fluid glucose concentrations has limited value. If the serous fluid glucose is less than 60 mg/dL or the glucose difference between the serum and fluid is greater than 30 mg/dL, an exudative process is identified. Only low fluid glucose levels are clinically significant, and a variety of disease processes are associated with them, particularly rheumatoid arthritis. Other conditions such as bacterial infections, tuberculosis, and malignant neoplasms may also present with decreased fluid glucose levels; however, normal serous fluid glucose values cannot rule out these disorders.

Amylase

The determination of simultaneous serum and fluid amylase levels, particularly in pleural and peritoneal fluids, is clinically useful and has become routine in many laboratories. A serous fluid amylase value that exceeds the established upper limit of normal (for serum specimens), or is 1.5 to 2 times the serum value, is considered abnormally increased (Kjeldsberg, 1986). These high fluid amylase levels are most often seen in effusions owing to pancreatitis, esophageal rupture (salivary amylase), gastroduodenal perforation, and metastatic disease.

Triglyceride

Because identification of a chylous effusion is clinically significant, determining the fluid's triglyceride level is an important adjunct when evaluating serous fluids. A milky appearance of an effusion does not specifically identify it as a chylous effusion because pseudochylous effusions can have a similar appearance. Therefore, fluid triglyceride levels are used as an additional determining factor. Serous fluid triglyceride values that exceed 110 mg/dL indicate a chylous effusion, whereas a fluid triglyceride value below 60 mg/dL precludes it as such. If the fluid triglyceride level is between 60 and 110 mg/dL, a lipoprotein electrophoresis

should be performed; the presence of chylomicrons identifies the effusion as a chylous effusion, whereas the absence of chylomicrons indicates a pseudochylous effusion. The cholesterol contents of chylous and pseudochylous effusions are usually not significantly different and, therefore, not clinically useful. Chylous effusions are associated with obstruction or damage to the lymphatic system. Neoplastic disease (e.g., lymphoma), trauma, tuberculosis, and surgical procedures often cause chylous effusions. Pseudochylous effusions are most often encountered with chronic inflammatory conditions (e.g., rheumatoid arthritis).

pH

Abnormally low pleural fluid pH measurements can help to identify patients with parapneumonic effusions (i.e., exudates owing to pneumonia or lung abscess) that require aggressive treatment. Parapneumonic effusions can involve both the parietal and visceral membranes, produce pus, and loculate in the pleural cavity. Studies show that if the pleural fluid pH is below 7.30, despite appropriate antibiotic therapy, the placement of drainage tubes is necessary for resolution of the effusion. In contrast, if the pleural fluid pH exceeds 7.30, the effusion completely resolves following antibiotic treatment alone. It is important to note that the collection of pleural fluid specimens for pH measurement requires the same rigorous sampling protocol as the collection of arterial blood gas specimens (i.e., an anaerobic sampling technique using a heparinized syringe, placing the specimen on ice, and immediately transporting the specimen to the laboratory for analysis). Pericardial and peritoneal fluid pH measurements currently have no clearly established clinical value.

Carcinoembryonic Antigen

The measurement of carcinoembryonic antigen (CEA), a tumor marker, is useful in evaluating pleural and peritoneal effusions from patients who have a previous history of or are currently suspected of having a CEA-producing tumor. When the CEA measurement is combined with a fluid cytology examination, the identification of malignant effusions is significantly increased.

Microbiologic Examination

Staining Techniques

The microbiologic examination includes the preparation of smears using a concentrated or cytocentrifuged specimen for the immediate identification of microorganisms. Depending on the suspected diagnosis, this may include Gram stain, an acid-fast stain, and other staining techniques. The sensitivity of these techniques depends on two factors: 1) the appropriate collection, processing, and handling of the fluid specimen and 2) the technical competence of the microscopist reading the smears. If either aspect is substandard, optimal results will not be obtained. In fluid specimens that have been allowed to clot, microorganisms may be caught in the clot matrix and obstructed from view; similarly, contamination of the specimen during its collection or delays in handling and processing can yield false positive results from in vivo bacterial proliferation. Because of the potential presence of stain precipitates, cellular components, and other debris, smears must be viewed by appropriately trained and experienced laboratorians. Under the best conditions, a Gram stain is positive in about 30 percent to 50 percent of bacterial effusions, whereas acid-fast stains are positive in only 10 percent to 30 percent of tuberculous effusions.

Culture

As with smear preparations, the larger the volume of pleural, pericardial, or peritoneal fluid used or the more concentrated the inoculum used for culture, the greater the chances of obtaining a positive culture. Both aerobic and anaerobic cultures should be performed. The sensitivity of a positive culture varies with the origin of the fluid and the organism present. Positive bacterial cultures are obtained in approximately 80 percent of all bacterial effusions. In contrast, peritoneal tuberculous (or mycobacterial) effusions culture positive in 50 percent to 70 percent of cases, pericardial effusions culture positive in about 50 percent of cases, and pleural tuberculous effusions culture positive in only about 30 percent of cases.

References

Kjeldsberg CR, Knight JA: Pleural and pericardial fluids. *In* Body Fluids (2nd ed.), Chicago, American Society of Clinical Pathologists Press, 1986, pp. 75–99.
Krieg AF, Kjeldsberg CR: Cerebrospinal fluid and other body fluids. *In* Henry JB (ed.): Clinical Diagnosis and Management of Laboratory Methods, Philadelphia, W. B. Saunders Company, 1991, pp. 463–473.

Bibliography

Glasser L: Extravascular biological fluids. *In* Kaplan LA, Pesce AJ (eds.): Clinical Chemistry, Theory, Analysis, and Correlation, St. Louis, C. V. Mosby Company, 1989, pp. 587–591.
Kalish RI, Cheskin HS, Blumenfeld TA: Body fluid specimens. *In* Slockbower JM, Blumenfeld TA (eds.): Collection and Handling of Laboratory Specimens, Philadelphia: J. B. Lippincott Company, 1983, pp. 114–124.
Kjeldsberg CR, Knight JA: Peritoneal fluid. *In* Body Fluids (2nd ed.), Chicago: American Society of Clinical Pathologists Press, 1986, pp. 105–115.

Study Questions

1. **Which of the following statements about serous fluid filled body cavities is true?**

   1. A parietal membrane is firmly attached to the body cavity wall.
   2. Serous fluid acts as a lubricant between opposing membranes.
   3. A serous membrane is composed of a single layer of flat mesothelial cells.
   4. The visceral and parietal membranes of an organ are actually a single continuous membrane.

      A. 1, 2, and 3 are correct.
      B. 1 and 3 are correct.
      C. 4 is correct.
      D. All are correct.

2. **Which of the following mechanisms is responsible for the formation of serous fluid in body cavities?**

   A. Ultrafiltration of the circulating blood plasma
   B. Selective absorption of the fluid from the lymphatic system
   C. Diuresis of solutes and water across a concentration gradient
   D. Active secretion by mesothelial cells that line the serous membranes

3. **Which of the following conditions enhances the formation of serous fluid in a body cavity?**

   A. Increased lymphatic absorption
   B. Increased capillary permeability
   C. Increased plasma oncotic pressure
   D. Decreased capillary hydrostatic pressure

4. **The pathologic accumulation of fluid in a body cavity is called**

   A. an abscess.
   B. an effusion.
   C. pleocytosis.
   D. paracentesis.

5. **Paracentesis and serous fluid testing are performed to**

   1. remove serous fluids that may be compressing a vital organ.
   2. determine the pathologic cause of an effusion.
   3. identify an effusion as a transudate or an exudate.
   4. prevent volume depletion owing to the accumulation of fluid in body cavities.

   A. 1, 2, and 3 are correct.
   B. 1 and 3 are correct.
   C. 4 is correct.
   D. All are correct.

6. **Thoracentesis refers specifically to the removal of fluid from the**

   A. abdominal cavity.
   B. pericardial cavity.
   C. peritoneal cavity.
   D. pleural cavity.

7. **Which of the following parameters best identifies a fluid as a transudate or an exudate?**

   A. Its color and clarity
   B. Its leukocyte and differential counts
   C. Its total protein and specific gravity measurements
   D. Its total protein ratio and lactate dehydrogenase ratio

8. **Chylous and pseudochylous effusions are differentiated by**

   A. a physical examination.
   B. their cholesterol concentrations.
   C. their triglyceride concentrations.
   D. their leukocyte and differential counts.

9. **Which of the following is most often associated with the formation of a transudate?**

   A. Pancreatitis
   B. Surgical procedures
   C. Congestive heart failure
   D. Metastatic neoplasm

10. **Match the type of serous effusion most often associated with each pathologic condition.**

	Pathologic Condition	Type of Serous Effusion
_____	A. Neoplasms	1. Exudate
_____	B. Hepatic cirrhosis	2. Transudate
_____	C. Infections	
_____	D. Rheumatoid arthritis	
_____	E. Trauma	
_____	F. Nephrotic syndrome	

11. **Each of the following laboratory findings on an effusion supports a specific diagnosis of disease EXCEPT**

    A. lupus erythematosus cells found during the microscopic examination.
    B. a serous fluid glucose concentration less than 60 mg/dL.
    C. microorganisms identified by Gram or acid-fast stain.
    D. malignant cells identified during the microscopic or cytologic examination.

12. **Abnormally low fluid pH measurements are useful in evaluating conditions associated with**

    A. pleural effusions.
    B. pleural and pericardial effusions.
    C. pericardial and peritoneal effusions.
    D. pleural, pericardial, and peritoneal effusions.

13. **A pleural or peritoneal fluid amylase level 2 times higher than the serum amylase level may be found in effusions resulting from**

    A. pancreatitis.
    B. hepatic cirrhosis.
    C. rheumatoid arthritis.
    D. lymphatic obstruction.

14. **A glucose concentration difference between the serum and an effusion that is greater than 30 mg/dL is associated with**

    A. pancreatitis.
    B. hepatic cirrhosis.
    C. rheumatoid arthritis.
    D. lymphatic obstruction.

15. **Each of the following will increase the chances of obtaining a positive stain or culture when performing microbiologic studies on infectious serous fluid EXCEPT**

    A. using a large volume of serous fluid for the inoculum.
    B. storing serous fluid specimens at refrigerator temperatures.
    C. using an anticoagulant in the serous fluid collection container.
    D. concentrating the serous fluid before preparing the smears for staining.

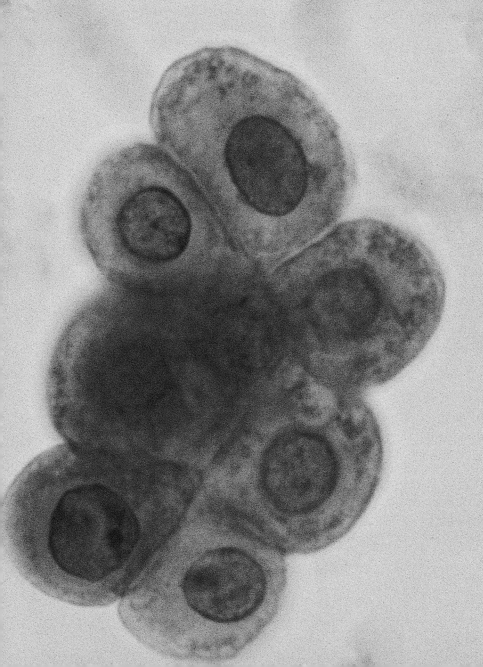

16

Case Studies

The purpose of this chapter is to help the student to develop problem-solving skills in clinical laboratory science. Hence, the student must not only learn the facts from the material presented in previous chapters but also actively participate in evaluating and correlating test results. Problem-solving involves understanding the physiologic process assessed by each test result, integrating the results obtained, and correlating the data with other clinical features (e.g., patient signs and symptoms). Problem-solving skills are also required to evaluate the quality of the laboratory data obtained and to make sound decisions regarding the validity of test results.

To help the student develop problem-solving skills, this chapter includes patient case studies. Each case study includes a brief patient history with appropriate test results obtained from the analysis of urine, blood, and other body fluid specimens. Using the information provided along with the knowledge obtained from previous chapters, the reader is asked to 1) identify and classify normal and abnormal findings; 2) account for discrepant results; 3) calculate ratios and indices; 4) suggest probable diagnoses; and 5) explain various physiologic and pathologic processes.

The body fluid analysis involved in each case study is called out at the top of each case to assist the reader in readily identifying those cases that will currently enhance his or her study of body fluids. Throughout this chapter, the following abbreviations are used:

Reagent Strip Result Key

Glu: neg, 50, 100, 250, 1000, 2000 mg/dL

Bili: neg, pos

Ket: neg, small, moderate, large

Blood: neg, trace, small, moderate, large

Pro: neg, trace, 30, 100, 300, 500 mg/dL

Urob: norm. 2, 4, 8, 12 mg/dL

Nitr: neg, pos

LE: neg, pos

Abbreviations

amt	amount
Bili	bilirubin
CaOx	calcium oxalate
CK	creatine kinase
CSF	cerebrospinal fluid
drp	drop
Epith	epithelial cells
GI	gastrointestinal
Glu	glucose
IVP	intravenous pyelogram
Ket	ketones
LD	lactate dehydrogenase
LE	leukocyte esterase
L/S	lecithin/sphingomyelin
mod	moderate
NA	not applicable
neg	negative
Nitr	nitrite
norm	normal
OFB	oval fat body
PG	phosphatidylglycerol
pos	positive
Pro	protein
RBC	red blood cell
RE	renal tubular cell
Refract	refractometer result
SE	squamous epithelial cell
slt	slightly
sm	small
Sp Grav	specific gravity
SSA	sulfosalicylic acid precipitation test
TE	transitional epithelial cell
UA	urinalysis
Urob	urobilinogen
UTI	urinary tract infection
WBC	white blood cell

CASE #1 URINALYSIS

. . . .

A large hospital and its outpatient clinic each has a laboratory area that performs routine urinalyses. Each laboratory performs daily quality assurance (QA) checks on reagents, equipment, and procedures. Because the control material used does not have sediment components, each laboratory sends a completed urinalysis specimen to the other laboratory for testing. After the urinalysis has been performed, the results are recorded, compared, and evaluated. The criterion for acceptability is that all parameters must agree within one grade.

RESULTS

One day all results were acceptable except those of the microscopic examination, which follow:

Hospital Laboratory	*Clinic Laboratory*
RBCs: 5 to 10 per HPF	RBCs: 25 to 50 per HPF
WBCs: 0 to 2 per HPF	WBCs: 0 to 2 per HPF
Casts: 0 to 2 hyaline per LPF	Casts: 5 to 10 hyaline per LPF

On investigation, it was found that the clinic's results were correct and that the hospital had a problem, which was immediately addressed and remedied.

. . . .

1. Which of the following conditions present in the hospital laboratory could cause the observed findings in this case?
    1. The urinalysis centrifuge had its brake left on.
    2. The urinalysis centrifuge was set for the wrong speed or time setting.
    3. The microscopic examination was performed on an unmixed or inadequately mixed specimen.
    4. The microscopic examination was performed using nonoptimized microscope settings for urine sediment viewing (e.g., there was not enough contrast to view low-refractile components).
    A. 1, 2, and 3 are correct.
    B. 1 and 3 are correct.
    C. 2 and 4 are correct.
    D. 4 is correct.
    E. All are correct.
2. Which of the following actions could prevent this from happening again?
    A. The microscope and centrifuge should be repaired.
    B. The laboratory should participate in a proficiency survey.
    C. A control material with sediment components should be employed daily.
    D. All results should be reviewed by the urinalysis supervisor before they are reported.

CASE #2 URINALYSIS

A routine urinalysis specimen from a patient suspected of having renal calculi is sent to the laboratory. During the microscopic examination, unusual crystals that resemble cholesterol plates are observed. The laboratorian is suspicious and performs a sulfosalicylic acid precipitation test (SSA for protein) and checks the specimen's specific gravity by refractometry. The patient care unit is contacted for a list of the patient's current medications. It is revealed that the patient had an intravenous pyelogram (IVP) 3 hours earlier. The patient is taking no medications except those given during the IVP procedure (i.e., demerol and xylocaine).

RESULTS

Physical Exam		Chemical Exam		Confirmatory Tests	Microscopic Exam	
Color:	yellow	Glu:	neg		RBCs:	0 to 2
Clarity:	cloudy	Bili:	neg		WBCs:	0 to 2
Odor:	NA	Ket:	neg		Casts:	neg
		Sp Grav:	1.020	Refract: >1.035	Epith:	Few TEs
		Blood:	neg		Crystals:	Mod *type*
		pH:	5.0			*undetermined*
		Pro:	neg	SSA: 4+ (delayed;		
		Urob:	norm	crystalline)		
		Nitr:	neg			
		LE:	neg			

1. Circle any abnormal or discrepant urinalysis findings.
2. What is the most likely identity of this crystal?
   A. Cystine
   B. Cholesterol
   C. Triple phosphate
   D. Uric acid—a rare form
   E. X-ray contrast media (e.g., renograffin)
3. Which specific gravity result best indicates the patient's renal ability to concentrate urine?
   A. Reagent strip result: 1.020
   B. Refractometer result: >1.035

CASE # 3 URINALYSIS

A 22-year-old woman is seen in the emergency room. She complains of a painful burning sensation when urinating (dysuria). She also states that she feels as if she has to urinate all the time. A midstream "clean catch" urine specimen is collected for a routine UA and culture.

RESULTS

Physical Exam		Chemical Exam		Microscopic Exam	
Color:	yellow	Glu:	neg	RBCs:	0 to 2
Clarity:	cloudy	Bili:	neg	WBCs:	10 to 25
Odor:	NA	Ket:	neg	Casts:	neg
		Sp Grav:	1.015	Bacteria:	mod
		Blood:	trace	Epith:	few SEs
		pH:	6.0		
		Pro:	trace		
		Urob:	norm		
		Nitr:	pos		
		LE:	pos		

1. Circle any abnormal or discrepant urinalysis findings.
2. Based on the results obtained, select the most probable diagnosis.
   A. A normal urinalysis
   B. An upper urinary tract infection (upper UTI)
   C. A lower urinary tract infection (lower UTI)
   D. A combined upper and lower UTI
3. Which single microscopic finding is most helpful in differentiating an upper UTI from a lower UTI?
   A. RBCs
   B. WBCs
   C. Casts
   D. Bacteria
   E. Epithelial cells
4. If the chemical screens for nitrite and leukocyte esterase were negative and all other results remained the same, would this change the initial diagnosis? Why or why not?

CASE # 4 URINALYSIS

A 30-year-old woman is seen by her physician. She has a temperature of 101°F and complains of nausea, headache, and flank (below the ribs and above the ileac crest) tenderness and pain. When asked, she states that urination is sometimes painful, that she must urinate much more frequently than usual, and that she has a sensation of urgency. A random, midstream "clean catch" urine specimen is collected for a routine UA and culture.

RESULTS

Physical Exam		Chemical Exam		Confirmatory Tests	Microscopic Exam	
Color:	yellow	Glu:	neg		RBCs:	0 to 2
Clarity:	cloudy	Bili:	neg		WBCs:	25 to 50
Odor:	NA	Ket:	neg		Casts:	0 to 2 granular
		Sp Grav:	1.010			2 to 5 WBC
		Blood:	trace		Bacteria:	mod
		pH:	6.5		Epith:	few SEs
		Pro:	30	SSA: 1+	Crystals:	few CaOx
		Urob:	norm			
		Nitr:	pos			
		LE:	pos			

1. Circle any abnormal or discrepant urinalysis findings.
2. The most probable diagnosis is
   A. a normal urinalysis.
   B. a yeast infection.
   C. an upper UTI.
   D. a lower UTI.
3. Another name for this condition is
   A. urethritis.
   B. acute cystitis.
   C. acute pyelonephritis.
   D. acute interstitial nephritis.
4. State two physiologic mechanisms that can lead to this condition.

CASE # 5 URINALYSIS

A 78-year-old man is admitted to the hospital because of complaints of moderate back and left rib pain and for the evaluation of anemia. On his admission to the hospital, routine admission blood work and a urinalysis are performed. The patient is found to be mildly anemic (normochromic, normocytic), with marked rouleaux formation noted on his blood smear. His red blood cell count, platelet count, hemoglobin, and hematocrit are all decreased. Radiographic studies showed lytic lesions in his lumbar vertebrae and ribs.

RESULTS

Physical Exam		Chemical Exam		Confirmatory Tests	Microscopic Exam	
Color:	yellow	Glu:	neg		RBCs:	0 to 2
Clarity:	clear	Bili:	neg		WBCs:	0 to 2
Odor:	NA	Ket:	neg		Casts:	0 to 2 hyaline
		Sp Grav:	1.025		Epith:	few TEs
		Blood:	neg		Crystals:	few uric acid
		pH:	5.0			
		Pro:	trace	SSA: 3+		
		Urob:	norm			
		Nitr:	neg			
		LE:	neg			

1. Circle any abnormal or discrepant urinalysis findings.
2. Explain the most probable cause for the discrepancy between the reagent pad test results for protein and the SSA test results.
3. A 24-hour urine collection reveals an increase in urine total protein. One would expect to see a markedly increased urinary excretion of which protein in this patient?
   A. Albumin
   B. Globulins
   C. Hemoglobin
   D. Tamm-Horsfall protein
4. The most probable diagnosis is
   A. orthostatic proteinuria.
   B. glomerulonephritis.
   C. nephrotic syndrome.
   D. multiple myeloma.
5. The proteinuria in this patient would be classified as
   A. glomerular proteinuria.
   B. tubular proteinuria.
   C. overflow proteinuria.
   D. postrenal proteinuria.

CASE # 6 URINALYSIS

A 36-year-old man with a history of diabetes mellitus is admitted to the hospital complaining of a decreased frequency of urination, a constant bloated feeling, weight gain, puffy eyes in the morning, and scrotal swelling. Mild edema of the patient's ankles, abdomen, and eyes is noted. Routine chemistry tests reveal hypoalbuminemia and hyperlipidemia (increased triglycerides and cholesterol).

RESULTS

Physical Exam	Chemical Exam		Confirmatory Tests	Microscopic Exam	
Color: colorless	Glu:	250		RBCs:	0 to 2
Clarity: clear	Bili:	neg		WBCs:	0 to 2
Odor: NA	Ket:	neg		Casts:	2 to 5 hyaline
A large amount of	Sp Grav:	1.010			0 to 2 fatty
white foam noted.	Blood:	mod			0 to 2 waxy
	pH:	5.0		Epith:	few TEs
	Pro:	500	SSA: 4+		few OFBs
	Urob:	norm		Bacteria:	neg
	Nitr:	neg			
	LE:	neg			

1. Circle any abnormal or discrepant urinalysis findings.
2. With this data, the most probable diagnosis is
   A. acute pyelonephritis.
   B. nephrotic syndrome.
   C. acute glomerulonephritis.
   D. lipiduria of unknown etiology.
3. The proteinuria in this patient should be classified as
   A. glomerular proteinuria.
   B. tubular proteinuria.
   C. overflow proteinuria.
   D. postrenal proteinuria.
4. What substance most accounts for the large amount of white foam observed?
   A. Fat
   B. Protein
   C. Glucose
   D. Casts
5. Explain the physiologic mechanism responsible for the edema exhibited in this patient.
6. In progressive renal disease with loss of glomerular filtering ability, which plasma protein is usually lost first? Explain why.

CASE # 7 URINALYSIS

A 30-year-old man is admitted to the hospital with headache and anorexia and excreting red urine. Examination reveals mild edema of the eyes and mild hypertension. A medical history reveals that the patient's daughter had strep throat one month previously and was treated successfully. Subsequently, the patient developed a sore throat that lasted a few days, but he did not seek treatment.

RESULTS

Physical Exam		Chemical Exam		Confirmatory Tests	Microscopic Exam	
Color:	red	Glu:	neg		RBCs:	25 to 50
Clarity:	cloudy	Bili:	neg		WBCs:	0 to 2
Odor:	NA	Ket:	neg		Casts:	2 to 5 granular
		Sp Grav:	1.010			0 to 2 RBC
		Blood:	mod			2 to 5 hyaline
		pH:	5.0		Epith:	few TEs
		Pro:	300	SSA: 3+	Bacteria:	neg
		Urob:	norm			
		Nitr:	neg			
		LE:	neg			

1. Circle any abnormal or discrepant urinalysis findings.
2. What is the most likely process by which red blood cells are entering the patient's urine?
3. At the patient's level of hematuria, is the blood present most likely contributing to the reagent strip protein test result?
   A. Yes
   B. No
4. From these data, select the most probable diagnosis.
   A. Acute cystitis
   B. Nephrotic syndrome
   C. Acute pyelonephritis
   D. Acute glomerulonephritis
5. The proteinuria in this patient would be classified as
   A. glomerular proteinuria.
   B. tubular proteinuria.
   C. overflow proteinuria.
   D. postrenal proteinuria.
6. Which of the following is considered the most specific indicator of glomerular disease and damage?
   A. Proteinuria
   B. TE cells
   C. RBC casts
   D. Granular casts

CASE # 8 URINALYSIS

A 51-year-old woman is admitted to the hospital for a vaginal hysterectomy. During surgery she is placed in the Simon's position (exaggerated lithotomy position) for 6 hours because of surgical complications. She receives two units of packed RBCs following surgery. Twenty four hours after surgery, a routine urinalysis, hemoglobin, hematocrit, and various chemistry tests are performed.

SERUM CHEMISTRY RESULTS

Creatine kinase (CK):	5800 U/L	(normal: 10 to 130 U/L)
Lactate dehydrogenase (LD):	1455 U/L	(normal: 150 to 320 U/L)
Haptoglobin:	175 mg/dL	(normal: 83 to 267 mg/dL)

URINE RESULTS

Physical Exam		Chemical Exam		Confirmatory Tests	Microscopic Exam	
Color:	brown	Glu:	neg		RBCs:	0 to 2
Clarity:	clear	Bili:	neg		WBCs:	2 to 5
Odor:	NA	Ket:	neg		Casts:	2 to 5 hyaline
		Sp Grav:	1.015			
		Blood:	large			
		pH:	5.5			
		Pro:	trace	SSA: trace		
		Urob:	norm			
		Nitr:	neg			
		LE:	neg			

1. Circle any abnormal or discrepant urinalysis findings.
2. In this case, if LD isoenzymes were measured, which isoenzyme(s) would you expect to be elevated?
   A. LD_1
   B. LD_2
   C. LD_3
   D. LD_4
   E. LD_5
3. In the patient's specimen, which substance is most likely causing the pigmenturia?
   A. Bilirubin
   B. Hemoglobin
   C. Myoglobin
   D. An unknown drug

CASE # 9 URINALYSIS

A 58-year-old male is seen in the emergency room complaining of intermittent severe pain that radiates from his right side to his abdomen and groin area (renal colic). He has a frequent need to urinate with little or no urine output. Other complaints include a "cold" that he has been self-treating with over-the-counter medications and vitamin supplements for more than a week.

RESULTS

Physical Exam		Chemical Exam		Confirmatory Tests		Microscopic Exam	
Color:	pink	Glu:	neg			RBCs:	10 to 25
Clarity:	slt cloudy	Bili:	neg			WBCs:	5 to 10
Odor:	NA	Ket:	neg			Casts:	0 to 2 hyaline
		Sp Grav:	>1.030	Refract:	1.035	Epith:	few TEs
		Blood	neg			Bacteria:	few
		pH:	5.5			Crystals:	many CaOx
		Pro:	trace	SSA:	trace		
		Urob:	norm				
		Nitr:	pos				
		LE:	neg				

1. Circle any abnormal or discrepant urinalysis findings.
2. For each discrepancy noted, list a test the laboratorian should perform to confirm or deny the cause of the test discrepancy.
3. Based on the information provided, which of the following is the most probable cause of the patient's condition?
   A. Renal calculi
   B. Urinary tract infection
   C. Acute glomerulonephritis
   D. Drug-induced acute interstitial nephritis
4. State at least three factors that could lead to the development of the patient's condition.

CASE # 10 URINALYSIS

An obese 58-year-old woman is seen by her physician. She complains of perineal itching and soreness. On pelvic examination, a white vaginal discharge is noted. A sample of the discharge is collected for culture. A midstream "clean catch" urine specimen is also collected for culture and routine urinalysis.

RESULTS

Physical Exam		Chemical Exam		Confirmatory Tests		Microscopic Exam	
Color:	yellow	Glu:	500	Clinitest:	500	RBCs:	0 to 2
Clarity:	cloudy	Bili:	neg			WBCs:	10 to 25; clumps
Odor:	NA	Ket:	neg			Casts:	0 to 2 hyaline
		Sp Grav:	1.015			Epith:	many SEs
		Blood:	neg			Bacteria:	neg
		pH:	5.0			Yeast:	mod
		Pro:	neg			Crystals:	few urates
		Urob:	norm				
		Nitr:	neg				
		LE:	pos				

1. Circle any abnormal or discrepant urinalysis findings.
2. What is the most likely cause of the patient's vaginitis?
3. Which two microscopic findings suggest that the urine tested is not from a midstream "clean catch" specimen?
4. Is the patient showing signs of renal damage or dysfunction?
   A. Yes
   B. No
5. Explain the physiologic mechanism most likely responsible for the presence of glucose in the patient's urine.
6. Select the diagnosis that best accounts for the glucosuria observed in this specimen.
   A. Normal; the glucose renal threshold was exceeded
   B. Insulin-dependent diabetes mellitus
   C. Non-insulin-dependent diabetes mellitus
   D. Glucose intolerance

CASE # 11 URINALYSIS

● ●

A 26-year-old man complains to his physician of weight loss, polydypsia, and polyuria. A routine urinalysis and plasma glucose level are obtained. The patient last ate 2 hours prior to specimen collection.

CHEMISTRY RESULTS

Plasma glucose: 230 mg/dL   (2-hour postprandial glucose: normal = 70 to 120 mg/dL; diabetic ≥ 140 mg/dL)

URINE RESULTS

Physical Exam		Chemical Exam		Confirmatory Tests		Microscopic Exam	
Color:	colorless	Glu:	> 2000	Clinitest (5 drp):	> 2000*	RBCs:	0 to 2
Clarity:	clear	Bili:	neg	Clinitest (2 drp):	≥ 5000	WBCs:	0 to 2
Odor:	NA	Ket:	small			Casts:	neg
		Sp Grav:	1.010				
		Blood:	neg				
		pH:	5.5				
		Pro:	neg				
		Urob:	norm				
		Nitr:	neg				
		LE:	neg				

*This test for reducing substances exhibited the pass-through effect.

● ●

1. Circle any abnormal or discrepant urinalysis findings.
2. Explain the pass-through effect observed when the Clinitest method was used to test the patient's urine.
3. Why is observing the pass-through effect so important?
4. Is the patient showing any signs of renal damage or dysfunction?
   A. Yes
   B. No
5. Select the diagnosis that best accounts for the glucosuria observed in this patient?
   A. Normal; the glucose renal threshold was exceeded
   B. Insulin-dependent diabetes mellitus
   C. Non-insulin-dependent diabetes mellitus
   D. Glucose intolerance

CASE # 12 URINALYSIS

A 14-day-old baby girl is admitted to the hospital with lethargy, diarrhea, vomiting, and difficulty in feeding. Physical examination reveals jaundice, an enlarged liver, cataract formation, and neurologic abnormalities (e.g., increased muscular tonus). No blood group incompatibility is found between the mother and the infant. The baby girl has lost 1.8 pounds since birth. The infant is fitted with a collection bag so that a urine specimen can be collected. The collection takes place over several hours, after which the baby's urine is sent to the laboratory for a routine urinalysis.

RESULTS

Physical Exam	Chemical Exam		Confirmatory Tests		Microscopic Exam	
Color: amber	Glu:	neg	Clinitest:	1000	RBCs:	0 to 2
Clarity: cloudy	Bili:	pos	Ictotest:	pos	WBCs:	0 to 2
Odor: NA	Ket:	neg			Casts:	0 to 2 hyaline
Yellow foam noted	Sp Grav:	1.025				0 to 2 granular
	Blood	neg			Epith:	few SEs
	pH:	8.0			Bacteria:	small
	Pro:	trace	SSA: 1+		Crystals:	mod triple
	Urob:	norm				phosphates
	Nitr:	neg				
	LE:	neg				

1. Circle any abnormal or discrepant urinalysis findings.
2. Which results may have been modified because of the specimen collection conditions?
3. What substance is most likely causing the yellow coloration of the foam?
4. What is the most likely explanation for the discrepancy in the glucose screening results?
5. What is a possible diagnosis for the patient? How should the laboratorian confirm this diagnosis?
6. Does the patient have a urinary tract infection? Why or why not?

CASE # 13 URINALYSIS

A 24-year-old man who had previously sustained a severe head injury in a car accident is seen by his physician. He complains of polydypsia and polyuria. Neurogenic diabetes insipidus is suspected and tests are performed to rule out other possibilities such as compulsive water ingestion.

RESULTS

Physical Exam		Chemical Exam		Microscopic Exam	
Color:	colorless	Glu:	neg	RBCs:	0 to 2
Clarity:	clear	Bili:	neg	WBCs:	0 to 2
Odor:	NA	Ket:	neg	Casts:	0 to 2 hyaline
		Sp Grav:	1.005		
		Blood:	neg		
		pH:	6.0		
		Pro:	neg		
		Urob:	norm		
		Nitr:	neg		
		LE:	neg		

1. Explain briefly the cause of polyuria in patients with diabetes insipidus.
2. Without fluid restrictions, the patient's urine osmolality is most likely
   A. less than 200 mOsm/kg.
   B. greater than 200 mOsm/kg.
3. The patient's polyuria should be classified as
   A. oncotic diuresis.
   B. psychosomatic diuresis.
   C. solute diuresis.
   D. water diuresis.
4. In neurogenic diabetes insipidus patients, if antidiuretic hormone (ADH) is given intravenously, the urine osmolality should
   A. remain unchanged.
   B. decrease.
   C. increase.
5. Which of the following tests could be used to evaluate the patient?
   A. The free-water clearance test
   B. The fluid deprivation test
   C. The glucose tolerance test
   D. The osmolar clearance test

Indicate whether each of the following statements is T (true) or F (false).
6. T F Patients with diabetes insipidus often have glucose present in the urine.
7. T F Patients with diabetes insipidus often have a high urine specific gravity.
8. T F Patients with diabetes insipidus often have urinary ketones present because of an inability to utilize the glucose present in the blood.
9. T F "Diabetes" is a general term referring to disorders characterized by copious production and excretion of urine.

CASE # 14 URINALYSIS

. . . .

A 48-year-old woman is admitted to a hospital for an emergency appendectomy. Owing to bleeding complications, she receives a unit of packed red blood cells following surgery. Two hours later, she develops fever, chills, and nausea. Two days following surgery, a routine urinalysis and a hemosiderin test (the Rous test) are performed.

RESULTS

Physical Exam		Chemical Exam		Confirmatory Tests		Microscopic Exam	
Color:	brown	Glu:	neg			RBCs:	0 to 2
Clarity:	slt cloudy	Bili:	neg			WBCs:	0 to 2
Odor:	NA	Ket:	neg			Casts:	2 to 5
		Sp Grav:	1.015				granular
		Blood:	large			Epith:	few SEs
		pH:	5.0				few TEs
		Pro:	trace	SSA:	trace	Crystals:	few
		Urob:	4				amorphous
		Nitr:	neg				urates
		LE:	neg				

Hemosiderin test: positive

. . . .

1. Circle any abnormal or discrepant urinalysis findings.
2. What is hemosiderin?
3. Explain how hemosiderin gets into the urine sediment.
4. What substance is most likely causing the brown color observed in the urine?
5. Explain the physiologic mechanism that leads to the increased urobilinogen in the patient's urine.
6. Owing to the intravascular hemolytic episode experienced by the patient, her serum bilirubin is significantly increased. Why is her urine bilirubin level still normal?

CASE # 15 URINALYSIS

A 23-year-old woman is seen in the emergency room with acute abdominal pain, nausea, and hypertension. She had an admission 1 year previously for intestinal complaints and neurologic symptoms that were compatible with depression. At that time, gastrointestinal (GI) and neurologic examinations were negative. The patient recently started oral contraceptives and states that she is taking no other medications. Routine hematology and chemistry tests are ordered, and all results are normal. A routine urinalysis is performed. One hour after testing the urine, the laboratorian notices that the urine has changed color significantly.

RESULTS

Physical Exam		Chemical Exam		Microscopic Exam	
Color:	yellow	Glu:	neg	RBCs:	0 to 2
(1 hour later — dark amber)		Bili:	neg	WBCs:	0 to 2
Clarity:	clear	Ket:	neg	Casts:	2 to 5 hyaline
Odor:	NA	Sp Grav:	1.015		0 to 2 granular
		Blood	neg	Epith:	few SEs
		pH:	5.0		few TEs
		Pro:	neg	Crystals:	few
		Urob:	norm		amorphous
		Nitr:	neg		urates
		LE:	neg		

Because of the observed color change, the laboratorian performs a Hoesch test.

Hoesch test: positive

1. Circle any abnormal or discrepant urinalysis findings.
2. What substance is most likely causing the color change observed in the patient's urine?
3. If the results of the Hoesch test were questionable, what test could be performed to confirm the presence of this substance?
4. Explain the physiologic process that results in this substance's appearing in the urine.
5. Based on the data provided, state the patient's most likely diagnosis.
6. In addition to the substance observed, this patient would most likely have increased levels of
   A. blood porphyrins.
   B. fecal porphyrins.
   C. urinary coproporphyrin.
   D. urinary δ-aminolevulinic acid.

CASE # 16 URINE AND FECAL ANALYSIS

A 45-year-old traveling salesman complains to his physician of diarrhea, weight loss, and back pain during the past month. Physical examination reveals a yellowing of the sclera of the eyes (jaundice), but no hepatomegaly or splenomegaly. Urine, blood, and fecal specimens (random and 72-hour) were collected for various tests, and the following results were obtained. A pancreatic tumor was identified by CT scan, and a biopsy of the tumor revealed pancreatic cancer.

URINE RESULTS

Physical Exam		Chemical Exam		Confirmatory Tests		Microscopic Exam	
Color:	amber	Glu:	neg			RBCs:	0 to 2
Clarity:	slt cloudy	Bili:	large	Ictotest:	pos	WBCs:	0 to 2
Odor:	NA	Ket:	neg			Casts:	0 to 2 hyaline
Yellow foam noted		Sp Grav:	1.015				2 to 5 granular
		Blood:	neg			Epith:	Few TEs
		pH:	5.5				
		Pro:	neg				
		Urob:	norm				
		Nitr:	neg				
		LE:	neg				

FECAL RESULTS

Fecal Macroscopic Exam	Fecal Microscopic Exam	Fecal Chemical Exam
Color: pale, clay-colored (acholic)	Leukocytes: absent	Fat: 10 g/d
Consistency: watery, greasy		
Form: bulky		

Microbiologic Exam

Stool cultures: negative for *Salmonella, Shigella, Campylobacter,* enteropathogenic *Escherichia coli,* or *Yersinia.*
Ova and parasites: negative for ova, cysts, and parasites.

BLOOD CHEMISTRY RESULTS

Xylose absorption test: normal

1. Circle any abnormal results.
2. This patient's fecal excretion should be classified as
   A. oncotic diuresis.
   B. osmotic diarrhea.
   C. secretory diarrhea.
   D. intestinal hypermotility.
3. What is the term for an increased amount of fat in the feces?

4. The most likely mechanism responsible for the patient's diarrhea is
   A. malabsorption.
   B. maldigestion.
   C. malexcretion.
   D. malsecretion.
5. Explain the physiologic mechanisms responsible for the increased fat and acholic stools excreted by the patient.
6. Why is the patient's urine urobilinogen result normal instead of decreased?

CASE # 17 FECAL ANALYSIS

A 23-year-old woman complains to her physician of headache, nausea, fever, and diarrhea over the previous week. She first experienced the diarrhea shortly after a summer picnic. She currently has five to six bowel movements each day. The stool does not appear bloody. A stool specimen is collected.

FECAL RESULTS

Fecal Macroscopic Exam

Color: brown
Consistency: watery

Fecal Microscopic Exam

Leukocytes: present

Fecal Chemical Exam

Sodium: 65 mEq/L
Potassium: 98 mEq/L
Osmolality: 340 mOsm/kg

Microbiologic Exam

Culture: *Salmonella* species present.
Ova and parasites: negative for ova, cysts, and parasites.

1. Circle any abnormal results.
2. Determine the calculated fecal osmolality using the formula:
   Osmolality $= 2 \times (Na_{fecal} + K_{fecal})$
3. Based on the difference between the observed and calculated osmolalities, this patient's condition would be classified as
   A. oncotic diuresis.
   B. osmotic diarrhea.
   C. secretory diarrhea.
   D. intestinal hypermotility.

CASE # 18 FECAL ANALYSIS

A 60-year-old woman is seen by her physician for a routine annual examination. Her only complaints are that she has a lack of stamina and she tires easily. Routine urinalysis and hematology tests are performed. She is sent home with instructions and supplies to collect three different fecal specimens for the detection of occult blood.

RESULTS

Urinalysis: normal

Fecal Occult Blood	Blood Hematology Results	Reference Range
Specimen #1 — positive	Hemoglobin: 9.8 g/dL	(female: 12 to 16 g/dL)
Specimen #2 — positive	Hematocrit: 36%	(female: 38% to 47%)
Specimen #3 — positive		

1. Circle any abnormal results.
2. Ingestion of which of the following substances can cause a false positive fecal occult blood test?
   1. Fish
   2. Bananas
   3. Cauliflower
   4. Vitamin C
      A. 1, 2, and 3 are correct.
      B. 1 and 3 are correct.
      C. 4 is correct.
      D. All are correct.
3. List at least two compounds other than hemoglobin that contain the heme moeity.
4. Why is guaiac the preferred indicator for fecal occult blood tests?
5. Which of the following could account for the occult blood results obtained?
   1. Ulcers
   2. Bleeding gums
   3. Hemorrhoids
   4. Colorectal cancer
      A. 1, 2, and 3 are correct.
      B. 1 and 3 are correct.
      C. 4 is correct.
      D. All are correct.
6. In this case, the data are suggestive of
   A. melena.
   B. creatorrhea.
   C. gastrointestinal bleeding.
   D. pancreatic cancer.

CASE # 19 SEMINAL FLUID ANALYSIS

A 36-year-old husband and his 32-year-old wife are undergoing evaluation for infertility. A seminal fluid specimen is collected at home and brought to the laboratory for routine testing.

SEMEN ANALYSIS

Physical Exam		Microscopic Exam	
Color:	gray	Motility:	70%
Volume:	4.5 mL	Concentration:	25×10^6 sperm/mL
Liquefaction:	50 min	Morphology:	70% normal
Viscosity:	0 (watery)	Viability:	60%
		Leukocytes:	0.8×10^6 cells/mL

1. Circle any abnormal or discrepant results.
2. Do any of the results obtained suggest improper specimen collection or laboratory error?
3. Are any of the results obtained associated with male infertility?
4. Based on these results, which chemical test should be performed to evaluate the functional integrity of the patient's seminal vesicles and ejaculatory ducts?

CASE # 20 AMNIOTIC FLUID ANALYSIS

A 32-year-old pregnant woman in her third pregnancy is seen by an obstetrician for the first time. The patient thinks she is around 33 weeks' gestation. She is from a third-world country and 3 months ago relocated to the United States with her husband and family. A patient history reveals that she has two children: a boy, 7 years old, and a girl, 5 years old. Both births were normal and uncomplicated; however, the patient states that her daughter had become extremely yellow shortly after her birth and was given a blood transfusion.

Routine prenatal blood work is performed. The mother is determined to be type O, Rh negative, and an antibody screen reveals the presence of an anti-Rh_0 (D). Her antibody titer is positive to a $1:32$ dilution. Her husband is determined to be type A, Rh positive. To assess and monitor the severity of the suspected hemolytic process taking place, weekly amniocenteses are scheduled.

AMNIOTIC FLUID RESULTS

33 Weeks' gestation		34 Weeks' gestation		35 Weeks' gestation	
ΔA_{450}:	0.200	ΔA_{450}:	0.245	Lecithin:	4.7 mg/dL
L/S Ratio:	1.1	L/S Ratio:	1.5	Sphingomyelin:	2.3 mg/dL
PG:	absent	PG:	absent	PG:	present

Spectrophotometer scan for ΔA_{450} determination:

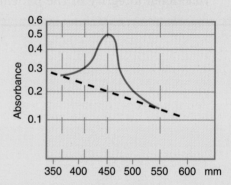

1. Calculate the ΔA_{450} for the amniotic fluid specimen obtained at 35 weeks' gestation.
2. Using the chart in Figure 12–4, determine the zone in which the ΔA_{450} value at 35 weeks' gestation resides.
3. Describe the clinical implications that accompany a result in this zone.
4. Using the values for lecithin and sphingomyelin provided at 35 weeks' gestation, calculate the L/S ratio.
5. Based on the fetal lung maturity tests performed *each* week, state if the fetal lungs are mature or immature.

CASE # 21 CEREBROSPINAL FLUID ANALYSIS

A 4-year-old girl is brought to the emergency room by her parents. She is lethargic, complains that her head hurts, and shows signs of stiffness in her neck. Her mother states that she has had "a temperature" for the last 2 days, and it is currently determined to be 104°C. She is admitted to the hospital, where blood is drawn and a lumbar puncture performed.

BLOOD CHEMISTRY RESULTS

Glucose, fasting: 90 mg/dL

CSF RESULTS

Physical Exam		Microscopic Exam		Chemical Exam	
Color:	colorless	Leukocyte count:	7300 cells/μL	Total protein:	130 mg/dL
Clarity:	cloudy (3+)	Differential count:		Glucose:	32 mg/dL
		Monocytes	7%	Lactate:	33 mg/dL
		Lymphocytes	6%		
		Neutrophils	87%		

Gram stain: results pending

1. Circle any abnormal results.
2. Calculate the CSF/plasma glucose ratio.
3. These results are most consistent with a preliminary diagnosis of
   A. viral meningitis.
   B. bacterial meningitis.
   C. Guillain-Barré syndrome.
   D. acute lymphocytic leukemia.
4. Does the CSF lactate value assist in the determination of a diagnosis for this patient?
5. If the Gram stain result is negative (i.e., no organisms are seen), should the diagnosis selected be changed? Why or why not?
6. Explain briefly the physiologic mechanisms that account for the CSF total protein and glucose values.

CASE # 22 CEREBROSPINAL FLUID ANALYSIS

A 39-year-old woman noticed numbness in her left leg and difficulty walking approximately 3 months ago. Since that time the numbness has seemed to come and go along with episodes of dizziness. More recently, she has experienced numbness on the right side of her face and "blurred" vision in her right eye that comes and goes. She gets tired easily and often feels unsteady while upright and walking. She is admitted to the hospital for tests.

BLOOD CHEMISTRY RESULTS

Glucose, fasting:	85 mg/dL		
Albumin:	4.6 g/dL	(Reference range:	3.5 to 5.0 mg/dL)
IgG:	1.4 g/dL	(Reference range:	0.65 to 1.50 g/dL)

CSF RESULTS

Physical Exam	Microscopic Exam		Chemical Exam	
Color: colorless	Leukocyte count:	3 cells/μL	Total protein:	45 mg/dL
Clarity: clear	Differential count:		Glucose:	72 mg/dL
	Monocytes	24%	Albumin:	28 mg/dL
	Lymphocytes	75%	IgG:	12.4 mg/dL
	Neutrophils	1%	Lactate:	18 mg/dL

Gram stain: no organisms seen

1. Circle any abnormal results.
2. Calculate the CSF/serum albumin index as follows:

$$\text{CSF/serum albumin index} = \frac{\text{Albumin}_{CSF}, \text{ mg/dL}}{\text{Albumin}_{serum}, \text{ g/dL}}$$

3. Why is the CSF/serum albumin index a good indicator of the integrity of the blood-brain barrier?
4. Calculate the CSF IgG index as follows:

$$\text{CSF IgG index} = \frac{\text{IgG}_{CSF}, \text{ mg/dL}}{\text{IgG}_{serum}, \text{ g/dL}} \times \frac{\text{Albumin}_{serum}, \text{ g/dL}}{\text{Albumin}_{CSF}, \text{ mg/dL}}$$

5. State a diagnosis that is consistent with the results obtained.
6. List two additional chemical tests, with the results expected, that could be used to confirm this diagnosis.

CASE # 23 SYNOVIAL FLUID ANALYSIS

A 51-year-old man presents with painful swelling in both knees. He is hospitalized, and an arthrocentesis is scheduled for the following morning. In the morning, a fasting blood sample is drawn for routine chemistry tests. Synovial fluid is aspirated from the patient's right knee and submitted to the laboratory.

BLOOD CHEMISTRY RESULTS

Glucose, plasma (fasting): 85 mg/dL   (Reference range: 60 to 105 mg/dL)
Uric acid: 12.7 mg/dL   (Reference range: 2.6 to 8.0 mg/dL)

SYNOVIAL FLUID RESULTS

Physical Exam		*Microscopic Exam*		*Chemical Exam*	
Color:	yellow	Leukocyte count:	43,000 cells/μL	Glucose:	55 mg/dL
Clarity:	cloudy	Differential count:		Uric acid:	12.4 mg/dL
Viscosity:	decreased	Monocytes	24%	Total protein:	4.0 g/dL
		Lymphocytes	13%	Lactate:	19 mg/dL
		Neutrophils	63%		

Crystals: many intracellular needle-shaped crystals; negative birefringence

Gram stain: no bacteria seen; many leukocytes present

1. Circle any abnormal results.
2. Calculate the plasma-synovial fluid glucose difference.
3. Based on the results obtained, this synovial fluid specimen should be classified as
   A. normal.
   B. noninflammatory (Group I).
   C. inflammatory (Group II).
   D. septic (Group III).
   E. hemorrhagic (Group IV).
4. What is the most likely identity of the crystals observed in the synovial fluid?
   A. Cholesterol
   B. Corticosteroid
   C. Hydroxyapatite
   D. Calcium pyrophosphate dihydrate
   E. Monosodium urate monohydrate
5. These results are most consistent with a diagnosis of
   A. gouty arthritis.
   B. pseudogout.
   C. rheumatoid arthritis.
   D. bacterial infection.
   E. traumatic arthritis, with previous corticosteroid injection.
6. If no crystals were observed in the microscopic examination, would the diagnosis change? Why or why not?

CASE # 24 SYNOVIAL FLUID ANALYSIS

A 37-year-old woman presents with persistent and painful swelling in her left knee several days following arthroscopic repair of a torn ligament (e.g., medial meniscus). A fasting blood sample is drawn for routine chemistry tests. Arthrocentesis is performed, and the synovial fluid is submitted to the laboratory.

BLOOD CHEMISTRY RESULTS

Glucose, plasma (fasting): 79 mg/dL   (Reference range: 60 to 105 mg/dL)
Uric acid: 6.2 mg/dL   (Reference range: 2.6 to 8.0 mg/dL)

SYNOVIAL FLUID RESULTS

Physical Exam		Microscopic Exam		Chemical Exam	
Color:	yellow	Leukocyte count:	97,000 cells/μL	Glucose:	35 mg/dL
Clarity:	cloudy	Differential count:		Uric acid:	5.9 mg/dL
Viscosity:	decreased	Monocytes	13%	Total protein:	5.3 g/dL
		Lymphocytes	5%	Lactate:	35 mg/dL
		Neutrophils	82%		
		Crystals:	none present		

Gram stain: gram-positive cocci present; many leukocytes present

1. Circle any abnormal results.
2. Calculate the plasma-synovial fluid glucose difference.
3. Based on the results obtained, this synovial fluid specimen should be classified as
    A.   normal.
    B.   noninflammatory (Group I).
    C.   inflammatory (Group II).
    D.   septic (Group III).
    E.   hemorrhagic (Group IV).
4. These results are most consistent with a diagnosis of
    A.   gouty arthritis.
    B.   pseudogout.
    C.   rheumatoid arthritis.
    D.   bacterial infection.
    E.   traumatic arthritis, with previous corticosteroid injection.

CASE # 25 SYNOVIAL FLUID ANALYSIS

   A 25-year-old professional football player is injured in an automobile accident. His recovery is complete except for persistent swelling in his left knee. This knee had been a chronic problem prior to the accident; the patient had a corticosteroid intra-articular injection 6 months previously. An arthrocentesis is scheduled along with the collection of a fasting blood sample for routine chemistry tests. The blood and synovial fluid are submitted to the laboratory.

BLOOD CHEMISTRY RESULTS

Glucose, plasma (fasting):   95 mg/dL   (Reference range: 60 to 105 mg/dL)
Uric acid: 5.7 mg/dL   (Reference range: 2.6 to 8.0 mg/dL)

SYNOVIAL FLUID RESULTS

Physical Exam		Microscopic Exam		Chemical Exam	
Color:	yellow	Leukocyte count:	950 cells/μL	Glucose:	80 mg/dL
Clarity:	slt cloudy	Differential count:		Uric acid:	5.9 mg/dL
Viscosity:	normal	Monocytes	65%	Total protein:	5.3 g/dL
		Lymphocytes	17%	Lactate:	21 mg/dL
		Neutrophils	18%		

Crystals: few needle-shaped crystals; negative birefringence

Gram stain: no bacteria seen; few leukocytes present

1.   Circle any abnormal results.
2.   Calculate the plasma-synovial fluid glucose difference.
3.   Based on the results obtained, this synovial fluid specimen should be classified as
     A.   normal.
     B.   noninflammatory (Group I).
     C.   inflammatory (Group II).
     D.   septic (Group III).
     E.   hemorrhagic (Group IV).
4.   Based on the results obtained, what is the most likely identity of the crystals observed in the synovial fluid?
     A.   Cholesterol
     B.   Corticosteroid
     C.   Hydroxyapatite
     D.   Calcium pyrophosphate dihydrate
     E.   Monosodium urate monohydrate
5.   These results are most consistent with a diagnosis of
     A.   gouty arthritis.
     B.   pseudogout.
     C.   rheumatoid arthritis.
     D.   bacterial infection.
     E.   traumatic arthritis, with previous corticosteroid injection.

CASE # 26 PLEURAL FLUID ANALYSIS

A 51-year-old man with a history of tuberculosis presents with a unilateral pleural effusion. A pleural fluid specimen is obtained by thoracentesis and sent to the laboratory for evaluation.

BLOOD CHEMISTRY RESULTS

Total protein:	7.0 g/dL	(Reference range: 6.0 to 8.3 g/dL)
Lactate dehydrogenase (LD):	520 U/L	(Reference range: 275 to 645 U/L)
Glucose, fasting:	75 mg/dL	(Reference range: 70 to 110 mg/dL)

PLEURAL FLUID RESULTS

Physical Exam		*Microscopic Exam*		*Chemical Exam*	
Color:	yellow	Leukocyte count:	1100 cells/μL	Total protein:	4.2 g/dL
Clarity:	cloudy	Differential count:		LD:	345 U/L
Clots present:	no	Mononuclear cells	93%	Glucose:	55 mg/dL
		Neutrophils	3%		

Gram stain: no organisms seen; leukocytes present

1. Calculate the fluid-to-serum total protein ratio.
2. Calculate the fluid-to-serum lactate dehydrogenase ratio.
3. Classify this pleural fluid specimen as a transudate or exudate and state two physiologic mechanisms that can cause this type of effusion.

CASE # 27 PERITONEAL FLUID ANALYSIS

A 48-year-old woman presents with ascites and pleural effusion. Blood is drawn, and a peritoneal fluid specimen is obtained by paracentesis and sent to the laboratory for evaluation.

BLOOD CHEMISTRY RESULTS

Total protein:	6.5 g/dL	(Reference range: 6.0 to 8.3 g/dL)
Lactate dehydrogenase (LD):	300 U/L	(Reference range: 275 to 645 U/L)
Glucose, fasting:	82 mg/dL	(Reference range: 70 to 110 mg/dL)
Liver function tests (ALT, AST, GGT, ALP):	normal	

PERITONEAL FLUID RESULTS

Physical Exam		*Microscopic Exam*		*Chemical Exam*	
Color:	yellow	Leukocyte count:	8 cells/μL	Total protein:	2.9 g/dL
Clarity:	clear			LD:	125 U/L
Clots present:	no			Glucose:	67 mg/dL

Gram stain: no organisms seen

Cytology examination: no malignant cells seen

1. Calculate the fluid-to-serum total protein ratio.
2. Calculate the fluid-to-serum lactate dehydrogenase ratio.
3. Classify this peritoneal fluid specimen as a transudate or exudate and state two physiologic mechanisms that can cause this type of effusion.

GLOSSARY OF TERMS

acholic stools: pale, gray, or clay-colored stools. They result when production of the normal fecal pigments—stercobilin, mesobilin, and urobilin—is partially or completely inhibited.

active transport: the movement of a substance (e.g., ion, solute) across a cell membrane and against a gradient, requiring the expenditure of energy.

acute interstitial nephritis (AIN): an acute inflammatory process that develops 3 to 21 days following exposure to an immunogenic drug (e.g., sulfonamides, penicillins) and results in injury to the renal tubules and interstitium. It is characterized by fever, skin rash, leukocyturia (particularly eosinophiliuria), and acute renal failure. Discontinuation of the offending agent can result in full recovery of renal function.

acute poststreptococcal glomerulonephritis: a type of glomerular inflammation occurring 1 to 2 weeks after a group A beta-hemolytic streptococcal infection. Onset is sudden, and the glomerular damage is immune mediated.

acute pyelonephritis: an inflammatory process involving the renal tubules, interstitium, and renal pelvis. It is most often due to a bacterial infection and is characterized by the sudden onset of symptoms, e.g., flank pain, dysuria, frequency of micturition, and urinary urgency.

acute renal failure (ARF): a renal disorder characterized by a sudden decrease in the glomerular filtration rate that results in azotemia and oliguria. It is a consequence of numerous conditions and can be categorized as prerenal (e.g., decrease in renal blood flow), renal (e.g., acute tubular necrosis), or postrenal (e.g., urinary tract obstruction). The disease course varies greatly, and survivors usually regain normal renal function.

acute tubular necrosis (ATN): a group of renal diseases characterized by the destruction of the renal tubular epithelium. It is classified into two types: ischemic ATN, resulting from decreased renal perfusion that results in tissue ischemia, and toxic ATN, resulting from the ingestion, inhalation, or injection of nephrotoxic substances.

afferent arteriole: a small branch of an interlobular renal artery that becomes the capillary tuft within a glomerulus.

albuminuria: the increased urinary excretion of the protein albumin.

aldosterone: a steroid hormone secreted by the adrenal cortex. It stimulates the absorption of sodium and the excretion of potassium in the distal tubules and is regulated by the renin-angiotensin-aldosterone system.

alkaptonuria: a rare recessively inherited disease characterized by excretion of large amounts of homogentisic acid (i.e., alkapton bodies) owing to a deficiency of the enzyme homogentisic acid oxidase.

aminoaciduria: the presence of increased amounts of amino acids in the urine.

amyloidosis: a group of systemic diseases

characterized by the deposition of amyloid, a proteinaceous substance, between cells in numerous tissues and organs.

antidiuretic hormone (ADH) (also called vasopressin): a hormone produced by the posterior pituitary that regulates the osmotic reabsorption of water by the collecting tubules. Without adequate ADH present, water is not reabsorbed.

anuria (also called anuresis): the absence or cessation of urine excretion.

aperture diaphragm: the microscope component that regulates the angle of light presented to the specimen. It is located at the base of the condenser and changes the diameter of the opening through which the source light rays must pass to enter the condenser.

arthritis: the inflammation of a joint.

arthrocentesis: a percutaneous puncture procedure used to remove synovial fluid from joint cavities.

ascites: the excessive accumulation of serous fluid in the peritoneal cavity.

ascorbic acid (also called vitamin C): a water-soluble vitamin; it is a strong reducing agent that readily oxidizes to its salt, dehydroascorbate.

ascorbic acid interference: the inhibition of a chemical reaction by the presence of ascorbic acid. As a strong reducing agent, ascorbic acid readily reacts with diazonium salts or hydrogen peroxide, removing these chemicals from intended reaction sequences. As a result, colorless dehydroascorbate is formed and no color change is observed.

azotemia: a condition characterized by increased amounts of nonprotein nitrogenous substances in the blood such as urea, creatinine, ammonia, uric acid, creatine, and amino acids. It is caused by decreased filtration and elimination of these substances by the kidneys.

bacteriuria: the presence of bacteria in urine.

baroreceptors: sensory nerve endings found in certain blood vessels that detect changes in blood pressure within these vessels. Baroreceptors are stimulated by the stretching of the vessel wall as pressure increases.

basement membrane: a trilayer structure located within the glomerulus along the base of the epithelium (podocytes) of the urinary (Bowman's) space. The size-discriminating component of the glomerular filtration barrier, the basement membrane limits the passage of substances to those with an effective molecular radius less than 4 nm. Using electron microscopy, three distinct layers are evident in the basement membrane: the lamina rara interna (next to the capillary endothelium), the lamina densa (centrally located), and the lamina rara externa (next to the podocytes).

bilirubin: a yellow-orange pigment resulting from heme catabolism. It causes a characteristic discoloration of urine, plasma, and other body fluids when present in the fluid in significant amounts. When exposed to air, bilirubin oxidizes to biliverdin, a green pigment.

biological hazard: a biological material or an entity contaminated with biological material that is potentially capable of transmitting disease.

birefringent (also called doubly refractile): the ability of a substance to refract light in two directions.

bladder: a muscular sac that serves as a reservoir for the accumulation of urine.

blood-brain barrier: the physiologic interface between the vascular system and the cerebrospinal fluid. Changes in the normal regulating conditions of the blood-brain barrier result in changes in the normal chemical and cellular composition of the cerebrospinal fluid.

Bowman's capsule: see **glomerulus**.

Bowman's space: see **urinary space**.

brightfield microscopy: type of microscopy that produces a magnified image that appears dark against a bright or white background.

calculi (also called stones): solid aggregates or concretions of chemicals, usually mineral salts, that form in secreting glands of the body.

casts: cylindrical bodies that form in the lumen of the renal tubules. Their core matrix is principally made up of Tamm-Horsfall mucoprotein, although other plasma proteins can be incorporated. Because casts are formed in the tubular lumen, any chemical or formed element present, e.g., cells, fat, and bacteria, can also be incorporated into its matrix. When excreted in the urine, casts are enumerated and classified by the type of inclusions present.

catabolism: a degradative process that converts complex substances into simpler components.

catheterized specimen: a urine specimen obtained using a sterile catheter (a flexible tube) that is inserted through the urethra and into the bladder. Urine flows directly from the bladder by gravity and collects in a plastic reservoir bag.

cerebrospinal fluid (CSF): the normally clear, colorless fluid found between the arachnoid and pia mater in the brain and spinal cord. It is formed primarily from plasma by selective secretions of the choroid plexus and, to a lesser extent, by intrathecal synthesis by ependymal cells of the ventricles.

Chemical Hygiene Plan (CHP): an established protocol developed by each facility for the identification, handling, storage, and disposal of all hazardous chemicals. It was established as a mandatory requirement for all facilities that deal with chemical hazards by the Occupational Safety and Health Administration (OSHA) in January 1990.

choroid plexus: the highly vascular folds of capillaries, nerves, and ependymal cells in the pia mater. Located in the four ventricles of the brain, the choroid plexus actively synthesizes cerebrospinal fluid.

chromatic aberration: the unequal refraction of light rays by a lens because the different wavelengths of light refract or bend at different angles. As a result, the image produced has undesired color fringes.

chronic glomerulonephritis: a slowly progressive glomerular disease that develops years after other forms of glomerulonephritis. It usually leads to irreversible renal failure, requiring dialysis or kidney transplantation.

chronic pyelonephritis: a renal inflammatory process involving the tubules, interstitium, renal calyces, and renal pelves, most often as a result of reflex nephropathies that cause chronic bacterial infections of the upper urinary tract. This chronic inflammation results in fibrosis and scarring of the kidney and eventually loss of renal function.

chronic renal failure (CRF): a renal disorder characterized by the progressive loss of renal function owing to an irreversible and intrinsic renal disease. The glomerular filtration rate decreases progressively. CRF concludes with end-stage renal disease, characterized by isosthenuria, significant proteinuria, variable hematuria, and numerous casts of all types, particularly waxy and broad casts.

chyle: a milky-appearing emulsion of lymph and chylomicrons (triglyceride) that originates from intestinal lymphatic absorption during digestion.

clarity (also called turbidity): the transparency of a urine specimen. Clarity varies with the amount of suspended particulate matter in the urine specimen.

clue cells: squamous epithelial cells with large numbers of bacteria adhering to them. They appear soft and finely granular with indistinct or "shaggy" cell borders. To be considered a clue cell, the bacteria do not need to cover the entire cell, but the bacterial organisms must extend beyond the cell's cytoplasmic borders. Clue cells are characteristic of bacterial vaginosis, a synergistic infection involving *Gardnerella vaginalis* and anaerobic bacteria.

collecting duct: the portion of a renal nephron following the distal convoluted tubule. Many distal tubules empty into a single collecting duct. The collecting duct traverses both the renal cortex and the medulla and is the site of final urine concentration. The collecting ducts terminate at the renal papilla, conveying the urine formed into the renal calyces of the kidney.

collecting duct cells: cuboidal or polygonal cells approximately 12 to 20 μm in diameter with a large, centrally located dense nucleus. These cells form the lining of the collecting tubules and become larger and more columnar as they approach the renal calyces.

collecting tubule: see **collecting duct.**

colligative property: a characteristic of a solution that depends only on the number of solute particles present, regardless of the molecular size or charge. The four colligative properties are freezing point depression, vapor pressure depression, osmotic pressure elevation, and boiling point elevation. These properties form the basis of methods and instrumentation used to measure the concentration of solutes in body fluids (e.g., serum, urine, fecal supernates). **(See freezing point osmometer and vapor pressure osmometer.)**

compound microscope: a microscope with two lens systems. The lens system closest to the specimen (objective) forms the initial image and the second lens system (eyepiece) further magnifies the image for viewing.

condenser: the microscope component that gathers and focuses the illumination light onto the specimen for viewing. It is a lens system (either a single lens or a combination of lenses) and is located beneath the microscope stage.

constipation: infrequent and difficult bowel movements, compared to an individual's normal bowel movement pattern. The fecal material produced is made up of hard, small, frequently spherical masses.

cortex: the outer portion of the kidney, approximately 1.4 cm thick and macroscopically granular in appearance. It is where the glomeruli and convoluted tubules are located.

countercurrent exchange mechanism: a passive exchange by diffusion of reabsorbed solutes and water from the nephron's medullary interstitium into the blood of its vascular blood supply (i.e., the vasa recta). A requirement of this process is that the flow of blood in the ascending and descending vessels of the U-shaped vasa recta be in opposite directions; hence the term *countercurrent.* The countercurrent exchange mechanism simultaneously supplies nutrients to the medulla and removes solutes and water reabsorbed into the blood. As a result, it assists in the maintenance of the medullary hypertonicity.

countercurrent multiplier mechanism: a process occurring in the loop of Henle of each nephron that establishes and maintains the osmotic gradient within the medullary interstitium. The medullary osmolality gradient ranges from being iso-osmotic (approximately 300 mOsm/kg) at its border with the cortex to approximately 1400 mOsm/kg at the inner medulla or papilla. A requirement of this process is that the flow of the ultrafiltrate in the descending and ascending limbs be in opposite directions; hence the name *countercurrent.* In addition, active sodium and chloride reabsorption in the ascending limb combined with passive water reabsorption in the descending limb are essential components of this process. The countercurrent multiplier mechanism accounts for approximately 50 percent of the solutes concentrated in the renal medulla.

creatinine clearance: a renal clearance test that measures the volume of plasma cleared of creatinine by the kidneys per unit of time. Reported in milliliters per minute, it is determined by the equation $C = U \times V/P$, in which U and P are the urine and plasma concentrations of creatinine, respectively, and V is the volume of urine excreted in a timed collection, usually 24 hours.

creatorrhea: the presence of undigested meat fibers in the feces.

critical value: a patient test result representing a life-threatening condition that requires immediate attention and intervention.

cryoscope: see **osmometer.**

crystals: entities formed by the solidification of urinary solutes. The solutes can be a single element, a compound, or a mixture and are arranged in a regular repeating pattern throughout the crystalline structure.

cystinosis: an inherited recessive disorder characterized by intracellular deposition of the amino acid cystine throughout the body. Cystine deposition within renal tubular cells results in their dysfunction and the development of extensive renal disease.

cystinuria: an autosomal recessive inherited disorder characterized by the inability to reabsorb the amino acids cystine, arginine, lysine, and ornithine in the renal tubules, as well as in the intestine. This results in the presence of cystine and the other dibasic amino acids in the urine, despite normal cystine metabolism. Because cystine is insoluble in an acid pH, it readily precipitates in the renal tubules, resulting in formation of calculi. The other dibasic amino acids are freely soluble and are easily excreted.

cytocentrifugation: a specialized centrifuge procedure used to produce a monolayer of the cellular constituents in various body fluids on a microscope slide. The slides are fixed and stained, providing a permanent preparation for cytologic studies.

darkfield microscopy: type of microscopy that produces a magnified image that appears brightly illuminated against a dark background. A special condenser presents only oblique light rays to the specimen. The specimen interacts with these rays (e.g., refraction, reflection), causing visualization of the specimen. It is used on unstained specimen preparations and is the preferred technique for identification of spirochetes.

decontamination: a process to remove a potential chemical or biological hazard from an area or entity (e.g., countertop, instrument, materials) and render the area or entity "safe." Various processes may be employed in decontamination, such as autoclaving, incineration, chemical neutralization, and disinfecting agents.

density: an expression of concentration in terms of the mass of solutes present per volume of solution.

diabetes insipidus: a metabolic disease characterized by polyuria and polydipsia owing to either defective antidiuretic hormone production (neurogenic) or lack of renal tubular response to antidiuretic hormone (nephrogenic).

diabetes mellitus: a metabolic disease characterized by the inability to metabolize glucose, resulting in hyperglycemia, glucosuria, and alterations in fat and protein metabolism. The cause is either defective insulin production or the formation of dysfunctional insulin by the pancreas. The disease is classified into types I or II, depending on age of onset, initial presentation, insulin requirements, and other factors.

diarrhea: an increase in the volume, liquidity, and frequency of bowel movements compared to an individual's normal bowel movement pattern.

diffuse: widely distributed.

disaccharidase deficiency: a lack of sufficient enzymes (disaccharidases) for the metabolism of disaccharides in the small intestine. This deficiency can be hereditary or acquired (e.g., resulting from diseases, drug therapy).

distal convoluted tubular cells: Oval to round cells approximately 14 to 25 μm in diameter with a small, central to slightly eccentric nucleus and a dense chromatin pattern. These cells form the lining of the distal convoluted tubules.

distal convoluted tubule: the portion of a renal nephron immediately following the loop of Henle. It begins at the juxtaglomerular apparatus with the macula densa, a specialized group of cells located at the vascular pole. The distal tubule is convoluted and after two to three loops becomes the collecting tubule (or duct).

distal tubule: the portion of the nephron that immediately follows the loop of Henle and precedes the collecting tubule or duct. It is subdivided into a straight portion that precedes the macula densa and a convoluted portion that begins at the macula densa and terminates with the collecting tubule.

diuresis: an increase in urine excretion. Various causes of diuresis include increased fluid intake, diuretic therapy, hormonal imbalance, renal dysfunction, and drug ingestion (e.g., alcohol, caffeine).

documentation: a written record. In the laboratory, it includes written policies and procedures, quality control, and maintenance records. It may encompass the recording of any action performed or observed including verbal correspondence, observations, and corrective actions taken.

dysuria: painful urination.

edema: the accumulation of fluid in the extracellular spaces of the tissues.

efferent arteriole: the arteriole exiting a glomerulus, the efferent arteriole is formed by the rejoining of the anastomosing capillary network within the glomerulus.

effusion: an accumulation of fluid in a body cavity as a result of a pathologic process.

Ehrlich's reaction: the development of a red- or magenta-colored chromophore as a result of the interaction of a substance (e.g., urobilinogen, porphobilinogen) with p-dimethylaminobenzaldehyde (also called Ehrlich's agent) in an acid medium.

-emia: of or relating to the blood.

endothelium: the layer of epithelial cells that line the vessels and serous cavities of the body.

epididymis: a long coiled tubular structure attached to the upper surface of each testis and continuous with the vas deferens. It is the site of final spermatozoa maturation and the development of motility. Spermatozoa are stored here until ejaculation.

epithelium: the layer of cells that covers the internal and external surfaces of the body.

erythroblastosis fetalis: a hemolytic disease of the newborn that results from a blood group incompatibility between the mother and the infant.

etiology: the study of factors that cause disease, such as genetic factors, infection, toxins, or trauma.

external quality assurance: the use of materials (e.g., specimens, kodachrome slides) from an external unbiased source to monitor and determine if quality goals (i.e., test results) are being achieved. Results are compared to the results from other facilities performing the same function. Proficiency surveys are one form of external quality assurance.

exudate: an effusion in a body cavity caused by increased capillary permeability or decreased lymphatic absorption. It is identified by a fluid-to-serum total protein ratio greater than 0.5, a fluid-to-serum lactate dehydrogenase ratio greater than 0.6, or both.

eyepiece (also called ocular): the microscope lens or system of lenses located closest to the viewer's eye. It produces the secondary image magnification of the specimen.

Fanconi syndrome: a complication of inherited and acquired diseases characterized by generalized proximal tubular dysfunction, resulting in aminoaciduria, proteinuria, glucosuria, and phosphaturia.

fasting specimen: a urine specimen collected after a fast and containing only those solutes and metabolites excreted during the fasting period.

fenestrated: pierced with openings.

field diaphragm: the microscope component that controls the diameter of the light beams that strike the specimen and hence reduces stray light. It is located at the light exit of the illumination source. With Köhler illumination, the field diaphragm is used to appropriately adjust and center the condenser.

first morning specimen: the first urine specimen voided after rising from sleep. The night before the collection, the patient voids before going to bed. Usually the first morning specimen has been retained in the bladder for 6 to 8 hours and is ideal to test for substances that may require concentration (e.g., protein) or incubation for detection (e.g., nitrites).

fluorescence microscopy: type of microscopy modified to visualize fluorescent substances. It employs two filters: one to select a specific wavelength of illumination light (excitation filter) that is absorbed by the specimen, and another filter (barrier filter) to transmit the different, longer-wavelength light emitted from the specimen to the eyepiece for viewing. The selection of these filters is determined by the fluorophore (natural or added) present in the specimen.

fluorescence polarization: an analytical technique based on the change in polarization observed in fluorescent light emitted compared to the incident polarized fluorescent light. The observed changes in the polarization of light directly result from the molecular size of the fluorophore-tagged complex. Large molecules cannot randomly orient as rapidly as small molecules. Hence, fluorophores tagged to large molecular complexes will emit more fluorescence in the same polarized plane as the initial incident light than will fluorophores tagged to molecular complexes.

focal: localized or limited to a specific area.

focal proliferative glomerulonephritis: a type of glomerular inflammation characterized by cellular proliferation in a specific part of the glomeruli (segmental) and limited to a specific number of glomeruli (focal).

focal segmental glomerulosclerosis (FSG): a type of glomerular disease characterized by sclerosis of the glomeruli. Not all glomeruli are affected, hence the term *focal,* and of those that are, only certain portions become diseased, hence the term *segmental.*

fractional collection (also called double-voided specimen): a urine specimen collected after a specific time interval. The patient voids at the beginning of the collection. This initial specimen may be tested (e.g., fasting specimen of a glucose tolerance test) or discarded. At the end of the time interval, the patient voids and collects this urine for testing (e.g., 2-hour postprandial [2 h PP] urine specimen for the detection of glucosuria). It is termed a double-voided specimen because, frequently, blood samples are drawn at the same time for comparison of the analyte of interest in the blood and urine.

free water clearance (also called solute-free water clearance): the volume of water cleared by the kidneys per minute in excess of that necessary to remove solutes. Denoted C_{H_2O} and reported in milliliters per minute, it is determined using the equation $C_{H_2O} = V \times C_{Osm}$. V is the volume of urine excreted in a timed collection (mL/min), and C_{Osm} is the osmolar clearance (mL/min).

freezing point osmometer: an instrument that measures osmolality based on the freezing point depression of a solution compared to that of pure water. It consists of a cooling bath that supercools the sample below its freezing point. Freezing of the sample is mechanically induced by a stir wire. As ice crystals form, a sensitive thermistor probe monitors the temperature until an equilibrium is obtained between the solid and liquid phases. This equilibrium temperature is the sample's freezing point, from which the osmolality of the sample is determined. One osmole of solute per kilogram of solvent (1 Osm/kg) depresses the freezing point of water by 1.86°C.

galactosuria: the presence of galactose in the urine.

glomerular filtration barrier: the structure within the glomerulus that determines the composition of the plasma ultrafiltrate formed in the urinary space by regulating the passage of solutes. The glomerular filtration barrier consists of the capillary endothelium, the basement membrane, and the epithelial podocytes, each coated with a "shield of negativity." Solute selectivity by the barrier is based on the molecular size and the electrical charge of the solute.

glomerular filtration rate (GFR): the rate of plasma cleared by the glomeruli per unit of time (mL/min). This rate is determined using clearance tests of substances that are known to be exclusively removed by glomerular filtration and that are not reabsorbed or secreted by the nephrons (e.g., inulin).

glomerular proteinuria: increased amounts of protein in urine because of a compromised or diseased glomerular filtration barrier.

glomerulonephritides (GN): a group of nephritic conditions characterized by damage and inflammation of the glomeruli. Causes are varied and include immunologic, metabolic, and hereditary disorders.

glomerulus (also called renal corpuscle): a tuft or network of capillaries encircled by and intimately related with the proximal end of a renal tubule (i.e., Bowman's capsule). The glomerulus is composed of four distinct structural components: the capillary endothelial cells, the epithelial cells (podocytes), the mesangium, and the basement membrane.

glucosuria: the presence of glucose in urine.

glycosuria: see **glucosuria.**

hematuria: the presence of red blood cells in urine.

hemoglobinuria: the presence of hemoglobin in urine.

hemosiderin: an insoluble form of storage iron. When renal tubular cells reabsorb hemoglobin, the iron is catabolized into ferritin (a major storage form of iron). Ferritin subsequently denatures to form insoluble hemosiderin granules (micelles of ferric hydroxide) that appear in the urine 2 to 3 days following a hemolytic episode.

hyaluronate: a high-molecular-weight polymer of repeating disaccharide units secreted by synoviocytes into the synovial fluid. It imparts the high viscosity to synovial fluid and serves as a lubricant for a joint. It is a salt or ester of hyaluronic acid.

hydramnios (also called polyhydramnios): an abnormally increased amount of amniotic fluid in the amniotic sac. It is often associated with central nervous system or gastrointestinal tract malformations of the fetus.

hydrometer: a weighted glass float with a long, narrow, calibrated stem used to measure the specific gravity of solutions. When placed in pure water (at a specific temperature), it displaces a volume of water equal to its weight, and the meniscus of the water intersects the calibrated stem at the value 1.000. When placed in a solution of greater specific gravity than water, the hydrometer displaces a smaller volume of liquid and the specific gravity is read from the calibrated stem.

hyperosmotic: see **hypertonic.**

hypersthenuric: the excretion of urine having a specific gravity greater than 1.010.

hypertonic: describing a solution or fluid having a higher concentration of osmotically active solutes compared to that of the blood plasma.

hypo-osmotic: see **hypotonic.**

hyposthenuric: the excretion of urine having a specific gravity less than 1.010.

hypotonic: describing a solution or fluid having a lower concentration of osmotically active solutes compared to that of the blood plasma.

IgA nephropathy: a type of glomerular inflammation characterized by the deposition of IgA in the glomerular mesangium. It often occurs 1 to 2 days following a mucosal infection of the respiratory, gastrointestinal, or urinary tract.

infectious waste disposal policy: a procedure outlining the equipment, materials, and steps used in the collection, storage, removal, and decontamination of infectious material and substances.

interdigitate: to interlock or interrelate.

interference contrast microscopy: type of microscopy in which the difference in optical light paths through the specimen is converted into intensity differences in the specimen image. Three-dimensional images of high contrast and resolution are obtained, without haloing. Two types available are modulation contrast (Hoffman) and differential interference contrast (Nomarski).

interstitial cells of Leydig: the cells located in the interstitial space between the seminiferous tubules of the testes. These cells produce and secrete the hormone testosterone.

ionic specific gravity: the density of a solution owing to ionic solutes only. Nonionizing substances such as urea, glucose, protein, and radiographic contrast media are not detectable using ionic specific gravity measurements (e.g., specific gravity by commercial reagent strips).

iso-osmotic: describing a solution or fluid having the same concentration of osmotically active solutes as that of the blood plasma.

isosthenuria: the excretion of urine having the same specific gravity (and osmolality) as the plasma. Because the specific gravity of protein-free plasma and the original ultrafiltrate is 1.010, the inability to excrete urine with a higher or lower specific gravity indicates significantly impaired renal tubular function.

jaundice: the yellowish pigmentation of skin, sclera, body tissues, and body fluids owing to the presence of increased amounts of bilirubin. Jaundice appears when plasma bilirubin concentrations reach approximately 2 to 3 mg/dL, i.e., two to three times the normal bilirubin concentrations.

juxtaglomerular apparatus: a specialized area located at the vascular pole of a nephron. It is composed of cells from the afferent and efferent arterioles, the macula densa of the distal tubule, and the extraglomerular mesangium. The juxtaglomerular apparatus is actually an endocrine organ and the primary producer of renin.

ketonuria: the presence of ketones (i.e., acetoacetate, β-hydroxybutyrate, acetone) in urine.

kidneys: the organs of the urinary system that produce urine. Normally, each individual has two kidneys. The kidneys' primary function is to filter the blood, removing waste products and regulating electrolytes, water, acid-base balance, and blood pressure.

KOH preparation: a preparation technique used to enhance the viewing of fungal elements. Secretions obtained using a sterile swab are suspended in saline. A drop of this suspension is placed on a microscope slide, followed by a drop of 10 percent KOH (potassium hydroxide). The slide is warmed and viewed microscopically. KOH destroys most formed elements with the exception of bacteria and fungal elements.

Köhler illumination: type of microscopic illumination in which a lamp condenser (located above the light source) focuses the image of the light source (lamp filament) onto the front focal plane of the substage condenser (where the aperture diaphragm is located). The substage condenser sharply focuses the image of the field diaphragm (located at or slightly in front of the lamp condenser) at the same plane as the focused specimen. As a result, the filament image does not appear in the field of view, and bright, even illumination is obtained. Köhler illumination requires appropriate adjustments of the condenser and both the field and aperture diaphragms.

leukocyturia: the presence of leukocytes, i.e., white blood cells, in the urine. cf. **pyuria**.

lipiduria: the presence of lipids in the urine.

liquefaction: the physical conversion of seminal fluid from a coagulum to a liquid following ejaculation.

loop of Henle: the tubular portion of a nephron immediately following and continuous with the proximal tubule. Located in the renal medulla, the loop of Henle is composed of a thin descending limb, a U-shaped segment (also called a hairpin turn), and thin and thick ascending limbs. The thick ascending limb of the loop of Henle (sometimes called the straight portion of the distal tubule) ends as the tubule enters the vascular pole of the glomerulus.

macula densa: a specialized and morphologically distinct area of the distal convoluted tubule. It is located at the vascular pole and is in intimate contact with the juxtaglomerular cells of the afferent arteriole.

malabsorption: the inadequate intestinal absorption of processed foodstuffs despite normal digestive ability.

maldigestion: the inability to convert foodstuffs in the gastrointestinal tract into readily absorbable substances.

maltese cross pattern: a design that appears as an orb divided into four quadrants by a bright maltese-style cross. When the microscopist uses polarizing microscopy, cholesterol droplets exhibit this characteristic pattern, which aids in their identification. Other substances, such as starch granules, can show a similar pattern.

maple syrup urine disease (MSUD): a rare autosomal recessive inherited defect or deficiency in the enzyme responsible for the oxidation of the branched-chain amino acids—leucine, isoleucine, and valine. As a result, these amino acids along with their corresponding α-keto acids accumulate in the blood, cerebrospinal fluid, and urine. The name derives from the subtle maple syrup odor of the urine from these patients.

material safety data sheet (MSDS): a written document provided by the manufacturer or distributor of a chemical substance listing information about that chemical's characteristics. An MSDS includes the chemical's identity and hazardous ingredients, its physical and chemical properties including reactivity, any physical or health hazards, and precautions for the safe handling, storage, and disposal of the chemical.

maximal tubular capacity (T_m): see **maximal tubular reabsorptive capacity** and **maximal tubular secretory capacity.**

maximal tubular reabsorptive capacity: denoted T_m, it is the maximal rate of *reabsorption* of a solute by the tubular epithelium per minute (mg/min). It varies with each solute and is dependent on the glomerular filtration rate.

maximal tubular secretory capacity: also denoted T_m, it is the maximal rate of *secretion* of a solute by the tubular epithelium per minute (mg/min). This rate differs for each solute.

mechanical stage: the microscope component that holds the microscope slide with the specimen for viewing. It is adjustable, front to back and side to side, to enable viewing of the entire specimen.

meconium: a dark green, gelatinous or mucus-like material representing swallowed amniotic fluid and intestinal secretions that is excreted by the near-term or full-term infant. The infant normally passes meconium as the first bowel movement shortly after birth.

medulla: the inner portion of the kidney. Macroscopically organized into pyramids, it is the location of the loops of Henle and the collecting tubules (or ducts).

melanuria: the increased excretion of melanin in the urine.

melena: the excretion of dark or black, pitchy-looking stools owing to the presence of large amounts (50 to 100 mL/d) of blood in the feces. The coloration is due to hemoglobin oxidation by intestinal and bacterial enzymes in the gastrointestinal tract.

membranoproliferative glomerulonephritis (MPGN): a type of glomerular inflammation characterized by cellular proliferation of the mesangium, with leukocyte infiltration and thickening of the glomerular basement membrane. Immunologically based, it is slowly progressive.

membranous glomerulonephritis (MGN): a type of glomerular inflammation characterized by the deposition of immunoglobulins and complement along the epithelial side (podocytes) of the basement membrane. It is associated with numerous immune-mediated diseases and is the major cause of nephrotic syndrome in adults.

meninges: the three membranes that surround the brain and spinal cord. The innermost membrane is the pia mater, the outermost membrane is the dura mater, and the centrally located membrane is the arachnoid mater.

meningitis: inflammation of the meninges.

mesangium: the cells that form the structural core tissue of a glomerulus, the mesangium lies between the glomerular capillaries (endothelium) and the podocytes (tubular epithelium). The mesangial cells derive from smooth muscle and have contractility characteristics and the ability to phagocytize and pinocytize.

mesothelial cells: flat cells that form a single layer of epithelium, which covers the surface of serous membranes (i.e., the pleura, pericardium, and peritoneum).

micturition: urination or the passing of urine.

midstream "clean catch" specimen: a urine specimen obtained after thorough cleansing of the glans penis in the male or the urethral meatus in the female. Following the cleansing procedure, the patient passes the first portion of the urine into the toilet, stops and collects the midportion in the specimen container, then passes any remaining urine into the toilet. Used for both routine urinalysis and urine culture, it is essentially free of contaminants from the genitalia and distal urethra.

minimal change disease (MCD): a type of glomerular inflammation characterized by the loss of the podocyte foot processes. Believed to be immune mediated, it is the major cause of nephrotic syndrome in children.

myoglobinuria: the presence of myoglobin in urine.

nephritis: inflammation of the kidney.

nephron: the functional unit of the kidney. Each kidney contains approximately 1.3 million nephrons. A nephron is composed of five distinct areas: the glomerulus, the proximal tubule, the loop of Henle, the distal tubule, and the collecting tubule or duct. Each region of the nephron is specialized and plays a role in the formation and final composition of urine.

nephrotic syndrome: a complication of numerous disorders characterized by the presentation of proteinuria, hypoalbuminemia, hyperlipidemia, lipiduria, and generalized edema.

nocturia: excessive or increased frequency of urination at night (i.e., the patient excretes greater than 500 mL per night).

numerical aperture (NA): a number that indicates the resolving power of a lens system. It is derived mathematically from the refractive index (N) of the optical medium (for air, N = 1) and the angle of light (μ) made by the lens: NA = N $\times$ sin μ.

objective: the lens or system of lenses located closest to the specimen. It produces the primary image magnification of the specimen.

occult blood: small amounts of blood, not visually apparent, in the feces.

Occupational Safety and Health Administration (OSHA): established by Congress in 1970, OSHA is a division of the U.S. Department of Labor that is responsible for defining potential safety and health hazards in the workplace, establishing guidelines to safeguard all workers from these hazards, and monitoring compliance with these guidelines. The intent is to alert, educate, and protect all employees in every environment to potential safety and health hazards.

oligoclonal bands: multiple discrete bands in the gamma region noted during electrophoresis of plasma or other body fluids (e.g., CSF).

oligohydramnios: a decreased amount of amniotic fluid in the amniotic sac.

oliguria: a significant decrease in the volume of urine excreted (less than 400 mL/d).

osmolality: an expression of concentration in terms of the total number of solute particles present per kilogram of solvent, denoted Osm/kg H_2O.

osmolar clearance: the volume of plasma water cleared by the kidneys each minute that contains the same amount of solutes that are present in the blood plasma (i.e., the same osmolality). Stated another way, osmolar clearance is the volume of plasma water necessary for the rate of solute elimination. Reported in milliliters per minute, it is determined by the equation $C = U \times V/P$, in which U and P are the urine and plasma osmolalities, respectively, and V is the volume of urine excreted in a timed collection, usually 24 hours.

osmometer: see **freezing point osmometer** and **vapor pressure osmometer.**

osmosis: the movement of water across a semipermeable membrane in an attempt to achieve an osmotic equilibrium between two compartments or solutions of differing osmolality (i.e., an osmotic gradient). This mechanism is passive, i.e., it requires no energy.

oval fat bodies: renal tubular epithelial cells or macrophages with inclusions of fat or lipids. Often these cells are engorged such that specific cellular identification is impossible.

overflow proteinuria: an increased amount of protein in urine owing to increased amounts of plasma proteins passing through a healthy glomerular filtration barrier.

paracellular: the transport of substances from one tissue space to another around cells via intercellular junctions.

paracentesis: a percutaneous puncture procedure used to remove fluid from a body cavity (e.g., the pleural, pericardial, or peritoneal cavity).

parcentered: describing objective lenses that retain the same field of view when the user switches from one objective to another of a differing magnification.

parfocal: describing objective lenses that remain in focus when the user switches from one objective to another of a differing magnification.

passive transport: the movement of a substance (e.g., an ion, a solute) across a cell membrane along a gradient (e.g., concen-

tration, charge). Passive transport does not require energy.

pathogenesis: the physiologic and biochemical mechanisms by which disease develops and progresses.

pericardiocentesis: a surgical puncture into the pericardial space for the aspiration of serous fluid.

pericardium: the serous membrane that surrounds the heart.

peritoneocentesis: a surgical puncture into the peritoneal space for the aspiration of serous fluid.

peritoneum: the serous membrane that lines the abdominal and pelvic walls (parietal) and the organs (visceral) that reside within.

peritubular capillaries: the network of capillaries (or plexus) that forms from the efferent arteriole and surrounds the tubules of the nephron in the renal cortex.

phase contrast microscopy: type of microscopy in which variations in the specimen refractive index are converted into variations in light intensity or contrast. Areas of the specimen appear light to dark with haloes of varying intensity related to the thickness of the component. Thin, flat components produce less haloing and the best-detailed images. It is ideal for viewing low-refractile elements and living cells.

phenylketonuria (PKU): an autosomal recessive inherited enzyme defect or deficiency characterized by the inability to convert phenylalanine to tyrosine. As a result, phenylalanine is converted to phenylketones, which are excreted in the urine.

pleocytosis: the presence of a greater than normal number of cells in the cerebrospinal fluid.

podocytes: the epithelial cells that line the urinary (Bowman's) space of the glomerulus. These cells completely cover the glomerular capillaries with large fingerlike processes that interdigitate to form a filtration slit. The name "podo," which is Greek for "foot," relates to the podocytes' footlike appearance when viewed in cross section. Collectively, the podocytes comprise the glomerular epithelium that forms Bowman's capsule.

polarizing microscopy: type of microscopy that illuminates the specimen with polarized light. It is used to identify and classify birefringent substances (i.e., substances that refract light in two directions) that shine brilliantly against a dark background.

polydipsia: intense and excessive thirst.

polyuria: the excretion of large volumes of urine (greater than 3 L/d).

porphobilinogen (PBG): an intermediate compound formed in the production of heme and a porphyrin precursor.

porphyria: the increased production of porphyrin precursors or porphyrins.

porphyrinuria: the presence of an increased amount of porphyrins or porphyrin precursors in urine.

postrenal proteinuria: an increased amount of protein in urine resulting from a disease process that adds protein to urine after its formation by the renal nephrons.

postural (orthostatic) proteinuria: an increased protein excretion in urine only when an individual is in an upright (orthostatic) position.

preventive maintenance: the performance of specific tasks in a timely fashion to eliminate equipment failure. These tasks vary with the instrument and include cleaning procedures, inspection of components, and component replacement when necessary.

procedure manual: a written document describing in detail all aspects of each policy and procedure performed in the laboratory. For example, it includes supplies needed, reagent preparation procedures, specimen requirements, mislabeled- and unlabeled-specimen protocols, procedures for the storage and disposal of wastes, technical procedures, quality control criteria, reporting formats, and references.

prostate gland: a lobular gland surrounding the male urethra immediately after it exits the bladder. It is an accessory gland of the male reproductive system. The prostate is testosterone dependent and produces a mildly acidic secretion rich in citric acid, enzymes, proteins, and zinc.

protective barriers: items used to eliminate exposure of the body to potentially infectious agents. These barriers include protective gowns, gloves, eye and face protectors, biosafety cabinets (fume hoods),splash shields, and specimen transport containers.

protein error of indicators: a phenomenon characterized by several pH indicators. These pH indicators undergo a color change in the presence of protein despite a constant pH. Described originally by Sorenson in 1909, the protein error of indicators now provides the basis of the protein screening tests employed on reagent strips.

proteinuria: the presence of an increased amount of protein in urine.

proximal convoluted tubular cells: large (approximately 20 to 60 μm in diameter), oblong or cigar-shaped cells with a small, often eccentric, nucleus (or they can be multinucleated) and a dense chromatin pattern; these cells form the lining of the proximal tubules.

proximal tubule: the tubular part of a nephron immediately following the glomerulus. The proximal tubule has both a convoluted portion and a straight portion, the latter becoming the loop of Henle after entering the renal medulla.

Prussian blue reaction (also called the Rous test): a chemical reaction used to identify the presence of iron. Iron-containing granules, e.g., hemosiderin, stain a characteristic blue color when mixed with a freshly prepared solution of potassium ferricyanide-HCl.

pseudochylous effusion: an effusion that appears milky but does not contain chylomicrons and has a low (less than 50 mg/dL) triglyceride content.

pseudoperoxidase activity: the action of heme-containing compounds (e.g., hemoglobin, myoglobin) to mimic true peroxidases by catalyzing the oxidation of some substrates in the presence of hydrogen peroxide.

pus: a protein-rich product of inflammation and cellular necrosis that consists of leukocytes and cellular debris.

pyuria: the presence of pus in urine. cf. **leukocyturia.**

quality assurance (QA): an established protocol of policies and procedures for all laboratory actions performed to ensure the quality of services (i.e., test results) rendered.

quality control (QC) materials: materials used to assess and monitor the accuracy and precision (i.e., analytical error) of a method.

random urine specimen: a urine specimen collected at any time, day or night, without prior patient preparation.

rapidly progressive glomerulonephritis (RPGN) (also called crescentic glomerulonephritis): a type of glomerular inflammation characterized by cellular proliferation into Bowman's space to form "crescents." Numerous disease processes can lead to its development, including systemic lupus erythematosus, vasculitis, and infections.

reflectance: the scattering or reflecting of light when it strikes a matte or unpolished surface. The intensity and wavelength of the reflected light will vary depending on the color of the surface and the wavelength of the incident light used.

refractive index: the ratio of light refraction in two differing media (N). It is mathematically expressed using either light velocity (V) or the angle of refraction ($\sin \theta$) in the two media, as $N_2/N_1 = V_1/V_2$ or $N_2/N_1 = \sin \theta_1/\sin \theta_2$. The refractive index is affected by the wavelength of light used, the solution's temperature, and the concentration of the solution.

refractometer: an instrument used to measure the specific gravity of liquids based on their refractive index.

refractometry: an indirect measurement of specific gravity based on the refractive index of light.

renal blood flow (RBF): the volume of blood that passes through the renal vasculature per unit of time. The RBF normally ranges from 1000 to 1200 mL/min.

renal clearance: the volume of plasma cleared of a substance by the kidneys per unit of time. Reported in milliliters per minute, it is determined by the equation $C = U \times V/P$, in which U and P are the urine and plasma concentrations of the substance, respectively, and V is the volume of urine excreted in a timed collection, usually 24 hours. The most common renal clearance test is the creatinine clearance test.

renal pelvis: the funnel-shaped structure located at the indented region of the kidney that receives the urine from the calyces and conveys it to the ureter.

renal phosphaturia: a rare hereditary disease characterized by the inability of the distal tubules to reabsorb inorganic phosphorus.

renal plasma flow (RPF): the volume of plasma that passes through the renal vasculature per unit of time. The RPF normally ranges from 600 to 700 mL/min.

renal proteinuria: increased amounts of protein in urine as a result of impaired renal function.

renal threshold level: the plasma concentration of a solute above which the amount of solute present in the ultrafiltrate exceeds the maximal tubular reabsorptive capacity (T_m). Once the renal threshold level has been reached, increased amounts of solute are excreted (i.e., lost) in the urine.

renal tubular acidosis (RTA): a renal disorder characterized by the inability of the renal tubules to secrete adequate hydrogen ions. Four types are recognized, and they can be inherited or acquired. Patients are unable to produce an acidic urine, regardless of the acid-base status of the blood plasma.

renin: a proteolytic enzyme produced and stored by the cells of the juxtaglomerular apparatus of the renal nephrons. Secretion of renin results in the formation of angiotensin and the secretion of aldosterone; thus, it plays an important role in the control of blood pressure and fluid balance.

resolution: the ability of a lens to distinguish two points or objects as separate. The resolving power (R) of a microscope is dependent on the wavelength of light used (λ) and the numerical aperture (NA) of the objective lens. The greater the resolving power, the smaller the distance distinguished between two separate points.

scybala: plural of scybalum. Dry, hard masses of fecal material in the intestine.

seminal fluid (also called **semen**): a complex body fluid that transports spermatozoa. It is composed of secretions from the testes, the epididymis, the seminal vesicles, and the prostate gland.

seminal vesicles: paired glands that secrete a slightly alkaline fluid, rich in fructose, into the ejaculatory duct. Most of the fluid in the ejaculate originates in the seminal vesicles.

seminiferous tubules: numerous coiled tubules located in the testes; the seminiferous tubules are collectively the site of spermatogenesis. Immature and immotile spermatozoa are released into the seminiferous tubular lumen and are carried by its secretions to the epididymis for maturation.

serous fluid: a fluid that has a composition similar to that of serum.

shield of negativity: a term describing the impediment produced by negatively charged components (e.g., proteoglycans) of the glomerular filtration barrier. Present on both sides of and throughout the filtration barrier, these negatively charged· components effectively limit the filtration of negatively charged substances from the blood (e.g., albumin) into the urinary space.

specific gravity: a measure of a solution's concentration based on its density. The solution's density is compared to the density of an equal volume of water at the same temperature. Specific gravity measurements are affected by both solute number and solute mass.

spherical aberration: the unequal refraction of light rays when they pass through different portions of a lens, such that the light rays are not brought to the same focus. As a result, the image produced is blurred or fuzzy and unable to be brought into sharp focus.

squamous epithelial cells: large (approximately 40 to 60 μm in diameter), thin, flagstone-shaped cells with a small, condensed, centrally located nucleus (or they can be anucleated) that form the lining of the urethra in the female and the distal urethra in the male.

STAT: an abbreviation for the Latin word *statim*, which means "immediately."

steatorrhea: the excretion of greater than 6 g/d of fat in the feces.

subarachnoid space: the space between the arachnoid and the pia mater.

suprapubic aspiration: a technique used to collect urine directly from the bladder by puncturing the abdominal wall and distended bladder using a sterile needle and syringe. It is used primarily to obtain sterile specimens for bacterial cultures from infants and occasionally from adults.

syndrome: a group of symptoms or characteristics that occur together, e.g., nephrotic syndrome, Fanconi syndrome.

synovial fluid: the fluid that fills joint cavities. It is formed by the ultrafiltration of plasma across the synovial membrane and by secretions from synoviocytes.

synoviocytes: cells of the synovial membrane. There are two types of synoviocytes: one type is actively phagocytic and synthesizes degradative enzymes, and the other type synthesizes and secretes hyaluronate.

systemic lupus erythematosus (SLE): an autoimmune disorder that affects numerous organ systems and is characterized by autoantibodies. It is a chronic disease, frequently insidious, often febrile, involving varied neurologic, hematologic, and immunologic abnormalities. Renal involvement, as well as pleuritis and pericarditis, is common. The clinical presentation is extremely varied and is associated with a constellation of symptoms such as joint pain, skin lesions, leukopenia, hypergammaglobulinemia, antinuclear antibodies, and LE cells.

Tamm-Horsfall protein: a mucoprotein produced and secreted only by renal tubular cells, particularly those of the thick ascending loops of Henle and the distal and collecting tubules.

technical competence: the ability of an individual to perform a skilled task correctly. It also includes the ability to evaluate results, such as recognizing discrepancies and absurdities.

test utilization: the frequency with which a test is performed on a single individual and how it is used to evaluate a disease process. Repeat testing of an individual is costly and may not provide additional or useful information. Sometimes a different test may provide more diagnostically useful information.

thoracentesis: a surgical puncture into the pleural space for the aspiration of serous fluid.

timed collection: a urine specimen collected throughout a specific timed interval. The patient voids at the beginning of the collection and discards this urine; then, all subsequent urine is collected. At the end of the time interval, the patient voids and includes this urine in the collection. This technique is used primarily for quantitative urine assays because it allows comparison of excretion patterns from day to day; the most common are 12-hour and 24-hour collections.

titratable acids: a term representing H^+ ions (acid) excreted in the urine as monobasic phosphate (e.g., NaH_2PO_4). The urinary excretion of these acids results in the elimination of H^+ ions and the reabsorption of sodium and bicarbonate. The titration of urine using a standard base (e.g., NaOH) to a pH of 7.4 (normal plasma pH) will quantitate the amount of H^+ ions excreted in this form; hence the name *titratable acids.*

transcellular: the transport of substances from one tissue space to another by passing through or across cells.

transitional (urothelial) epithelial cells: round or pear-shaped cells with an oval to round nucleus and abundant cytoplasm. They form the lining of the renal calyces, renal pelves, ureters, and bladder. These cells vary considerably in size, ranging from 20 to 40 μm in diameter depending on their location in the three principal layers of this epithelium, i.e., the superficial layer, the intermediate layers, and the basal layer.

transudate: an effusion in a body cavity caused by increased hydrostatic pressure (i.e., blood pressure) or decreased plasma oncotic pressure. It is identified by a fluid-to-serum total protein ratio of less than 0.5 *and* a fluid-to-serum lactate dehydrogenase ratio of less than 0.6.

tubular proteinuria: increased amounts of protein in urine owing to impaired or altered renal tubular function.

tubular reabsorption: the movement of substances (by active or passive transport) from the tubular ultrafiltrate into the peritubular blood or the interstitium by the renal tubular cells.

tubular secretion: the movement of substances (by active or passive transport) from the peritubular blood or the interstitium into the tubular ultrafiltrate by the renal tubular cells.

turnaround time: to the laboratorian, it is the time that elapses from receipt of the specimen in the laboratory to the reporting of that specimen's test results. To physicians and nursing personnel, a broader time frame is assigned.

tyrosinuria: the presence of the amino acid tyrosine in the urine.

Universal Precautions (UP): a policy describing the procedures to employ when obtaining, handling, storing, or disposing of all blood, body fluid, or body substances regardless of patient identity or patient health status. All body substances should be treated as potentially infectious.

urea cycle: a passive process occurring throughout the nephron that establishes and maintains a high concentration of urea in the renal medulla. This process accounts for approximately 50 percent of the solutes concentrated in the medulla. With the countercurrent exchange mechanism, the urea cycle helps establish and maintain the high medullary osmotic gradient. Because urea can passively diffuse into the interstitium, as well as back into the lumen fluid, the selectivity of the tubular epithelium in each portion of the nephron plays an integral part in the urea-cycling process.

ureter: a fibromuscular tube, approximately 25 cm long, that emerges from the renal pelvis of each kidney and extends down to connect to the base of the bladder. Peristaltic activity by smooth muscle moves the urine through the ureters down into the bladder.

urethra: a canal connecting the bladder to the exterior of the body. It is approximately 4 cm long in the female and approximately 24 cm long in the male.

-uria: of or relating to urine.

urinary space: the area in which the ultrafiltrate of plasma first forms in the nephron. This space, also known as Bowman's space, is located between the podocytes of the glomerulus and the specialized epithelium (Bowman's capsule) of the proximal end of the renal tubule that surrounds the glomerulus.

urinary system: the structures involved in the formation, storage, and excretion of urine. It includes the kidneys, ureters, bladder, and urethra.

urinary tract infection (UTI): the invasion and the proliferation of microorganisms in the kidney or urinary tract.

urine: a fluid, composed of water and metabolic waste products, secreted by the kidneys. It begins as an ultrafiltrate of plasma that is modified as it passes through the renal nephrons. The composition of urine remains unchanged after passing from the renal pelvis of the kidneys into the ureters.

urine preservative: a procedure or chemical substance used to prevent composition changes in a voided urine specimen (e.g., loss or gain of chemical substances, deterioration of formed elements). The most common form of urine preservation is refrigeration.

urinometer: see **hydrometer.**

urobilin: an orange-brown pigment derived from the spontaneous oxidation of colorless urobilinogen.

urobilinogen: a colorless tetrapyrrole derived from bilirubin. It is produced in the intestinal tract by the action of anaerobic bacteria and is later partially reabsorbed. The majority of the reabsorbed urobilinogen is reprocessed by the liver and re-excreted in the bile; the remainder passes to the kidneys for excretion in the urine. The portion of urobilinogen that is not reabsorbed becomes oxidized to the orange-brown pigment urobilin in the large intestine, which accounts for the characteristic color of feces.

urobilins: orange-brown pigments that impart to feces its characteristic color. Specifically, they are stercobilin, mesobilin, and urobilin, which result from spontaneous intestinal oxidation of the colorless tetrapyrroles stereobilinogen, mesobilinogen, and urobilinogen.

urochrome: a lipid-soluble yellow pigment that is continuously produced during endogenous metabolism. Present in plasma and excreted in the urine, urochrome gives urine its characteristic yellow color.

uroerythrin: a pink (or red) pigment in urine that is thought to derive from melanin metabolism. Uroerythrin deposits on urate crystals to produce a precipitate described as "brick dust."

vapor pressure osmometer: an instrument that measures osmolality based on the vapor pressure depression of a solution as compared to that of pure water. The dew point of the air in a closed chamber containing a small amount of a sample is measured and compared to that obtained using pure water. A calibrated microprocessor converts the change in the dew point observed into osmolality, which is read directly from the instrument readout.

vasa recta: the vascular network of long U-shaped capillaries that forms from the peritubular capillaries and surrounds the loops of Henle in the renal medulla.

ventricles: the four fluid-filled cavities in the brain lined with ependymal cells. The choroid plexus is located here.

viscosity: a measure of fluid flow or its resistance to flow. Low-viscosity fluids (e.g., water) flow freely and will form discrete droplets when expelled drop by drop from a pipette. In contrast, high-viscosity fluids (e.g., corn syrup) flow less freely and will not form discrete droplets; rather, they momentarily form threads or strings as they are expelled from a pipette.

xanthochromia: the pink, orange, or yellowish discoloration of supernatant cerebrospinal fluid following centrifugation.

yeast infection: an inflammatory condition that results from the proliferation of a fungi, most commonly *Candida* species.

ANSWERS TO STUDY QUESTIONS

Chapter 1

1. D
2. D
3. D
4. B
5. A
6. A. 7
   B. 3
   C. 5
   D. 2
   E. 1
   F. 4
7. D
8. B
9. B
10. C
11. A
12. C
13. B
14. C
15. C
16. B
17. D
18. A
19. A
20. A. 2
    B. 3
    C. 6
    D. 5
    E. 4

Chapter 2

1. D
2. B
3. A
4. A
5. C
6. C
7. D
8. B
9. B
10. B
11. D
12. D
13. C
14. A
15. A. 3
    B. 1
    C. 2
    D. 3
    E. 3
    F. 2
16. C
17. A
18. C
19. D
20. B

Chapter 3

1. B
2. B
3. D
4. A
5. C
6. A
7. C
8. C
   A
   A
   A
   C
   B
   A
9. D
10. C

Chapter 4

1. A. 10
   B. 7
   C. 6
   D. 5
   E. 1
   F. 4
   G. 3
   H. 2
   I. 8
   J. 9
   K. 11
2. C
3. A
4. C
5. A
6. A
7. D
8. A
9. A
10. D
11. D
12. A
13. A
14. C
15. C
16. A
17. C
18. A
19. C
20. D
21. B
22. D
23. C
24. A
25. B
26. C
27. C
28. D
29. A
30. B
31. A

Chapter 5

. . . .

1. A
2. B
3. A
4. C
5. C
6. C
7. C
8. A
9. B
10. C
11. D
12. C
13. D
14. C
15. B
16. D

17. B
18. A
19. A
20. C
21. B
22. B
23. B
24. A. Yes
    B. Yes
    C. Hypo-osmotic
25. C
26. B
27. D
28. D
29. D

30. A. 42 mL/min (Note that the plasma and urine creatinine results must first be converted to the same units).
    B. 58 mL/min
    C. Yes

31. A
32. B
33. A
34. C

35. C
36. A
37. D

Chapter 6

. . . .

1. D
2. D
3. A
4. C
5. A. 2, 3
    B. 8
    C. 4, 7
    D. 7 (4)
    E. 6 (4)
    F. 3, 7
    G. 1
    H. 2
    I. 5
6. A
7. D
8. B
9. A
10. A

11. A. 1
    B. 2
    C. 1
    D. 2
    E. 2
    F. 1
    G. 1
    H. 2
    I. 2
    J. 2
    K. 1
    L. 1
12. D
13. A

14. A. 5
    B. 3
    C. 1
    D. 1, 2
    E. 5
    F. 1, 4
15. D
16. B
17. A
18. A. 1
    B. 1
    C. 3
    D. 2
    E. 1

19. C
20. D
21. A
22. A
23. D
24. C
25. C
26. A
27. B
28. D

Chapter 7

. . . .

1. C
2. A
3. B
4. C
5. D
6. C
7. B
8. C
9. B
10. B
11. A
12. D
13. B
14. A
15. B
16. B
17. D
18. D
19. D
20. B
21. D
22. A
23. D
24. A. 3
    B. 2
    C. 3
    D. 1
    E. 4
    F. 2
    G. 1
    H. 2
    I. 3

25. A
26. A
27. C
28. B
29. D
30. D
31. B
32. D
33. B
34. D
35. C
36. C
37. D
38. B
39. D
40. C
41. B
42. D
43. C
44. D
45. D
46. A
47. B
48. A
49. D
50. D
51. C
52. D

Chapter 8

1. D	24. A. 3
2. D	B. 1 (2)
3. C	C. 3 (2)
4. B	D. 1 (2)
5. A	E. 1
6. C	F. 1
7. D	G. 1
8. D	H. 1
9. B	I. 3 (2)
10. C	J. 1
11. D	K. 1
12. B	25. A. 8
13. A. 4	B. 6
B. 3	C. 4
C. 1	D. 5
D. 2	E. 1
E. 5	F. 9
14. B	G. 7
15. A	26. A
16. C	27. A
17. A	28. B
18. A	29. A
19. D	30. D
20. C	31. B
21. B	32. A
22. A	33. A
23. B	34. C
	35. A

Chapter 9

1. A	15. B	29. C
2. B	16. C	30. A
3. A	17. B	31. D
4. D	18. A	32. C
5. D	19. A	33. A
6. A	20. A	34. A
7. D	21. B	35. D
8. C	22. B	36. A
9. B	23. D	37. D
10. A	24. B	38. D
11. D	25. B	39. C
12. C	26. C	40. C
13. D	27. C	41. B
14. D	28. B	42. A

Chapter 10

1. B	9. A	17. C
2. A	10. B	18. C
3. B	11. C	19. A
4. D	12. C	20. A
5. D	13. B	21. D
6. D	14. C	22. D
7. A	15. B	23. B
8. B	16. A	24. B

Chapter 11

1. B	7. D
2. D	8. C
3. A	9. D
4. C	10. C
5. A. 4	11. B
B. 7	12. D
C. 3	13. C
D. 5	14. D
E. 6	15. B
F. 8	16. D
6. B	17. A

Chapter 12

1. C	6. B	11. B
2. C	7. D	12. D
3. D	8. D	13. D
4. C	9. B	
5. A	10. A	

Chapter 13

1. A	9. C	17. A
2. B	10. A	18. A
3. A	11. B	19. D
4. D	12. D	20. B
5. A	13. A	21. A
6. B	14. C	22. D
7. A	15. B	23. C
8. C	16. C	24. B

Chapter 14

. . . .

1. B	7. B	13. B
2. A	8. A	14. B
3. A	9. D	15. A
4. C	10. D	16. C
5. D	11. D	17. A
6. C	12. C	

Chapter 15

. . . .

1. D	10. A. 1
2. A	B. 2
3. B	C. 1
4. B	D. 1
5. A	E. 1
6. D	F. 2
7. D	11. B
8. C	12. A
9. C	13. A
	14. C
	15. B

Chapter 16

. . . .

Case #1

1. E
2. C

Case #2

1. Abnormal findings—
    Physical exam: cloudy
    Microscopic exam: unidentified crystals
   Discrepant results—specific gravity by refractometer and reagent strip do not agree
2. E
3. A

Case #3

1. Abnormal findings—
    Physical exam: cloudy
    Chemical exam: blood trace; protein trace; nitrite pos; LE pos
    Microscopic exam: WBCs 10 to 25; bacteria mod

2. C
3. C
4. No, the nitrite and the LE by reagent strip are screening tests and have limitations:
   1) the amount of these substances present may be below the sensitivity of the test;
   2) the bacteria or WBCs present may not produce or contain these substances; and
   3) interfering substances can cause false negative results.

Case #4

1. Abnormal findings—
    Physical exam: cloudy
    Chemical exam: blood; protein/SSA; nitrite; LE
    Microscopic exam: WBCs 25 to 50; 2 to 5 WBC casts; bacteria mod
2. C
3. C
4. Two different mechanisms: the movement of bacteria from the lower urinary tract to the kidneys (ascending infection), or bacteria in the blood localizing in the kidneys (hematogenous infection).

Case #5

1. Abnormal findings—
    Chemical exam: protein
   Discrepant results—protein results by reagent strip and SSA do not agree
2. Protein(s) other than albumin are present.
3. B
4. D
5. C

Case #6

1. Abnormal findings—
    Physical exam: a large amount of foam is present.
    Chemical exam: glucose; blood; protein
    Microscopic exam: fatty casts; waxy casts; oval fat bodies
2. B
3. A
4. B
5. Severe proteinuria results in hypoproteinemia. As blood protein is lost, the intra-

vascular oncotic pressure decreases and fluid moves into the tissues.

6. Albumin, because of its size (it is small enough to pass through the glomerular filtration barrier if the shield of negativity is removed) and its high plasma concentration (compared to other plasma proteins).

Case #7

1. Abnormal findings—
   Physical exam: color, clarity
   Chemical exam: blood; protein
   Microscopic exam: RBCs; granular casts; RBC casts
2. Normally RBCs are too large to pass through the glomerular filtration barrier. However, nephrogenic strains of streptococcus form immune complexes, which deposit on the glomerular membrane—called acute poststreptococcal glomerulonephritis—causing damage to the barrier and the passage of RBCs.
3. B
4. D
5. A
6. C

Case #8

1. Abnormal urine findings—
   Physical exam: color
   Chemical exam: blood; protein
   Abnormal blood results—CK and LD
2. E
3. C

Case #9

1. Abnormal findings—
   Physical exam: color, clarity
   Chemical exam: Sp Grav; protein, nitrite
   Microscopic exam: RBCs; WBCs; many CaOx cells
   Discrepant results—reagent strip blood and microscopic exam
2. Check for ascorbic acid, which can produce false negative blood tests by reagent strip (depending on the brand of test strips used).
3. A

4. Factors that influence renal calculi formation:
   1) an increase in concentration of the chemical salts
   2) changes in the urinary pH
   3) a urinary stasis
   4) the presence of a foreign body seed

Case #10

1. Abnormal findings—
   Physical exam: clarity
   Chemical exam: glucose; LEs
   Microscopic exam: WBCs; yeast; many SEs (indicates that specimen is not a "clean catch")
2. a yeast infection
3. yeast and many SEs
4. B
5. The blood glucose level is high and the amount of glucose passing through the filtration barrier exceeds the renal tubular capacity to reabsorb it—i.e., the Tm for glucose reabsorption is exceeded. Therefore, the additional glucose remains in the tubular fluid and is excreted in the urine.
6. C

Case #11

1. Abnormal findings—
   Chemical exam: glucose; ketone
2. Very high glucose concentrations cause the Clinitest reaction to rapidly turn to orange (indicates a high concentration) and continue to change color. At the appropriate read time, the reaction mixture best matches the green and blue colors that represent a low glucose concentration.
3. If the entire Clinitest reaction is not observed, the pass-through effect would not be seen and a falsely low glucose result may be reported out.
4. B
5. B

Case #12

1. Abnormal findings—
   Physical exam: color; clarity; yellow foam

Chemical exam: bilirubin; pH; protein
Microscopic exam: bacteria
Discrepant results—the glucose by reagent strip and the Clinitest do not agree
2. Color; clarity; pH; bacteria; crystals
3. Bilirubin
4. A reducing substance other than glucose is
also present.
5. Galactosemia. Presence of galactose can
be confirmed by carbohydrate thin-layer
chromatography. Confirm with cell culture
to detect the specific enzyme deficiency.
6. No, the few bacteria present are probably
a result of the length of time and the type
of specimen collection. The negative and
normal WBCs, LEs, and nitrite support
this conclusion.

Case #13

1. Because of damage to the hypothalmus or
posterior pituitary, antidiuretic hormone
(ADH) production is partially or totally
deficient. Therefore, tubular reabsorption
of water does not occur, resulting in polyuria.
2. A
3. D
4. C
5. B
6. F
7. F
8. F
9. T

Case #14

1. Abnormal findings—
Physical exam: color; clarity
Chemical exam: blood; protein; urobilinogen
Microscopic exam: granular casts
2. Hemosiderin is a storage form of iron that
results from ferritin denaturation.
3. Free hemoglobin passes through the filtration barrier and is reabsorbed primarily
by the proximal renal tubule (and to a
lesser degree by the distal tubules). The
tubular cells catabolize the hemoglobin to
ferritin and subsequently denature it to
form hemosiderin. When these renal cells

are sloughed, hemosiderin is found in the
urine.
4. Two sources are possible: the degradation
(oxidation) of hemoglobin and the oxidation of urobilinogen to urobilin.
5. A hemolytic episode causes the formation
and excretion into the intestine of an increased amount of bilirubin. As a result,
an increased amount of urobilinogen is
formed and absorbed into the enterohepatic circulation. The increased amount
of urobilinogen absorbed is excreted in the
urine.
6. Intravascular hemolysis results in primarily an increased amount of *un*conjugated
bilirubin in the blood. It *cannot* be excreted in the urine because it is not water-
soluble and because it is tightly bound
to albumin, preventing it from passing
through the glomerular filtration barrier.

Case #15

1. Abnormal findings—
Physical exam: color change
Chemical exam: the Hoesch test
2. Porphobilinogen
3. The Watson-Schwartz test
4. An enzyme deficiency in the pathway of
hemoglobin synthesis causes an increased
production of heme precursors, i.e., δ-
aminolevulinic acid and porphobilinogen,
which are water-soluble and excreted in
the urine. Porphobilinogen becomes oxidized, causing the color change observed
in this urine.
5. Acute intermittent porphyria
6. D

Case #16

1. Urine abnormal findings—
Physical exam: color; clarity; yellow
foam
Chemical exam: bilirubin; protein; urobilinogen
Microscopic exam: granular casts
Fecal abnormal findings—color; consistency; form; fat content
2. B
3. Steatorrhea

4. B

5. An obstruction, most likely of the common bile duct owing to pancreatic cancer, is preventing bile and pancreatic enzymes from entering the intestine. Consequently, fat digestion is impaired, resulting in increased fecal fat excretion. The feces becomes pale in color (i.e., acholic) because the amount of bilirubin entering the intestine is decreased; hence the amount of urobilins (i.e., urobilin, stercobilin, mesobilin) that give fecal matter its normal color are decreased.

6. The sensitivity of the reagent strip urobilinogen test is limited. These tests are not able to accurately detect the absence of or decreased amounts of urobilinogen.

Case #17

1. Fecal abnormal findings—consistency; leukocytes; *Salmonella* sp. present
2. 326 mOsm/kg
3. C

Case #18

1. Abnormal findings—hemoglobin and hematocrit low; fecal occult blood positive
2. A
3. Myoglobin and cytochromes
4. Guaiac is preferred because of its sensitivity level. Its use reduces the number of false positive results obtained that are due to dietary factors.
5. D
6. C

Case #19

1. Abnormal seminal fluid findings—sperm concentration
Discrepant results—viability (60%) and motility (70%) contradict each other
2. Yes, a laboratory error is suspected because the viability (60%) and motility (70%) determinations contradict each other.
3. Yes, low concentrations of sperm are associated with infertility.
4. Fructose level; low fructose levels are associated with azospermia.

Case #20

1. At 450 nm: $0.200 - 0.500 = 0.300$
2. Zone III
3. The fetus is severely affected and the child should be delivered immediately if the lungs are mature.
4. $4.7 \div 2.3 = 2.0$
5. 33 weeks' gestation—immature
34 weeks' gestation—immature
35 weeks' gestation—immature

Case #21

1. Abnormal CSF findings—cloudy; leukocyte count and differential; total protein; glucose; lactate
2. 0.36
3. B
4. Yes, the high lactate level (greater than 30 mg/dL) combined with a low glucose value is associated with bacterial meningitis.
5. No, Gram stain results are not 100% sensitive owing to numerous factors.
6. Increased CSF protein—an inflammatory process involving the meninges impairs reabsorption of protein from the CSF back into the blood.
Increased CSF glucose—owing to decreased transport across the blood-brain barrier plus increased glycolysis within the central nervous system.

Case #22

1. Abnormal CSF findings—total protein; IgG
2. 6.1
3. Albumin is not produced intrathecally; therefore, increased CSF albumin levels indicate changes to the blood-brain barrier that allow increased amounts of albumin to pass.
4. 1.46
5. Multiple myeloma
6. 1) CSF protein electrophoresis, which reveals oligoclonal banding in approximately 90% of patients with multiple myeloma.
2) A positive myelin basic protein test on CSF indicates an active demyelinating process consistent with multiple myeloma.

Case #23

1. Abnormal findings—blood uric acid; synovial fluid clarity; viscosity; leukocyte count and differential; crystals; glucose; total protein
2. 30 mg/dL
3. C
4. E
5. A
6. No, the microscopic examination for crystals is not 100% sensitive and is dependent upon numerous factors. For example, sometimes the synovial fluid is removed from an area of the synovium that does not contain crystals, or only a few crystals are present, which can be missed during the microscopic exam.

Case #24

1. Abnormal findings—synovial fluid clarity; viscosity; leukocyte count and differential; glucose; total protein; lactate; Gram stain
2. 44 mg/dL
3. D
4. D

Case #25

1. Abnormal findings—synovial fluid clarity; leukocyte count; crystals; glucose; total protein
2. 15 mg/dL
3. B
4. B
5. E

Case #26

1. 0.60
2. 0.66
3. Exudates result from inflammatory processes that increase the permeability of the capillary endothelium in the parietal membrane or decrease the absorption of serous fluid by the lymphatic system.

Case #27

1. 0.45
2. 0.42
3. Transudates result from a systemic disorder that causes either an increase in hydrostatic pressure (i.e., blood pressure) or a decrease in the plasma oncotic pressure in the parietal membrane capillaries.

NOMOGRAM FOR THE DETERMINATION OF BODY SURFACE AREA OF CHILDREN AND ADULTS

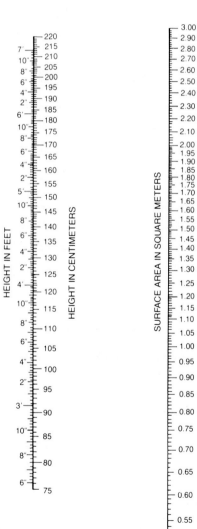

From Boothby WM, Sandiford RB: Boston M. & S.J. 185:337, 1921.

*According to the SI system, mass is the preferred term; weight is more commonly used in the United States.

APPENDIX B

....

AN EXAMPLE OF A MATERIAL SAFETY DATA SHEET*

SAFETY DATA SHEET

Regulated by: OSHA 29 CFR 1910.1200, USA/ WHMIS, Canada/ EC Directive

===

Miles, Inc. Diagnostics Division 511 Benedict Tarrytown, NY, 10591 USA	EMERGENCY TELEPHONE 1-219-264-8400 (Miles) 1-800-424-9300 (Chemtrec) Technical Information 1-219-264-8400 (Ames)	HMIS HAZARD RATING	Health: 2 Fire: 0 Reactivity: 2 Personal : B Protection

===

SECTION 1: IDENTIFICATION

Product Name: CLINITEST Reagent Tablets (foil wrapped)

Product Number: 2159

Date Prepared: 06-10-92   **New:**   **Revised:** X

===

SECTION 2: HAZARDOUS INGREDIENTS in PRODUCT

CAS#	COMPONENT	AMOUNT	EXPOSURE LIMITS/TOX DATA
1310-73-2	Sodium Hydroxide	35%	2 mg/m3 PEL-C 2 mg/m3 TLV-C LD50 oral rat-140-340 mg/kg
7758-98-7	Copper Sulfate	3%	1 mg/m3 PEL-TWA (Cu) 1 mg/m3 TLV-TWA (Cu) LD50 oral rat-300 mg/m3

European Community Risk and Safety Phrases:: R35, S26, S27, S37/39

===

SECTION 3: PHYSICAL DATA

Appearance and Odor: Solid pale blue tablets with no markings. When wet or dissolved, material is very caustic.

pH: N/A-when dry, Wet-very caustic   **Specific Gravity (H2O=1):** N/D

Boiling Point (F): N/A   **Vapor Pressure:** N/A

Melting Point (F): N/A   **Evaporation Rate:** N/A

Solubility in Water: Completely Soluble

===

N/D = Not Determined   N/A = Not Applicable
2159TAB

Page 1 of 6

* Material Safety Data Sheet for Clinitest reagent tablets. Courtesy of Miles Inc., Elkhart, IN.

472

SAFETY DATA SHEET

<u>Product Name:</u> CLINITEST Reagent Tablets (foil wrapped)

SECTION 4: CRITICAL HAZARDS

<u>MAN:</u> Corrosive, when wet or dissolved can cause severe burns to the eyes and skin. Clinitest tablets are highly sensitive to moisture from air or water. Moisture may cause a chemical reaction and glass bottle could explode.

<u>ENVIRONMENT:</u> None determined.
==
SECTION 5: EMERGENCY FIRST AID PROCEDURES

<u>Emergency and First Aid Procedures:</u> Call a Physician Immediately and arrange
for transport to nearest ER (EMERGENCY ROOM).

While awaiting the physician or transport to ER:

<u>Inhalation:</u> If not breathing, give artificial respiration. If breathing is difficult, give oxygen. Get immediate medical attention.

<u>Ingestion:</u> Wash out mouth with water provided the person is conscious. Give one or two glasses of milk or water to dilute. DO NOT induce vomiting. Get immediate medical attention.

<u>Skin Contact:</u> Immediately remove any contaminated clothing. Wash the contact area thoroughly with water for at least 15 minutes. Get prompt medical attention. Wash clothing before reuse.

<u>Eye Contact:</u> In case of contact flush eyes with copious amounts of water for at least 15-20 minutes. Raise eye lids several times to be sure material is rinsed out. Transport to hospital to see an ophthalmologist.
==

SECTION 6: FIRE AND EXPLOSION HAZARD DATA

<u>Flash Point (Method Used):</u> None

<u>Flammable Limits:</u>   <u>LEL:</u> N/A   <u>UEL:</u> N/A

<u>Extinguishing Media:</u> CO2 preferred on small fires in surrounding area. Water on tablets will cause a chemical reaction.

<u>Special Fire Fighting Procedures:</u> It is always best to wear self-contained breathing apparatus. Wet tablets are corrosive - prevent contact.

<u>Unusual Fire and Explosion Hazards:</u> Exposed tablets contacted with water could generate sufficient heat to ignite surrounding combustible material.
==

N/D = Not Determined   N/A = Not Applicable
2159TAB

SAFETY DATA SHEET

Product Name: CLINITEST Reagent Tablets (foil wrapped)

SECTION 7: SPILL OR LEAK PROCEDURES

Steps to be taken in case material is released or spilled:
Wear appropriate protective equipment. Take up spilled tablets and dissolve one at a time in an open container. CAUTION! Resulting solution will be very caustic. Handle as a concentrated solution of sodium hydroxide. Wipe spill area with damp paper towels and properly dispose.
===

SECTION 8: HANDLING AND STORAGE

Store at temperature and conditions as indicated on the Product Labels. Keep containers closed. Excessive moisture may cause a chemical reaction and a bottle explosion may occur.

Corrosive! Prevent contact with the eyes, skin and clothing. Keep tablets dry, tablets are highly sensitive to moisture from air or water.
===

SECTION 9: PERSONAL PROTECTION

Ventilation: Use general room ventilation.

Respiratory Protection: None required.

Protective Gloves: Standard laboratory chemical rubber or latex gloves are recommended for handling spilled or broken tablets.

Eye Protection: Chemical safety goggles and/or face shield recommended for handling spilled or broken tablets. Contact lenses should not be worn in the laboratory.

Other Protective Equipment/Clothing: None required.
===

N/D = Not Determined   N/A = Not Applicable
2159TAB

SAFETY DATA SHEET

Product Name: CLINITEST Reagent Tablets (foil wrapped)

SECTION 10: REACTIVITY DATA

Stability: Unstable: Stable: X

Conditions to Avoid: Stable if kept dry. Moisture will start a chemical reaction
                      which will release gas and heat.
Materials to Avoid: Avoid accidental contact with moisture/water. Avoid acids,
                      flammable liquids, organics, and metals.

Hazardous Decomposition Products: Decomposition in water will produce a caustic
                                   solution and heat.

Hazardous Polymerization: Will Occur: Will Not Occur: X

Conditions to Avoid: None determined
===

SECTION 11: TOXICOLOGICAL INFORMATION

CHRONIC EFFECTS OF OVEREXPOSURE: Repeated contact with dilute sodium hydroxide
solutions may cause dermatitis.

Carcinogen or Suspected Carcinogen:
     None of the components are listed as a carcinogen or suspected carcinogen.

Medical Conditions Aggravated by Exposure:
     Pre-existing skin diseases and conditions.

ACUTE EXPOSURE EFFECTS:

INHALATION: Corrosive! Inhalation of dusts or mists may cause severe respiratory
irritation with possible pulmonary edema.

INGESTION: Corrosive! Swallowing may cause gastrointestinal burns and damage.

SKIN CONTACT: Corrosive! Contact may cause severe chemical burns and tissue
destruction.

EYE CONTACT: Corrosive, May cause severe chemical burns and possible blindness.
===

N/D = Not Determined   N/A = Not Applicable
2159TAB

SAFETY DATA SHEET

Product Name: CLINITEST Reagent Tablets (foil wrapped)

SECTION 12: ECOLOGICAL INFORMATION

Ecological effects of this mixture have not been determined.

This product contains 3% copper sulfate which has been known to harm aquatic plants. The reported EC10 Salmo gairdeneri (rainbow trout embryo, larvae) 16.5 ug/L/28 days.; death and deformity.

===

SECTION 13: DISPOSAL

Primary Container Type: The product is foil wrapped tablets in a box.

Waste Disposal Method: Each disposal facility must determine proper disposal methods to comply with Local, State and Federal Environmental Regulations.
===

SECTION 14: TRANSPORTATION (IATA Regulations)

PROPER SHIPPING NAME: Sodium Hydroxide, Solid

TECHNICAL NAME: same

UN NUMBER: UN1823

HAZARD CLASS AND PACKAGING GROUP: 8, II

LABEL(s): Corrosive   Pass: IATA 814   Cargo: IATA 816

UNIT VOLUME: 100 tablets

PRIMARY CONTAINER TYPE: Foil wrapped tablets

SALES UNIT: 100 foil wrapped tablets per box.
===

N/D = Not Determined   N/A = Not Applicable
2159TAB

SAFETY DATA SHEET

Product Name: CLINITEST Reagent Tablets (foil wrapped)

SECTION 15: OTHER REGULATORY INFORMATION

SARA 311/312: Hazard Categories for SARA Section 311/312 Reporting:
    Acute health

SARA 313 This Product Contains the Following Chemicals Subject to Annual Release
Reporting Requirements Under the SARA Section 313 (40 CFR 372):
            Copper compound 3% (Copper Sulfate)

===: :==== :========

SECTION 16: OTHER INFORMATION

None

==

Prepared by: _____

==

    The opinions expressed herein are those of qualified experts within Miles Inc.. We
believe that the information contained herein is current as of the date of this
Material Safety Data Sheet. Since the use of this information and these opinions
and the conditions of use of the product are not within the control of Miles Inc.,
it is the users obligation to assure safe use of the product.

N/D = Not Determined   N/A = Not Applicable
2159TAB

APPENDIX C

CELL COUNTS USING A HEMACYTOMETER

Manual methods using a hemacytometer are most often used to perform cell counts on cerebrospinal fluid, synovial fluid, seminal fluid, pleural fluid, pericardial fluid, and peritoneal fluid. In these body fluids, the number of erythrocytes and leukocytes may be low, and other cells and cellular debris are frequently present. An electronic cell counter may produce erroneous results for body fluid cell counts. The background count of most electronic counters can be equal to or higher than the actual number of cells present in the body fluid; in addition, all particles of an appropriate size, including macrophages, mesothelial cells, tumor cells, and cellular debris, are counted. Because of the high viscosity of body fluids, particularly synovial fluid, and the possibility of fibrin clots, both of which interfere with electronic counters, special sampling procedures may need to be performed. On the other hand, manual cell counts are time-consuming, require special technical skills, have poor reproducibility, and are subject to numerous errors; therefore, it is imperative that they be performed by technically proficient laboratorians.

Diluents

Body fluids that are clear usually do not require a dilution, and the fluid can be mounted directly onto a hemacytometer for cell counting. In contrast, fluids that are visibly cloudy or bloody must be diluted to obtain accurate cell counts. For slightly cloudy fluids, a 1:10 dilution is usually sufficient; moderately cloudy fluids are diluted 1:20; and extremely cloudy or bloody fluids often require a 1:100 dilution.

The diluent selected depends on the cell counts requested and the body fluid being evaluated. Isotonic solutions such as normal saline are required for erythrocyte counts, whereas dilute acetic acid solutions are widely used for leukocyte counts. Acetic acid provides two functions: it lyses any erythrocytes present, and it enhances the microscopic visualization of leukocytes. Leukocyte counts on cerebrospinal, seminal, pleural, pericardial, and peritoneal fluids are routinely diluted using acetic acid solutions; however, these diluents should not be used with synovial fluid. Because of the high hyaluronate and protein content in synovial fluid, acetic acid causes the formation of mucin clots and the clumping of cells, both of which interfere with accurate cell counting. Instead, synovial fluid should be diluted with normal saline, hypotonic saline, or a hyaluronidase buffer solution. The latter solution is specifically formulated to prevent the development of mucin clots and can include the stain toluidine blue O to aid in the visualization and identification of cellular elements. For leukocyte counts on synovial fluid, a hypotonic saline solution can be used to lyse any erythrocytes present. Table C–1 summa-

TABLE C–1.   DILUENTS FOR BODY FLUID SPECIMENS

DILUENT	CONCENTRATION	PREPARATION	USE
Isotonic saline (0.85%)	8.5 g/L	Dissolve 0.85 g NaCl in 100 mL reagent grade water* (Type I or II).	Total, white blood cell, and red blood cell counts
Hypotonic saline (0.30%)	3.0 g/L	Dissolve 0.30 g NaCl in 100 mL reagent grade water (Type I or II).	Synovial fluid: white blood cell counts
Dilute acetic acid†	3%**	Dilute 3 mL glacial acetic acid to 100 mL with reagent grade water (Type I or II). (*Caution: always add acid to water.*)	White blood cell counts
Hyaluronidase buffer solution††	0.1 g/L	Dissolve 10 mg hyaluronidase (Type 1–S, Sigma Chemical Co.), 40 mg dextrose, and 8 mg toluidine blue O in 100 mL of 0.067 mol/L phosphate buffer. Phosphate buffer (0.067 mol/L): Solution A—Dissolve 2.279 g monobasic potassium phosphate (MW 136.09) in 250 mL Type I water in a volumetric flask. Solution B—Dissolve 4.756 g dibasic sodium phosphate (MW 141.96) in 500 mL Type I water in a volumetric flask. Combine 13 mL solution A, 87 mL solution B, and 13 mL absolute methanol. Buffer solution is stable for 3 months at 2–5°C.	Synovial fluid: total, white blood cell and red blood cell counts
Seminal fluid diluent		Dissolve 5 g sodium bicarbonate and 1 mL 35% v/v formalin (and 25 mg trypan blue, optional) in 100 mL reagent grade water (Type I or II).	Sperm counts

* For specifications, see NCCLS: "Preparation and testing of reagent grade water in the clinical laboratory," 11(13):7–10, 1991.
† Solutions of dilute acetic acid cause the formation of mucin clots and cell clumping when used with synovial fluid specimens.
** Other concentrations of acetic acid are also used, e.g., 5%, 10%.
†† From Kjeldsberg CR, Knight JA: Body Fluids (2nd ed.), Chicago, American Society of Clinical Pathologists Press, 1986, p. 154.

rizes the diluents commonly used with body fluids and their preparations.

Pretreatment of Synovial Fluid Specimens

Because synovial fluid is highly viscous, it is difficult to pipette accurately and can result in an uneven distribution of cells in the counting chamber. The pretreatment of synovial fluid with hyaluronidase will reduce the viscosity of the fluid and eliminate these problems. The laboratorian can pretreat synovial fluid as follows:

1. Prepare a 0.5 g/L solution of hyaluronidase by dissolving 50 mg hyaluronidase (Type 1-S, Sigma Chemical Co.) in 100 mL 0.067 mol/L phosphate buffer (see Table C–1 for the buffer solution's preparation).
2. For each milliliter of synovial fluid, add 1 drop of the hyaluronidase solution (0.5 g/L).
3. Mix well and allow the fluid to stand for 5 minutes.
4. Use the treated synovial fluid undiluted

for cell counts, or, if necessary, dilute using saline or a 0.1 g/L hyaluronidase buffer solution (see Table C–1 for solution preparation).

Pretreatment of Mucoid Seminal Fluid Specimens

To reduce the viscosity of mucoid seminal fluid specimens that fail to liquify adequately after 60 minutes, one of the following solutions can be used. The effect these substances may have on sperm function or on the biochemistry of the seminal plasma is currently not known (WHO, 1992). Make a 1:1 dilution using the semen specimen and one of the following solutions.

1. α-amylase (150 U/mL)
2. Alevaire (Breon Laboratories, Inc.), a mucolytic agent
3. Bromelin (1 g/L)
4. Plasmin (0.35 to 0.50 casein units/mL)
5. Chymotrypsin (150 USP/mL)

Cell Count Procedure

1. Mix body fluid specimens well for 1 to 2 minutes before filling a hemacytometer chamber with undiluted fluid or preparing a dilution of the specimen. While the specimen is mixing, clean the hemacytometer to remove any dust present, which can interfere with the placement of the coverslip.
2. Erythrocyte and total cell counts must be performed first because, for the leukocyte count, body fluids are usually exposed to acetic acid, which destroys erythrocytes while enhancing leukocyte identification. Body fluids with low cell counts (i.e., clear fluids) are evaluated undiluted.
3. Leukocyte counts can be performed using isotonic diluents, but frequently the fluid is exposed to glacial acetic acid or acetic acid diluents to enhance the visualization of leukocytes and the lysis of any erythrocytes present. (This modification cannot be used with synovial fluid specimens.) Body fluids with low cell counts (i.e., clear

fluids) are evaluated undiluted. The following procedure can be used to enhance the visualization of leukocytes in undiluted fluid specimens:
   a. Rinse the inside of a disposable Pasteur pipette with glacial acetic acid, allow it to drain completely, and wipe off the outside and end of the pipette carefully with gauze. *CAUTION:* Glacial acetic acid is caustic. Safety glasses, gloves, and a gown should be worn and a hood used when working with glacial acetic acid.
   b. Place the prerinsed pipette into the well-mixed body fluid and allow the pipette to fill approximately 1 inch of its length by capillary action. Place a finger over the open end of the pipette and remove the pipette containing sample from the body fluid.
   c. Mix the fluid sample with the acid in the pipette by holding the pipette in a horizontal position and removing your finger from the top. Rotate the pipette carefully for 10 to 20 seconds. Be careful not to allow fluid to drip out of either end of the pipette.
   d. The fluid can now be used to fill a hemocytometer. Allow 3 to 5 minutes for the cells to settle and the erythrocytes to lyse.
4. Dilutions of body fluid specimens should be made using a quantitative technique. Calibrated automatic pipettes (e.g., Pipetman, Eppendorf) can be used to make manual dilutions, or commercial diluting systems (e.g., Unopettes) can be employed. Viscous fluids, such as synovial fluid and seminal fluid, must be diluted manually using a positive displacement pipette because its accuracy is not affected by high-viscosity fluids. Cerebrospinal, pleural, pericardial, and peritoneal fluids and "pretreated" synovial fluid can be diluted using commercial diluting systems or manually using either an air or a positive displacement pipette. The use of Thoma red blood cell and white blood cell pipettes is not recommended for two reasons: these pipettes represent a biohazard because they require mouth suction using an aspi-

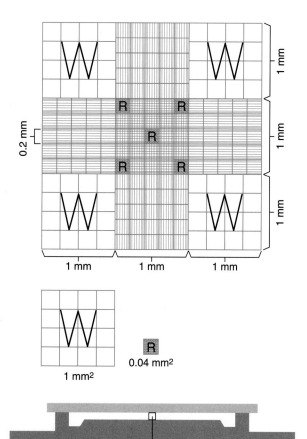

rator tube, and they produce inaccurate dilutions with highly viscous fluids (e.g., seminal fluid, synovial fluid).

5. Using a disposable pipette, fill both sides of an "improved" Neubauer hemacytometer (Fig. C–1) with well-mixed, undiluted or appropriately diluted body fluid.

6. Allow the chamber to remain undisturbed for 3 to 5 minutes for the cells to settle (and the erythrocytes to lyse, depending on the diluent used).

7. Examine the hemacytometer chambers microscopically for an even distribution of cells without overlap or clumping. If either overlapping or clumping is present, the hemacytometer should be cleaned, the specimen mixed well, and the chambers refilled, or a new dilution should be made.

8. The number of squares counted in each chamber depends on the total number of cells present. The more cells that are counted, the more accurate is the cell count. Therefore, it is important that the dilution used is not excessive and that an adequate number of cells are present. For fluids with extremely low cell counts, additional squares can be counted; conversely, for fluids with a high cell count, fewer squares may be counted. Regardless of the variation used, the calculation must be adjusted appropriately for the volume of body fluid actually counted. The following format is routinely used in clinical laboratories:

a. With *cerebrospinal, synovial, pleural, pericardial, and peritoneal fluids,* the laboratorian should count all the cells present in the four large corner squares and the center square in *both* chambers of the hemacytometer. See the "W" squares in Figure C–1. The number of cells counted on each side should agree within 10% to 20%. (Total area counted = 10 mm^2)

b. With *seminal fluid,* the laboratorian should follow this format:

1) For spermatozoa counts, count all sperm present in five red blood cell squares, i.e., the four corner squares and the center square within the central large square on one side of the hemacytometer. See the "R" squares in Figure C–1. Count the same area in the second chamber of the hemacytometer. The number of sperm counted on each side should agree within 10% to 20%. (Total area counted = 0.20 mm^2) An alternative method is to count two large "W" squares.

2) For round cell or white cell counts, count the round cells present in the four large corner squares and the center large square on one side of the hemacytometer. See the "W" squares in Figure C–1. Count the same area in the second chamber of the hemacytometer. The number of cells counted on each side should agree within 10% to 20%. (Total area counted = 10 mm^2)

Calculations

When using the hemacytometer, the total number of cells counted is multiplied by both a dilution factor (which accounts for any dilution made before filling the counting chambers) and a volume factor (which accounts for the volume actually counted in the chamber) to obtain the number of cells present in each μL (or mm^3) of fluid. This number is multiplied by a conversion factor to obtain the cell count per liter of fluid. Regardless of the number of squares counted or the dilution used, all hemacytometer calculations use the following general formula:

$$\frac{\text{Cells}}{\text{counted}} \times \frac{\text{Dilution}}{\text{factor}} \times \frac{\text{Volume}}{\text{factor}} = \frac{\text{Cells}}{\mu L(mm^3)}$$

$$\frac{\text{Cells}}{\mu L(mm^3)} \times \frac{10^6 \mu L}{L} = \text{Cells} \times 10^6/L$$

Unit conversion factor

To calculate the "volume factor," the actual volume of fluid counted in mm^3 (μL) must be determined. This volume is determined by multiplying the area counted by the depth (0.1 mm) between the coverslip and chamber. Subsequently, the "volume factor" is equal to 1 divided by the volume counted in mm^3 (μL).

$$\text{Volume factor} = \frac{1}{\text{area} \times \text{depth}}$$

For example, if 5 large squares are counted (5 × 1 mm^2), the area is 5 mm^2, the depth is 0.1 mm, and the volume of fluid counted is 0.5 mm.^{3} Hence, the volume factor is 2, i.e., 1 divided by 0.5.

Following are some examples of cell counts in body fluid specimens using a hemacytometer and undiluted fluid or diluted fluid and the appropriate calculation.

Example A:

An *undiluted* cerebrospinal fluid specimen is mounted on a hemacytometer and the five large squares are counted in *both* chambers, i.e., 10 mm^2. A total of 30 cells are counted.

$$30 \times 1 \times \frac{1}{(10 \times 0.1)} = 30 \text{ cells}/\mu L$$

Cells counted, Dilution factor, Volume factor

$$\frac{30 \text{ cells}}{\mu L} \times \frac{10^6 \mu L}{L} = 30 \times 10^6 \text{ cells/L}$$

Example B:

A synovial fluid specimen is diluted 1:20 and is mounted on a hemacytometer for counting. The four large corner squares and the center square are counted in one chamber, i.e., 5 mm^2. A total of 58 cells are counted.

$$58 \times 20 \times \frac{1}{(5 \times 0.1)} = 2320 \text{ cells}/\mu L$$

Cells counted, Dilution factor, Volume factor

$$\frac{2320 \text{ cells}}{\mu L} \times \frac{10^6 \mu L}{L} = 2320 \times 10^6 \text{ cells/L}$$

Example C:

A seminal fluid specimen is diluted 1:20 and is mounted on a hemacytometer for counting. The four small corner squares and the center square ("R" squares) within the large central square are counted in one chamber, i.e., 5 × 0.04 mm^2 = 0.2 mm^2. A total of 37 cells are counted. Note that spermatozoa counts are reported as the number of spermatozoa per milliliter.

$$37 \times 20 \times \frac{1}{(0.2 \times 0.1)} = 37,000 \text{ cells}/\mu L$$

Cells counted, Dilution factor, Volume factor

$$\frac{37,000 \text{ cells}}{\mu L} \times \frac{10^3 \mu L}{mL} = 37 \times 10^6 \text{cells/mL}$$

Often a total cell count (including both erythrocytes and leukocytes) and a leukocyte count may be performed on a body fluid, and the erythrocyte count is then calculated as the difference between these two counts.

References

. . . .

Kjeldsberg CR, Knight JA: Laboratory methods. *In* Body Fluids (2nd ed.), Chicago, American Society of Clinical Pathologists Press, 1986, p. 154.

National Committee for Clinical Laboratory Standards. Preparation and Testing of Reagent Grade Water in the Clinical Laboratory. Approved Guideline. NCCLS Document C3-A2 (ISBN 1-56238-127X), *11*(13): 7–10, 1991.

World Health Organization (WHO). Laboratory Manual for the Examination of Human Semen and Semen-Cervical Mucus Interaction (3rd ed.), New York, Cambridge University Press, 1992, p. 5.

Bibliography

. . . .

Brown B: Hematology: Principles and Procedures (6th ed.), Philadelphia, Lea & Febiger, 1993, p. 87–97.

Turgeon ML: Clinical Hematology, Theory and Procedures, Boston, Little, Brown & Co., Inc., 1988, pp. 342–393.

APPENDIX D

REFERENCE RANGES

URINE (RANDOM SPECIMEN) REFERENCE RANGES

PHYSICAL EXAMINATION

Component	Result
Color	Colorless to amber (varies with state of hydration, diet, health)
Clarity	Clear
Specific gravity	1.002 to 1.035 (physiologically possible 1.002 to 1.040)
Osmolality	275 to 900 mOsm/kg H_2O (physiologically possible 50 to 1400 mOsm/kg H_2O)
Volume	600 to 1800 mL/d (varies with state of hydration, diet, health)

CHEMICAL EXAMINATION

Component	Result
Bilirubin	Negative
Glucose	Negative
Ketones	Negative
Leukocyte esterase	Negative
Nitrite	Negative
pH	4.5 to 8.0
Protein	Negative
Urobilinogen	≤ 1 mg/dL

MICROSCOPIC EXAMINATION*

Component	Number	Magnification
Red blood cells	0 to 3	Per high-power field
White blood cells	0 to 8	Per high-power field
Casts	0 to 2 hyaline	Per low-power field
Epithelial cells		
Squamous	Few	Per low-power field
Transitional	Few	Per high-power field
Renal	Few	Per high-power field
Bacteria and yeast	Negative	Per high-power field

* Using the UriSystem for standardized microscopic analysis.

FECAL REFERENCE RANGES

PHYSICAL EXAMINATION

Color	Brown
Consistency	Firm, formed
Form	Tubular, cylindrical

CHEMICAL EXAMINATION

Fat, quantitative (72-hour specimen)

Total fat	<6 g/d
	$<20\%$ of stool
Osmolality	285 to 430 mOsm/kg H_2O
Potassium	30 to 140 mEq/L
Sodium	40 to 110 mEq/L

MICROSCOPIC EXAMINATION

Fat, qualitative

Neutral fat	Few globules present per high-power field
Total fat	<100 fat globules per high-power field
	Globule diameter: ≤ 4 microns
Leukocytes (qualitative)	None present
Meat and vegetable fibers (qualitative)	Few

SEMINAL FLUID REFERENCE RANGE

PHYSICAL EXAMINATION

Appearance	Gray-white, opalescent, opaque
Volume	2.0 to 5.0 mL
Viscosity	Discrete droplets (watery) within 60 minutes

CHEMICAL EXAMINATION

pH	7.2 to 7.8
Acid phosphatase (total)	≥ 200 U per ejaculate at 37°C (*p*-nitrophenylphosphate)
Citric acid (total)	≥ 52 μmol per ejaculate
Fructose (total)	≥ 13 μmol per ejaculate
Zinc (total)	≥ 2.4 μmol per ejaculate

MICROSCOPIC EXAMINATION

Motility	50% or more with moderate to rapid linear (forward) progression
Concentration	20 to 250×10^6 spermatozoa/mL
Morphology	50% or more have normal morphology
Viability	50% or more are alive
Leukocytes (white blood cells)	Less than 1×10^6/mL

AMNIOTIC FLUID REFERENCE RANGES

PHYSICAL EXAMINATION

Color	Colorless to pale yellow
Clarity	Clear to slightly turbid*

CHEMICAL EXAMINATION

ΔA_{450} determination

27 weeks' gestation	<0.065
30 weeks' gestation	<0.052
35 weeks' gestation	<0.035
40 weeks' gestation	<0.022
Lecithin/sphingomyelin ratio (mature)	>2.0

* The amount of turbidity increases with gestational age.

CEREBROSPINAL FLUID REFERENCE RANGE*

PHYSICAL EXAMINATION

Color　　　　　　Colorless
Clarity　　　　　Clear

CHEMICAL EXAMINATION

Component	Conventional Units	Factor	SI Units
Electrolytes			
Calcium	2.0 to 2.8 mEq/L	0.5	1.00 to 1.40 mmol/L
Chloride	115 to 130 mEq/L	1.	115 to 130 mmol/L
Lactate	10 to 22 mg/dL	0.111	1.1 to 2.4 mmol/L
Magnesium	2.4 to 3.0 mEq/L	0.5	1.2 to 1.5 mmol/L
Potassium	2.6 to 3.0 mEq/L	1.	2.6 to 3.0 mmol/L
Sodium	135 to 150 mEq/L	1.	135 to 150 mmol/L
Glucose	50 to 80 mg/dL	0.5551	2.8 to 4.4 mmol/L
Total protein	15 to 45 mg/dL	10.	150 to 450 mg/L
Albumin	10 to 30 mg/dL	10.	100 to 300 mg/L
IgG	1 to 4 mg/dL	10.	10 to 40 mg/L

Protein Electrophoresis	Percentage of Total Protein
Prealbumin	2% to 7%
Albumin	56% to 76%
α_1-Globulin	2% to 7%
α_2-Globulin	4% to 12%
β-Globulin	8% to 18%
γ-Globulin	3% to 12%

MICROSCOPIC EXAMINATION

Leukocyte Count	Conventional Units	Factor	SI Units
Neonates (<1 year old)	0 to 30 cells/μL	10^6	0 to 30 $\times$ 10^6 cells/L
1 to 4 years old	0 to 20 cells/μL	10^6	0 to 20 $\times$ 10^6 cells/L
5 to 18 years old	0 to 10 cells/μL	10^6	0 to 10 $\times$ 10^6 cells/L
Adults (>18 years old)	0 to 5 cells/μL	10^6	0 to 5 $\times$ 10^6 cells/L

Differential Cell Count	Percentage of Total Protein
Neonates	
Lymphocytes	5% to 35%
Monocytes	50% to 90%
Neutrophils	0% to 8%
Adults	
Lymphocytes	40% to 80%
Monocytes	15% to 45%
Neutrophils	0% to 6%

For cerebrospinal fluid specimens obtained by lumbar puncture.

SYNOVIAL FLUID REFERENCE RANGE*

PHYSICAL EXAMINATION

Total volume	0.1 to 3.5 mL
Color	Pale yellow
Clarity	Clear
Viscosity	High, forms strings 3 to 6 cm long
Clots spontaneously	No

CHEMICAL EXAMINATION

Glucose	Equivalent to plasma values†
Uric acid	Equivalent to plasma values†
Total protein	1 to 3 g/dL
Lactate	9 to 33 mg/dL**
Hyaluronate	0.3 to 0.4 g/dL

MICROSCOPIC EXAMINATION

Erythrocyte count	<2000 cells/μL
Leukocyte count	<200 cells/μL
Differential cell count	
Monocytes and macrophages	Approximately 60%
Lymphocytes	Approximately 30%
Neutrophils	Approximately 10%
Crystals	None present

* *Values given are for fluid obtained from the knee.*

† *Synovial fluid values are equivalent to plasma values if obtained from a fasting patient.*

** *Normal lactate values are assumed to be similar to those of blood and cerebrospinal fluid; actual reference intervals have yet to be established (Kjeldsberg CR, Knight JA: Synovial fluid. In Body Fluids (2nd ed.), Chicago, American Society of Clinical Pathologists Press, 1986, pp. 129–152).*

INDEX

Note: Page numbers in *italics* indicate illustrations; those followed by t refer to tables.